CLINICAL
OBSTETRICS &
GYNAECOLOGY

SECOND EDITION

DEDICATION

This book is dedicated to the millions of women
worldwide who will suffer disability, lose their
babies, or lose their lives through the want
of adequate reproductive healthcare.

for Elsevier
Commissioning Editor: Pauline Graham
Development Editor: Lulu Stader
Project Manager: Anne Dickie and Nayagi Athmanathan
Designer: Stewart Larking
Illustration Manager: Merlyn Harvey
Illustrators: Ian Ramsden and Graeme Chambers

CLINICAL OBSTETRICS & GYNAECOLOGY

SECOND EDITION

EDITED BY

BRIAN A. MAGOWAN
MB, CHB, FRCOG, DipFetMed

Consultant Obstetrician and Gynaecologist
The Borders General Hospital
Melrose UK

PHILIP OWEN
MB, BCH, MD, MRCOG

Consultant Obstetrician and Gynaecologist
Department of Obstetrics
Princess Royal Maternity Unit
Glasgow, UK

JAMES DRIFE
MD FRCOG FRCPED FRCSED HONFCOGSA

Professor of Obstetrics and Gynaecology, University of Leeds
Honorary Consultant Obstetrician and Gynaecologist
The Leeds Teaching Hospitals NHS Trust
Leeds UK

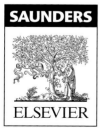

SAUNDERS

ELSEVIER

Edinburgh • London • New York • Oxford • Philadelphia • St Louis • Sydney • Toronto 2009

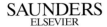

SAUNDERS
ELSEVIER

An imprint of Elsevier Limited

First Edition 2004 © Elsevier Limited.
© 2009 Elsevier Limited. All rights reserved.

First edition 2004

ISBN: 978 0 7020 3069 7
International Edition ISBN: 978 0 7020 3075 8

British Library Cataloguing in Publication Data
A catalogue record for this book is available from the British Library

Library of Congress Cataloging in Publication Data
A catalog record for this book is available from the Library of Congress

Note

Printed in China

So much has changed since the first edition of this book that we have involved a comprehensive group of experts to ensure that this new edition is up to date and relevant.

What remains constant, however, is the many challenges that obstetrics and gynaecology offer. From the ethics of assisted conception treatments through the global importance of contraception, the challenges of gynaecological cancer care and the dilemmas of prenatal diagnosis, to mention but a few, there are many issues with which to become familiar.

What has not changed since the last edition is the fact that over half a million women worldwide are still dying each year from treatable pregnancy complications. Ninety-nine percent of these women live in under-resourced countries and the hurdles to improving their care are immense. These hurdles, however, are ours to overcome — medically, socially, politically and financially.

Wherever you study or practise obstetrics and gynaecology, a sound knowledge of the clinical aspects will underpin your understanding of this specialty and maximize your ability to learn about and contribute to the care of women. This book is aimed at providing you with that knowledge.

BM, PO, JD

Contributors

Dr Susan Brechin
Consultant in Sexual & Reproductive
Health, NHS Grampian
Centre for Contraception and
Reproductive Health
Aberdeen

Dr Janet Brennand
Consultant in Fetal & Maternal Medicine
The Queen Mother's Hospital
Glasgow

Dr Audrey Brown
Consultant in Sexual and Reproductive
Healthcare
Sandyford Initiative
Glasgow

Professor Alan D Cameron
The Ian Donald Fetal Medicine Unit
The Queen Mother's Hospital
Glasgow

Dr Sharon Cameron
Consultant Gynaecologist
The Simpson Centre for Reproductive
Health
Royal Infirmary of Edinburgh
Edinburgh

Dr Dan Clutterbuck
Consultant in Genitourinary Medicine
NHS Lothian University Hospitals
Division
Edinburgh

Mr Simon Crawford
Consultant Gynaecological Surgeon
Princess Anne Hospital
Southampton University Hospitals NHS
Trust
Southampton

Dr Sarah Creighton
Consultant Gynaecologist
University College Hospital
London

Professor James Drife
Department of Obstetrics and
Gynaecology,
Leeds General Infirmary
Professor, Academic Unit Obstetrics
and Gynaecology, University of Leeds
Leeds

Dr Colin Duncan
Clinical Senior Lecturer in Obstetrics
and Gynaecology
The University of Edinburgh
The Queen's Medical Research
Institute
Edinburgh

Dr David R FitzPatrick
Senior Clinical Scientist and Honorary
Consultant Geneticist
MRC Human Genetics Unit
Western General Hospital
Edinburgh

Dr Siona Gaffney
Specialist Registrar in Obstetrics and
Gynaecology
University Hospital North Tees
Stockton on Tees

Dr Janice Gibson
Consultant Obstetrician and
Subspecialist in Maternal
and Fetal Medicine
The Southern General Hospital
Glasgow

Dr Kate Grady
Consultant Anaesthetist
South Manchester University Hospital
Manchester

Professor Janesh Gupta
Professor of Obstetrics and
Gynaecology
Birmingham Women's Hospital, BMI
Priory Hospital,
BMI Birmingham Hospital
Birmingham

Dr Katriona Hill
Specialist Registrar in Obstetrics and
Gynaecology,
The Simpson Centre for Reproductive
Health
Royal Infirmary of Edinburgh
Edinburgh

Mr Kim Hinshaw
Consultant Obstetrician and
Gynaecologist
City Hospitals Sunderland NHS
Foundation Trust
Sunderland

Professor Khalid S Khan
Professor of Obstetrics,
Gynaecology and Clinical
Epidemiology, University of
Birmingham
Honorary Consultant,
Birmingham Women's NHS Foundation
Trust
Birmingham

Dr Ian Laing
Consultant Neonatologist and
Associate Patient
Services Director
The Simpson Centre for Reproductive
Health
Royal Infirmary of Edinburgh
Edinburgh

Dr Pallavi Latthe
Consultant Obstetrician and
Gynaecologist, Subspecialist
Urogynaecologist
Birmingham Women's NHS
Foundation Trust
Birmingham

Professor Tina Lavender
Professor of Midwifery and Women's
Health
University of Central Lancashire
Liverpool

Professor Mary Ann Lumsden
Professor of Gynaecology, Head of
Section of Reproductive
and Maternal Medicine
University of Glasgow
Glasgow

Dr Brian A Magowan
Consultant Obstetrician and
Gynaecologist
The Borders General Hospital
Melrose

Professor Gary Mires
Undergraduate Teaching Dean,
Consultant Obstetrician
School of Medicine
Division of Maternal and Child Health
Sciences
Ninewells Hospital and Medical
School
Dundee

Professor Deirdre J Murphy
Department of Obstetrics &
Gynaecology
Trinity College Dublin & Coombe
Women & Infants University Hospital
Dublin

Dr Catherine Nelson-Piercy
Consultant Obstetric Physician
Guy's & St Thomas' Hospital and
Queen Charlotte's Hospital, Imperial
Healthcare Trust
London

Dr Anthony Nicoll
Consultant Obstetrician and Honorary
Senior Lecturer
Ninewells Hospital
Dundee

Professor Jane Norman
Chair of Maternal and Fetal Health
University of Edinburgh Centre for
Reproductive Biology
The Queens Medical Research Institute
Edinburgh

Dr Philip Owen
Consultant Obstetrician and
Gynaecologist
Department of Obstetrics
Princess Royal Maternity Unit
Glasgow

Dr Ian Ramsay
Consultant Obstetrician and
Urogynaecologist
Forth Valley Acute Hospitals Trust
Department of Obstetrics and
Gynaecology
Stirling Royal Infirmary
Stirling

Dr Jane E Ramsay
Consultant Obstetrician and
Gynaecologist
Ayrshire Maternity Unit
Crosshouse Hospital
Kilmarnock

Mr Anthony Rutherford
Consultant in Reproductive Medicine
and Gynaecological Surgery
Leeds Teaching Hospitals NHS Trust,
Leeds

Dr Philip Savage
Consultant in Medical Oncology
Charing Cross Hospital
London

Dr Andrew Thomson
Consultant in Obstetrics and
Gynaecology
Royal Alexandra Hospital
Paisley

Professor Derek Tuffnell
Consultant Obstetrician, Bradford
Royal Infirmary
Honorary Visiting Professor in
Obstetrics,
Bradford University
Bradford

Dr Nynke Van de Broek
Senior Clinical Lecturer Sexual and
Reproductive Health
Honorary Consultant Obstetrician and
Gynaecologist
Liverpool School of Tropical Medicine
Liverpool

Contents

Contents

1 Clinical pelvic anatomy

Introduction

A thorough understanding of pelvic anatomy is essential for clinical practice. Not only does it facilitate an understanding of the process of labour, it also allows an appreciation of the mechanisms of sexual function and reproduction, and establishes a background to the understanding of gynaecological pathology. Congenital abnormalities are discussed in Chapter 4.

Obstetric anatomy

The bony pelvis

The girdle of bones formed by the sacrum and the two innominate bones has several important functions **(Fig. 1.1)**. It supports the weight of the upper body, and transmits the stresses of weight bearing to the lower limbs via the acetabulae. It provides firm attachments for the supporting tissues of the pelvic floor, including the sphincters of the lower bowel and bladder, and it forms the bony margins of the birth canal, accommodating the passage of the fetus during labour.

The birth canal is bounded by the true pelvis, i.e. that part of the bony girdle which lies below the pelvic brim – the lower parts of the two innominate bones and the sacrum. These bones are bound together at the sacroiliac joints, and at the symphysis pubis anteriorly. The brim is outlined by the promontory of the sacrum, the sacral alae, the iliopectineal lines, and the symphysis. The pelvic outlet is bounded by bone and ligament including the tip of the sacrum, the sacrotuberous ligaments, the ischial tuberosities, and the subpubic arch (of rounded 'Norman' shape) formed by the fused rami of the ischial and pubic bones. In the erect posture the pelvic brim is inclined at an angle of 65–70° to the horizontal. Because of the curvature of the sacrum, the axis of the pelvis (the pathway of descent of the fetal head in labour) is a J-shaped curve **(Fig. 38.4)**.

The change in the cross-sectional shape of the birth canal at different levels is fundamentally important in understanding the mechanics of labour. The canal can be envisaged initially as a sector of a curved cylinder of about 12 cm diameter **(Fig. 1.2)**. The stresses of weight bearing at the brim level in the average woman tend to flatten the inlet a little, reducing the anteroposterior diameter, but increasing the transverse diameter. In the lower pelvis, the counterpressure through the necks of the femora tends to compress the pelvis from the sides, reducing the transverse diameters of this part of the pelvis (Figs 38.2 and 38.3). At an intermediate level, opposite the third segment of the sacrum, the canal retains a circular cross-section. With this picture in mind, the 'average' diameters of the pelvis at brim, cavity, and outlet levels can be readily understood **(Table 1.1)**.

The distortions from a circular cross-section, however, are very modest. If, in circumstances of malnutrition or metabolic bone disease, the consolidation of bone is impaired, more gross distortion of pelvic shape is liable to occur, and labour is likely to involve mechanical difficulty. This is termed cephalopelvic disproportion. The changing cross-sectional shape of the true pelvis at different levels – transverse oval at the brim and anteroposterior oval at the outlet – usually determines a fundamental feature of labour, i.e. that the ovoid fetal head enters the brim with its longer (anteroposterior) diameter in a transverse or oblique position, but rotates during descent to bring the longer head diameter into the longer anteroposterior diameter of the outlet before the time of birth. This rotation is necessary because of the relatively large size of the human fetal head at term, which reflects the unique size and development of the fetal brain (Fig. 43.1).

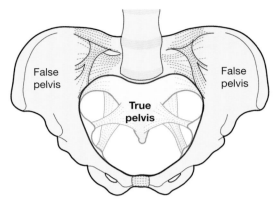

Fig. 1.1 The 'true' and 'false' pelvis.

Table 1.1		
Average pelvic diameters		
		Diameter
Level	**Direction**	**Size**
Inlet	Anteroposterior	11.5 cm
	Transverse	13 cm
Cavity	All diameters	12 cm
Outlet	Anteroposterior	12.5 cm
	Transverse intertuberous	11 cm
	Interspinous	10.5 cm

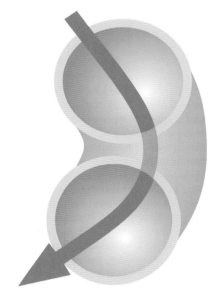

Fig. 1.2 The birth canal resembles a curved cylinder.

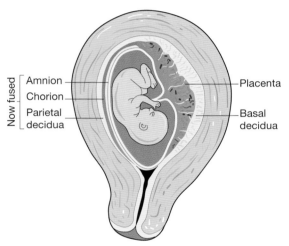

Fig. 1.3 The uterus and developing fetus at 12 weeks' gestation.

In most affluent countries, marked pelvic deformation is rare. Pelvimetry using X-rays, CT, or MRI scans can be used to measure the pelvic diameters but is of limited clinical value in predicting the likelihood of a successful vaginal delivery. Mechanical difficulty in labour is assessed by close observation of the progress of dilatation of the cervix, and of descent, assessed by both abdominal and vaginal examination.

The pelvic organs during pregnancy

The uterus

The uterus is a remarkable organ, composed largely of smooth muscle, the myometrium, which increases in weight during pregnancy from about 40 g to around 1000 g as the myometrial muscle fibres undergo both hyperplasia and hypertrophy **(Fig. 1.3)**. It provides a 'protected' implantation site for the genetically 'foreign' fertilized ovum, accommodates the developing fetus as it grows, and finally expels it into the outside world during labour.

Whereas the body of the uterus is formed from a thick layer of plain muscle, the cervix, which communicates with the upper vagina, is largely composed of denser collagenous tissue. This forms a rigid collar, retaining the fetus in utero as the myometrium hypertrophies and stretches. The junctional area between the body and cervix is known as the isthmus, which, in late pregnancy and labour, undergoes dilatation and thinning, forming the lower segment of the uterus. It is through this thinned area that the uterine wall is incised during caesarean section.

The uterine arteries, branches of the anterior division of the internal iliac arteries, become tortuous and coiled within the uterine wall **(Fig. 1.4)**. Innervation of the uterus is derived from both sympathetic and parasympathetic systems, and the functional significance of the motor pathways is incompletely understood. Drugs which stimulate alpha-adrenergic receptors activate the myometrium,

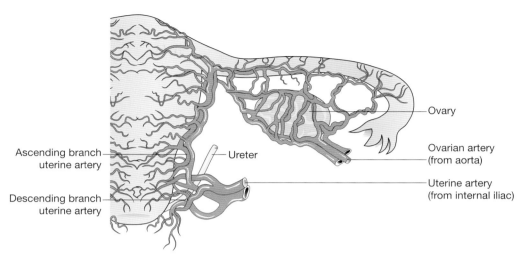

Fig. 1.4 The blood supply of the uterus, fallopian tube and ovary (posterior view).

whereas beta-adrenergic drugs have an inhibitory effect, and both beta-agonists and alpha-antagonists have been used in attempts to inhibit premature labour (see p. 302). Afferent fibres from the cervix enter the cord via the pelvic splanchnic (parasympathetic) nerves (S2,3,4). Pain stimuli during labour from the fundus and body of the uterus travel via the hypogastric (sympathetic) plexus, and enter the cord at the level of the lower thoracic segments.

The cervix

This becomes more vascular and softens in early pregnancy. The mucous secretion from the endocervical glands becomes thick and tenacious, forming a mechanical barrier to ascending infection. In late pregnancy the cervix 'ripens' – the dense mesh of collagen fibres loosens, as fluid is taken up by the hydrophilic mucopolysaccharides which occupy the interstices between the collagen bundles. This allows the cervix to become shorter as its upper part expands.

Additional changes

The ligaments of the sacroiliac and symphyseal joints become more extensible under the influence of pregnancy hormones. As a result, the pelvic girdle has more 'give' during labour. The increased mobility of the joints may result in backache or symphyseal pain.

The urinary tract in pregnancy

Frequency of micturition is often noticed in early pregnancy. As pregnancy advances, the ureters become dilated, probably due to the relaxing effect of progesterone on the smooth muscle wall, but also in part due to the mechanical effects of the gravid uterus. The urinary tract is therefore more vulnerable to ascending infection (acute pyelonephritis) in comparison to non-pregnancy.

The perineum

This term usually refers to the area of skin between the vaginal orifice and the anus. The underlying musculature at the outlet of the pelvis, surrounding the lower vagina and the anal canal, is important in the maintenance of bowel and urinary continence, and in sexual response. The muscles intermesh to form a firm pyramidal support, the perineal body, between the lower third of the posterior vaginal wall and the anal canal **(Fig. 1.5)**. The tissues of the perineal body are often markedly stretched during the expulsive second stage of labour and may be torn as the head is delivered. Injury to the anal sphincters may lead to impaired anal continence of faeces and/or flatus. Poor healing of an episiotomy or tear is liable to result in scarring, which may cause dyspareunia (pain during intercourse).

Anatomical points for obstetric analgesia

Pudendal nerve block

Knowledge of the pudendal nerves is important in obstetrics because they may be blocked to minimize pain during instrumental delivery, and because their integrity is vital for visceral muscular support and for sphincter function. These nerves, which innervate the vulva and perineum, are derived from the second, third and fourth sacral roots **(Fig. 1.2)**. On each side the nerve passes behind the sacrospinous ligament close to the tip of the ischial spine, and re-enters the pelvis along with the pudendal blood vessels in the pudendal canal. After giving off an inferior rectal branch, they divide into the perineal nerves and the dorsal nerves of the clitoris. Motor fibres of the pudendal nerve supply the levator ani, the superficial and deep perineal

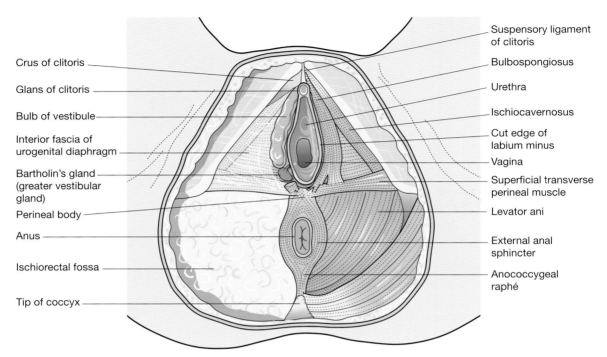

Crus of clitoris

Glans of clitoris

Bulb of vestibule

Interior fascia of
urogenital diaphragm

Bartholin's gland
(greater vestibular
gland)

Perineal body

Anus

Ischiorectal fossa

Tip of coccyx

Suspensory ligament
of clitoris

Bulbospongiosus

Urethra

Ischiocavernosus

Cut edge of
labium minus

Vagina

Superficial transverse
perineal muscle

Levator ani

External anal
sphincter

Anococcygeal
raphé

Fig. 1.5 The perineum. A view from below the pelvic outlet, showing the intermeshing muscles.

muscles, and the voluntary urethral sphincter. Sensory fibres innervate the central areas of the vulva and perineum. The peripheral skin areas are supplied by branches of the ilioinguinal nerve, the genitofemoral nerve, and the posterior femoral cutaneous nerve **(Fig. 1.6)**. The pudendal nerve can be blocked by an injection of local anaesthetic just below the tip of the ischial spine, as described on page 347.

Spinal block

The spinal cord ends at the level of L1–2. A spinal injection at the level of the L3–4 space will produce excellent analgesia up to around the level of the T10 nerve root or above, depending on the position of the patient and the volume of local anaesthetic used.

Epidural block

The epidural space, between the dura and the periosteum and ligaments of the spinal canal, is about 4 mm deep. Epidural injection of local anaesthetic blocks the spinal nerve roots as they traverse the space.

Gynaecological anatomy

The uterus

The uterus has the shape of a slightly flattened pear, and measures 7.5 × 5.0 × 2.5 cm. Its principal named parts are the fundus, the cornua, the body, and the cervix **(Fig. 1.7)**.

It forms part of the genital tract, lying in close proximity to the urinary tract anteriorly, and the lower bowel behind. All three tracts traverse the pelvic floor in the hiatus between the two bellies of the levator ani muscle. Clinically this means that a problem in one tract can readily affect another **(Fig. 1.8)**.

The uterine cavity is around 6 or 7 cm in length, and forms a flattened slit, with the anterior and posterior walls in virtual contact. The wall has three layers: the endometrium (innermost); the myometrium; and the peritoneum (outermost).

Endometrium

The endometrium is the epithelial lining of the cavity. The surface consists of a single layer of columnar ciliated cells, with invaginations forming uterine mucus-secreting glands within a cellular stroma. It undergoes cyclical changes in both the glands and stroma, leading to shedding and renewal about every 28 days.

There are two layers – a superficial functional layer which is shed monthly, and a basal layer which is not shed, and from which the new functional layer is regenerated. The epithelium of the functional layer shows active proliferative changes after a menstrual period until ovulation occurs, when the endometrial glands undergo secretory changes. Permanent destruction of the basal layer will result in amenorrhoea. This fact forms the basis for ablative techniques for the treatment of menorrhagia.

The normal changes in endometrial histology during the menstrual cycle, described on page 55, are determined by changing secretion of ovarian steroid hormones. If the

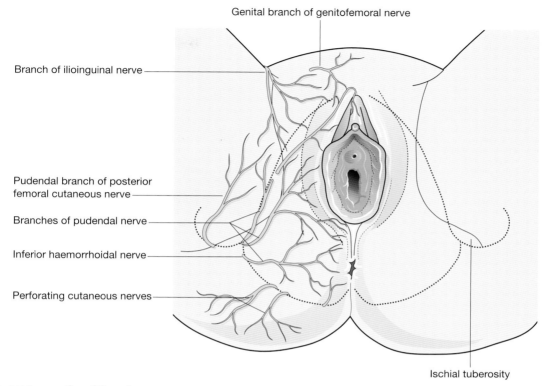

Genital branch of genitofemoral nerve

Branch of ilioinguinal nerve

Pudendal branch of posterior femoral cutaneous nerve

Branches of pudendal nerve

Inferior haemorrhoidal nerve

Perforating cutaneous nerves

Ischial tuberosity

Fig. 1.6 Innervation of the vulva.

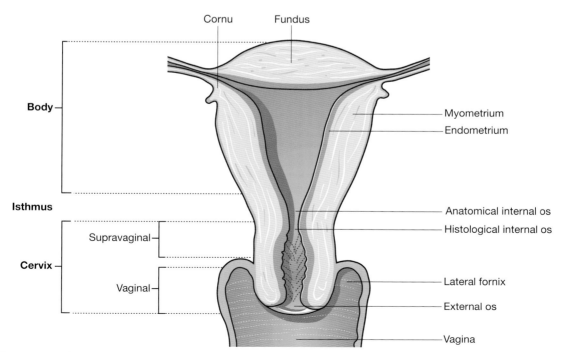

Cornu   Fundus

Body

Myometrium
Endometrium

Isthmus

Anatomical internal os
Histological internal os

Supravaginal

Cervix

Vaginal

Lateral fornix

External os

Vagina

Fig. 1.7 Coronal section of the uterus.

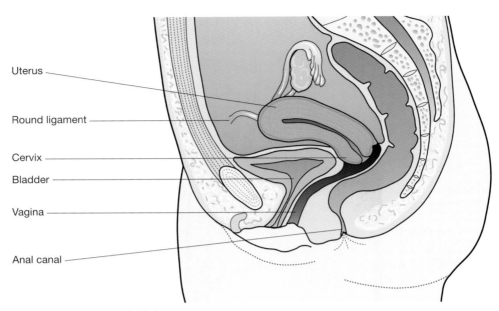

Fig. 1.8 Female pelvic organs: sagittal view.

endometrium is exposed to sustained oestrogenic stimulation, whether endogenous or exogenous, it may become hyperplastic. Benign hyperplasia may precede malignant change.

Myometrium

The smooth muscle fibres of the uterine wall do not form distinct layers. While the outermost fibres are predominantly longitudinal, continuous with the musculature of the uterine tubes above and the vaginal wall below, the main thickness of the uterine wall is formed from a mesh of criss-crossing spiral strands. The individual muscle cells contain filaments of actin and myosin, which interact to generate contractions. During labour the propagation of contractile excitation throughout the uterine wall is facilitated by the formation of 'gap junctions' between adjacent muscle cells. As a result, the spread of excitation resembles that in a syncytium.

Peritoneum

The posterior surface of the uterus is completely covered by peritoneum, which passes down over the posterior fornix of the vagina into the pouch of Douglas. Anteriorly the peritoneum is reflected off the uterus at a much higher level onto the superior surface of the bladder.

The cervix

The cervix connects the uterus and vagina, and projects into the upper vagina. The 'gutter' surrounding this projection comprises the vaginal fornices – lateral, anterior and posterior. The cervix is about 2.5 cm long; the shorter part of it, which lies above the fornices, is termed the supravaginal part. The endocervical canal is fusiform in shape between the external and internal os. After childbirth the external os loses its circular shape and resembles a transverse slit. The epithelial lining of the canal is a columnar mucous membrane with an anterior and posterior longitudinal ridge, from which shallow palmate folds extend; hence the name arbor vitae.

There are numerous glands secreting mucus which becomes more abundant and less viscous at the time of ovulation in mid-cycle. The vaginal surface of the cervix is covered with stratified squamous epithelium, similar to that lining the vagina. The squamocolumnar junction (histological external os) commonly does not correspond to the anatomical os, but may lie either above or external to the anatomical os. This 'tidal zone', within which the epithelial junction migrates at different stages of life, is termed the transformation zone. The ebb and flow of the squamocolumnar junction is influenced by oestrogenic stimulation. In the newborn female, and in pregnancy particularly, outgrowth of the columnar epithelium is very common, forming a bright pink 'rosette' around the external os. This appearance has been misnamed an 'erosion', but the epithelial covering, though delicate, is intact. In cases where the cervix has undergone deep bilateral laceration during childbirth, the resulting anterior and posterior lips tend to evert, exposing the glandular epithelium of the canal widely. This appearance is termed 'ectropion'.

Clinical aspects

The transformation zone is typically the area where precancerous change occurs. This can be detected by microscopic assessment of a cervical cytological smear. If the duct of a cervical gland becomes occluded, the gland distends with mucus to form a retention cyst (or Nabothian follicle). Multiple follicles are not uncommon, giving the cervix an irregular nodular feel and appearance. The body of the uterus is usually angled forward in relation to the

Fundus of anteverted uterus

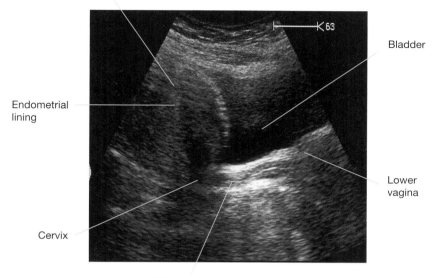

Bladder

Endometrial lining

Lower vagina

Cervix

Upper vagina

Fig. 1.9 Transabdominal scan of the bladder, uterus and vagina.

cervix (anteflexion), while the uterus and cervix as a whole lean forward from the upper vagina (anteversion). In about 15% of women the uterus leans backwards towards the sacrum, and is described as retroverted. The cervical os then faces down the long axis of the vagina, rather than at right angles to it. In most instances retroversion is an asymptomatic variant of normality.

It is especially important to distinguish retroversion from anteversion before introducing a sound or similar instrument into the uterine cavity, to avoid perforation of the uterine wall. After the menopause the uterus and cervix gradually become atrophic, and cervical mucus is scanty. The amount of cervix projecting into the vagina also diminishes.

Because the uterus lies immediately behind the bladder, and between the lower parts of the ureters, particular care must be taken not to damage these structures during hysterectomy **(Fig. 1.9)**. The endometrium and uterine cavity can be examined by hysteroscopy. The tubal ostiae can be seen **(Fig. 1.10)**. Because the anterior and posterior walls are normally in contact, the cavity must be inflated with gas or fluid to obtain an adequate view of the surfaces.

The uterine attachments and supports

Structures attached to the uterus include **(Fig. 1.11A,B)**:

- round ligament
- ovarian ligament
- uterosacral ligament or fold
- cardinal ligament/transverse cervical ligament (of Mackenrodt).

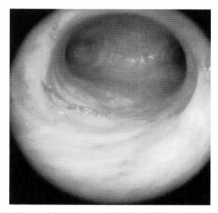

Fig. 1.10 Normal hysteroscopic view of the endometrial cavity, showing both tubal ostia.

The broad ligament is merely a double fold of peritoneum extending laterally from the uterus towards the pelvic side-wall. The hilum of the ovary arises from its posterior surface. The portion of the fold lateral to the ovary and tube is termed the infundibulopelvic ligament. Between the leaves of this fold, the uterine and ovarian blood vessels form an anastomotic loop. The ovarian ligament forms a ridge on the posterior leaf of the broad ligament, from the cornu of the uterus to the medial pole of the ovary. Developmentally it is part of the gubernaculum of the ovary, in continuity with the round ligament, which curves round anteriorly from the cornu towards the inguinal canal, through which it passes. The uterosacral ligaments pass upwards and backwards

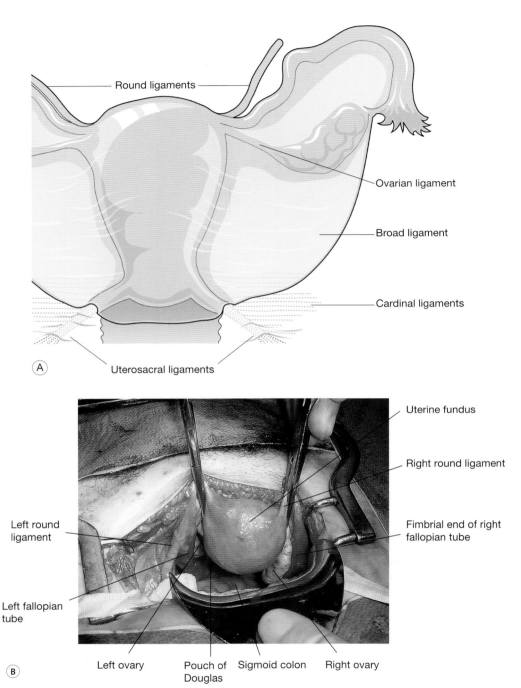

Round ligaments

Ovarian ligament

Broad ligament

Cardinal ligaments

(A) Uterosacral ligaments

Uterine fundus

Right round ligament

Left round ligament

Fimbrial end of right fallopian tube

Left fallopian tube

(B)

Left ovary Pouch of Sigmoid colon Right ovary
Douglas

Fig. 1.11 The uterus and appendages. (A) Schematic view of the uterine ligaments seen from behind. **(B)** View of the uterus, fallopian tubes and ovaries at abdominal hysterectomy.

from the posterior aspect of the cervix towards the lateral part of the second piece of the sacrum. In their lower part they contain plain muscle along with fibrous tissue and autonomic nerve fibres. In their upper part they dwindle to shallow peritoneal folds. The ligaments divide the pouch of Douglas from the pararectal fossa on each side.

The main ligaments providing support to the internal genital organs are the cardinal ligaments. The traditional name 'transverse cervical ligaments' is a misnomer. The cardinal ligaments are essentially dense condensations of connective tissue around the venous and nerve plexuses and arterial vessels which extend from the pelvic sidewall

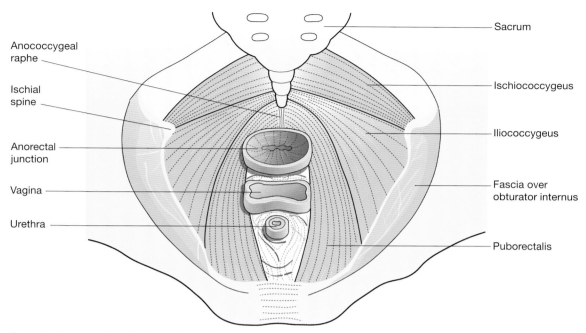

Anococcygeal
raphe

Ischial
spine

Anorectal
junction

Vagina

Urethra

Sacrum

Ischiococcygeus

Iliococcygeus

Fascia over
obturator internus

Puborectalis

Fig. 1.12 The urogenital diaphragm from above.

towards the genital tract. Medially they are firmly fused with the fascia surrounding the cervix and upper part of the vagina. They pass upwards and backwards towards the root of the internal iliac vessels. These condensations of fibrous and elastic tissue, together with plain muscle fibres, are sometimes referred to as the parametrium. They support the upper vagina and cervix, helping to maintain the angle between the axis of the vagina and that of the anteverted uterus. Inferiorly they are continuous with the fascia on the upper surface of the levator muscles.

The pelvic diaphragm

Below the level of the cardinal ligaments, the pelvic organs are supported by a sloping shelf of muscle on each side, formed by the levator ani muscle **(Fig. 1.12)**. The disposition of the muscle bundles is comparable to that of the abdominal musculature. Near to the midline there is a longitudinal muscle bundle, the puborectalis (cf. the rectus abdominis). Laterally the muscle sheets (iliococcygeus and ischiococcygeus) are oblique/transverse. The most medial fibres of puborectalis are inserted into the upper part of the perineal body. The succeeding fibres turn medially behind the anorectal flexure, and are inserted into the anococcygeal raphe and the tip of the coccyx, along with the fibres of ilio- and ischiococcygeus. Thus all three visceral tubes reach the body surface via a hiatus between the medial margins of puborectalis, and all are supported from behind by the sling action of the muscle when it contracts. Innervation is from the pudendal nerve (S2,3,4). The fascia on the upper surface of the pelvic diaphragm blends with the

lower part of the cardinal ligaments. The fascia on the inferior surface of levator ani forms the roof of the ischiorectal fossa.

The main blood supply of the uterus is from the uterine arteries, which are branches of the internal iliac vessels **(Fig. 1.13)**. Each passes medially in the base of the broad ligament above the ureter, and ascends along the lateral aspect of the uterus, forming an anastomotic loop in the broad ligament with the ovarian artery (see **Fig. 1.4**). The uterine veins form a plexus in the parametrium below the uterine arteries, draining into the internal iliac veins. The principal lymph drainage is to iliac and obturator glands on the pelvic sidewall. From the fundus and cornua, lymph drains via the ovarian pathway to aortic nodes, while a few lymphatics in the round ligaments drain into the inguinal nodes **(Fig. 1.14)**. The uterus is supplied by sympathetic and parasympathetic nerves, the exact functional significance of which is uncertain.

Congenital abnormalities of the uterus

Most of the female genital tract develops from the two paramesonephric (Müllerian) ducts, the caudal portions of which approximate in the midline and fuse to form the uterus, cervix, and upper part of the vagina. The upper divergent portions of the ducts form the uterine tubes.

Congenital abnormality can result from:

- failure of or incomplete fusion
- failure of canalization
- asymmetrical maldevelopment.

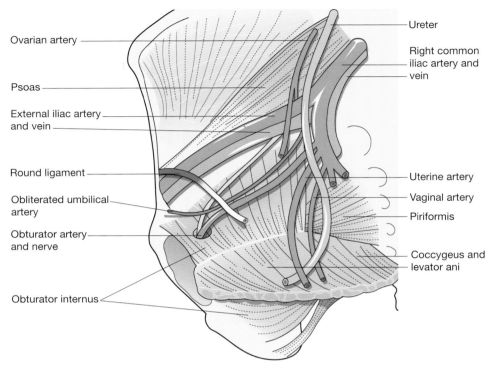

Ovarian artery

Psoas

External iliac artery
and vein

Round ligament

Obliterated umbilical
artery

Obturator artery
and nerve

Obturator internus

Ureter

Right common
iliac artery and
vein

Uterine artery

Vaginal artery

Piriformis

Coccygeus and
levator ani

Fig. 1.13 The lateral pelvic sidewall.

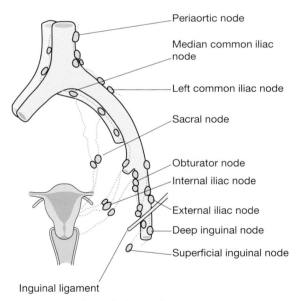

Periaortic node

Median common iliac
node

Left common iliac node

Sacral node

Obturator node

Internal iliac node

External iliac node

Deep inguinal node

Superficial inguinal node

Inguinal ligament

Fig. 1.14 Lymphatic drainage of the uterus. The lymph
channels follow the blood supply.

The diagrams in Figure 4.5 illustrate some of abnormalities which may be encountered. Failures of canalization are likely to present at puberty, as menstrual blood has no way to escape. Incomplete fusion is associated with late miscarriage, preterm labour, and malpresentation. Because of the intimate association during development, congenital abnormality of the female genital tract is commonly associated with abnormality of the urinary tract.

The vulva

The term vulva generally encompasses all the external female genitalia, i.e. the mons pubis, the labia majora and minora, the clitoris, and the structures within the vestibule – the external urinary meatus and the hymen. The mons pubis is a thickened pad of fat, cushioning the pubic bones anteriorly. The labia majora contain fatty tissue overlying the vascular bulbs of the vestibule and the bulbospongiosus muscles. The skin of the labia majora bears secondary sexual hair on the lateral surfaces only. There are abundant sebaceous, sweat, and apocrine glands. The folds of the labia minora vary considerably in size, and may be concealed by the labia majora or may project between them. They contain no fat, but are vascular and erectile during sexual arousal; the skin contains many sebaceous glands. Anteriorly the folds bifurcate before uniting to form a hood above the clitoris and a frenulum along its dorsal surface. Posteriorly the labia minora are linked by a fine ridge of skin, the fourchette.

The labia minora and the fourchette form the boundaries of the vestibule. Between the fourchette and the posterior part of the hymen there is a crescentic furrow termed the navicular fossa. The urethral meatus lies within the vestibule, close to the anterior margin of the vaginal orifice.

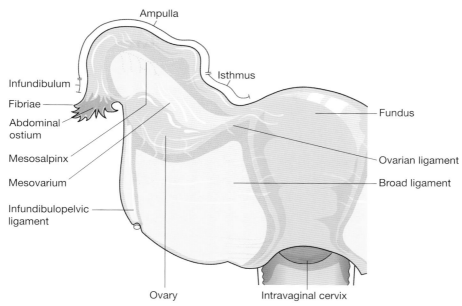

Ampulla

Isthmus

Infundibulum

Fibriae

Abdominal ostium

Mesosalpinx

Mesovarium

Infundibulopelvic ligament

Fundus

Ovarian ligament

Broad ligament

Ovary

Intravaginal cervix

Fig. 1.15 Posterior view of the uterus and broad ligament.

There are pairs of small mucus-secreting paraurethral glands in the lower part of the posterior wall of the urethra. These rudimentary tubules are homologous with the glands in the male prostate. If they become infected and blocked, they may form a paraurethral abscess, cyst, or urethral diverticulum. Two mucus-secreting glands, known as Bartholin's glands (or greater vestibular glands), lie posterolateral to the vaginal orifice on each side, embedded in the posterior pole of the vascular vestibular bulb (see **Fig. 1.5**). Their ducts open near the lateral limits of the navicular fossa. The glands only become palpable, and the duct orifices become visible, if infection is present.

Blood supply

The main sources of the vascularity of the vulva are branches of the internal pudendal arteries. There are also branches from the superficial and deep external pudendal arteries.

Nerve supply

The main sensory supply to the vulva is via the pudendal nerves. Peripheral parts of the vulvar skin are supplied by filaments from the iliohypogastric and ilioinguinal nerves, and from the perineal branches of the posterior cutaneous nerves of the thigh (see **Fig. 1.6**). The pudendal nerve provides motor fibres to all the muscles of the perineum, including the voluntary urinary and bowel sphincters, as well as the levator ani.

Lymph drainage

The main pathway of drainage is to the superficial inguinal glands, and on through the deep inguinal to the external iliac glands. Some lymphatics from the deeper structures of the vulva pass with vaginal lymphatics to the internal iliac nodes.

The fallopian tubes

The tube extends on each side from the cornu of the uterus within the upper border of the broad ligament for about 10 cm. The tubes and ovaries together are commonly described as the uterine appendages, or adnexa **(Fig. 1.15)**.

The tube can be divided into four parts **(Fig. 1.16)**. The interstitial (intramural) part forms a narrow passage through the thickness of the myometrium. The isthmus, extending out from the cornu for about 3 cm, is also narrow. The ampulla is thin-walled, 'baggy', and tortuous; its lateral portion is free from the broad ligament, and droops down behind it towards the ovary. Near its lateral limit the abdominal ostium is constricted, but opens out again to form the infundibulum. This trumpet-shaped expansion is fringed by a ring of delicate fronds (or fimbriae), one of which is attached to the surface of the ovary.

The walls of the tubes include outer longitudinal and inner circular layers of smooth muscle. The delicate lining (endosalpinx), containing columnar ciliated and secretory cells, has longitudinal folds in the isthmic segment, which change into a highly intricate branching pattern in the ampulla.

Tubal function

At the time of ovulation the fimbriae clasp the ovary in the area where the stigma (or point of follicular rupture) is forming. Usually, therefore, the ovum is discharged into the infundibulum (funnel) and is carried by tubal peristalsis into

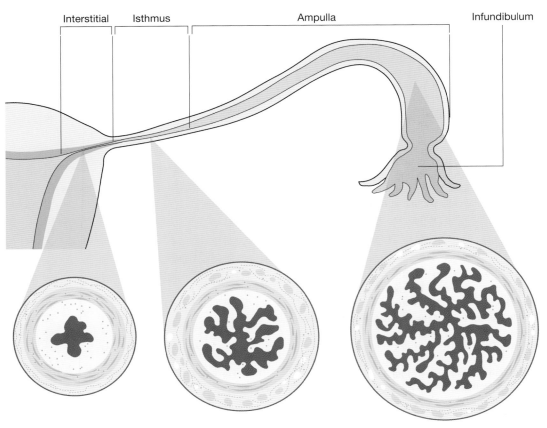

Fig. 1.16 The oviduct, showing the structure of the mucosal layer.

the ampulla of the tube, which is where fertilization occurs. Transit of the zygote to the site of implantation in the uterus takes several days.

Sterilization is effected by occluding both tubes, preferably in the narrow isthmic portion, using clips, sutures, rings, or diathermy.

Patency of the tubes can be tested by injecting a watery dye (methylthioninium chloride [methylene blue]) through the cervix, and observing spill from the abdominal ostia by laparoscopy. The contours of the uterine cavity and tubal lumen may also be demonstrated with radio-opaque fluid during a hysterosalpingogram.

The vagina

The vagina, which links the external and internal parts of the female genital tract, has a dual function: it forms the coital canal, affording access for spermatozoa to reach the cervix, and, with the cervix, it forms the soft-tissue birth canal. It lies in close proximity to the urethra and bladder anteriorly, and to the anal canal and rectum posteriorly. All three canals traverse the pelvic floor, passing between the medial (puborectalis) portions of the levator ani muscles. The insertion of these muscle fibres into the anococcygeal raphe creates a sling behind the bowel so that, at the junction of the lower rectum and the anal canal, a sharp angle is created which is opened when the muscle relaxes. Other muscle fibres are inserted into the perineal body near its apex, creating a similar sling which angulates the axis of the vagina at that level. In turn, the anterior vaginal wall in the area of the bladder neck receives support.

There are differences in the anatomy of the vagina above and below this level. The lower third of the vagina is closely invested by the superficial and deep muscles of the perineum. It:

■ incorporates the urethra in its anterior wall
■ is separated from the bowel by the perineal body
■ has a rich arterial blood supply from branches of the vaginal arteries, and from both external and internal pudendal vessels.

The upper two-thirds of the vagina, above the levator shelf:

■ is not invested by muscles, but is wide and capacious
■ is in apposition with the bladder base anteriorly, and with the rectum (and, above that, the pouch of Douglas) posteriorly

- is supported laterally and at the vault by the parametrium (cardinal and uterosacral ligaments). During sexual arousal the smooth muscle fibres within the parametrium elevate the vaginal vault and cervix, thereby elongating the vagina, and straightening its long axis.

Vaginal structure

The vaginal walls form an elastic fibromuscular tube with a multilayered structure. The lining of stratified squamous epithelium is corrugated into transverse folds (or rugae), which facilitates stretching during childbirth. The epithelium contains no glands, but during the reproductive years the more superficial cells contain abundant glycogen. This polysaccharide is broken down by lactobacilli which form the normal flora of the vagina, producing lactic acid. This accounts for the low pH in the vaginal lumen (average pH 4.5).

Between the epithelium and the muscle there is a layer of areolar tissue containing an extensive venous plexus. Vascular engorgement during sexual arousal, analogous to erection in the male, is most marked in the lower part of the vagina, encroaching on the vaginal lumen as the rugae distend. The vasocongestive response also results in increased transudation into the vaginal lumen.

The smooth muscle layers (outer longitudinal, inner circular) are not distinct, and an interlacing pattern is usual. Deep to the muscle there is another extensive plexus of veins, within the outer vaginal fascia.

The ovary

The ovaries are attached on each side to the posterior surface of the broad ligaments through a narrowed base termed the hilum. The ovaries are also attached to the cornua of the uterus by the ovarian ligaments. Developmentally these are the upper portions of the gubernacula ovarii, and they are responsible for drawing the ovaries down into the pelvis from the posterior wall of the abdominal cavity. Typically, each ovary lies in an ovarian fossa, a shallow peritoneal depression lateral to the ureter, near the pelvic sidewall. The position may vary, however, and when the uterus is retroverted, one or both ovaries may lie in the pouch of Douglas.

The ovaries are ovoid in shape, with an irregular surface and a firm, largely solid, stroma which can be divided indistinctly into an outer cortex and an inner medulla. The surface epithelium of cuboidal coelomic cells forms an incomplete layer, beneath which is a fibrous investment – the tunica albuginea. The germ cells from which the ova are derived are embedded in the substance of the ovaries.

The ovarian blood vessels and nerves enter through the hilum from the broad ligament. The ovarian arteries are direct branches of the aorta. Within the broad ligaments they form an anastomotic loop with branches of the uterine arteries.

Anatomy of the lower urinary tract

The descending ureters are narrow thick-walled muscular tubes which cross into the pelvis close to the bifurcation of the common iliac arteries. They lie immediately under the peritoneum of the pelvic sidewall, behind the lateral attachment of the broad ligaments. Curving medially and forwards, they pass through the base of the broad ligaments below the uterine arteries, about 2 cm lateral to the supravaginal part of the cervix, a short distance above the lateral fornices of the vagina.

Approaching the bladder, the ureters pass medially in front of the upper vagina, and enter the bladder base obliquely at the upper angles of the trigone.

The wall of the ureter is composed of three elements: an external fibrous sheath, layers of smooth muscle, and a lining of transitional epithelium. There may be partial or complete duplication of one or both ureters. An ectopic ureter is one that opens anywhere but the trigone of the bladder, and this may even be into the vagina or the vestibule. Urinary incontinence inevitably results.

The bladder

The urinary reservoir, lined with transitional epithelium, has the shape of a tetrahedron when empty, but the mesh of smooth muscle in the bladder wall can readily distend to contain a volume of half a litre or more. This muscle coat (the detrusor muscle) is thus normally relaxed and capable of considerable stretching without a contractile response. If urinary outflow during micturition is chronically impeded, however, the detrusor muscle becomes irritable and ultimately hypertrophic, producing prominent trabecular bands visible at cystoscopy.

The bladder is covered with peritoneum on its superior surface only. The peritoneum is reflected onto the anterior abdominal wall at a varying level, dependent on the degree of bladder filling. The oblique passage of the terminal part of each ureter through the bladder wall creates a one-way valve, which normally prevents urinary backflow from the bladder. This protects the kidneys from ascending infection. The triangular area within the bladder base defined by the two ureteric orifices and the internal urethral orifice is termed the trigone. Over this area the epithelium remains smooth, even when the bladder is empty.

The urethra

The female urethra is about 4 cm long. Below the bladder neck it is embedded in the anterior vaginal wall, and the smooth muscle layers of the two structures intermingle. The urethral tissues also reflect the vascularity and turgidity of the vagina itself. Many of the urethral muscle fibres near the bladder neck are longitudinal and continuous with those of the bladder above, forming a funnel which opens out when these fibres contract, flattening the angle between the bladder base and the upper urethra. There are also abundant elastic fibres at this level, whose action helps to restore urethral closure after micturition. Around the lower part of the urethra there is a fusiform collar of voluntary muscle – the external urethral sphincter. This segment of the urethra passes through the perineal membrane, which keeps it in a stable position. The upper urethra, on the other hand, shares the mobility of the bladder neck. The urethra is lined by transitional epithelium in its upper part, and by squamous epithelium below.

Nerve supply

Apart from the external sphincter, the efferent nerve supply controlling bladder function is from the pelvic parasympathetic system (S2,3,4), which provides the main motor fibres to the detrusor muscle. Afferent fibres conveying the normal sensations of bladder filling also return through the parasympathetic pathway, though some sympathetic sensory fibres convey the feelings of bladder overdistension via the hypogastric plexus. At the level of the second, third and fourth sacral segments of the spinal cord, the sensory and motor parasympathetic nerves form spinal reflex arcs, which are moderated by interaction with higher centres in the brain. Urinary continence depends upon a variety of factors. These include the elastic fibres surrounding the bladder neck which normally maintain urethral closure; and the tone or reflex contraction of the levator ani muscles which, through their insertion into the perineal body, elevate the urethrovesical junction, creating an angulation at the junction of the mobile (upper) and fixed (lower) portions of the urethra. The turgidity of spongy tissue underlying the urethral epithelium also assists in occluding the urethra, as does the action of the voluntary sphincter.

Key points

- Without understanding the anatomy of the pelvis it is impossible to understand the mechanisms of labour.
- The cross-sectional shape of the birth canal is different at different levels. At the pelvic brim it is oval in shape, and the widest part of this oval is in the lateral plane from one side to the other. The outlet is also oval, with the widest part in the anteroposterior plane. The head enters the pelvic brim in the transverse position, as the inlet is widest in this plane, but rotates 90° at the pelvic floor to the anteroposterior plane before delivery. The shoulders also follow the same rotation.

2

Human embryogenesis

Introduction

In obstetric practice it is common to use 280 days (40 weeks) from the first day of the last menstrual period (LMP) to estimate the delivery date of a full-term pregnancy. This period has also become a convenient but inaccurate description of the number of weeks of 'pregnancy'. This is an obvious source of confusion since embryologists refer to the number of gestational days, i.e. days since fertilization, when discussing early human development. Since conception requires male and female gametes to be in the same place (the ampulla of the fallopian tube) at the same time (within a few hours of ovulation and within 6 days of intercourse), it can be approximated to:

- ≈14 days after the first day of the LMP, i.e. an estimate of the day of ovulation in a woman with a regular 28-day cycle
- the day of ovulation as judged by a change in basal body temperature, serum luteinizing hormone (LH), and/or oestrogen-to-progesterone ratios
- 6 days prior to the rapid increase in chorionic gonadotrophin levels that is associated with implantation of the embryo.

In most pregnancies, only the first of these options is available, and thus 8 weeks of 'pregnancy' implies 42 gestational days (GD).

Nomenclature

Embryology is cursed with a dense, classically based nomenclature. Attempts at standardization have often led to the same structure having at least two different names (e.g. yolk sac and umbilical vesicle; branchial and pharyngeal arches) and/or the same structure changing its name at different stages of development (e.g. allantois → urachus → medial umbilical ligament). This complexity can be disheartening, so only the most up-to-date terms will be used and these will be related to the mature tissues wherever possible. Some transient structures are important

Box 2.1

Axis formation

Axis formation occurs in the early undifferentiated embryo to determine which end will be the head and which the tail (rostrocaudal axis), which is the front and which is the back (dorsoventral axis), and to which side the heart will loop (left–right axis) **(Fig. 2.1)**. In other vertebrates much of this information is coded by RNA and protein gradients in the cytoplasm of the fertilized egg or by the site of sperm entry. The nature of these signals in human embryos is not well understood. From a medical point of view, failure to form either the rostrocaudal or the dorsoventral axis would result in early embryonic lethality. Complete reversal of the left–right axis (situs inversus) can be a coincidental finding in healthy adults.

Kartagener's syndrome is a genetic condition where situs inversus is associated with recurrent chest infections due to abnormal respiratory cilia. Identification of the molecular basis of this condition as a ciliopathy has elucidated the mechanism by which the left–right axis is formed. The primitive node is a specialized region at the caudal end of the primitive streak which is lined with ciliated cells. The nodal cilia function to sweep secreted signalling molecules to one side of the embryo, thus beginning a cascade of transcription which establishes left–right asymmetry.

in understanding malformations and these will be highlighted.

To start with the title of this chapter, the transition from embryonic to fetal life is at ≈56 GD (i.e. ≈10 weeks post-LMP). This is an arbitrary but useful boundary that is based on the fact that 90% of adult structures are recognizable at this stage. One of the most important concepts in embryogenesis is the establishment of the three main embryonic axes: (1) rostrocaudal (more correctly termed anteroposterior in early embryogenesis); (2) dorsoventral; (3) left–right **(Box 2.1, Fig. 2.1)**.

Fertilization to implantation (0–6 GD)

In vitro fertilization has greatly increased our understanding of the early cellular and molecular events in human embryogenesis **(Fig. 2.2)**. Sadly for the male

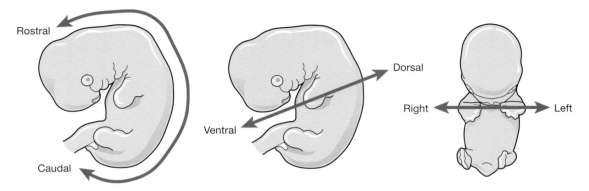

Fig. 2.1 The rostral–caudal, dorsal–ventral and left–right embryonic axes.

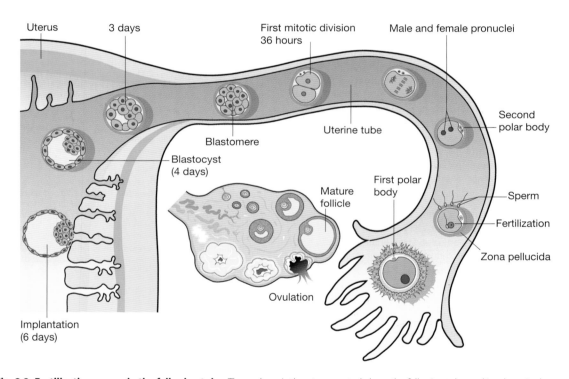

Fig. 2.2 Fertilization occurs in the fallopian tube. The embryo is then transported along the fallopian tube and implants in the uterine wall around 6 GD.

ego, the sperm has only three essential roles in embryogenesis:

1. to stimulate a change in the zona pellucida that prevents further sperm entering the cell
2. to deliver a paternally imprinted haploid genome (see **Box 2.2**) in order to reconstitute a diploid chromosome number
3. to stimulate the second meiotic division in the egg with subsequent production of the second polar body.

In contrast to the sperm, the egg is a complex cell with many subcompartments, each with a critical role. At the most basic level the egg carries a maternally imprinted haploid genome **(Box 2.2)**. It also determines the orientation of at least one of the 'axes' in the early embryo **(Box 2.1)**, and it provides all the RNA and protein synthesis requirements until the embryonic genome becomes transcriptionally active at 2–3 days post-fertilization.

The first mitotic division occurs 36 hours after fertilization. The next four mitoses are at intervals of ≈17 hours and produce a ball of cells called a blastomere. After the fifth mitotic division the blastomere becomes polarized as a sphere with a single-cell-layered wall (trophoblast) and an inner cell mass. The inner cell mass of this blastocyst contains the cells that will form the embryo itself. The 128 cells that are present following the seventh mitotic division still occupy the same volume as the initial fertilized egg, i.e. there has been no physical growth. The embryo sheds the zona pellucida at about this time, a process termed fancifully as 'hatching'. Over these first 5 days the embryo is transported along the fallopian tube and becomes attached to the uterine wall around 6 GD.

Implantation and formation of the germ layers (7–18 GD)

At implantation the trophoblast buries itself in the endometrium. The embryo thus gains access to the maternal circulation and behaves as an efficient paracytic organism which enables a very rapid period of growth. The inner cell mass begins to differentiate and the embryo takes on the appearance of a disc consisting of two layers of morphologically distinct cells: the epiblast (the dorsal region) and the hypoblast (the ventral region, **Fig. 2.3A**). This is the first real evidence of embryonic polarity. The largest embryonic cavity at this stage is the umbilical vesicle which is lined with hypoblast cells. The amniotic cavity begins to form by 9 GD and is lined with epiblast cells.

By day 16 the embryonic disc takes on an oval shape and a second axis (rostrocaudal or head–tail axis) becomes apparent. This is accompanied by a process known as gastrulation, during which cells from the epiblast migrate towards a groove in the caudal end of the disc known as the primitive streak **(Fig. 2.3B)**. The migrating cells pass though the primitive streak and form a new embryonic compartment or 'germ layer' called the mesoderm. The dorsal epiblast now becomes the embryonic ectoderm and the hypoblast is replaced by embryonic endoderm. The embryo now has three 'germ' layers

---

Box 2.2

Imprinting

The male and female gamete both contain 23 chromosomes, one copy of each autosomal chromosome (numbered 1–22 in decreasing order of size) and one sex chromosome (X in egg and X or Y in sperm). The DNA sequence of each pair of chromosomes is essentially identical, but the maternal copy we inherit functions differently from the paternal copy; indeed, they can be considered antagonistic. For example, the short arm of chromosome 11 contains the gene insulin-like growth factor type 2 (IGF2). Although there are two copies of IGF2 in each cell, only one is ever active and this is always on the paternally inherited chromosome 11. IGF2 produces a protein which promotes fetal growth (the 'male' drive) but is silenced on the maternal copy (the 'female' drive). This particular mechanism probably evolved to balance the conflict between the advantage to the male of having a large offspring at birth against the risk to the mother of delivering such a large offspring.

Differential gene activation is the result of the silencing of one copy of a gene via covalent modifications of both the DNA itself (methylation) and histone proteins (acetylation) which are intimately associated with the double-stranded DNA molecule. These parent-of-origin-specific modifications are known as 'genomic imprinting'. Beckwith–Wiedemann syndrome is caused by specific genetic mutations that result in a fetus having two active copies of IGF2. This result is an infant that is large for gestational age and who is prone to tumour formation, particularly Wilms' tumour. Several other examples of imprinting mutations are known.

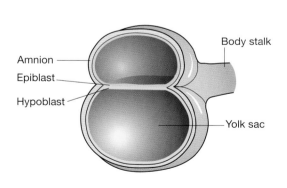

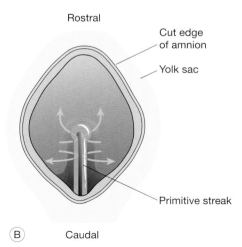

A

B

Rostral

Cut edge of amnion

Yolk sac

Amnion

Epiblast

Hypoblast

Body stalk

Yolk sac

Primitive streak

Caudal

Fig. 2.3 Formation of the germ layers. (A) The inner cell mass takes on the appearance of a disc comprising two layers of morphologically distinct cells: the epiblast (the dorsal region) and the hypoblast (the ventral region). **(B)** Gastrulation is the process where cells from the epiblast migrate towards and through the primitive streak – a groove that forms in the caudal end of the disc – to form the mesoderm and to replace the hypoblast with the embryonic endoderm.

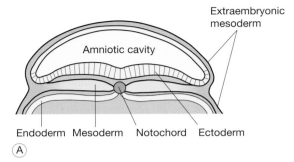

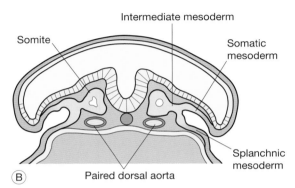

Fig. 2.4 Formation of the neural tube. The notochord – a strip of specialized midline mesodermal cells – induces a midline groove on the ectodermal surface **(A)** The edges of this groove will fuse to form the neural tube **(B)** Failure of this tube to close rostrally results in anencephaly, and failure caudally leads to spina bifida.

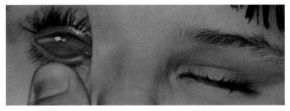

Fig. 2.5 Anophthalmia. The eye socket is empty.

bounded by the umbilical vesicle ventrally and the amniotic cavity dorsally.

Organogenesis (19–56+ GD)

The outline of organogenesis given here is necessarily brief and is divided into five main areas:

1. neural tube and brain
2. gut tube and derivatives
3. heart and liver
4. craniofacial structures
5. limbs and skeletal muscle.

Neural tube and brain

Formation of the neural tube and primitive brain is the first evidence of organogenesis. It begins at 19 GD, when a midline groove forms on the dorsal ectodermal surface, rostral to the primitive streak. This change in the surface ectoderm is induced by a strip of specialized midline mesodermal cells called the notochord **(Fig. 2.4)**. Two important paired structures form on either side of this groove:

- the neural folds
- the somites.

The neural folds grow rapidly and begin to fuse across the midline in the cervical region to form the neural tube by 22 GD. At the same time, paired segmental condensations of the mesoderm (somites) are beginning to form blocks of tissue on either side of the midline (paraxial mesoderm). A new pair of somites appears every 6.6 hours in a rostrocaudal direction. The somites are critical for establishing the adult body plan and their formation is an example of repeated segment (metameric) pattern formation during embryogenesis **(Box 2.3)**.

Fusion of the neural tube proceeds rapidly in both rostral and caudal directions. This apparently simple tube will give rise to the entire central nervous system (CNS). At

Box 2.3

Pattern formation

Pattern formation is a molecular concept whereby the future fate of a group of cells is determined by specific patterns of gene expression or activity prior to any morphological change being detected. The most striking patterns involve the activation of specific transcription factors induced by gradients of signalling molecules within the embryo. The best-known example involves *Hox* gene determination of the identity of individual somites along the rostrocaudal axis. Later in development *Hox* genes also play a role in patterning the limb bud. However, many other classes of transcription factors are vital for pattern formation.

Defects in these patterning processes underlie many types of malformation. For example, mutations in one allele of the transcription factor *PAX6* result in failure of

iris formation (aniridia) and homozygous mutations cause complete absence of the eye (anophthalmia; **Fig. 2.5**), whereas mutations in the related gene *PAX9* cause the absence of particular teeth (hypodontia). Mutation in a single gene can produce a specific syndrome characterized by a particular combination of malformations. This suggests that the mutated gene may be used at different stages of development and in different tissues. Other malformation combinations may be the result of deletion of a chromosomal region that causes adjacent genes to be lost, e.g. WAGR syndrome is caused by a deletion on chromosome 11p13 and is characterized by aniridia and Wilms' tumour as a consequence of both *WT1* and *PAX6* mapping to 11p13.

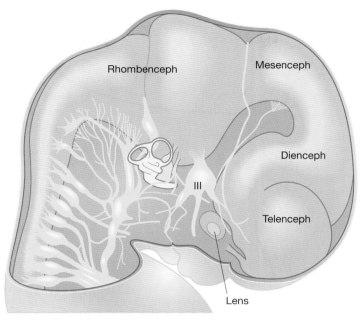

Fig. 2.6 Development of the CNS. The main brain segments – forebrain (telencephalon and diencephalon), midbrain (mesencephalon) and hindbrain (rhombencephalon) – are shown in a 48–51 GD human embryo. Cranial nerves I and III are also visible at this stage and are indicated, as is the lens that is located within the optic vesicle.

either end of the embryo the neural tube remains open for a short time, and these openings are referred to as the rostral and caudal neuropores. The rostral neuropore closes by 23 GD, and failure of this process results in one of the most severe of human malformations, anencephaly. The caudal neuropore is the last part of the neural tube to close at 26 GD, and failure of this closure leads to spina bifida .

The rostral half of the neural tube is more complex and forms the future brain. The caudal part forms the spinal cord. In common with many other embryological structures, the formation of the CNS is best viewed as a tube which is segmented along the rostrocaudal long axis, each linear segment then differentiates dorsoventrally to produce the final adult form. At day 26 the CNS is a tube with four main segments:

1. forebrain – prosencephalon
2. midbrain – mesencephalon
3. hindbrain – rhombencephalon
4. spinal cord.

The forebrain

The prosencephalon is initially subdivided into three segments. The most rostral is the telencephalon medium, then come the D1 and D2 compartments of the diencephalon. All three segments surround the future third ventricle **(Fig. 2.6)**. D1 will give rise to the bilateral optic evaginations by day 28 (see Craniofacial structures, below) and D2 will form the thalamus, hypothalamus, pineal gland

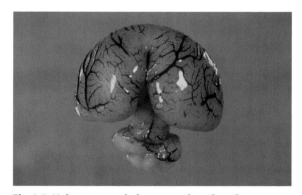

Fig. 2.7 Holoprosencephaly occurs when there is failure of division between the two future cerebral hemispheres. The condition is associated with profound cerebral impairment.

and part of the pituitary (neurohypophysis). The telencephalon medium forms as a rostral out-pouching of the third ventricle. By day 32 a midline crest separates the two future cerebral hemispheres. Failure of this process results in a malformation called holoprosencephaly **(Fig. 2.7)**. Subsequent development of telencephalic structures is complex and mostly occurs during fetal and postnatal life. In addition to the cerebral hemispheres the telencephalon gives rise to the caudate and lentiform nuclei (derivatives of the corpus striatum) and the connections between the hemispheres derived from the lamina

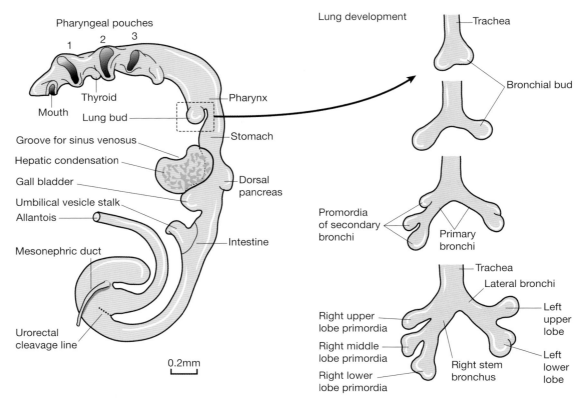

Fig. 2.8 Development of the gut tube and its derivatives. In the left panel is a drawing of the developing gut. Initially, the primitive gut is simply a concavity within the embryo lined with embryonic endoderm, with a large direct connection to the umbilical vesical. As development progresses, the gut becomes a tube with a fundamental role in the development of the gastrointestinal tract, the thyroid and pituitary glands, the lungs, the pancreas, the bile ducts and gall bladder, and the urogenital system. The right panel shows the development of the lungs – from top to bottom – at 28 days; at 32 days; at 33 days; and at the end of the 5th week.

terminalis (anterior commissure, hippocampal commissure and corpus callosum).

The midbrain

The mesencephalon is less complicated than the forebrain. It segments dorsally to form the superior and inferior colliculi (roles in integrating visual and auditory signals, respectively) and ventrally to form the tegmentum (oculomotor nuclei of cranial nerves III and IV). This typifies a general pattern within the neural tube, where dorsal grey matter has a sensory function and ventral grey matter has a motor function. Later in development the cerebral peduncles occupy a significant proportion of the midbrain.

The hindbrain

The rhombencephalon is highly segmented into eight regions known as rhombomeres. The exact function of each rhombomere is not clear but they appear to have a role in forming the motor components of cranial nerves V, VII, IX and X. More rostrally the rhombencephalon forms the pons and the cerebellum. Like the cerebral hemispheres, the

cerebellum continues to develop throughout intrauterine life.

The spinal cord

The spinal cord itself is unsegmented along the rostrocaudal axis. The adjacent somites produce the repeated pattern of spinal nerve roots that is seen in adult life. The cord is patterned in the dorsoventral axis and maintains the dorsal/sensory, ventral/motor pattern for grey matter function mentioned above.

Gut tube and its derivatives

Initially, the primitive gut is simply a concavity within the embryo that is lined with embryonic endoderm and is open to the umbilical vesicle **(Fig. 2.8)**. As development progresses, the gut becomes a tube with a fundamental role in the development of many organs. The most important of these, in rostrocaudal order, are:

- the thyroid and pituitary glands
- the lungs

- the pancreas
- the bile ducts and gall bladder (covered in the section on Heart and liver, below)
- the urogenital system.

All these structures arise as invaginations of the gut tube endoderm into the underlying mesoderm. The gut tube, like the neural tube, is strictly patterned along the rostro-caudal long axis with complex dorsoventral specification. Morphogenesis broadly proceeds in rostrocaudal temporal sequence, again like the neural tube.

Thyroid and pituitary glands

The tongue develops from a bud of tissue on the ventral wall of the gut tube. Just caudal to this, the thyroid primordium is evident from day 20 as a midline ventral invagination of endoderm. The base of the invagination hypertrophies and differentiates to form the thyroid gland itself. By 40 GD the thyroid gland lies at the level of the second and third tracheal cartilage. Terms such as 'descended' are used in morphogenesis; however, most commonly, differential growth of surrounding tissue, rather than active burrowing of the structure, results in the change in position within the embryo. The stalk of the thyroid invagination (thyroglossal duct) usually regresses, apart from a small pit at the base of the tongue, called the foramen caecum. Remnants of the thyroglossal ducts can persist in the form of ectopic thyroid tissue and thyroglossal cysts.

The pituitary is formed by the meeting of two different invaginations, one from the dorsal wall of the rostral gut tube (Rathke's pouch) and the other from the floor of the dien-cephalon. Neoplastic change in the stalk of the former results in the rare hormone-secreting tumour craniopharyngioma.

The lungs

The respiratory diverticulum is first seen as an invagina-tion of the ventral wall of the gut tube at 26 GD. This di-verticulum elongates so that the trachea lies immediately ventral to the oesophagus. The development of each of these structures is intimately related, and developmental problems may result in tracheo-oesophageal fistulae and/ or oesophageal atresia. The development of the airways proceeds by a process known as branching morphogen-esis, in which there is bifurcation of the invaginating tube-like structures at regular intervals. The earliest branching events show evidence of the left–right asymmetry apparent in adult life **(Fig. 2.8)**.

The pancreas

The pancreas develops as separate dorsal and ventral in-vaginations in the gut tube, caudal to the developing stom-ach. The ventral pancreas develops in the same region as the hepatic ducts and gall bladder (see below), and their ductal systems are connected. The dorsal pancreas is larg-er and its duct drains directly into the duodenum. At some point after 42 GD the dorsal and ventral pancreas fuse and the ducts of both structures anastomose.

The urogenital system

The development of the renal, adrenal, gonadal, geni-tal and anorectal systems are closely related. The paired primitive kidney (mesonephros) develops from intermediate mesoderm on either side of the gut tube. The mesonephros is connected to a specialized midline region of the caudal gut (the cloaca) via the metamerically patterned mesone-phric (Wolffian) ducts. At the caudal end of the mesonephric duct is a diverticulum called the ureteric bud that induces the surrounding mesenchyme to form the mature kidney (metanephros) **(Fig. 2.9)**. Failure of this process results in renal agenesis. The primitive gonad develops at the rostral end of the mesonephric duct at the level of the stomach. At 46 GD a second paired-duct system, the paramesonephric (Müllerian) duct, forms parallel to the mesonephric duct **(Fig. 2.10)**. In male embryos, a cascade of gene activation initi-ated by SRY protein causes the primitive gonad to become a testis and the mesonephric duct forms the vas deferens; the paramesonephric duct regresses. In female embryos, the primitive gonad becomes the ovary, the mesonephric duct regresses, and the paramesonephric ducts form the fallopian tubes, uterus and upper vagina. This sexually di-morphic development occurs during late embryogenesis and early fetal life, and molecular analysis of this system has been very useful in understanding intersex states (Ch. 5). The mesonephros regresses in both sexes.

The cloaca separates dorsally to form the rectum and ventrally to form the bladder, urethra and the lower part of the vagina. The external genitalia develop from swellings on the ectodermal surface of the embryo: the midline genital tubercle which forms the penis and clitoris; the paramedial genital fold which forms part of the penile urethra and the labia minora; and the paired lateral genital swellings which form the scrotum and labia majora. Development of the external genitalia is a late event and it is often difficult for a non-expert to correctly assign the sex of a mid-gestation fetus by external morphology.

Heart and liver

The heart and liver are derived from a condensation of mesenchyme that forms by day 20 in the very rostral part of the embryo, between the forebrain and the en-doderm. This mesenchyme forms the heart tube, which then shows highly programmed regional growth over the next 2 days to become asymmetrically looped. This 'car-diac looping' is the first evidence of a left–right axis in the embryo. The heart tube (like the neural tube and gut tube) is highly organized along its long axis to form, in a caudorostral direction, the atria, the left ventricle, the right ventricle and the conotruncal region. The subsegmen-tal growth of the heart tube continues until four cham-bers are recognizable but retain a common connection **(Fig. 2.11)**. Separation of the chambers and the formation of AV valves is dependent on the fusion of ridges of tis-sue within the heart (the endocardial cushions). Failure of this process results in a heart malformation not infrequently

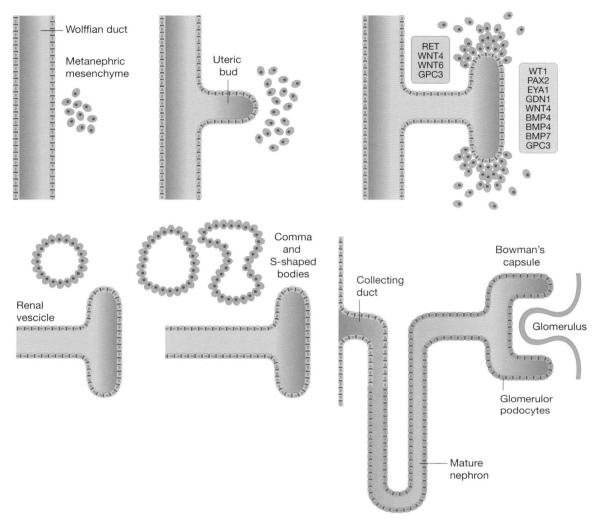

Fig. 2.9 Development of the kidney. The ureteric bud forms as an outpouching of the Wolffian (mesonephric duct) and induces a particular set of genes in the surrounding mesenchyme which leads to a cascade of branching morphogenesis in the bud and differentiation of the mesenchyme to form comma and S-shaped bodies which are precursors of the glomeruli of the mature kidney (metanephros).

found in Down syndrome, an AV canal defect. The aorta at this stage consists of a ventral root that feeds four paired vessels (aortic arches) which supply the rapidly growing pharyngeal arches (see below). A combination of regression and differential growth of these arches eventually shapes the mature thoracic aorta. The right side of the fourth arch, for example, becomes the right subclavian artery, whereas the left side of the fourth arch becomes part of the aortic arch.

The first evidence of liver formation is on day 22 as a condensation of mesenchyme in the cardiac region overlying a thickened region of gut endoderm (hepatic plate). The ductal system of the liver and the gall bladder is derived from an invagination of the hepatic plate, whereas the hepatocytes are mesenchymal in origin.

Craniofacial structures

The face develops around the primitive oral cavity at the rostral end of the gut tube. The major early morphogenic events involve:

- the paired sensory placodes
- the facial processes.

The paired sensory placodes

The otic, nasal and optic placodes are defined thickenings on the surface ectoderm. The otic placode is the first to appear at 20 GD on the lateral wall of the hindbrain. This placode gradually invaginates to become the otic cyst and then undergoes complex morphogenesis to form the semicircular canals and cochlea. The external ear develops from mounds of tissue (auricular hillocks) on the first and second pharyngeal arches (see below). The middle ear develops from the tissue between these arches. The nasal placode is first evident on the fronto-nasal process by 30 GD and invaginates to form the nasal air passages. The optic placode is induced at ≈28 GD by signals emanating from the bilateral optic evagination (optic stalks) arising from the diencephalon. The optic placode invaginates to form the optic vesicle that will ultimately become the lens of the eye **(Fig. 2.12)**. The cupped end of the optic stalk becomes the neural retina, and the stalk itself, the optic nerve. Failure of any part of this process will result in anophthalmia.

The facial processes

By 22 GD paired tubes of tissue form ventral to the hind-brain. These 'pharyngeal arches' have a fundamental role in the morphogenesis of the head and neck. There are usually only three pharyngeal arches visible in the embryo, and the cells that form the arches contain a significant number of migratory neural crest cells **(Box 2.4)**. The first pharyngeal arch is the most important in face development, and through differential growth this tube of tissue becomes C-shaped; the top arm forms the maxillary process and the bottom arm the mandibular process **(Fig. 2.13)**. The upper lip is formed at ≈40 GD by fusion of the maxillary process with the midline unpaired fronto-nasal process. Failure to fuse results in unilateral or bilateral cleft lip **(Fig. 2.14A)**. The lower jaw is formed by fusion of the mandibular processes in the midline. The secondary palate forms from outgrowths of palatal shelves from the maxillary process within the oral cavity. These initially grow down beside the tongue and then elevate to fuse in the midline. Failure to do so results in cleft palate **(Fig. 2.14B)**.

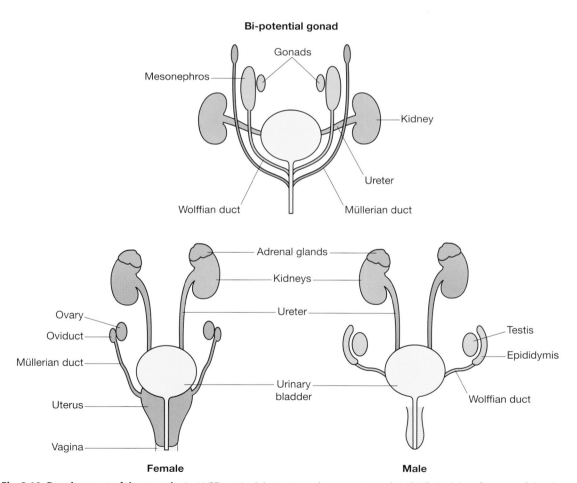

Fig. 2.10 Development of the gonads. At 46 GD a paired duct system, the paramesonephric (Müllerian) duct, forms parallel to the mesonephric duct. In male embryos, a cascade of gene activation initiated by SRY protein causes the primitive gonad to become a testis and the mesonephric duct to form the vas deferens; the paramesonephric duct regresses. In female embryos, the primitive gonad becomes the ovary, the mesonephric duct regresses, and the paramesonephric ducts form the fallopian tubes, uterus and upper vagina.

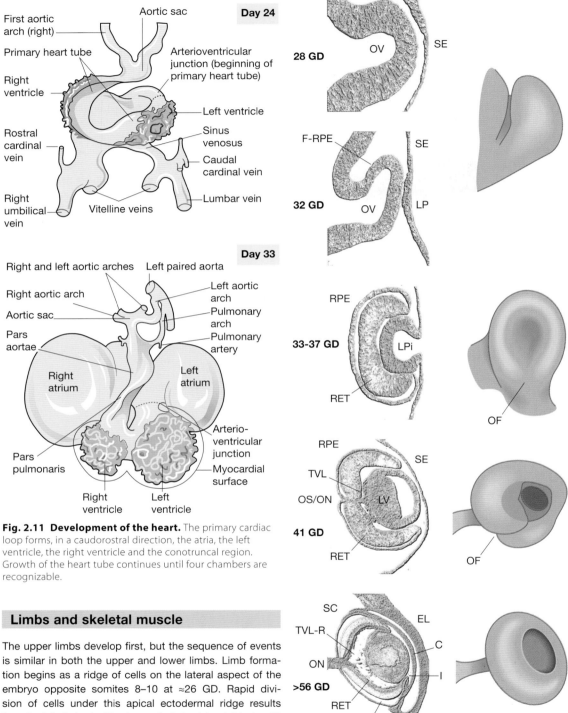

Fig. 2.11 Development of the heart. The primary cardiac loop forms, in a caudorostral direction, the atria, the left ventricle, the right ventricle and the conotruncal region. Growth of the heart tube continues until four chambers are recognizable.

Limbs and skeletal muscle

The upper limbs develop first, but the sequence of events is similar in both the upper and lower limbs. Limb formation begins as a ridge of cells on the lateral aspect of the embryo opposite somites 8–10 at ≈26 GD. Rapid division of cells under this apical ectodermal ridge results in paired limb buds (the lower limb bud is visible by 28 GD). These limb buds elongate and a terminal hand plate becomes apparent by 33 GD. By 41 GD finger rays can be seen. The fingers are then formed by a remarkable process of apoptosis, or programmed cell death, in the interdigital spaces **(Fig. 2.15)**. Failure of this process results in syndactyly. The molecular signals that pattern the hand plate are reminiscent of those that pattern the

Fig. 2.12 Development of the eye. (A) The invaginating lens placode becomes separated from the surface ectoderm. **(B,C)** The retina is formed from an outpouching of the forebrain (the optic cup). C = cornea, GD = gestational days, (F-)RPE = (future) retinal pigment epithelium, I = iris, LP = lens placode, LPi = lens pit, LV = lens vesicle, OF = optic fissure, OV = optic vesicle, RET = retina, SE = surface ectoderm.

Box 2.4

Neural crest cells

Neural crest cells are migratory cells that originate in the dorsal region neural fold throughout the length of the embryo. They have many important functions including the formation of pigment cells, enteric glial cells and the adrenal medulla. Cranial neural crest cells make major contributions to the facial skeleton, the musculature and the outflow tract of the heart. Much of the mesenchyme of the pharyngeal arches is of neural crest origin. Several human conditions are the result of failure of normal migration of neural crest cells. One of the best studied of these is Waardenburg syndrome, which is characterized by sensorineural deafness, heterochromia iridis (different-coloured eyes), Hirschsprung's disease and patchy depigmentation of the skin. The same condition can be caused by mutations in two different transcription factors, *PAX3* and *MITF*, which appear to be critical to neural crest cell survival in the embryo.

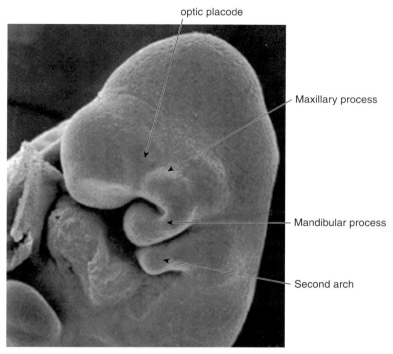

optic placode

Maxillary process

Mandibular process

Second arch

Fig. 2.13 Face development. By 22 GD, paired tubes of tissue form ventral to the hindbrain – the 'pharyngeal arches'. The first pharyngeal arch becomes C-shaped. The top arm of the 'C' forms the maxillary process, and the bottom arm the mandibular process.

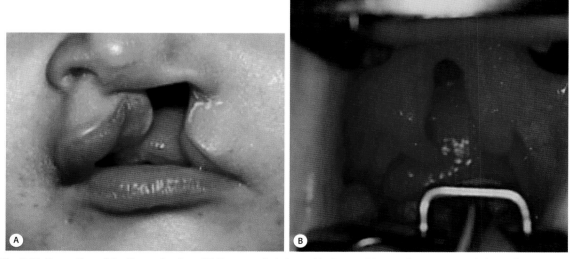

Fig. 2.14 Formation of the lips and palate. (A) The upper lip is formed by fusion of the maxillary process with the midline unpaired frontonasal process. Failure of this process results in unilateral or bilateral cleft lip. **(B)** The lower jaw is formed by fusion of the mandibular processes in the midline. Failure of this process results in cleft palate.

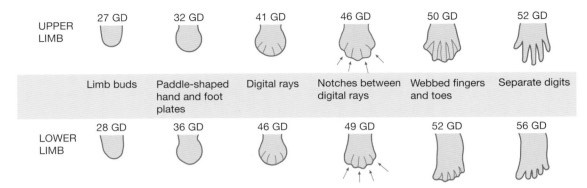

Fig. 2.15 The development of the hands and feet between the 4th and 8th week.

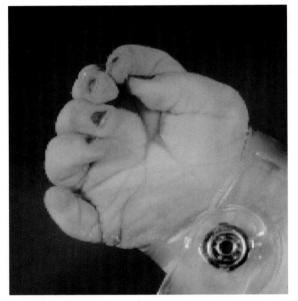

Fig. 2.16 Extra digit (polydactyly). This results from the failure of normal pattern formation in the hand plate.

neural tube, as well as other structures in the embryo **(Box 2.3)**. Failure of this patterning can lead to polydactyly **(Fig. 2.16)**.

The cells that form the muscle of the trunk and the limbs are also patterned and migrate from the paraxial mesoderm of the somites. Their fate is determined by their somite of origin. Other tissues derived from the paraxial mesoderm include the vertebrae and the dermis.

Key *point*

- Embryology is very helpful when learning normal human anatomy. An adequate understanding of developmental processes is crucial to understand birth defects and to develop strategies to prevent or treat malformations.

3

History and examination

Introduction

In general, history and examination cannot be divided neatly into different specialties, and questions relating to obstetrics and gynaecology should form part of the assessment of any woman presenting to any specialty. There may be embarrassment and recrimination, for example, when a suspected appendicitis turns out to be a pelvic infection secondary to an unsuspected intrauterine contraceptive device. Similarly, not all problems presenting to obstetricians and gynaecologists are obstetrical or gynaecological in nature. It is therefore important to take a full history and perform an appropriate examination in all cases. The key points of gynaecological and obstetrical history and examination are emphasized below.

Gynaecological history

A gynaecological history should follow the usual model for history-taking with questions about the presenting complaint, its history and associated problems. It should include a past medical history and information about prescription and non-prescription drugs used, and any known allergies. After questions about social circumstances and activities, and family history, the history is completed with a general systemic enquiry. However, during a gynaecological history there are specific key areas to be expanded upon. These include menstrual, fertility, pelvic pain, urogynaecological and obstetric histories.

Menstrual history

The pattern of bleeding

The simple phrase 'tell me about your periods' often elicits all the information required. The bleeding pattern of the menstrual cycle is expressed as a fraction, such that a cycle of 4/28 means the woman bleeds for 4 days every 28 days. A cycle of 4–10/21–42 means the woman bleeds for between 4 and 10 days every 21 to 42 days. Asking the shortest time between the start of successive periods, the longest time between periods, and the average time between periods helps determine the cycle characteristics.

Bleeding too little

Amenorrhoea is the absence of periods. Primary amenorrhoea is when someone has not started menstruating by the age of 16. Secondary amenorrhoea means that periods have been absent for longer than 6 months. Oligomenorrhoea means the periods are infrequent, with a cycle of 42 days or more.

The climacteric is the peri-menopausal time when periods become less regular and are accompanied by increasing menopausal symptoms. The menopause is the time after the last ever period, and can only therefore be assessed retrospectively.

Irregular periods, oligomenorrhoea or amenorrhoea, suggest anovulation or irregular ovulation. Specific questions about weight, weight change, acne, greasy skin, hirsutism, flushes or galactorrhoea may help identify the nature of the ovarian dysfunction.

Bleeding too much

It is very difficult to find out how heavy someone's periods are. If menstrual blood loss is accurately measured, an average of 35 ml of blood is lost each month. Heavy menstrual bleeding (previously known as menorrhagia) is defined as loss of more than 80 ml during regular menstruation. Some women will complain of very heavy periods with a normal blood loss, while others will not complain in the presence of heavy menstrual bleeding. Asking how often pads or tampons have to be changed and using pictorial charts can provide more objective information. Whether menstrual loss is excessive, however, is a largely subjective assessment.

Specific symptoms can indicate abnormally heavy menstruation. Although small pieces of tissue are normal, blood clots are not. 'Flooding' is when menstrual blood soaks through all protection. It is both abnormal and distressing. Symptoms of anaemia may also be present. A history of the menstrual cycle since menarche (the first period) can reveal changes in the bleeding pattern. However, an emphasis on the effect on lifestyle and treatments tried previously is particularly important.

Bleeding at the wrong time

It is important to ask specifically about bleeding, brown, or bloody discharge between periods (intermenstrual bleeding [IMB]), or after intercourse (postcoital bleeding [PCB]). These symptoms can point to abnormalities of the cervix or uterine cavity. Postmenopausal bleeding (PMB) is defined as bleeding more than 1 year after the last period. Undiagnosed abnormal bleeding requires further investigation.

Fertility history

Last menstrual period (LMP)

This question is vital and should be followed with whether that period came at the expected time and was of normal character. As well as alerting to the possibility of pregnancy, the information is important because some investigations need to be performed at specific times of the menstrual cycle.

Contraception

It is useful to establish whether the woman is sexually active, perhaps with something like 'Are you currently in a physical sexual relationship?' and then 'Are you using any contraception at present?' A further discussion about fertility issues, unprotected intercourse and risk factors for certain diseases may be appropriate. A contraceptive history should include any problems with chosen contraceptives and why they were stopped. Questions may be followed up with 'Are you hoping for a pregnancy?' if the situation is not clear.

If there are any infertility issues, their duration and the results of any investigation or treatment may be of relevance. If the woman is postmenopausal, enquiry should be made about past or current use of hormone replacement therapy and whether she has any symptoms attributable to the menopause.

Cervical smears

Women between the ages of 20 and 64 are invited for cervical screening every 3 to 5 years. The date of the woman's last smear should be noted, and when it was recommended that she have her next smear. Any previous abnormalities should also be noted, and whether she has had any colposcopic investigation or treatment. If she is over 50, it may be relevant to discuss breast screening.

Pelvic pain history

Painful periods

Dysmenorrhoea is a common problem and its effects on lifestyle is important. The cramping pain of primary dysmenorrhoea is at its most intense just before and during the early stages of a period. Young women are particularly affected and the pain has usually been present from the time of the first period. It is not usually associated with structural abnormalities and may improve with age or after a pregnancy. Secondary dysmenorrhoea is when menstruation has not tended to be painful in the past, and is more likely to indicate pelvic pathology. In particular, progressive dysmenorrhoea, where the intensity of the pain increases throughout menstruation, may suggest endometriosis.

Pelvic pain

The relationship of pelvic pain to the menstrual cycle is important. Pain immediately prior to or during periods is more likely to be of gynaecological origin. 'Mittelschmerz' is a cramping pelvic pain that can be midline or unilateral. It occurs 2 weeks before a period and is caused by ovulation. Intermittent discomfort may suggest some scarring or ovarian pathology but it is more commonly non-gynaecological. It is vital to take a urinary and lower gastrointestinal history as urinary tract infection or irritable bowel syndrome may present with pelvic pain. Any pain is likely to be worse if the person is anxious, stressed or depressed. Chronic pelvic pain is particularly affected by psychosomatic factors, and recognizing this during history-taking is important.

Pain on intercourse

There are two main types of dyspareunia, superficial and deep. They can be differentiated by asking 'Is it painful just as he begins to enter or when he is deep inside?' Deep dyspareunia is associated with pelvic pathology such as scarring, adhesions, endometriosis or masses that restrict uterine mobility. Superficial dyspareunia can arise from local abnormalities at the introitus or from inadequate lubrication. It can also be due to a voluntary or involuntary contraction of the muscles of the pelvic floor referred to as 'vaginismus' – see chapter 12.

Vaginal discharge

Discharge can be normal or be associated with cervical ectopy and, particularly if offensive or irritant, can indicate infection. It can also suggest neoplasia of the cervix or endometrium. Enquire about the duration, amount, colour, smell and relationship to cycle.

Urogynaecological history

Urinary incontinence

A good initial question to ask is 'Do you ever leak urine when you don't intend to?' If so, find out what provokes it, how it affects her lifestyle and what steps she takes to avoid it. 'Do you ever not make it to the toilet in time?' can help identify urge incontinence as can a history of frequency and small volumes passed after desperation. Incontinence after exercise, coughing, laughing or straining can suggest stress incontinence. It can be difficult to differentiate stress incontinence and urge incontinence, however, as there is often a mixed picture.

Other urinary symptoms

Enquiry should be made about frequency and nocturia. If present, small volumes and an inability to interrupt the flow may suggest detrusor instability. If large volumes are passed, ask about thirst and fluid intake. A history of dysuria or haematuria may suggest bladder infection or pathology. 'Strangury' is the constant desire to pass urine and suggests urinary tract inflammation.

Prolapse

Prolapse may be associated with vaginal discomfort, a dragging sensation, the feeling of something 'coming down' and possibly backache. Although the uterus, anterior vaginal wall and posterior vaginal wall can prolapse, it is difficult to separate these by history. Bladder and bowel function should be explored, including a question about the need to digitally manipulate the vagina in order to be able to void.

Gynaecological examination

Signs of gynaecological disease are not limited to the pelvis. A full examination may reveal anaemia, pleural effusions, visual field defects or lymphadenopathy in gynaecological conditions. However, passing a speculum, taking a cervical smear and performing a bimanual pelvic examination are the key skills to acquire. A great deal of sensitivity is required in their use.

Passing a speculum

Preparation

The patient should empty her bladder and remove sanitary protection. The examination room should be quiet and have a private area for the patient to undress. It should contain an examination couch with a modesty sheet and good adjustable lighting. A female chaperone should always be present. The examination requires full explanation and verbal consent.

Stand on the right of the patient with gloves, speculum and lubricating gel immediately to hand. The patient should lie back, bend her knees, put her heels together and let her knees fall apart. The light should be adjusted to give a good view of the vulva and perineum and the modesty sheet should cover the patient's abdomen and thighs.

Inspection

Inspect the hair distribution and vulval skin. Hair extending towards the umbilicus and onto the inner thighs can be associated with disorders of androgen excess, as can clitoromegaly. The vulva can be a site of chronic skin conditions such as eczema and psoriasis, specific conditions such as lichen sclerosis and warts, cysts of the Bartholin's glands (history box), and cancers. Ulceration may imply herpes, syphilis, trauma or malignancy.

 History

Caspar Bartholin the Younger (1655–1738) was a Danish anatomist and son of Thomas Bartholin the Elder, also an anatomist; he was the first to describe the vulvovestibular glands.

Look at the perineum **(Fig. 3.1)** and gently part the labia to inspect the introitus. Perineal scars are usually secondary to tears or episiotomy during childbirth. A red papule around the urethral opening is usually a prolapsed area of urethral mucosa. A white, plaque-like discharge may suggest thrush, and pale skin with punctate red areas implies atrophic vaginitis. Asking the woman to cough may reveal demonstrable stress incontinence or the bulge of a prolapse.

Speculum examination

Disposable speculums tend to be all one size, but smaller and larger metal speculums are available if required. Ensure the speculum is warmed, working normally, and lubricated with gel. Hold the speculum so that its blades are oriented in the same direction as the vaginal opening. Part the labia and slowly insert the speculum, rotating it gently until the blades are horizontal **(Fig. 3.2)**.

If the patient is in the lithotomy position at the edge of the couch, the speculum can be turned downwards to avoid pressure on the clitoris. If the patient is lying on the couch itself, it is usually easier to rotate the speculum upwards. It should be inserted fully in a slightly posterior direction, before firmly, but gently, opening to visualize the cervix **(Fig. 3.3)**. The speculum can be closed a little when the cervix pops into view.

If the cervix is not visible, it is often because the speculum has not been inserted far enough before opening. If this is not the case, the cervix is either above or below the blades. As most uteri are anteverted, it is usually below the blades, and the speculum should be angled more

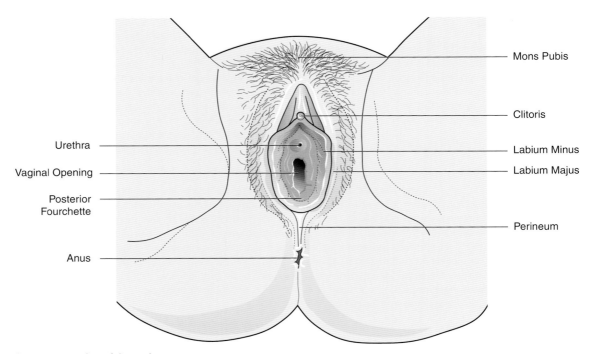

Fig. 3.1 Inspection of the perineum.

Mons Pubis

Clitoris

Labium Minus

Labium Majus

Perineum

Urethra

Vaginal Opening

Posterior Fourchette

Anus

posteriorly before reopening. Otherwise, gently insert a finger to determine its position.

Inspect the vagina for atrophic vaginitis and discharge. A creamy or mucousy discharge is normal. A yellow-greenish frothy discharge is seen with *Trichomonas vaginalis* and a grey-green fishy discharge suggests bacterial vaginosis. There may be a purulent cervical discharge with gonorrhoea, and an increased mucousy discharge may occur with chlamydial cervicitis. Swabs, if required, should be taken from the vaginal fornices (high vaginal) or the cervical canal (endocervical).

The cervical os is small and round in the nulliparous and bigger and more slit-like in parous women. Threads from an IUCD may be present. Translucent lumps or cysts around the os are Nabothian follicles (history box), but warts and tumours can sometimes be seen. An ectopy is red, as the epithelium of the cervical canal extends onto the surface of the paler outer cervical epithelium. It varies across the cycle and should be looked on as normal, although it may be associated with contact bleeding or increased discharge.

♭ History

Small retention cysts in the cervix ('Nabothian follicles') were originally described by the French surgeon Guillaume Desnoues in 1681, but attributed to Martin Naboth, Professor of Chemistry at Leipzig, in 1707.

The speculum should be opened further and withdrawn beyond the cervix before rotation back again, closure and removal.

Taking a cervical smear

Smears should ideally be performed in the mid to late follicular phase and not during menstruation. Confirm the woman's details and ensure you have ascertained all the information required for the request form. Run the speculum under warm water to provide appropriate lubrication, and visualize the cervix.

The most commonly used technique involves using liquid-based cytology and a broom-type sampling device. Insert the central bristles of the broom-like device into the endocervical canal deep enough to allow the shorter bristles to fully contact the ectocervix. Push gently and rotate the broom in a clockwise direction five times **(Fig. 3.4)**.

Immediately put the broom into the container of preserving solution and rinse as quickly as possible by rotating ten times while pushing against the side of the container. Discard the broom, tighten the lid, and label the container with the patient's details. Complete and check the cytology request form, ensuring that all the information required is provided, and marry this, or the computer-generated barcode if the form is completed electronically, to the container for transport to the laboratory. Inform the woman how long the result will take and how it will be delivered.

A bivalve speculum holds open the vaginal walls and obscures any cystocele or rectocele. A univalve speculum

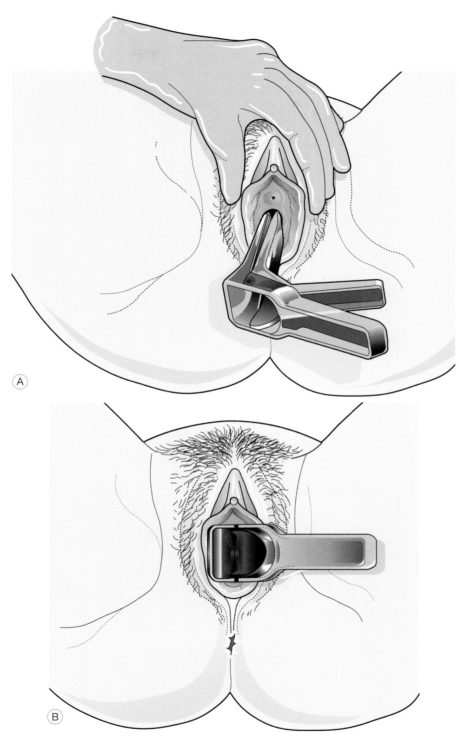

Fig. 3.2 A–C Insertion of a bivalve (Cuscoe's) speculum.

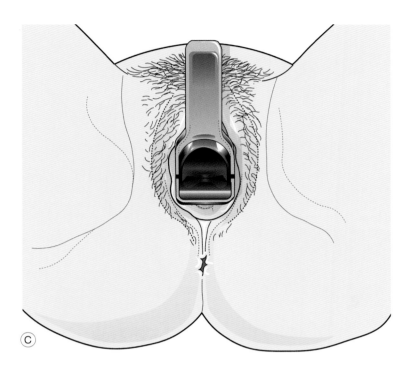

Fig. 3.2—cont'd

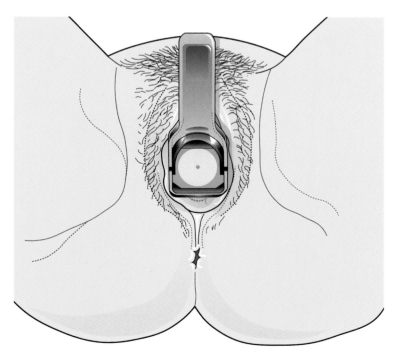

Fig. 3.3 Visualization of the cervix.

can demonstrate these. The patient lies in the left-lateral position with her knees drawn up. The lubricated blade of the speculum is used to hold back the anterior vaginal wall. Coughing will show a bulge of the posterior wall if a rectocele is present. When the posterior wall is held back, coughing will demonstrate the bulge of a cystocele and/or uterine descent (**Figs 3.5** and **Fig 3.6**).

Pelvic examination (Fig. 3.7)

Apply lubricating gel to the gloved fingers of the right hand. Part the labia with the index and middle fingers of the left hand. Gently slip the right index finger into the vagina. If comfortable, slip the middle finger in below the index finger, making room posteriorly to avoid the sensitive urethra. The cervix feels like the tip of a nose and protrudes into the top of the vagina.

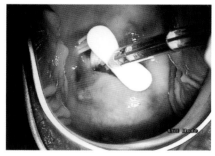

Fig. 3.4 Taking a cervical smear.

Feel the cervix and record irregularities or discomfort. 'Cervical excitation' is when touching the cervix causes intense pain and it implies active pelvic inflammation. The dimple of the os can be felt and the firmness of the uterine body lies above or below the cervix. A vaginal cyst may be an embryological duct remnant, and vaginal nodules may represent endometriosis.

Assess the position of the uterus. It is usually anteverted with the cervix posterior and the uterine body anterior. If the uterus is retroverted, the cervix is anterior and the uterine body lies posteriorly. The fingers should be manipulated behind the cervix to lift the uterus. With the left hand above the umbilicus, feel through the abdomen for the moving uterus **(Fig. 3.8)**. If the uterus cannot be palpated, the hand should be moved gradually down until the uterus is between the fingers **(Fig 3.9A)**.

Assess the mobility, regularity and size of the uterus. The adhesions of endometriosis, infection, surgery or malignancy fix the uterus and make bimanual examination more uncomfortable. Asymmetry of the uterus may imply fibroids. Uterine size is often related to stage of pregnancy. A normally sized uterus feels like a plum. At 6 weeks a pregnant uterus feels like a tangerine, at 8 weeks an apple, at 10 weeks an orange and at 12 weeks a grapefruit. At 14 weeks the uterus can be felt on abdominal palpation alone.

Feel for adnexal masses in the vaginal fornices lateral to the cervix on each side. Push up the tissues in the adnexa and, starting with a hand above the umbilicus, bring it down to the appropriate iliac fossa, trying to feel a mass

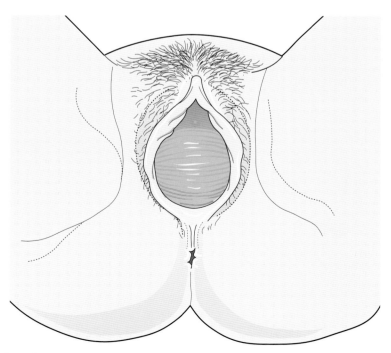

Fig. 3.5 The bulge of a prolapse.

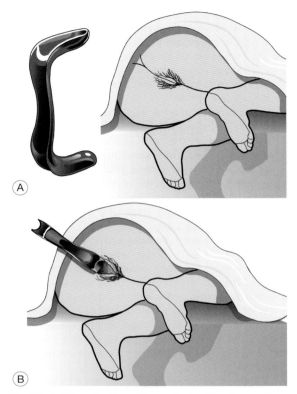

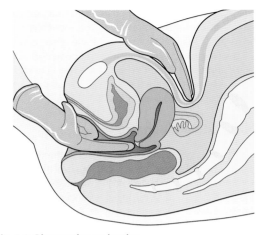

Fig. 3.8 Bimanual examination.

Fig. 3.6 A,B Examination with a univalve (Sims') speculum (history box).

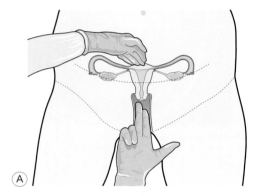

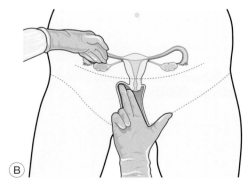

Fig. 3.9 Examination of the uterus and adnexa.

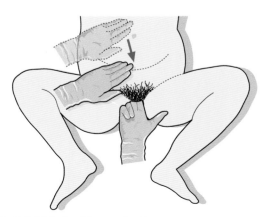

Fig. 3.7 Digital pelvic examination.

bimanually **(Fig. 3.9B)**. In thin women the ovaries can just be felt, but a definite adnexal mass is abnormal and should be investigated further. As large adnexal masses tend to move to the midline, it can be difficult to differentiate a large ovarian cyst from a large uterus.

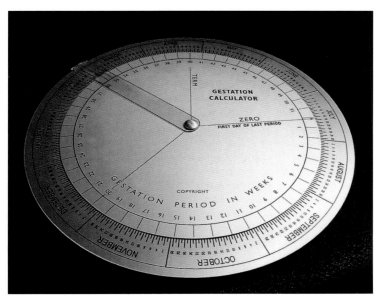

Fig. 3.10 Gestational wheel.

Obstetrical history

An obstetrical history follows the usual model for history-taking. However, as with gynaecological histories, there are several unique things to be covered. A history from a pregnant woman starts with calculating the gestation and putting this pregnancy in the context of previous pregnancies. The presenting complaint is next and this encompasses a record of what is happening now, risk factors and symptom progression. It is followed by a complete history of this pregnancy and previous pregnancies. After this, medical, gynaecological, drug, social and family histories are expanded. However, these are often straightforward as pregnant women are usually young and healthy.

Establishment of the estimated day of delivery (EDD)

Term is between 37 and 42 weeks' gestation, but the actual EDD is 40 weeks after day 1 of the last menstrual period (LMP). This can cause confusion as gestation is calculated from the LMP, not conception. When someone is 12 weeks' pregnant she conceived 10 weeks ago. Gestational wheel calculators allow the easy calculation of EDD and current gestation from the LMP **(Fig. 3.10)**. In the absence of a calculator, Naegele's rule (history box) can be used. To calculate the EDD, subtract 3 months from the LMP and add 10 days.

 History

Naegele's rule was devised by Franz Karl Naegele (1778–1851), a German obstetrician.

These methods assume a regular 4-week cycle. If this is not the case, the EDD may require adjustment. With a regular 5-week cycle, the true EDD will be 1 week later than calculated. An ultrasound scan (USS) is used to confirm the final EDD. However, scans have an associated error that increases with gestation, and in the early second trimester this is approximately plus or minus 1 week. In general, the EDD from the LMP is used, unless the USS date differs by more than a week.

Obstetrical summary

Parity is a summary of a woman's obstetrical history and two numbers are used to document this. Added together, the numbers give the number of previous pregnancies. Someone who is para 0+0 has not been pregnant before. The first number is the total number of live births, plus the number of stillbirths after 24 weeks' gestation. The second number is the number of pregnancies before 24 weeks in which the baby was not born alive.

A woman who is para 3+3 has been pregnant six times. The first '3' might represent a normal term delivery, a live birth at 23 weeks after which the baby died, and a stillbirth at 25 weeks' gestation. The other three pregnancies may have been a spontaneous miscarriage at 23 weeks, an early ectopic pregnancy and a first-trimester pregnancy termination. The numbers relate to pregnancies rather than babies, so that the mother of twins would be para 1+0. A woman who is primiparous is 'pregnant and para 0'. A parous woman is 'pregnant and para 1' (or more).

What is happening now?

The next stage is the presenting complaint and its history. Assuming there is a specific problem, the history should include when it was first noticed, its progress, management and associated symptoms. It may also be useful to ask about important risk factors, for example a past history of placental abruption, chronic hypertension, smoking or pre-eclampsia.

Remember that there are two patients. The fetus should be assessed by asking about movements, and any recent tests of fetal well-being. Fetal movements are first felt around 20 weeks, a time referred to as the 'quickening' but can be as early as 16 weeks. Normally, there are several movements each hour but they are more frequently noticed when concentrated on. Kick charts usually involve noting the time when 10 movements have occurred.

History of this pregnancy

This pregnancy should now be covered in detail. The first thing to ask about is pre-conceptual folic acid, followed by the diagnosis of pregnancy and problems such as bleeding and vomiting or pain in the first trimester. The next thing to ask about is the booking appointment, results of investigations, including USS and prenatal screening tests. Then cover subsequent antenatal care, including clinics, parentcraft and any day unit assessment. The reason for and outcome of any additional USS should be reported. Any concerns, problems identified or emergency attendance at hospital should be documented along with plans for the rest of the pregnancy and delivery.

Past obstetric history

Each of the woman's previous pregnancies should be discussed chronologically. Information required includes the date, the gestation and outcome. If the pregnancy ended in the first or second trimester, the diagnosis and management, including any operative procedures, should be recorded. For other pregnancies, information about the method of delivery, the reason for an operative delivery, the sex, weight, health and method of feeding of the baby should be obtained. In particular, any pregnancy and postnatal complication should be highlighted.

Medical history

The medical history should include previous operations, hospitalizations and medical problems. Continuing medical problems are of great importance because they may have an effect on the pregnancy and make complications more likely or complex. In addition, pregnancy may have an effect on medical problems, resulting in their deterioration, improvement or an alteration in management.

Gynaecological history

All or some of the gynaecological topics may be important in the history. Infertility treatment, particularly the use of assisted reproductive technologies such as intracytoplasmic sperm injection (ICSI), may suggest the need for additional counselling and tests. The date of the last cervical smear is relevant.

Drug history

It is important to record drugs taken, both over-the-counter and prescribed, and the reasons for their use. The need to continue the drug, or change its dose, as well as any possible teratogenic effects should be considered.

Family history

In a pregnant woman, it is a family history of fetal abnormalities, genetic conditions or consanguinity that is particularly important. In addition, some obstetrical conditions such as twins, pre-eclampsia, gestational diabetes and obstetric cholestasis may have a familial element.

Social history

It is important to assess the facilities for the forthcoming baby and determine whether further support is required. The woman's occupation and her plans for working during the pregnancy should be noted. It is also important to ask about smoking, drinking and other drugs of misuse.

Systemic enquiry

Often, the systemic enquiry will be covered in the history of the presenting complaint. Remember, however, that many symptoms are more common in pregnancy, including urinary frequency, shortness of breath, tiredness, headache, nausea and breast tenderness.

Low-risk versus high-risk pregnancy

The key to good antenatal care is to recognize which women are more likely to develop problems in pregnancy before they happen. Clearly, all women can develop problems, but women at extremes of age and weight, those with pre-existing medical conditions like diabetes, hypertension and epilepsy, those with significant past or family histories of obstetric problems, and those who smoke heavily, misuse drugs or have poor social circumstances are all more likely to develop problems. In these 'high-risk' pregnancies, antenatal care should be tailored to meet the increased needs of the woman and fetus.

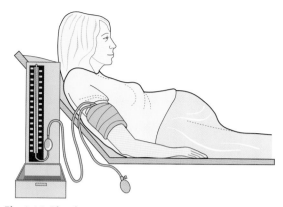

Fig. 3.11 Blood pressure measurement.

Obstetrical examination

In an obstetrical examination the areas to focus on should be guided by the clinical history. It is only by becoming familiar with examination findings in normal pregnancy that deviations from normal can be fully appreciated. In the hyperdynamic circulation of pregnancy, for example, cardiac murmurs are common. The vast majority of these are flow murmurs, but previously unrecognized pathological murmurs occasionally become apparent. Likewise, in normal pregnancy, skin changes and increasing oedema are common.

A systematic approach is preferable. Starting with the hands and working up to the head and down to the abdomen and legs will avoid missing important signs. Examination of the skin, sclera, conjunctiva, retina, thyroid, liver, and tendon reflexes may reveal important abnormalities that may otherwise be missed. There are three elements of obstetrical examination, however, that are particularly important: blood pressure assessment, abdominal palpation and vaginal examination.

Blood pressure assessment

The pregnant woman should lie in a semirecumbent position at an approximately 30° angle and time should be taken to ensure that she is relaxed. The room should be quiet, and any tight clothing on her arm removed. The blood pressure should be taken from her right arm, supported at the level of the heart **(Fig. 3.11)**.

An appropriately sized cuff should be used, as too small a cuff will overestimate the blood pressure. The best cuffs have an indication of acceptable arm circumference on them. Ideally, the cuff bladder should cover 80% of the arm circumference and the width of the bladder should be 40% of the arm circumference. Problems occur if the bladder length is less than 67% (this usually means the arm circumference is more than 34 cm). In such cases a large or thigh cuff should be used.

Place the centre of the cuff bladder directly over the brachial artery on the inner side of the right upper arm, at the same level as the sternum at the fourth intercostal space. Apply the cuff all round, evenly and firmly but not tightly, with the connecting tubes pointing upwards and the antecubital fossa free. Palpate the brachial artery in the antecubital fossa and place the bell end of the stethoscope over it without undue pressure.

Rapidly pump the pressure in the sphygmomanometer cuff to 20–30 mmHg above the point where brachial artery pulsation ceases. Let the air out at 2–3 mmHg per second. The systolic blood pressure is the point where the first clear tapping sound is heard. Read the top of the meniscus or needle to the nearest 2 mmHg. The diastolic blood pressure is the point where the Korotkoff (history box) sounds first become muffled (phase IV) rather than where they disappear (Korotkoff V). Ideally, the record should detail which phase was used, and if there is uncertainty, the measurement can be repeated.

 History

Nikolai Sergeivich Korotkov (1874–1920) was a Russian physician who devised a method of measuring diastolic blood pressure by applying the stethoscope to the brachial artery during the deflation of a sphygmomanometer cuff.

Abdominal palpation

Ensure the patient has privacy, is comfortable and relaxed. Although pregnant women should avoid lying flat on their back for any period of time as this can compress major vessels, the woman should be examined in the recumbent position.

Initially the abdomen is inspected. During inspection look for the distended abdomen of pregnancy and note asymmetry, fetal movements and tense stretching. The skin may reveal old or fresh striae gravidarum, a midline pigmented linea nigra and any scars from previous surgery. The most common scars to see are the Pfannenstiel (history box) scar of previous pelvic surgery, the small subumbilical and suprapubic scars of laparoscopy, and the gridiron incision of a previous appendicectomy.

History

The Pfannesteil incision is a curved suprapubic incision described by Herman Johannes Pfannesteil in 1900. It is lower than the Joel Cohen incision, which is 3 cm below a line joining the anterior superior iliac spines.

The next stage is palpation. This begins with the symphysiofundal height (SFH) **(Fig. 3.12)**. The uterus is palpated with the palm of the left hand, moving it upwards and pressing with the lateral border. There is a 'give' at the fundus. Hold the end of a tape measure, measuring-side

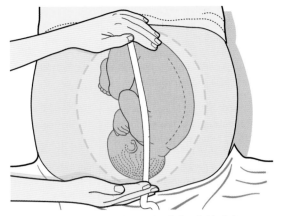

Fig. 3.12 Measurement of symphysiofundal height.

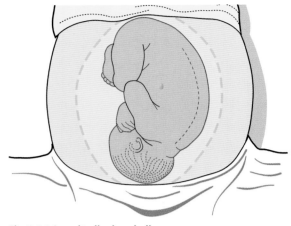

Fig. 3.14 Longitudinal cephalic.

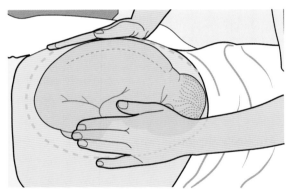

Fig. 3.13 Palpation of the lie and liquor volume.

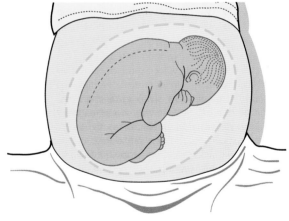

Fig. 3.15 Oblique breech.

(i.e. centimetre-side) down, at the fundus and mark the tape at the upper border of the pubic symphysis.

At 20 weeks' gestation, the uterus comes up to around the umbilicus and the SFH is ≈20 cm. Each week the uterus grows 1 cm, so that at 28 weeks it is ≈28±2 cm and at 32 weeks it is ≈32±2 cm. Metric measurement is therefore a reasonable guide to the size for gestation, and is useful in identifying those that are large or small for dates.

The next stage is to feel the uterus using gentle pressure of both hands, noting any irregularities, any tender areas and the two fetal 'poles', head and bottom. The 'lie' of the fetus refers to the axis of the poles in relation to the mother. It is usually longitudinal but can be transverse or oblique. The presentation refers to the part of the baby that is entering the pelvis. Generally it is a head (cephalic) or a bottom (breech) but it can be the back or limbs **(Figs. 3.13–3.16)**. In twins, it should be possible to feel at least three fetal poles.

The 'engagement' of the head refers to how far into the pelvis it has moved **(Figs. 3.17–3.21)**. This may be palpated by turning to face the woman's feet and pushing suprapubically, trying to ballot the head between the fingers. The descent can be likened to a setting sun and is recorded as fifths palpable. It is 'engaged' when the maximum diameter

of the fetal head has passed through the pelvic brim. Therefore at three-fifths (3/5) palpable it is not engaged but at two-fifths (2/5) palpable it is.

An attempt should be made to get an impression of the liquor volume, particularly if the SFH is abnormal. In oligohydramnios, fetal parts can often be felt easily, while in polyhydramnios the uterus is usually tense and fetal parts are difficult to feel. Also feel for the back of the fetus. It is firmer than the limbs (the side of most movements) and lies to one side. This helps work out the position of the fetus and where to pick up the fetal heart, it runs at a rate of 110–150 bpm and is heard over the shoulder.

The fetal heart is heard using a USS transducer or a Pinard stethoscope **(Figs 3.22** and **3.23)** (history boxes). To use a Pinard stethoscope, place the funnel over the anterior shoulder of the fetus and an ear at the other end, and listen carefully without holding on. It can be tricky, and is rather like listening to a clock ticking behind a waterfall. At the end of the examination ensure that the woman is comfortable, cover her abdomen, and help her to sit up.

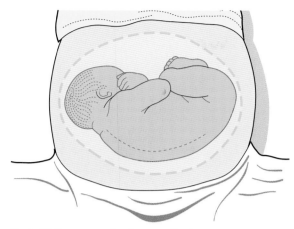

Fig. 3.16 Transverse (back presenting).

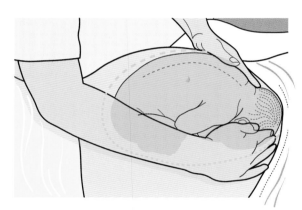

Fig. 3.17 Palpation of the descent of the fetal head.

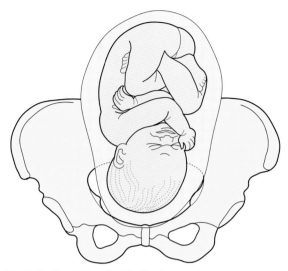

Fig. 3.18 Head 5/5 palpable (free).

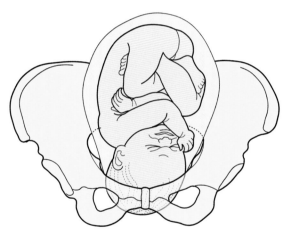

Fig. 3.19 Head 4/5 palpable.

 History

The Doppler phenomenon was first noted by an Austrian mathematician, Christian Doppler (1803–1853), in relation to the change in pitch of an approaching and receding sound source. Ultrasonic Doppler was first used in medicine to study cardiac function in 1957, and the use of ultrasound to image internal structure was pioneered in obstetrics by Ian Donald (1910–1987), Professor of Midwifery in Glasgow.

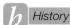 *History*

Pinard's stethoscope was invented in France in 1816 by René-Théophile-Hyacinthe Laennec (1781–1826). It consisted of a wooden tube and was monaural. His device was similar to the common ear trumpet, a historical form of hearing aid; indeed, his invention was almost indistinguishable in structure and function from the trumpet, which was commonly called a 'microphone'.

Obstetrical vaginal examination

Vaginal examination is the cornerstone of intrapartum management, but is also a key skill in antenatal assessment. It is used in the diagnosis of pre-labour rupture of membranes and to assess pre-labour cervical change.

Although the diagnosis of membrane rupture is often made from the clinical history, a speculum examination is important for three reasons. The first is to look for evidence of liquor in the vagina. The technique is similar to gynaecological speculum examination with careful aseptic technique. A pool of fluid, sometimes containing white flecks of vernix, can usually be seen in the posterior vagina or coming from the cervix on coughing. The second is to allow a high vaginal swab to be taken, looking particularly for pathogenic bacteria, notably group B β-haemolytic streptococci. The third is to allow a visual inspection of the cervix to avoid digital examination.

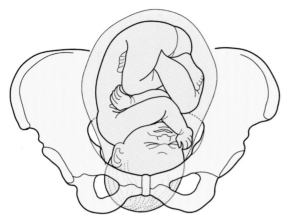

Fig. 3.20 Head 2/5 palpable (engaged).

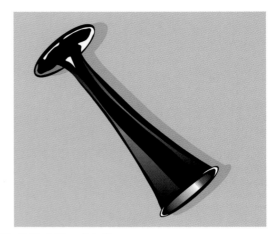

Fig. 3.22 A Pinard stethoscope.

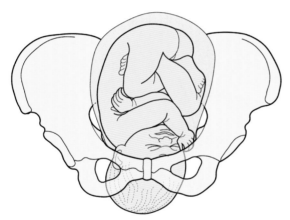

Fig. 3.21 Head 0/5 palpable (fully engaged).

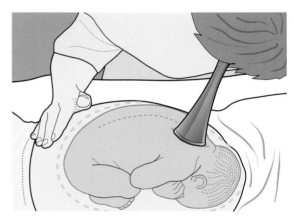

Fig. 3.23 Using the Pinard stethoscope.

Digital examination assesses pre-labour cervical change in preterm and post-term pregnancies. This helps determine those at risk of preterm delivery and is useful in the management of labour induction. After abdominal palpation, the vaginal examination is performed in the same way as a gynaecological examination. In addition, however, it is important to note the ischial spines posterolaterally, as the 'station', or degree of descent, is made with reference to this point.

Feel for the cervix and note its position. Is it anterior or posterior and difficult to reach? Note its length. The cervix shortens from 3–4 cm until it is flush with the fetal head and does not protrude into the vagina. This is called effacement. What is its consistency? Is it soft like a cheek or hard like a nose? Feel for the os and how much it is dilated. Note if it is closed or whether one or two fingers can be inserted. The station of the presenting part is determined as above.

The cervix is assessed by the modified Bishop's score (see Table 40.2). As the cervix ripens, it becomes softer, shorter, more anterior and more dilated, and the fetal head descends. As the onset of spontaneous labour approaches, the Bishop's score increases.

Key *points*

- Taking a history is never the same for any two patients, and many questions will follow from previous answers.
- Always ensure the woman is comfortable and an appropriate chaperone is present during the examination.

4

Paediatric gynaecology

Introduction

Puberty should transform a girl into a fertile woman, and its social importance is so great that any deviation from normality may be the cause of considerable embarrassment and anxiety. This chapter describes normal puberty and outlines the management of both delayed puberty and precocious puberty. There is also a short discussion about sexual abuse.

Normal puberty

Puberty encompasses:

- an adolescent growth spurt
- the acquisition of secondary sexual characteristics
- the onset of menstruation (menarche)
- the establishment of ovulatory function.

Endocrine changes

Puberty begins with the reactivation of the hypothalamo-pituitary–ovarian axis, which has lain dormant from the 3rd or 4th month of postnatal life. During childhood the hypothalamus and pituitary are highly sensitive to suppression by low levels of gonadal steroids. With the onset of puberty, this extreme sensitivity is lost.

The first recognized endocrine event is the appearance of sleep-related, pulsatile release of gonadotrophins. As puberty progresses, these extend throughout the 24 hours of the day. These gonadotrophins lead to production of ovarian oestrogen, which initiates the physical changes of puberty. Changes in the ovaries are evident at an early stage. In normal girls, before any physical signs of puberty are apparent, ultrasonography demonstrates a progressive increase in the size of ovarian follicles, such that after the age of 8½ years a multicystic appearance of the ovaries (defined as more than six follicles greater than 4 mm in diameter, in each ovary) can often be demonstrated.

Signs of puberty

The external signs of puberty usually (but not always) occur in a specific order **(Fig. 4.1)**. The onset of the adolescent growth spurt is an early feature of puberty in girls and this may enable a girl to temporarily outstrip an older brother in height. This acceleration in growth is dependent on growth hormone as well as gonadal steroids.

Almost at the same time, the subareolar breast bud appears (thelarche). Breast development, which is primarily under the control of ovarian oestrogens, is described in five stages **(Fig. 4.2)**. The appearance of the breast bud is followed shortly afterwards by pubic and axillary hair (pubarche), mainly under the influence of ovarian and adrenal androgens **(Fig. 4.3)**. Menarche is a late feature in the course of puberty.

Age of menarche

Since the turn of the 20th century the average age for the onset of puberty has become progressively younger. In 1900 the average age of the menarche was approximately 15.5 years, while currently it is 12.8 years. This has been attributed to improvement in socioeconomic conditions, nutrition and general health. This trend appears to have slowed or ceased in Western Europe and the USA during the past 30 years, as might be expected once nutrition and child care had reached an optimum level.

Influence of body weight

It had previously been proposed that the menarche was closely related to the attainment of a critical body weight, which in the USA and Europe was approximately 48 kg. Further analysis suggested that the significant component of body weight was body fat, which during the adolescent growth spurt increases to about 22% of body weight. This converts a lean body weight-to-fat ratio of 5:1 at the initiation of the growth spurt to one of 3:1 at the menarche. Factors which delay the attainment of a critical body weight may delay the menarche. These include:

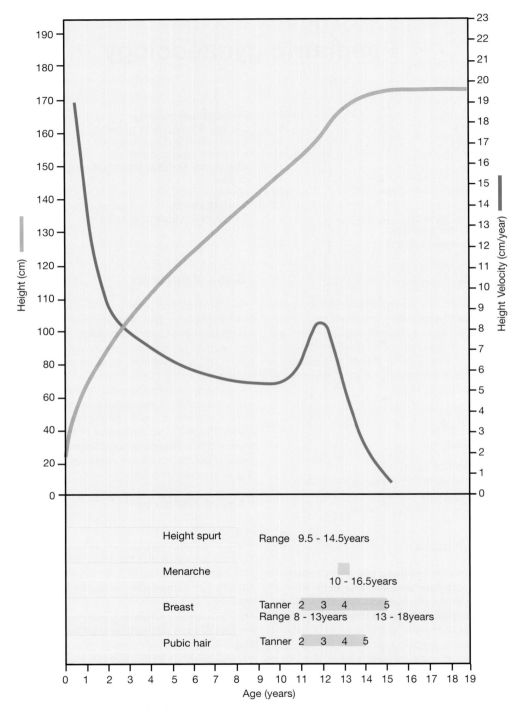

Fig. 4.1 Schematic representation of puberty.

- Malnutrition.
- Slow growth before and after birth.
- Twins, who have a later menarche than singletons of the same population.
- Athletic training, as it results in an increased proportion of lean body mass at the expense of adipose tissue. For

each year of premenarcheal training, the menarche is delayed by 5 months.
- Eating disorders. Anorexia nervosa in particular can cause both primary and secondary amenorrhoea and a halt in pubertal progress.

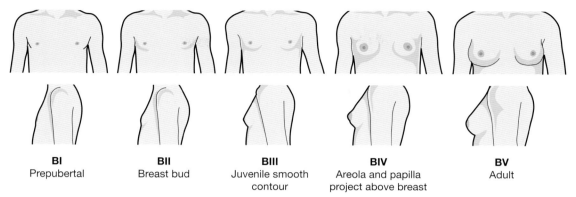

Fig. 4.2 Tanner stages of breast development. (History box)

BI	BII	BIII	BIV	BV
Prepubertal	Breast bud	Juvenile smooth contour	Areola and papilla project above breast	Adult

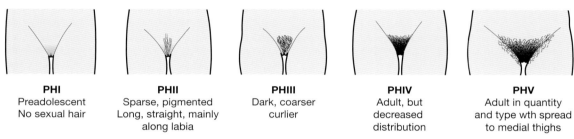

Fig. 4.3 Tanner stages of pubic hair development.

PHI	PHII	PHIII	PHIV	PHV
Preadolescent No sexual hair	Sparse, pigmented Long, straight, mainly along labia	Dark, coarser curlier	Adult, but decreased distribution	Adult in quantity and type wth spread to medial thighs

History

James Mourilyan Tanner (b.1920), a British paediatrician, described Tanner's stages of puberty in girls based on breast size, shape and pubic hair distribution. He also described Tanner's stages for male genitalia development.

- Environmental factors may also play a role. Urban communities tend to have an earlier menarche than rural communities, as do girls from social class I when compared to girls from social classes II and III.

Progression through puberty

95% of normal girls attain stage 2 breast development (the appearance of the subareolar breast bud) by the age of 13.2 years. 50% will complete all stages of puberty in 2–3 years, while 97% will do so in 5 years.

The bone age, which is an index of physiological maturation, correlates closely with the menarche. It can be measured by an X-ray of the hand. 80% of girls begin to menstruate at a bone age of 13–14 years.

After the menarche, menstrual cycles tend to be irregular as ovulation is initially infrequent. Most girls take several months or even a year or so to establish a regular cycle.

Delayed puberty

Definition

Delayed puberty in girls may be defined as the absence of physical manifestations of puberty by the age of 13 years. Primary amenorrhoea is defined as no menstruation by the age of 14 years accompanied by failure to develop secondary sexual characteristics. It is also defined as no menstruation by the age of 16 years in the presence of normal sexual development, and this is discussed further in Chapter 7. In some instances a girl may enter puberty but the normal progression is not maintained. This is described as arrested puberty.

Causes of delayed puberty

These features of delayed puberty fall into three main categories **(Table 4.1)**.

Constitutional delay

Constitutional delay – in other words the girl is normal but inherently late in entering puberty – is the commonest cause of delayed puberty. Although these individuals are usually of short stature, and have usually been shorter than their peers for years, their height is generally appropriate

Table 4.1

Differential features of delayed puberty

	Stature	Gonadotrophins	Gonadal steroids	Karyotype
Constitutional delay	Short	Pre-pubertal	Low	Normal
Hypogonadotrophic hypogonadism	Normal	Low	Low	Normal
Primary gonadal failure:				
Turner syndrome and variants	Short	High	Low	XO and variants
Gonadal dysgenesis	Normal	High	Low	XX or XY

for their bone age. All stages of development are delayed. They may be considered to be physiologically immature, with a functional deficiency of gonadotrophin-releasing hormone for their chronological age, but not for their stage of physiological development. There is frequently a history of delayed menarche in their mothers.

In these patients, bone age shows a better correlation with the onset and progression of puberty than does chronological age. On attaining a bone age of 11–13 years they can be expected to enter puberty.

Hypogonadotrophic hypogonadism

This arises from a defect of gonadotrophin-releasing hormone (GnRH) secretion, and consequently of follicle-stimulating hormone (FSH) and luteinizing hormone (LH). It may be associated with:

- Conditions affecting body weight, such as chronic systemic disease, malnutrition or anorexia nervosa.
- Central nervous system tumours, which may lead to interference with GnRH synthesis or secretion, or with its stimulation of the pituitary gonadotrophs. The most common of these rare conditions is craniopharyngioma.
- Isolated gonadotrophin deficiency is very rare. Such patients are generally of appropriate height for chronological age, in contrast to patients with central nervous system tumours, who usually have associated growth hormone deficiency, and to those with constitutional delay, who are short for chronological age. The commonest form is Kallmann's syndrome (history box), in which anosmia arising from agenesis or hypoplasia of the olfactory bulbs is associated with GnRH deficiency.

h *History*

Kallmann's syndrome was described in 1944 by Franz Josef Kallmann, a German-American geneticist, although others – such as the Spanish physician Aureliano Maestre de San Juan (1828–1890) – had noticed a correlation between anosmia and hypogonadism in 1856.

Primary gonadal failure (hypergonadotrophic hypogonadism)

Although gonadal dysgenesis may occur in isolation, it is most commonly associated with chromosomal anomalies, particularly Turner syndrome (history box). Gonadal failure may also occur following chemotherapy or radiotherapy, as the result of germ cell damage.

  History

Henry Hubert Turner (1892–1970), an endocrinologist from Illinois, described a syndrome in 1938 characterized by sexual infantilism, short stature and webbing of the neck. The same condition was described in Europe as Bonnieve–Ullrich syndrome by Otto Ullrich in 1930.

Other causes

These include hyperprolactinaemia and hypothyroidism.

Investigation and management of delayed or arrested puberty

The scheme of investigation follows logically from the differential diagnosis discussed above:

1. Plasma FSH, LH, oestradiol, prolactin and thyroid function tests
2. Karyotype
3. X-ray for bone age
4. Cranial CT or MRI scan.

Management after results
Constitutional delay

Often, reassurance and continued observation are sufficient. It is important to reassure the parents as well as the girl herself. Where psychological problems arise as a result of comparison with her peers, treatment may be indicated. This may take the form of 3 months' therapy with low-dose estradiol, 2 μg daily. If necessary, this can be repeated.

Hypogonadotrophic hypogonadism

In those with low weight, restoration of weight usually results in spontaneous onset of puberty. Those with central nervous system tumours require appropriate neurosurgical treatment.

Where the defect lies at the hypothalamic level, for example with Kallmann's syndrome, pulsatile administration of GnRH via an infusion pump results in progress through all stages of puberty in the course of 12 months. It is, however, a very demanding form of treatment and in most cases replacement therapy with estradiol is usually employed for physical maturation. Pulsatile GnRH treatment, however, is necessary if ovulation induction is required.

Primary gonadal failure

Girls with pure Turner syndrome or complete ovarian dysgenesis will usually be infertile, although there are reports of successful pregnancies achieved with ovum donation. They will require hormone replacement therapy throughout their lives until the age of 50. The first stage in treatment is to achieve apparently normal progress through puberty, and this is achieved by estradiol replacement therapy. It is commenced at a low dose (2 μg daily) until breast development is adequate. It is important not to begin with higher doses as this may result in poor breast development. Subsequently, higher doses of 10–20 μg daily may be introduced and a progestogen added to avoid unopposed oestrogen stimulation of the endometrium. Commonly, ongoing oestrogen replacement is with the combined oral contraceptive pill, although hormone replacement therapy can also be used.

Precocious puberty

The appearance of signs of sexual maturation prior to the age of 8 years constitutes precocious puberty.

Causes of precocious puberty

Constitutional

80% of cases are constitutional, with the normal sequence of pubertal development occurring at an early age. The growth spurt is a striking feature, but frequently it is the occurrence of menstruation which brings the girl to medical attention. Caution should be exercised in accepting blood loss as menstrual in origin before excluding a local lesion, such as a foreign body or even neoplasia of the vagina or cervix.

Intracranial lesions

This is the next most likely cause, particularly in younger girls. An intracranial lesion resulting from encephalitis, meningitis or hydrocephaly, or a small space-occupying lesion, may trigger premature reactivation of the hypothalamo-pituitary–ovarian axis.

Feminizing tumours

Feminizing tumours of the ovary or adrenal may give rise to vaginal bleeding without signs of pubertal development.

Other causes

Other possible causes are hypothyroidism, and the very rare McCune–Albright syndrome, (history box) in which cystic cavities develop in the long bones (polyostotic fibrous dysplasia) and café-au-lait skin pigmentation is evident.

 History

Fuller Albright (1900–1969), an endocrinologist from Massachusetts, described this monostotic form of fibrous dysplasia of bone with associated patchy skin pigmentation and sexual precocity.

Investigation and management of precocious puberty

1. Plasma FSH, LH, oestradiol and thyroid function tests.
2. X-ray of the hand to determine bone age, which is advanced in the constitutional and cerebral forms.
3. Ultrasound scan of the abdomen and pelvis.
4. Radiological skeletal survey of the long bones. Changes in the McCune–Albright syndrome may be restricted to one side of the body.
5. Cranial CT or MRI scan.

Ultrasound examination by an experienced sonographer has become the mainstay of diagnosis. In the constitutional and cerebral forms, the ovaries will show the multicystic appearance previously described in normal puberty. It will also distinguish between a follicular cyst, which may be expected to subside spontaneously, and a predominantly solid oestrogen-secreting granulosa/theca cell tumour of the ovary, which will require surgical removal.

With precocious puberty the aims of treatment are:

1. to arrest or induce regression of the physical signs of puberty, and in particular menstruation, for obvious social reasons
2. to avert the rapid advance in bone age, as premature fusion of the epiphyses would compromise the final height of the child.

The introduction of GnRH agonists, which suppress gonadotrophin secretion, has revolutionized the treatment of constitutional and cerebral precocious puberty. Preparations are available which may be used intranasally or as a depot injection, and treatment can be continued for 2–3 years without significant side-effects.

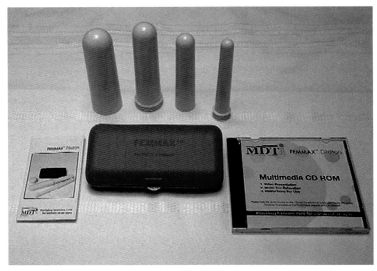

Fig. 4.4 Dilators can be used to create a vagina providing the uterus, if present, is non-functioning. (Courtesy of Medical Devices Technology International Ltd.)

Abnormal genital tract development

Vagina

There may be horizontal septae, vertical septae, or the vagina may be absent.

Horizontal septae

There may be cryptomenorrhoea with cyclical pain and a haematocolpos. If obstruction is caused simply by the hymen (blood looks blue behind it), then a cruciate incision, usually under anaesthesia, is all that is required. If the septum looks pink rather than blue, the situation is potentially more serious and should be referred to a specialist surgeon. If the septum is in the low or mid portion of the vagina, total excision and resuturing is necessary. If the septum is high, a combined abdominal and vaginal approach may be required. Pregnancy rates are excellent with low septae but only around 25% for those higher in the vagina.

Vertical septae

These may be associated with abnormal uterine development. Although presentation may be with dyspareunia, infertility or occasionally in advanced labour, the septum is often asymptomatic. It can be surgically removed.

Vaginal atresia

This is associated with an absent, or only a rudimentary, uterus and is known as the Rokitansky syndrome. Presentation is at puberty with amenorrhoea (or cryptomenorrhoea) in the presence of normal secondary sexual characteristics. If the uterus is non-functioning, it is possible to create a vagina with regular use of vaginal dilators **(Fig. 4.4),** or by one of a variety of surgical techniques. Surrogacy is an option for childbearing.

Uterus

Abnormal uterine shapes **(Fig. 4.5)** are usually asymptomatic but may present with primary infertility, recurrent pregnancy loss, or menstrual dysfunction (oligomenorrhoea, dysmenorrhoea or menorrhagia). In pregnancy, there may be miscarriage, preterm labour, or abnormal fetal lie.

Unicornuate uterus With this there is a higher miscarriage rate and risk of preterm labour.

Bicornuate uterus This may carry a pregnancy to an adequately advanced gestation, and the chance of this probably increases with successive pregnancies. A 'Strassman' procedure will correct the defect, but the benefits for pregnancy are unproven. A bicornuate uterus may be asymmetrical with one side hypoplastic. Pregnancy in the hypoplastic horn carries a risk of rupture.

Septate uterus If it is appropriate to remove the septum, a hysteroscopic approach is probably the most appropriate.

Sexual abuse

This is the involvement of dependent sexually immature children and adolescents in sexual activity they do not truly comprehend, to which they are unable to give informed consent and which violates social taboos or family roles. The abuser is usually male and well known to the child and family. It may present to the medical services acutely, following injury or allegation, or may be suggested by precociousness and other behavioural disorders.

There are numerous pitfalls to the clinical examination, and a depth of experience is required if the results of an examination are to stand up in court. Early senior multidisciplinary help is essential in this highly emotive area where

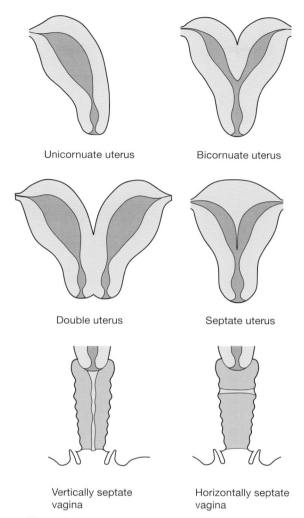

Unicornuate uterus

Bicornuate uterus

Double uterus

Septate uterus

Vertically septate vagina

Horizontally septate vagina

Fig. 4.5 Common genital tract malformations.

incorrect interpretation of the signs may have major consequences. The use of a colposcope is important and photographic records are extremely useful.

The history should be carefully taken and documented, and the social work team involved if appropriate. Swabs (which may include swabs for DNA analysis) should be taken with a 'secure chain of evidence' in case required for a later legal action. Particular attention should be paid to bleeding, bruising or any other area of injury, particularly lacerations at the posterior fourchette and perineal abrasions.

A normal hymen has a number of different shapes (annular, crescentic, fimbriated, septate, sleeve or funnel shaped) and these should not be confused with tears **(Fig. 4.6A,B)**. Notches and clefts can be highly suggestive of penetrating injury, but may be normal if associated with an intravaginal ridge above them **(Fig. 4.6C)**; they are very rare in the posterior segment in non-abused girls. 'Straddle injuries',

caused by falling astride an object such as a fence, very rarely affect the hymen and there is much more likely to be bruising anterior to the vagina or laterally (e.g. labia majora). It is also rare for tampon use to cause hymenal injury (although it may increase the diameter slightly), and there are no reported cases of congenital absence of the hymen. Conversely, a normal pre-pubertal hymen does not exclude abuse.

Paediatric vaginal discharge

Such a symptom raises the possibility of, but does not necessarily imply, sexual abuse.

Non-microbial causes

Threadworms are possible. Foreign body insertion is rare.

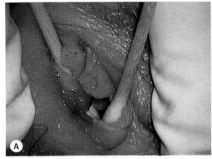

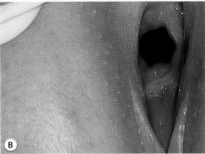

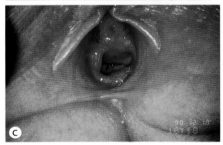

Fig. 4.6 It is essential to differentiate normal hymenal views from those that are pathological. (A) Acute tearing. **(B)** Partial-thickness tear at the posterior margin. **(C)** Concavities in the hymen. The correct differentiation of a tear from the normal appearance requires a suitably experienced opinion.

Microbial causes

Investigation is difficult to interpret as there are few data on the commensal profile of children. In those with discharge, the group A streptococcus is commonly found, followed by *Haemophilus influenzae* and *Candida* species. The bowel flora is also common. *Gardnerella* and *Trichomonas vaginalis* are probably not commensals. Swabs should also be checked for *Chlamydia trachomatis* and *Neisseria gonorrhoeae*.

Vaginal bleeding in the pre-pubertal girl always needs specialist referral and may require examination of the vagina, which is usually done under a general anaesthetic.

Key *points*

- Delayed puberty, the absence of physical manifestations of puberty by the age of 13 years, is most commonly a variant of normality referred to as 'constitutional delay'. It may, however, be caused by hypogonadotrophic hypogonadism, Turner syndrome, or gonadal dysgenesis. It may be worth checking gonadotrophin levels and a karyotype.
- Precocious puberty, the appearance of signs of sexual maturation prior to the age of 8 years, may also be constitutional but is also associated with intracranial lesions, feminizing tumours and the very rare McCune–Albright syndrome.

5

Disorders of sex development (DSD)

Introduction

Disorders of sex development (DSD) are a group of conditions where the development of chromosomal, gonadal or anatomical sex is atypical. Individuals may present with a blend of male and female characteristics, for example a baby with ambiguous genitalia at birth or an adolescent girl with primary amenorrhoea who on investigation is found to have an XY karyotype. The term DSD is a recently adopted classification which replaces the older terms of intersex, hermaphroditism, pseudohermaphroditism and sex reversal. This older nomenclature is confusing to clinicians and can be felt as pejorative by patients.

Definitions

The prosaic definition of 'sex' is: 'a species dimorphism, represented at different planes by chromosomes and the genes they carry, gonads, sex ducts, external genitalia, bodily habitus, secondary sex characters and behaviour or psychological attitudes'. 'Phenotypic sex' is the apparent sex, judged by external characteristics. Older terms no longer in regular use include 'gonadal sex', referring to whether there is a testes or ovary present, and 'karyotypic sex', referring to the chromosome status. 'Sexual orientation' refers to the direction of erotic interest, and 'gender identity' refers to a person's self-representation as male or female. Psychosexual development is highly complex and is influenced by many factors, including chromosomes, pre- and postnatal exposure to hormones, and brain structure, as well as social influences and family dynamics.

Causes of gender identity disorder or gender dissatisfaction in the absence of atypical sex development are not discussed in this chapter.

Some fundamental principles

1. In the normal fetus the chromosomal complement of the zygote determines whether the gonad becomes a testis or ovary. The first step in the pathway to a male or female phenotype is dependent on the SRY gene (sex-determining region of the Y chromosome). This gene, helped by other testes-determining genes, causes the gonad to begin development into a testis.
2. Ovarian development was in the past considered a 'default' development due solely to the absence of SRY; however, recently, ovarian-determining genes have also been found.
3. All fetuses have Müllerian and Wolffian ducts and the potential to develop male or female internal and external genitalia.
4. This process can go wrong at any stage, leading to the birth of a baby with a DSD.
5. DSD can be diagnosed at birth but can also present at adolescence.
6. All babies should be assigned to a sex of rearing. In the presence of a DSD this is decided by the parent and a multidisciplinary specialized team. Birth registration can be delayed until agreement is reached.
7. Medical management includes genital surgery to reinforce the chosen sex of rearing, but this is a controversial and topical issue.

Normal sex differentiation

The chromosomes

Chromosomal complement is the only sex characteristic of the early conceptus. Central to the accumulation of knowledge of sex chromosome anomalies was the discovery of the nuclear chromatin body, a microscopic blob found under the nuclear membrane of all female cells. It is now clear that one X chromosome is necessary for cell viability, but once ovarian differentiation has been initiated the second X has no function and condenses to form the Barr body **(Fig. 5.1)** (history box). More than two X chromosomes will mean that there are additional bodies – the formula being 'X chromosomes – 1 = number of Barr bodies' (see **Fig. 5.2**).

---

h **History**

Murray Llewellyn Barr (1908–1995), a Canadian physician whose main interest was cytological research as it applies to sex anomalies and mental retardation, discovered that the extra X chromosome in the female formed a dark spot when stained.

The Y chromosome

It has long been known that the short arm of the Y chromosome controls testicular development, but identification of the gene has proved a long task. Studies were based on cases in which the gonads and other sex features were contrary to the chromosomes, so-called 'sex reversal'. It is now clear that a gene called SRY (sex-determining region of Y) is responsible. It encodes a DNA-binding protein which probably influences other genes to produce differentiation of the primitive gonadal streak into testis. The detail of SRY's mode of action is now the focus of attention. A very few XX males do not have SRY, so some other genetic material must, in certain circumstances, be able to induce testicular differentiation.

Mixed chromosomes

It is not uncommon for lymphocytes to have mixed sex chromosome complements. This can be due to mosaicism arising from post-fertilization mitotic errors or very rarely to chimaerism, when the cell-mix derives from two separate acts of syngamy (union of gametes). Syngamy may result from dispermic conceptions – one sperm fertilizing the ovum nucleus and another uniting with an unextruded second polar body (see **Fig. 5.3**) – or from dizygous twins with transfer of tissue soon after conception.

Genital differentiation

Hormone production by the testes normally determines the phenotypic sex. First, Sertoli cells develop and produce anti-Müllerian hormone (AMH), which promotes the regression of Müllerian structures. Then, Leydig cells appear and, at around 8 weeks, under the stimulation of human chorionic gonadotrophin (hCG), start to secrete testosterone. This causes development of the Wolffian structures (the vas deferens, seminal vesicles and epididymis). Peripheral conversion of testosterone to dihydrotestosterone requires the enzyme 5-alpha-reductase and virilizes the external genitalia. At 12 weeks the fetus is recognizably

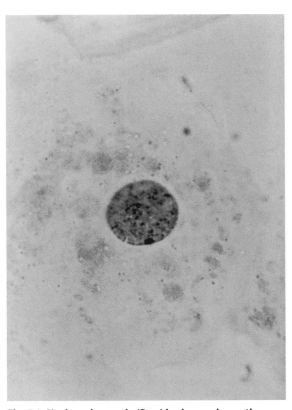

Fig. 5.1 Nuclear chromatin (Barr) body seen beneath nuclear membrane close to 6 o'clock.

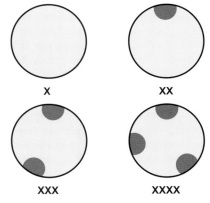

Sex chromatin
in relation to"**X**" chromosomes

X · XX · XXX · XXXX

Fig. 5.2 Sex chromatin in relation to X chromosomes. Barr bodies are peripheral blobs consisting of nuclear chromatin. There is always one less Barr body than the number of X chromosomes.

male and masculinization of the genitalia is said to be complete by 14 weeks. The penis, similar in size to the clitoris at 14 weeks, then enlarges from around 20 weeks until birth.

The ovarian cortex develops at 12 weeks and by 13.5 weeks primordial follicles are present. As AMH is not produced, the Müllerian ducts develop into the uterus, fallopian tubes and upper portion of the vagina. Without androgens the urogenital sinus develops into the female external genitalia, forming the clitoris, labia and lower vagina. The Wolffian structures regress at around 10 weeks due to the absence of testosterone. By 15 weeks the urogenital and Müllerian parts of the vagina meet and fuse and this 'vaginal plate' develops a lumen around 20 weeks (see Fig. 2.10 p. 23).

Incidence of DSD

The incidence of DSD is unknown but current estimates are in the region or 1 to 2 cases per 1000. For practical purposes it is enough to realize that one GP can expect to have a dozen or so cases on his or her list, perhaps not all identified; most will be chromosomal. The problems of these conditions, however, are of such complexity and sensitivity that they assume a clinical importance quite disproportionate to incidence or mortality rates.

Classification of DSD

The new DSD terminology along with previously used terms is listed in Table 5.1. DSD also allows inclusion of conditions such as Turner syndrome and Rokitansky syndrome where there is a disorder of sex development which was not previously included in the intersex classification. There is a significant overlap in many of the physical and psychological difficulties experienced by these differing groups of patients and inclusion allows rationalization and improvement of clinical service provision.

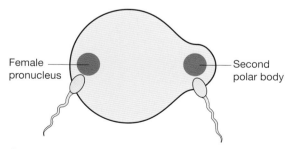

Fig. 5.3 Dispermic conception. Very rarely, an unextruded second polar body may be fertilized in addition to the haploid ovum nucleus; if the sperms involved are of different sexes, an XX/XY chimaera will result.

Sex chromosome DSD

Turner syndrome results from a complete or partial absence of one X chromosome. It is the commonest chromosomal anomaly in females, occurring in 1 out of 2500 phenotypic female births. Although there can be variation amongst affected women, most have clinical features falling into the following three categories.

- short stature
- ovarian dysgenesis
- internal and external dysmorphic features which may be associated with lymphoedema.

Clinical features associated with Turner syndrome include:

- inflammatory bowel disease
- sensorineural and conduction deafness
- renal anomalies
- cardiovascular disease, both structural (e.g. coarctation) and atherosclerotic
- low bone density
- endocrine dysfunction, e.g. autoimmune thyroid disease.

The most common chromosome complement in Turner syndrome is monosomy 45,X or the presence of an abnormal X chromosome such as isochromosome X, a partial deletion or a ring X. Mosaicism is also common and includes 45,X/46,XX and 45,X/46,XY. An accurate karyotype is important as it allows some prediction of clinical severity. Ring karyotype is associated with a more severe phenotype, whereas mosaics generally have a milder phenotype with up to 40% entering spontaneous puberty. If there is a Y chromosome, or fragment of a Y present, then there is a higher incidence of gonadal

Table 5.1	
New DSD terminology along with previously used terms	
New terminology	**Old terminology**
Disorders of sex development (DSD)	Intersex
46,XY DSD	Male pseudohermaphrodite Undervirilization of an XY male Undermasculinization of an XY male
46,XX DSD	Female pseudohermaphrodite Overvirilization of an XX female Masculinization of an XX female
Ovotesticular DSD	True hermaphrodite
46,XX testicular DSD	XX male or XX sex reversal
46,XY complete gonadal dysgenesis	XY sex reversal
Sex chromosome DSD, e.g. Turner syndrome	Sex chromosomal anomalies

tumours and the streak gonads should be removed prophylactically.

Although the majority of individuals with Turner syndrome are diagnosed during childhood or adolescence, about 10% are not diagnosed until adulthood. The focus of paediatric care is on short stature, whereas adult women are generally more concerned with oestrogen replacement and fertility prospects. Pregnancy is possible, but in general ovum donation is required.

Women with Turner syndrome should be looked after by clinicians experienced in this condition and regular monitoring for associated problems such as deafness and heart disease is essential.

46,XX DSD

The commonest condition in this group is congenital adrenal hyperplasia (CAH). CAH is also the commonest DSD, with an incidence of 1 in 14,000 worldwide. It usually presents with ambiguous genitalia in the neonate.

The name is derived from hyperplasia in the adrenal gland, which arises from the overproduction of steroids **(Fig. 5.4)**. Affected individuals have an enzyme block in the steroidogenic pathway in the adrenal gland, with over 90% being a deficiency in 21-hydroxylase; this enzyme converts progesterone to deoxycorticosterone in the aldosterone biosynthetic pathway, and 17-hydroxyprogesterone (17-OHP) to deoxycortisol in the cortisol biosynthetic pathway. The resultant low levels of cortisol continue to drive the negative feedback loop, leading to increased levels of androgen precursors and, in turn, to elevated testosterone production.

Excessive testosterone levels in a female fetus will lead to virilization of the external genitalia. The clitoris is enlarged and the labia are fused and scrotal in appearance. The upper vagina joins the male-type urethra and opens as one channel onto the perineum. The chromosomes are XX and the ovaries are normal, as are the internal structures, including the fallopian tubes, uterus and upper vagina.

Approximately 75% of children with 21-hydroxylase CAH will have a 'salt-losing' variety, which affects the ability to produce aldosterone. This represents a life-threatening situation, and those children who are salt-losing often become dangerously unwell within a few days of birth. Affected individuals require lifelong steroid replacement, such as hydrocortisone, along with fludrocortisone for salt losers. Traditional management comprises feminizing genital surgery during the first year of life to reduce the size of the clitoris and open up the lower vagina. Recent research, however, has confirmed that childhood clitoral surgery can reduce clitoral sensation and is detrimental to adult sexual function. In addition, vaginal surgery usually needs revising at adolescence. This has caused adult patients and some clinicians to question the need for universal feminizing surgery. This issue is hotly debated and further research in this area is ongoing.

CAH is an autosomal recessive condition and molecular genetics now allows prenatal diagnosis in families where an affected child has already been born. Prenatal therapy is possible with dexamethasone, as this crosses the placenta and should therefore reduce the drive mediated by the low cortisol levels. Studies of this are ongoing.

46,XY DSD

Complete androgen insensitivity syndrome (CAIS)

CAIS is the most frequently occurring of this rare group of conditions, with an incidence of 1 in 40,000 to 1 in 90,000 births. Until recently this condition was called 'testicular feminization syndrome'; however, this name is both stigmatizing and inaccurate. CAIS is due to an abnormality of the androgen receptor, which is completely or partially unable to respond to androgen stimulation. In a fetus with CAIS, testes form normally due to the action of the *SRY* gene. At the appropriate time, these testes secrete AMH, leading to the regression of the Müllerian ducts. CAIS women do not therefore have a uterus. Testosterone is also produced at the appropriate time; however, due to the inability of the

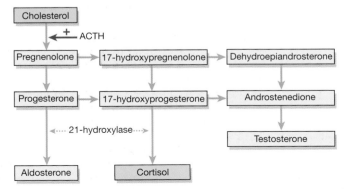

Fig. 5.4 Synthesis of steroid hormones. Deficiency of the enzyme 21-hydroxylase leads to a build-up of precursors, particularly the weak androgens dehydroepiandrosterone and androsterone.

androgen receptor to respond, the external genitalia do not virilize and instead undergo female development. The result is a female (both physically and psychologically) with no uterus, and testes are found at some point in their line of descent through the abdomen from the pelvis to the inguinal canal. During puberty, breast development will be normal, but the effects of androgens are not seen, and pubic and axillary hair growth is minimal. Around two-thirds of women with CAIS have inherited the androgen receptor gene mutation from their mother (i.e. X-linked inheritance), with the remaining one-third thought to be new mutations.

The commonest presentation is with primary amenorrhoea, although children can also present before puberty with an inguinal hernia found to contain a testis. The diagnosis is made on clinical examination with typical findings in association with an XY karyotype. However, the genetic mutation responsible can be identified in up to 90% and appropriate referral for genetic testing should be considered. Psychological support is the initial mainstay of treatment, with full disclosure of diagnosis, including karyotype, mandatory. In the past the karyotype was often concealed from the patients, leading to secrecy, stigma and isolation. Well-organized patient peer support groups have a valuable role, but the patient needs to be aware of her diagnosis if she is to access these.

Gonadectomy is usually recommended post-puberty due to the small risk of malignancy associated with intra-abdominal testes. After gonadectomy, oestrogen replacement is necessary to maintain bone density and general well-being. The vagina is blind-ending and usually short. Vaginal self-dilation has good success rates in creating a vagina adequate for intercourse and reconstructive vaginal surgery is rarely required.

Ongoing psychological input from a suitably trained professional who has clinical experience with DSD is a vital part of long-term management.

Partial forms of androgen insensitivity also occur, leading to a spectrum of clinical features. Presentation in this situation is often at birth with ambiguous genitalia, and careful assessment by a specialized team is required to determine the most appropriate sex of rearing.

5-alpha-reductase deficiency

5-alpha-reductase deficiency leads to failure of peripheral conversion of testosterone to dihydrotestosterone. This condition has an autosomal recessive inheritance. Presentation can be with ambiguous genitalia at birth but can also be with increasing virilization at puberty of a female child due to the large increase in circulating testosterone. Clinical management is complex and requires a specialized team. If the child is pubertal, her input into any decision is essential, as is informed consent for any medical or hormonal treatment offered.

Ovotesticular DSD

Ovotesticular states – previously termed true hermaphrodites – involve the presence of ovarian and testicular tissue in the same individual, either as separate gonads or as 'ovotestes'. The majority of cases have a 46,XX karyotype. Occasionally, an abnormal karyotype is found, but only rarely is this XX/XY – the karyotype which might be expected. It is commoner amongst the Bantu of South Africa.

As the proportion of ovarian and testicular tissue varies, there is no classical clinical picture. Other forms of DSD have fairly standard clinical patterns and can be confirmed by specific tests: ovotesticular states are suspected by excluding these other diagnoses and are confirmed by histological evidence of both types of gonadal tissue – often a rather major undertaking.

46,XY complete gonadal dysgenesis

This condition is also known as Swyer syndrome. The chromosomes are XY but the gonads are streak gonads and do not function. 10–20% of women with this syndrome have a deletion in the DNA-binding region of the *SRY* gene. Nevertheless, in approximately 80–90% of cases, the *SRY* gene is normal and mutations in other testis-determining factors are probably implicated. As the gonads do not become testes, no testosterone or AMH is produced and development is phenotypically female. The external genitalia are unambiguously female at birth and the uterus, vagina and fallopian tubes are normal. The condition usually first becomes apparent in adolescence with delayed puberty and amenorrhoea. A high incidence of gonadoblastoma and germ cell malignancies in the dysgenetic gonad has been reported, and current practice is to proceed to a gonadectomy once the diagnosis is made. Management is otherwise in line with other cases of ovarian failure and involves induction of puberty with oestrogen in order to develop secondary sexual characteristics and long-term combined replacement therapy with oestrogen and progesterone. Pregnancy is possible with a donated egg.

Summary

DSD may present at birth with ambiguous genitalia in conditions such as CAH and partial androgen insensitivity syndrome. Presentation can also occur at adolescence with primary amenorrhoea or failure to go into puberty in conditions such as CAIS and gonadal dysgenesis. More rarely, presentation is with virilization at puberty with 5-alpha-reductase deficiency.

In all such cases management should be by a multidisciplinary team, the key members of which are an endocrinologist, psychologist and surgeon. For children, the surgeon is most commonly a paediatric urologist; at adolescence, a gynaecologist may also become involved. Careful clinical assessment is essential, and is supported by specialist imaging as well as biochemical and genetic investigation. For newborns with DSD, the decision must be taken as to the most appropriate sex of rearing. Factors taken into consideration will include diagnosis, clinical findings, future fertility potential, and the opinions of the family. If the diagnosis is made later in childhood or at adolescence, the sex of rearing is already determined and is not usually re-assigned. The diagnosis of CAH in a neonate is a medical emergency due to the risk of a salt-losing crisis. However, the allocation of sex of rearing should not be rushed into and, as noted above, birth registration can be deferred until an agreed decision has been made.

Management and Prospects

The most controversial aspect of management is the role of feminizing genital surgery in children with ambiguous genitalia assigned to a female sex of rearing. Parents can be more worried about the immediate appearance and find it more difficult to look at the long term issues. It is important that parents and clinicians are aware of the impact on future sexual function when making a decision about irreversible genital surgery for their child.

Key *points*

- Gender can be defined according to the chromosomes, gonads, genital sex or psychological status of an individual.
- The female state is neutral: development of the male requires a Y chromosome, testosterone production and functioning androgen receptors.
- Disorders of sex development (DSD) are complex conditions where there is a blend of sexual characteristics in an individual.
- Presentation can be prenatally (following prenatal diagnosis), at birth or during adolescence.
- Management should be undertaken by a multidisciplinary specialist team.

6

The normal menstrual cycle

Introduction

Evolutionary aspects

Humans are one of the few species which have a monthly reproductive cycle. Most mammals ovulate less frequently than once a month – for example, sheep ovulate once a year and rabbits ovulate in response to coitus. In these species insemination usually leads to pregnancy, but in normal humans there is only a 30% chance of conception at each ovulation. The high frequency of ovulation in our species compensates for our relatively low fertility.

Overview of the cycle

The menstrual cycle can be described by referring to either the uterus or the ovary. The endometrial cycle results from the growth and shedding of the uterine lining – the endometrium. At the end of the menstrual phase, the endometrium thickens again – the proliferative phase. After ovulation, endometrial growth stops and the glands become more active and full of secretions – the secretory phase.

These endometrial changes are controlled by the ovarian cycle. The average duration of the ovarian cycle is 28 days and it is composed of:

- a follicular phase
- ovulation
- a postovulatory or luteal phase.

If the cycle is prolonged, the follicular phase lengthens (longer time to ovulation) but the luteal phase remains constant at 14 days. Fundamental to the normal menstrual cycle are:

- an intact hypothalamo-pituitary–ovarian endocrine axis
- the presence of responsive follicles in the ovaries
- a functional uterus.

Endocrine control of the menstrual cycle

Control of follicular maturation and ovulation is exercised by the hypothalamo-pituitary–ovarian axis **(Fig. 6.1)**. The hypothalamus controls the cycle, but it can itself be influenced by higher centres in the brain, allowing factors such as anxiety or stress to affect the cycle. The hypothalamus acts on the pituitary gland by secreting gonadotrophin-releasing hormone (GnRH), a decapeptide which is secreted in a pulsatile manner. The pulses are secreted approximately every 90 minutes. GnRH travels through the small blood vessels of the pituitary portal system to the anterior pituitary, where it acts on the pituitary gonadotrophs to stimulate the synthesis and release of follicle-stimulating hormone (FSH) and luteinizing hormone (LH). Although there are two gonadotrophins, it appears that there is a single releasing hormone for both.

FSH is a glycoprotein which stimulates growth of follicles during the 'follicular phase' of the cycle. FSH also stimulates sex hormone secretion, predominantly of oestradiol, by the granulosa cells of the mature ovarian follicle.

LH is also a glycoprotein. LH also stimulates sex hormone production (testosterone, which is subsequently converted by the action of FSH into oestradiol). LH plays an essential role in ovulation. It is the mid-cycle surge of LH which triggers rupture of the mature follicle with release of the oocyte. Postovulatory production of progesterone by the corpus luteum is also under the influence of LH.

Both FSH and LH and the other two glycoprotein hormones – thyroid-stimulating hormone (TSH) and human chorionic gonadotrophin (hCG) – are composed of two protein subunits, the alpha chain and the beta chain. The amino acid sequence of the alpha subunit is common to all four glycoproteins, but the beta chains are distinctive to each hormone. Sensitive assays for these hormones therefore have to be specific for the beta chain.

The cyclical activity within the ovary which constitutes the ovarian cycle is maintained by the feedback mechanisms which operate between the ovary, the hypothalamus, and the pituitary. These are described in the next section.

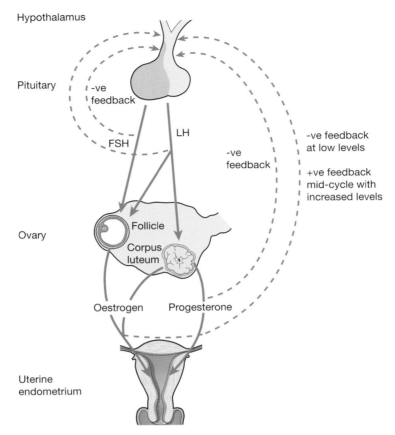

Fig. 6.1 Hypothalamo-pituitary–ovarian–uterine axis.

The ovarian cycle

Follicular phase

Days 1–8

At the start of the cycle, levels of FSH and LH rise in response to the fall of oestrogen and progesterone at menstruation. This stimulates development of 10–20 follicles. The follicle which is most sensitive to FSH is the 'dominant 'follicle, and is the one destined to reach full maturation and ovulation. This dominant follicle appears during the mid-follicular phase, whilst the remainder undergo atresia. With growth of the dominant follicle, oestrogen levels increase.

Days 9–14

As the follicle increases in size, localized accumulations of fluid appear among the granulosa cells and become confluent, giving rise to a fluid-filled central cavity called the antrum **(Fig. 6.2)**, which transforms the primary follicle into a Graafian follicle (history box) in which the oocyte occupies an eccentric position, surrounded by two to three layers of granulosa cells termed the cumulus oophorus.

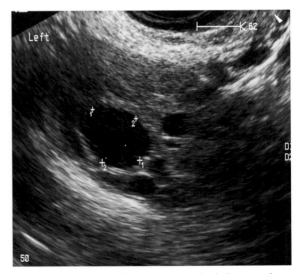

Fig. 6.2 A dominant follicle on transvaginal ultrasound scan.

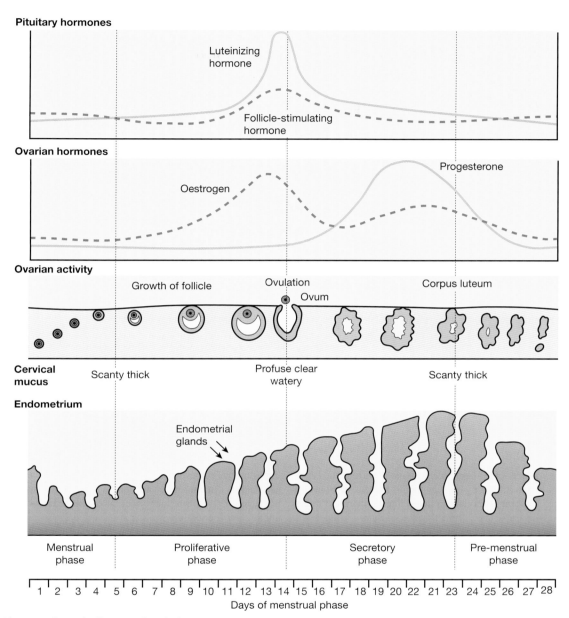

Fig. 6.3 Schematic diagram of ovulation.

 History

Regnier de Graaf (1641–1673) was a Dutch physician and anatomist who realized the reproductive function of the ovarian follicle. From the observation of pregnancy in rabbits, he concluded that the follicle contained the oocyte, although he never observed it. Others, including Fallopius (1523–1562), had noticed the follicles previously but failed to recognize its reproductive significance.

Associated with follicular maturation, there is a progressive increase in the production of oestrogen (mainly oestradiol) by the granulosa cells of the developing follicle. As the oestrogen level rises, the release of both gonadotrophins is suppressed (negative feedback), which serves to prevent hyperstimulation of the ovary and the maturation of multiple follicles.

The granulosa cells also produce inhibin. This has been implicated as a factor in the restriction of the number of follicles undergoing maturation.

Ovulation

Day 14

Ovulation is associated with rapid enlargement of the follicle, followed by protrusion from the surface of the ovarian cortex and rupture of the follicle with extrusion of the oocyte and adherent cumulus oophorus **(Fig. 6.3)**. Some women

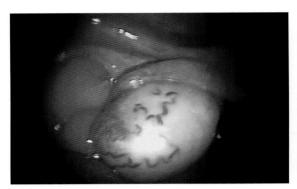

Fig. 6.4 Laparoscopic view of corpus luteum.

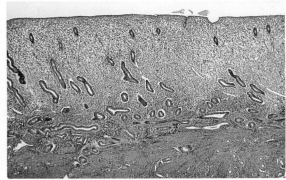

Fig. 6.5 Proliferative endometrium.

can identify the time of ovulation because they experience a short-lived pain in one or other iliac fossa. Ultrasound studies have shown that this pain – known as 'mittelschmerz' – actually occurs just before follicular rupture.

The final rise in oestradiol concentration is thought to be responsible for the subsequent mid-cycle surge of LH and, to a lesser extent, of FSH – positive feedback. Immediately before ovulation there is a precipitous fall in oestradiol levels and an increase in progesterone production. Ovulation follows within 18 hours of the mid-cycle surge of LH.

Luteal phase

Days 15–28

The remainder of the Graafian follicle which is retained in the ovary is penetrated by capillaries and fibroblasts from the theca. The granulosa cells undergo luteinization and these structures collectively form the corpus luteum **(Fig. 6.4)**. This is the major source of the sex steroid hormones, oestrogen and progesterone, secreted by the ovary in the postovulatory phase.

Establishment of the corpus luteum results in a marked increase in progesterone secretion and a second rise in oestradiol levels. Progesterone levels peak 1 week after ovulation (day 21 of 28-day cycle). Tests of serum progesterone at this time may be used in fertility investigations to confirm the occurrence of ovulation.

During the luteal phase gonadotrophin levels reach a nadir and remain low until the regression of the corpus luteum, which occurs at days 26–28. If conception and implantation occur, the corpus luteum does not regress, because it is maintained by hCG secreted by the trophoblast. The detection of the presence of hCG in a sample of urine forms the basis of pregnancy testing. If, however, conception and implantation have not occurred successfully, the corpus luteum regresses, progesterone levels fall, and menstruation ensues. The consequent fall in the levels of sex hormones allows the FSH and LH levels to rise and initiate the next cycle.

The uterine cycle

The cyclical production of sex hormones by the ovary induces important changes in the uterus. These involve the endometrium and cervical mucus.

The endometrium

The endometrium is composed of two layers: a superficial layer which is shed in the course of menstruation and a basal layer which does not take part in this process but which regenerates the superficial layer during the subsequent cycle.

The junction between these layers is marked by a change in the character of the arterioles supplying the endometrium. The portion traversing the basal endometrium is straight, but thereafter its course becomes convoluted, giving rise to the spiral section of the arteriole. This anatomical configuration assumes importance in the physiological shedding of the superficial layers of the endometrium.

Proliferative phase

During the follicular phase in the ovary, the endometrium is exposed to oestrogen secretion. After menstruation, the secretion of oestradiol from the ovary brings about repair and regeneration of the endometrium. With ongoing exposure to oestradiol there is ongoing growth and proliferation of glands and blood vessels. At this stage – the 'proliferative' phase – the glands are tubular and arranged in a regular pattern, parallel to each other **(Fig. 6.5)**.

Secretory phase

After ovulation, progesterone production induces secretory changes in the endometrial glands, preparing the endometrium for implantation **(Fig. 6.6)**. This is first evident as the appearance of secretory vacuoles in the glandular epithelium below the nuclei. This swiftly progresses to secretion of material into the lumen of the glands, which become tortuous and their margins appear serrated.

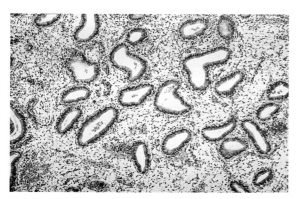

Fig. 6.6 Secretory endometrium.

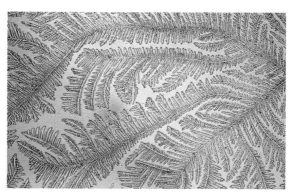

Fig. 6.7 Cervical mucus – ferning.

Menstrual phase

Normally, the luteal phase of the ovary lasts for 14 days, at the end of which regression of the corpus luteum is associated with a decline in ovarian oestrogen and progesterone production. This fall is followed by intense spasmodic contraction of the spiral section of the endometrial arterioles, giving rise to ischaemic necrosis, shedding of the superficial layer of the endometrium and bleeding.

The vasospasm appears to be due to local production of prostaglandins. Prostaglandins may also account for the increased uterine contractions at the time of the menstrual flow. The failure of menstrual blood to clot has been ascribed to the presence of local fibrinolytic activity in the endometrial blood vessels which reaches a peak at the time of menstruation.

Cervical mucus

The glands of the cervix secrete cervical mucus. This changes in quantity and character throughout the cycle in response to sex hormones from the ovary.

■ Early in the follicular phase the cervical mucus is scant
■ Later in the follicular phase the increasing oestrogen levels induce changes in the composition of the mucus (becomes more stretchy). This change is described by the term 'spinnbarkheit'. The water content increases progressively so that just before ovulation occurs the mucus has become watery and is easily penetrated by the spermatozoa. This mid-cycle mucus has a characteristic fern-like pattern when examined microscopically **(Fig. 6.7)**.
■ After ovulation the progesterone secreted by the corpus luteum counteracts the effect of the oestrogen, and the mucus becomes thick and impermeable. This prevents entry of further spermatozoa. This effect on mucus is one of the ways by which the progestogen-only methods of contraception exert their contraceptive effect.

These changes can be monitored by the woman herself, if she is using the 'rhythm method' of contraception. In the clinic the changes can be monitored by examining cervical mucus under the low power of a microscope.

Other cyclical changes

Although the purpose of the cyclical changes in ovarian hormones is to affect the genital tract, these hormones circulate throughout the body and can affect other organs.

Basal body temperature

A rise in basal body temperature of approximately 0.5°C occurs following ovulation and is sustained until the onset of menstruation. This is due to the thermogenic effect of progesterone acting at the hypothalamic level. Should conception occur, the elevation in basal body temperature is maintained throughout pregnancy. A similar effect can be induced by the administration of progestogens.

Breast changes

The human mammary gland is very sensitive to oestrogen and progesterone. Breast swelling is often the first sign of puberty, in response to the small increase in ovarian oestrogen. Oestrogen and progesterone act synergistically on the breast, and, during the normal cycle, breast swelling occurs in the luteal phase, apparently in response to increasing progesterone levels. The swelling is probably due to vascular changes and is not due to changes in the glandular tissue.

Psychological changes

Some women notice changes in mood during the menstrual cycle, with an increase in emotional lability in the late luteal phase. Such changes may be directly due to falling levels of progesterone, although mood changes are not always closely synchronized with hormonal fluctuations. The dividing line between normal cyclical changes and the premenstrual syndrome is unclear **(see Ch.17)**.

Key *points*

- At the start of the cycle, levels of FSH and LH rise and these stimulate the development of 10–20 follicles. A single dominant follicle matures, secreting oestrogen, and the remainder undergo atresia. As the oestrogen level rises, the release of both gonadotrophins is suppressed (negative feedback), which serves to prevent multiple follicles from maturing and ovulating.
- The very high preovulatory oestradiol level stimulates a positive-feedback mid-cycle surge of LH, which triggers ovulation. The remainder of the ruptured follicle becomes the corpus luteum, and secretes progesterone.
- Progesterone brings about secretory changes in the endometrium that are necessary for successful implantation.
- If conception and implantation occur, the corpus luteum is maintained by hCG secreted by the trophoblast. If, however, conception and implantation have not occurred successfully, the corpus luteum regresses, the levels of sex hormones fall, and menstruation ensues.

7

Amenorrhoea

Introduction

Amenorrhoea may be defined as the failure of menstruation to occur at the expected time.

It may be considered in two categories:

1. Primary amenorrhoea – when menstruation has never occurred.
2. Secondary amenorrhoea – when established menstruation ceases for 6 months or more.

Primary amenorrhoea

Failure to menstruate by the age of 16 is referred to as primary amenorrhoea. The likely cause of primary amenorrhoea depends on whether secondary sexual characteristics are present or not. If secondary sexual characteristics are absent, then the cause is most likely delayed puberty (see p. 43). If pubertal development is normal, then an anatomical cause should be suspected.

The main 'anatomical' causes are:

- Congenital absence of the uterus. This is due to a failure of the Müllerian ducts to develop.
- Imperforate hymen. With this condition, menstrual blood is retained within the vagina (a haematocolpos) causing cyclical lower abdominal pain each month at the time of menstruation (cryptomenorrhoea). Inspection of the vulva reveals a distended hymenal membrane through which dark blood may be seen, and treatment by incision, usually under anaesthesia, is all that is required (Fig. 7.1).

Failure to menstruate may also be physiological delay – in other words, the development is normal but there is an inherent delay in the onset of menstruation. There is often a family history of the same delay in the mother. A progestogen challenge test is useful to identify constitutional menstrual delay. A progestogen (e.g. norethisterone) is given orally for 5 days, and withdrawal should lead to a vaginal bleed. If such a bleed occurs, it is reasonable to offer reassurance that spontaneous menstruation is likely to occur. An abdominal ultrasound may be reassuring to confirm that the uterus and ovaries are normal.

Low body weight and excessive exercise are also associated with primary amenorrhoea. The other causes listed in **Table 7.1** are rare, although a few are outlined under the 'secondary amenorrhoea' discussion below (see chapters 4 and 5).

Secondary amenorrhoea

Secondary amenorrhoea means the cessation of established menstruation. It is defined as no menstruation for 6 months in the absence of pregnancy. A full list of causes is given in **Table 7.2**, but the commonest are weight loss, polycystic ovary syndrome (PCOS) and hyperprolactinaemia. The more common conditions are discussed below.

Causes

Physiological

The commonest causes of amenorrhoea during the reproductive phase of life are physiological – pregnancy and lactation. Pregnancy should therefore be excluded in all sexually active women presenting with amenorrhoea.

The high postpartum level of prolactin associated with breast feeding suppresses ovulation and gives rise to lactational amenorrhoea. The mechanism is probably related to reduced gonadotrophin-releasing hormone (GnRH) production as a result of changes in the sensitivity of the hypothalamic–pituitary axis to oestrogen. Amenorrhoea usually persists throughout the time that the infant is fully breastfed, but with the introduction of supplementary feeding, and therefore reduction in the frequency of suckling, prolactin levels fall and ovarian activity is resumed. This hypo-oestrogenic state may lead to atrophic vaginitis, and occasionally to painful intercourse.

Hypothalamic

Hypothalamic amenorrhoea ('hypogonadotrophic hypogonadism') is frequently associated with stress – for example, leaving home for higher education – and in such cases the condition usually resolves spontaneously. Physical stress in the form of athletic training can also result in suppression

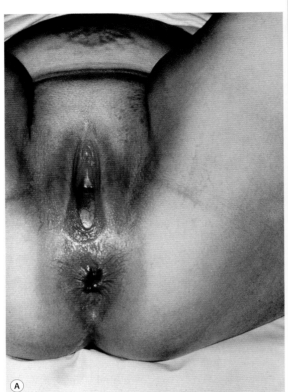
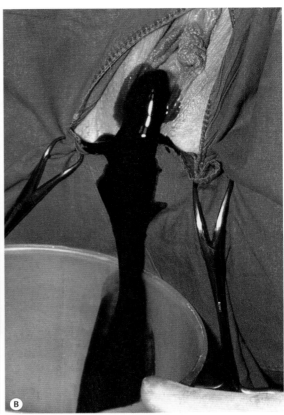

Fig. 7.1 **Imperforate hymen (A) before and (B) after incision.**

Table 7.1		
Causes of primary amenorrhoea		
System	**Problem**	**Incidence**
Chromosomal	XO – Turner syndrome	Rare
	46,XY DSD	Rare
	Ovotesticular DSD	Rare
Hypothalamic	Physiological delay	Common
	Weight loss/anorexia/ heavy exercise	Common
	Isolated GnRH deficiency	Rare
	Congenital CNS defects	Rare
	Intracranial tumours	Rare
Pituitary	Partial/total hypopituitarism	Rare
	Hyperprolactinaemia	Rare
	Pituitary adenoma	Rare
	Empty sella syndrome	Rare
	Trauma/surgery	Rare
Ovarian	True agenesis	Rare
	Premature ovarian failure	Rare
	Radiation/chemotherapy/ autoimmune	Rare
	Polycystic ovaries	Not uncommon
	Virilizing ovarian tumours	Rare
Other endocrine	Primary hypothyroidism	Rare
	Adrenal hyperplasia	Rare
	Adrenal tumour	Rare
Uterine/vaginal	Imperforate hymen	Not uncommon
	Uterovaginal agenesis	Rare

Table 7.2

Causes of secondary amenorrhoea

System	Problem	Incidence
Physiological	Pregnancy	Common
	Lactation	Common
	Menopause	Common
Hypothalamic	Weight loss/anorexia	Common
	Heavy exercise	Common
	Stress	Common
Pituitary	Hyperprolactinaemia	Not uncommon
	Partial/total hypopituitarism	Rare
	Trauma/surgery	Rare
Ovarian	Polycystic ovary syndrome	Common
	Premature ovarian failure	Uncommon
	Surgery/radiotherapy/ chemotherapy	Uncommon
	Resistant ovary syndrome	Rare
	Virilizing ovarian tumours	Rare
Other endocrine	Primary hypothyroidism	Rare
	Adrenal hyperplasia	Rare
	Adrenal tumour	Rare
Uterine/vaginal	Surgery – hysterectomy	Common
	Endometrial ablation	Common
	Progestogen intrauterine device	Common
	Asherman's syndrome	Rare

of the hypothalamo-pituitary–ovarian axis. There are low levels of pituitary gonadotrophins in association with low levels of prolactin and oestrogen.

If hypothalamic amenorrhoea is not related to low body weight (see below), treatment will depend on whether or not the woman wants to conceive. If pregnancy is not desired, oestrogen replacement therapy is advisable, and is conveniently provided in the form of the oral contraceptive pill. If the woman wishes to become pregnant, ovulation may be induced with pulsatile GnRH therapy or exogenous gonadotrophins (p. 72).

The hypothalamus is also sensitive to changes in body weight, and weight loss, even to only 10–15% below the ideal, may be associated with amenorrhoea. Anorexia nervosa should be considered. Restoration of the body weight results in the return of ovulatory function, although there may be a significant time interval between the attainment of the ideal body weight and the resumption of ovarian activity. Ovulation induction therapy is not recommended prior to the restoration of body weight, as pregnancy, if it occurs, carries the risk of growth restriction of the fetus and increased perinatal mortality.

Pituitary

Prolactin stimulates breast development and subsequent lactation. The secretion of prolactin, a polypeptide hormone produced by the lactotrophs of the anterior pituitary, is inhibited by dopamine from the hypothalamus. High levels of prolactin, which may be either physiological (during lactation) or pathological (see below), in turn suppress ovarian activity by interfering with the secretion of gonadotrophins.

Mildly elevated prolactin levels are common and can be due to stress (e.g. of venepuncture). Sustained higher levels can result in amenorrhoea and galactorrhoea unrelated to

Box 7.1

Causes of hyperprolactinaemia

Pituitary adenoma

- Microadenomas
- Macroadenomas

Secondary to other causes

- Primary hypothyroidism
- Chronic renal failure
- Pituitary stalk compression
- PCOS
- Drugs (phenothiazines, haloperidol, metoclopramide, cimetidine, methyldopa, antihistamines and morphine)
- Idiopathic

pregnancy. Galactorrhoea occurs in <50% of those with hyperprolactinaemia, and <50% of those with galactorrhoea have an elevated prolactin level. The causes of hyperprolactinaemia are given in **Box 7.1**.

Adenomas occur in the lateral wings of the anterior pituitary and are usually soft and discrete with a pseudocapsule of compressed tissue **(Fig. 7.2)**. If the prolactin is more than 1000 mU/l, then imaging with CT or (ideally) MRI should be carried out. A microadenoma is less than 10 mm in diameter and a macroadenoma more than 10 mm. Visual fields should be checked as optic chiasma compression may lead to bitemporal hemianopia. One-third of adenomas regress spontaneously and less than 5% of microadenomas become macroadenomas. Serum levels correlate well with tumour size, so that if the tumour is relatively large and the prolactin level only modestly elevated, then pituitary stalk compression from a non-secreting macroadenoma or other tumour is possible

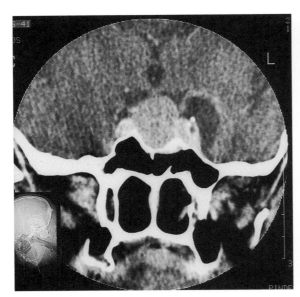

Fig. 7.2 CT scan of a pituitary macroadenoma.

(e.g. a craniopharyngioma). It is possible that apparently idiopathic hyperprolactinaemia may be caused by microadenomas which are too small to be picked up by an MRI scan.

All patients should have pituitary imaging before treatment. This treatment is usually with a dopamine agonist, either bromocriptine or cabergoline, which suppresses the prolactin level and also induces regression of the prolactinoma. Transnasal transsphenoidal microsurgical excision of an adenoma is only rarely required.

Ovarian

Premature ovarian failure

The menopause (with cessation of ovarian function) normally occurs around the age of 50. The term 'premature ovarian failure' is usually used to describe cessation of ovarian function before the age of 40. As in the natural menopause, failure is usually due to depletion of primordial follicles in the ovaries.

Premature ovarian failure occurs in 1% of women and may be due to surgery, viral infections (e.g. mumps), cytotoxic drugs or radiotherapy. It may also be idiopathic and is occasionally associated with chromosomal abnormality (XO mosaics or XXX). A low oestrogen level, very high follicle-stimulating hormone (FSH) and the absence of any menstrual activity are poor prognostic signs for recovery. Pregnancy by in vitro fertilization (IVF) with donor oocytes may be possible. There is an association with other autoimmune disorders. Hormone replacement therapy is required to relieve postmenopausal symptoms and minimize the risk of osteoporosis.

Polycystic ovary syndrome (PCOS)

Polycystic ovary syndrome is associated with menstrual disturbance, and is the most common form of anovulatory infertility. It is estimated to affect up to 10% of women. It

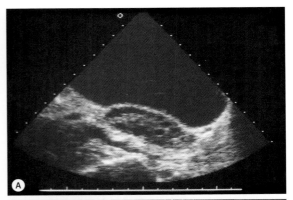

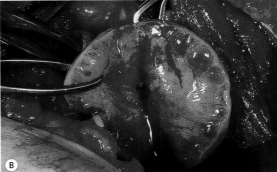

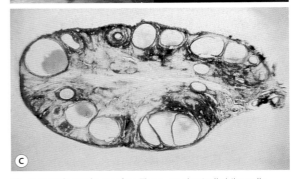

Fig. 7.3 Polycystic ovaries. These are classically bilaterally enlarged with multiple peripherally situated cysts 'like a ring of pearls' in a dense stroma: **(A)** ultrasound scan; **(B)** surgical dissection; **(C)** pathological preparation.

is characterized by the presence of at least two out of the following three criteria:

- oligo- or amenorrhoea
- ultrasound appearance of large-volume ovaries (>10cm^3) and/or multiple small follicles (12 or more <10mm) **(Fig. 7.3)**
- clinical evidence of excess androgens (acne, hirsutism) or biochemical evidence (raised testosterone).

The aetiology of the condition is unknown, but recent evidence suggests that the principal underlying disorder is one of insulin resistance, with the resultant hyperinsulinaemia stimulating excess ovarian androgen production. Associated with the prevalent insulin resistance, there is a

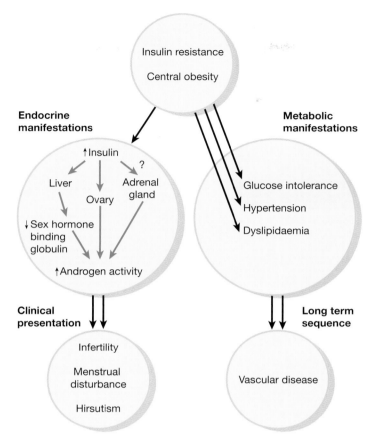

Fig. 7.4 Pathogenesis of polycystic ovary syndrome. Polycystic ovary syndrome can be considered to be a disorder primarily of insulin resistance, with the resultant hyperinsulinaemia stimulating excess ovarian androgen production. There may also be dyslipidaemia and a predisposition to later non-insulin-dependent diabetes and cardiovascular disease. ? = uncertain relationship between insulin and the adrenal gland.

characteristic dyslipidaemia and a predisposition to non-insulin-dependent diabetes and cardiovascular disease in later life. PCOS may therefore be considered to be a systemic metabolic condition rather one primarily of gynaecological origin **(Fig. 7.4)**.

Treatment depends on whether the presenting problem has been menstrual irregularity, hirsutism or infertility. The combined oral contraceptive pill has been used to regulate the menses. Hirsutism may also be treated with the combined oral contraceptive pill since it suppresses ovarian androgen production or with the anti-androgen cyproterone acetate. Clomifene is used to induce ovulation in women with anovulatory infertility (p. 73). If clomifene does not work, ovulation may be induced by injections of gonadotrophins, or by laparoscopic laser or diathermy to the ovary.

The cornerstone to management, however, is weight reduction, which reduces insulin resistance, corrects the hormone imbalance and promotes ovulation. Ongoing research is evaluating the possible role of insulin-sensitizing agents (e.g. metformin) as a therapeutic option in the management of anovulation and other symptoms of PCOS.

Long term, there is an increased risk of endometrial hyperplasia and endometrial carcinoma as a consequence of the effects of anovulation with unopposed oestrogen stimulation of the endometrium. There is also an increased risk of non-insulin-dependent diabetes mellitus and cardiovascular disease. Individuals may gain benefit from early screening for cardiovascular risk factors, particularly hypertension and glucose intolerance.

Other endocrine causes

These are rare. Women with thyrotoxicosis may have amenorrhoea. Primary hypothyroidism is also associated with amenorrhoea, as thyrotrophin-releasing hormone stimulates prolactin secretion. The most common of the rare adrenal problems is late-onset congenital adrenal hyperplasia. This is usually due to a deficiency of the enzyme 21-hydroxylase **(Fig. 5.4)**, and treatment with a low dose of corticosteroids is usually sufficient to re-establish ovulatory function by suppressing adrenal function. Androgen-secreting adrenal tumours can also occur.

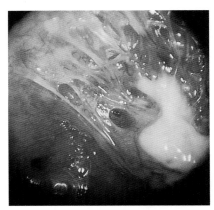

Fig. 7.5 Rarely, adhesions can form within the uterine cavity. If so severe that they obstruct the menstrual flow, the condition is referred to as Asherman's syndrome.

 History

Asherman's syndrome was first described in 1894 by Heinrich Fritsch and further characterized by the gynaecologist Josephen Asherman (1889–1968). It is also known as Fritsch syndrome, or Fritsch–Asherman syndrome.

Uterine

Excessive uterine curettage – usually at the time of miscarriage, termination of pregnancy or secondary postpartum haemorrhage – may remove the basal layer of the endometrium and result in the formation of uterine adhesions (synechiae), a condition known as Asherman's syndrome **(Fig. 7.5)** (history box). It may rarely also result from severe postpartum infection. Treatment involves breaking down the adhesions through a hysteroscope with or without inserting an IUD to deter reformation.

Summary of clinical management

Initial management:

- Exclude pregnancy.
- Ask about perimenopausal symptoms (e.g. flushings, vaginal dryness).
- Take a history including weight changes, drugs, medical disorders and thyroid symptoms.
- Carry out an examination, looking particularly at height, weight, visual fields and the presence of hirsutism or virilization. Also carry out a pelvic examination, unless this is contraindicated.
- Check serum for LH, FSH, prolactin, testosterone, thyroxine and thyroid-stimulating hormone (TSH).
- Arrange a transvaginal ultrasound scan, looking for polycystic ovaries.
- Review with the results **(Table 7.3)**.

Table 7.3		
Further management based on test results		
Ultrasound scan	A scan showing large-volume ovaries (>10 cm³) and/or multiple small follicles (12 or more <10 mm)	If pregnancy desired, clomifene or gonadotrophins. If pregnancy not desired, consider the combined oral contraceptive pill
Elevated PRL level	If PRL >1000 mU/l on at least two occasions, the diagnosis is hyperprolactinaemia	Arrange MRI or CT of the pituitary. Treat with dopamine agonist
Elevated FSH	If FSH >30 U/l, repeat 6 weeks later. If still elevated and the patient >40 years old, the patient is menopausal. If less than 40, the diagnosis is premature ovarian failure	Consider HRT. Pregnancy with oocyte donation is possible
Abnormal TFTs	If the TFTs are abnormal, treat as appropriate	

FSH, follicle-stimulating hormone; HRT, hormone replacement therapy; LH, luteinizing hormone; PRL, prolactin; TFTs thyroid function tests.

If the tests listed in **Table 7.3** are normal, consider the following causes:

- weight loss
- depression, emotional disturbance and extreme exercise
- Asherman's syndrome
- idiopathic amenorrhoea.

In the majority of patients who present with secondary amenorrhoea, investigations will fail to demonstrate any significant endocrine abnormality – idiopathic amenorrhoea. It is probable that there is a disturbance of the normal feedback mechanisms of control. Undue sensitivity of the hypothalamus and pituitary to the negative feedback suppression of endogenous oestrogen may result in impaired gonadotrophin secretion which is inadequate to stimulate follicular development, and results in cycle initiation failure. Those requiring ovulation usually respond well to an anti-oestrogen such as clomifene.

> ### Key *points*
>
> - The commonest causes of primary amenorrhoea (when menstruation has never occurred) are physiological delay, weight loss, heavy exercise and an imperforate hymen.
> - Secondary amenorrhoea is said to have occurred when established menstruation ceases for 6 months or more. Outside pregnancy, lactation and the menopause, the commonest causes are the polycystic ovary syndrome, stress, weight loss and hyperprolactinaemia.
> - Polycystic ovary syndrome is the commonest cause of anovulatory infertility.

8

Infertility

Introduction

Infertility is a condition that affects approximately one in six couples at some stage in their lives. The cause may be related to a problem with the man, woman or both. In view of the intimate nature of the problem, infertility is often associated with personal distress and embarrassment; effective treatment, however, is now available to help an increasing proportion of these couples.

Definitions

Infertility can be defined as the inability of the couple to conceive within 2 years of beginning regular unprotected sexual intercourse. A couple can have primary infertility – no previous pregnancies within the relationship – or secondary infertility, where the couple has had at least one pregnancy.

Infertility is rarely absolute, and most couples have a degree of subfertility. Around 84% of the normal fertile population will conceive within 1 year, and 92% by the end of 2 years. Cumulative pregnancy rates and live birth rates are the terms used to express the chance of conception within a given time interval. **Figure 8.1** illustrates the cumulative pregnancy rate for the normal fertile population.

Fecundability is the percentage of women exposed to the risk of a pregnancy for one menstrual cycle who will subsequently produce a live-born infant (normal range – 15–28%). Fecundability usually diminishes slightly with each passing month of not conceiving.

Age and fertility

Normal fertility declines as the woman's age increases. A woman is born with a finite number of oocytes, around one million. This falls to approximately 250,000 at puberty, and by the time the menopause is reached the number of oocytes has fallen to below 1000. During her reproductive life a woman will release only 500 mature oocytes – a form of pre-conceptual natural selection – while the remaining oocytes undergo atresia or apoptosis. The rate of oocyte loss is relatively constant throughout early life until around the age of 37 years, when the rate of loss accelerates. At the menopause, which occurs at an average age of 51, there are no functioning oocytes.

The decline in fertility is directly related to the declining oocyte population and the eggs' inherent quality. There is a small, but noticeable, fall in monthly fecundity rates from the age of 31 years, a more pronounced decrease from the age of 36 years, and a very steep decline over the age of 40 years. In addition, there is a substantial increase in spontaneous miscarriage rates with advancing maternal age. Although older men are less fertile, the effect of age on men is less pronounced than in women.

Causes of infertility

The causes of infertility can be classified simply, as outlined in **Figure 8.2**. In some couples, more than one problem can be identified.

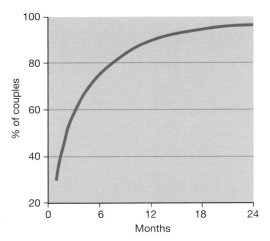

Fig. 8.1 **Cumulative pregnancy rates in the normal fertile population.**

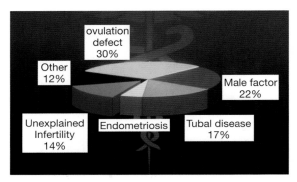

Fig. 8.2 **Causes of infertility** (From Taylor & Collins 1992, with permission.)

Diagnosis

The diagnosis of infertility is a process of exclusion, identifying those patients where the cause is clear, those in whom there is a possible cause, and those in whom the cause is essentially unexplained. The aim of investigation should be to reach a diagnosis as soon as possible, using only tests that are of proven value.

History and examination

Factors that provide clues to the aetiology are outlined in **Tables 8.1** and **8.2**. Other important factors to be noted are the woman's age and the duration of infertility – generally, the longer the period of infertility, the poorer is the prognosis. The order in which the investigations are performed varies depending on whether the couple has primary or secondary infertility, with an earlier assessment of tubal patency in the latter. Early assessment is also indicated if a

Table 8.1

Examination of a woman

Examination	Reason
Height and weight for body mass index (BMI)	High or low BMI associated with lower fertility
Body hair distribution	Hyperandrogenism
Galactorrhoea	Hyperprolactinaemia
Uterine structural abnormalities	May be associated with infertility
Fixed or tender uterus	Endometriosis or pelvic inflammatory disease associated with tubal damage

Table 8.2

Examination of a man

Examination	Reason
Scrotum	Varicocele
Size (volume) of the testes	Small testes associated with oligospermia
Position of the testes	Undescended testes
Prostate	Chronic infection

specific abnormality is suspected from the history, and for an older patient.

Examination of the woman

Height and weight should be recorded and used to calculate the body mass index (BMI), using the formula: weight $(kg)/height (m)^2$. The normal range is between 19 and 25. A change of weight of greater than 10% in the preceding year may cause a disturbance of the menstrual pattern and anovulation. A BMI at either extreme is detrimental to fertility (see later).

Increased body hair is associated with hyperandrogenism, most commonly because of polycystic ovary syndrome. Breast examination may demonstrate galactorrhoea, which is associated with hyperprolactinaemia. Pelvic examination is important to look for signs of structural abnormalities, infection, and pathological processes such as endometriosis or pelvic inflammatory disease.

Examination of the man

Examination of the man is not essential in the absence of any relevant history. If, however, the semen analysis is abnormal, examination of the genitalia may be helpful, looking specifically at size (volume), consistency and position of the testes, the outline of the epididymis (for the presence of the vas deferens), and finally the scrotum for any evidence of swellings.

Investigations and their interpretation

The investigations should be arranged in a logical manner with reference to the history, along with appropriate general health screening **(Box 8.1)**. Additional tests may be necessary, depending on the clinical circumstances **(Box 8.2)**.

Male factors

Classification

Male factor infertility can be a problem of sperm production, sperm function, or sperm delivery. Sperm production may be completely absent (azoospermia) in, for example, testicular failure. More commonly a patient may present with a reduced count of sperm of normal appearance (oligospermia). Additionally, a high proportion of the sperm may be poorly motile, lacking the normal forward progressive movement (asthenospermia), or may appear morphologically defective (teratospermia) with abnormalities of the head, midpiece or tail.

Normal sperm function – the ability of the sperm to reach, bind, and fertilize the oocyte – is more difficult to

Table 8.3

WHO criteria for semen analysis

Volume	>2 ml
pH	7–8
Concentration	>20 × 10⁶/ml
Motility	>50% forward >25% with rapid linear progress
Morphology	>15% normal
Alive	>50%
Antisperm antibodies (MAR test)	Negative
WCC	<1 × 10⁶

Reproduced with permission from WHO.

demonstrate. At present there are no reliable methods of measuring sperm function, other than monitoring the proportion of sperm moving and assessing the speed of their progress. Antisperm antibodies can affect sperm motility.

Problems with sperm delivery may be caused by absence or blockage of the vas deferens or epididymis. It may also be related to impotence, premature ejaculation, or a physical inability to have normal sexual intercourse.

Semen analysis

This provides information about spermatogenesis and an aspect of sperm delivery, but gives little information about sperm function. The World Health Organization (WHO) has produced a normal range of values for semen **(Table 8.3)**. The values, however, are empirical and do not reflect a cut-off point below which pregnancy will not occur. Only in the 5% of patients that present with azoospermia can an absolute male cause be confirmed. Even if the sperm density is less than 5 million/ml, 19% will father a child, compared to a pregnancy rate of 43% in women whose partners have a count greater than 5 million/ml. A similar picture exists when the other variables, motility and morphology, are considered. Only when motility is below 20% and morphology falls below 15% does the basic semen analysis have any significant predictive value. In conclusion, the basic semen analysis (with the exception of azoospermia) is of little prognostic value.

A man's sperm count varies considerably, and in the presence of one abnormal result a second count should be arranged. As spermatogenesis takes approximately 3 months to complete, the samples ought to be produced at least 3 months apart. Samples should be produced by masturbation or after intercourse into a non-lubricated condom after a period of abstinence of between 3 and 5 days. The sample should be analysed in an accredited laboratory, with careful assessment of morphology using strict definitions of abnormality (Kruger criteria), as morphology is also closely associated with the sperm's ability to fertilize.

Tests of sperm function

Sperm function tests are no longer used in routine clinical practice, with more emphasis now placed on the identification of the number of abnormal/normal sperm as part of the routine analysis. Some sperm function tests, such as the ability of sperm to swim through culture medium, are employed in specialized Reproductive Medicine Units, where more complicated treatment may be contemplated.

The postcoital test involves asking the couple to have sexual intercourse timed to the woman's mid-cycle. Then, 6–12 hours later, a sample of endocervical mucus is taken, looking for the presence or absence of sperm. Some studies have shown a positive correlation between the finding of motile sperm in the mucus and the chance of subsequent pregnancy. The use of this test, however, is controversial, as other studies have shown that the finding of a positive or negative result does not alter the chance or timing of a pregnancy. As a result, most centres have abandoned this procedure.

Antibodies can develop against sperm in response to injury or infection of the testis and epididymis. Men who have had a vasectomy and attempted reversal are the commonest group in whom antisperm antibodies are identified. The antibodies can be serum (IgG) or bound (IgA), and attach principally to the tail, midpiece or head of the sperm. Tests used to detect antisperm antibodies include the mixed agglutination reaction (MAR) test, and the immunobead test. Levels between 17% and 49% are likely to be associated with a fall in fertility, and levels greater than 50% are thought to significantly affect fertility.

Female factors

Ovulation

Ovulation is an 'all or nothing' phenomenon, with usually one oocyte released per ovulatory cycle.

Causes of anovulation

Ovarian failure is found in about 50% of patients with primary amenorrhoea, and 15% of those presenting with secondary amenorrhoea. Most patients with primary amenorrhoea will have an established diagnosis before presenting to an infertility clinic. The cause may be genetic, e.g. Turner syndrome (45,XO), or autoimmune. In those presenting with secondary amenorrhoea and ovarian failure there may be an obvious cause, such as previous ovarian surgery, abdominal radiotherapy or chemotherapy. There will also be a proportion of patients in whom no reason can be identified – idiopathic premature menopause.

Weight-related anovulation Weight plays an important part in the control of ovulation. A minimum degree of body fat (generally believed to be around 22% of body weight) is needed to maintain ovulatory cycles. Substantial weight loss leads to the disappearance of the normal 24-hour secretory pattern of luteinizing hormone-releasing hormone (LHRH), which reverts to the nocturnal pattern seen in pubescent girls. As a result, the ovaries develop a multifollicular appearance on ultrasound. Prolonged exercise can, by increasing the muscle bulk and decreasing the body fat, have the same effect, and it is not uncommon for women athletes or ballerinas to be amenorrhoeic. Excessive weight can also have an adverse effect on ovulation. This probably results from excess oestrone, generated in the adipose tissue from androgens, interfering with the normal feedback mechanism to the pituitary gland.

Excess weight has been shown to have a profound affect on female fertility, with a significant reduction in the chance of a successful pregnancy: it reduces the chance of conception, increases the risk of miscarriage, as well as substantially increasing the risk of obstetric complications during the pregnancy and at delivery. The distribution of the fat is important, with central (visceral) fat having a bigger impact than peripheral fat distribution. The waist–hip ratio, which more reliably picks up visceral fat distribution, seems a more reliable guide to the impact of fat on fertility than is the body mass index (BMI).

Polycystic ovary syndrome 50% of patients presenting with anovulatory infertility will have polycystic ovary syndrome (PCOS) – see Chapter 7.

Luteinized unruptured follicle syndrome In certain patients the oocyte may be retained following the luteinizing hormone (LH) surge, the so-called 'luteinized unruptured follicle syndrome' (LUF). Repeated pelvic ultrasound scans fail to show the expected collapse of the follicle at ovulation, and the follicle persists into the luteal phase. As no longitudinal studies have shown this to be a persistent finding in the same patient, however, there is uncertainty regarding its relevance to fertility.

Hyperprolactinaemia Hyperprolactinaemia is diagnosed in 10–15% of cases of secondary amenorrhoea. About one-third of these patients will have galactorrhoea, and occasionally there may be some evidence of visual impairment (bitemporal hemianopia) due to pressure on the optic chiasma from pituitary adenoma.

Tests of ovulation

There is only one true test that proves ovulation has occurred, and that is pregnancy. However, there are a number of investigations that imply that ovulation has taken place:

- History: over 90% of women with regular menstrual cycles will ovulate spontaneously.
- LH kit: this picks up the mid-cycle surge of LH that starts the cascade reaction leading to ovulation.
- Mid-luteal phase progesterone: this is the most commonly used test of ovulation. A luteal phase progesterone value of greater than 28 nmol/l is found in conception cycles, and as a result this value is generally regarded as evidence of satisfactory ovulation. However, it is important to time the blood sample carefully – between 7 and 10 days before the next menstrual period. This can only be determined with some knowledge of the length of the patient's normal menstrual cycle.

Other tests Less commonly employed tests include serial ultrasound scans to monitor the growth, and subsequent disappearance, of a Graafian follicle. A luteal phase endometrial biopsy looking for appropriately timed secretory changes is no longer considered of value. Basal body temperature was previously considered to be of value as there is a rise of 0.5°C if ovulation has occurred (due to progesterone) but in practice this is now rarely used.

Testing ovarian reserve

Ovarian reserve is defined as the number of viable oocytes in the ovary. This is particularly important in women contemplating more complex fertility treatment, and may provide a guide to their response to treatment. Checking the level of follicle-stimulating hormone (FSH) at the beginning of the menstrual cycle is probably the most commonly employed test. A raised FSH taken between days 2 to 5 of the menstrual cycle indicates impaired ovarian reserve, and likely poor response to ovarian stimulation. Other methods that appear to be more reliable include:

- Measuring the antral follicle count – the number of small developing follicles seen in the ovary on ultrasound.
- Measuring the ovarian volume – this is an indication of ovarian activity, as ovaries decrease in size with advancing age and decline in oocyte numbers.
- Measuring the concentration of anti-Müllerian hormone (AMH). AMH is produced in small developing follicles, and, unlike FSH, can be measured reliably throughout the menstrual cycle.

Although tests of ovarian reserve may be important in identifying those patients who may not respond well to fertility treatment, there is limited information on their value in predicting overall fertility.

Further investigations

Pelvic ultrasound is very useful in defining ovarian morphology, and is more reliable than pelvic examination in picking up other pelvic pathology such as fibroids, ovarian cyst, and uterine polyps.

Chlamydia serology has been used as a screening test for tubal pathology. Those with a positive antibody titre are more likely to have tubal pathology, because of the association between chlamydial infection and salpingitis.

Serum testosterone measurement is indicated if there is evidence of hirsutism, to exclude more sinister disorders such as androgen-secreting tumours of the ovary or adrenal gland. Thyroid function tests are commonly performed, as approximately 7% of women in this age group will have a thyroid disorder, which may have an impact on a pregnancy if not appropriately treated.

A progestogen challenge test may be useful in patients with a history of amenorrhoea and normal levels of FSH and prolactin. It is used to determine whether the patient is clinically oestrogenized. This acts as a guide to what would be the most appropriate medication to use to induce ovulation. Medroxyprogesterone acetate, 5 mg daily for 5 days, is usually sufficient to induce a withdrawal bleed. If the bleeding is normal the patient is well oestrogenized, whereas if it is absent or scanty the patient is relatively poorly oestrogenized. The presence of a withdrawal bleed also demonstrates the presence of endometrium and the patency of the genital tract.

Tubal patency
Classification

The fallopian tube can be blocked distally – at the fimbrial end – or, less commonly, at the proximal end – the cornu. In addition, the tubo-ovarian relationship may be disrupted by peritubal adhesions. Fimbrial disease has varying degrees of severity:

- agglutination of the fimbria to produce a narrowed opening – known as a phimosis
- complete agglutination to form a hydrosalpinx (fluid-filled tube).

In addition, tubal damage can also involve the endosalpinx, with intraluminal adhesions and flattening of the mucosal folds. Microsurgery to relieve tubal blockage, therefore, may not restore tubal function.

The important features for fertility prognosis appear to be:

- degree of dilatation of the fallopian tube
- extent of the fibrosis of the wall of the tube
- damage to the endosalpinx.

Tests of tubal patency

In the absence of a positive history suggestive of pelvic pathology, a negative physical examination, and a negative *Chlamydia* antibody titre, the least invasive method for assessing tubal patency should be employed.

Hysterosalpingography (HSG) HSG is the simplest method to assess tubal patency. It involves inserting a cannula into the cervix and passing radio-opaque fluid into the uterine cavity and fallopian tubes, demonstrating their outline **(Fig. 8.3)**. The test is performed under X-ray control on an outpatient basis. If the HSG is normal, the diagnosis can be relied upon in 97% of cases. However, if the HSG is abnormal, the diagnosis can only be relied upon in 34% of cases (false positive rate 66%), and a laparoscopy is required to confirm the nature of the abnormality.

Hysterosalpingo-contrast sonography (HyCoSy) This technique involves a standard pelvic ultrasound scan at which galactose-containing ultrasound contrast medium is inserted into the uterine cavity, outlining any abnormalities such as submucosal fibroids and endometrial polyps, before passing down the fallopian tubes to confirm tubal patency. The technique offers a similar level of diagnostic accuracy to HSG.

Diagnostic laparoscopy Diagnostic laparoscopy remains the 'gold standard' investigation. It provides a direct view

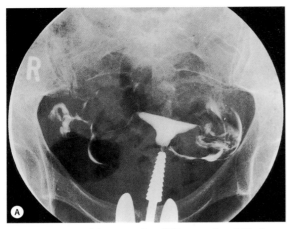 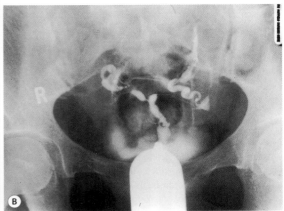

Fig. 8.3 Hysterosalpingography of (A) normal and (B) abnormal uteri. In (B) the radio-opaque dye does not leak from the fallopian tubes, thus indicating a blockage.

of the pelvic organs, and also offers the possibility to treat minor pathology discovered during the investigation. Methylthioninium chloride (methylene blue) dye is inserted through a cannula in the cervix to demonstrate tubal patency. Hysteroscopy is often carried out at the same time, looking at the uterine cavity. The diagnostic laparoscopy requires admission to hospital, usually as a day case, and a general anaesthetic. As such it is the most invasive and expensive investigation performed on the woman. For this reason, some doctors prefer to use a hysterosalpingogram as a first-line assessment.

Selective salpingography If HSG or laparoscopy detects a proximal blockage, further investigation is required. The blockage could simply be related to muscular spasm, or to genuine pathology. A fine guidewire is inserted into the internal tubal ostium under direct fluoroscopic control or by direct vision using a hysteroscope. This may dislodge a small plug of amorphous debris, restoring patency. This technique appears to increase the likelihood of pregnancy in women with proximal tubal damage.

Salpingoscopy More detailed investigation of the interior of the fallopian tube is now possible but is only really necessary if the question of tubal surgery is raised. A fine telescope, called a salpingoscope, can be passed down an operating laparoscope and inserted into the ampullary portion of the fallopian tube. Approximately 50% of patients with macroscopically damaged fallopian tubes will have fine intratubal adhesions. If present, these adhesions adversely affect the outcome of surgery.

Falloposcopy More recently, advances in fibreoptics have allowed the development of a very fine instrument, a falloposcope, with a diameter of less than 1 mm, which can be inserted into the fallopian tube via the uterine cavity. Falloposcopy appears to be effective in detecting tubal pathology, and can be performed on an outpatient basis. The equipment is fragile and expensive, however, and its use is limited to a small number of centres, mainly as a research tool.

It is important to note that all of these techniques are useful in demonstrating patency, but none is capable of directly assessing tubal function.

Treatment

Approximately one-fifth of couples with subfertility conceive spontaneously during investigation or while awaiting treatment. For those in whom investigations reveal no true cause, many will require no more than a careful explanation of their chances of conception. However, age and length of infertility must be taken into account when adopting such a conservative approach. Before considering active treatment the couple should be counselled about general health matters such as smoking, alcohol intake, and diet. It is appropriate to recommend folic acid to the woman as routine prevention of neural tube defects. Where the diagnosis is established, specific treatments can be employed.

Anovulation

There are various ways of inducing ovulation, depending on the underlying cause. Successful ovulation induction should be continued for long enough to give the optimum chance for conception – generally 12 months.

Hyperprolactinaemia is treated with a dopamine agonist, either bromocriptine or cabergoline.

Excess or decreased body weight should be treated by dietary adjustments. Although ovulation can generally be induced by exogenous gonadotrophins, this should be avoided, particularly if the patient is underweight, as there is an increased risk of pregnancy complications. Patients with moderate obesity often show resistance to treatment with clomifene citrate and gonadotrophins, requiring much higher doses to induce ovulation.

Anovulation in oestrogenized patients

Most of these patients have polycystic ovary syndrome (85% of patients presenting with oligomenorrhoea and 25% of those with amenorrhoea). First-line treatment in this condition is oral anti-oestrogen therapy, usually with clomifene citrate.

Clomifene citrate, a derivative of the weak non-steroidal oestrogen triphenylethylene, is formulated as a mixture of two isomers, enclomifene and zuclomifene, the former being the important isomer for ovulation induction. Its mode of action is to increase the plasma FSH concentration, mainly by competitively blocking the negative feedback effects of endogenous oestradiol on the hypothalamus. FSH is the principal hormone needed for follicular recruitment and development.

Initially, a dose of 25–50 mg daily for 5 days is given at the beginning of a cycle (days 2–6). If there is no response, the dose is increased to a maximum of 100 mg daily for 5 days. Rarely, in obese patients, the dose may be increased to 150 mg daily for 5 days. It is important to monitor the response to treatment as there is a small risk of a multiple pregnancy. In monitoring the response to treatment with clomifene, serum progesterone will not indicate whether more than one follicle has developed and serial ultrasound scans of follicular growth may be more useful.

Ovulation can be achieved successfully in approximately 80% of cycles, with cumulative pregnancy rates of up to 81% after 12 months' treatment. Unfortunately, there is a disappointingly high miscarriage rate in patients treated for PCOS, perhaps related to the high background level of LH. There is an increased risk of multiple pregnancy (7% twins; 1% triplets or greater), mostly confined to patients with PCOS.

Side-effects while using clomifene citrate include:

- hot flushes (11%)
- pelvic discomfort (7%)
- nausea (2%)
- breast discomfort (2%).

These are seldom severe, and simple explanation and reassurance are all that is required. More significant problems include visual disturbances (1.5%) and cholestatic jaundice (rare). In both these situations the drug should be discontinued and not used again. Some women do not respond to oral ovulation-induction agents such as clomifene. These patients require treatment with exogenous gonadotrophins.

Exogenous gonadotrophins are derived from two sources: extracted from postmenopausal women's urine or, more recently, created in vitro by genetically engineered mammalian cells. Although the original urinary-derived gonadotrophins contained an equal mixture of FSH and LH (75 IU per ampoule), refinement of the extraction techniques has resulted in highly purified FSH compounds (greater than 99% of protein content is FSH). The recombinant genetically engineered FSH preparations attain similar levels of purity.

All these medications require parenteral administration, by either subcutaneous or intramuscular injection. Around 4% of women undergoing gonadotrophin treatment will develop ovarian hyperstimulation syndrome and this will be severe in 0.5%. The incidence of multiple pregnancy with gonadotrophin treatment is around 20%. The aim is to achieve development of a single follicle using a low-dose regimen, starting at one ampoule (75 IU) daily for 10 days, and then increasing the dose, if necessary, by small increments until satisfactory follicular growth occurs. Response is monitored by ovarian ultrasound, sometimes combined with serum oestradiol measurement.

When the Graafian follicle reaches maturity, ovulation is induced by administering human chorionic gonadotrophin (hCG) (5000 IU). This replaces the normal LH surge. Gonadotrophin therapy is highly successful in restoring normal fertility in patients with hypothalamic amenorrhoea (see below), but patients with PCOS resistant to clomifene are less successfully treated; they are more prone to multifollicular development, have a lower chance of pregnancy, a higher rate of miscarriage and, if the patient does conceive, there is a greater chance of a multiple pregnancy.

If standard ovulation-induction treatment fails in patients with PCOS, laparoscopic ovarian diathermy can be tried. The ovarian capsule is pierced four times for 5 seconds with a needle point diathermy. Although both ovaries are usually treated, recent evidence suggests that only one ovary needs to be punctured. Encouraging results have been reported, with spontaneous ovulation returning in up to 71% of cycles, without the risk of hyperstimulation or multiple pregnancy. In patients where spontaneous ovulation does not occur, most become more responsive to clomifene or gonadotrophin therapy. Unfortunately, the effect is time-limited, with chronic anovulation returning in 50% of patients within 2 years. There is also a risk of iatrogenic adhesion formation.

Initial evidence suggested that metformin, an oral antidiabetic drug, which works by increasing peripheral utilization of glucose in the presence of endogenous insulin, may be of value in helping induce ovulation in obese patients with PCOS. More recent work has concluded that metformin does not have a significant impact when used either alone or in combination with clomifene. It remains uncertain whether there is any value in using metformin in conjunction with gonadotrophins in IVF treatment.

Anovulation in oestrogen-deficient women

Women who have a low FSH, normal prolactin, and either a low serum oestradiol or a negative progestogen withdrawal test (hypogonadotrophic hypogonadism) need exogenous gonadotrophins (see above) or pulsatile LHRH treatment. Exogenous gonadotrophin treatment in this group of patients is less prone to side-effects such as multiple pregnancy, but, nevertheless, careful monitoring as described above is necessary.

Pulsatile LHRH treatment is an alternative to gonado-trophin therapy in patients with hypothalamic disorders of gonadotrophin regulation. Pulsatile doses of LHRH are given either intravenously or subcutaneously at intervals of 60–90 minutes using a small pump. Ovulation occurs in about 90% of cycles, restoring fertility to normal rates. This treatment minimizes the risk of multiple follicular develop-ment and, as a result, there is a lower risk of multiple preg-nancy (10%). Patients with PCOS respond poorly to this treatment, with ovulation rates of around 40% and preg-nancy rates of <10%.

Tubal disease

There are two treatments for tubal disease: surgery and in-vitro fertilization (IVF). IVF is described later in this chapter.

Tubal surgery

Surgery was the principal treatment for occlusive tubal disease but, as the results of IVF have improved, it is per-formed less frequently.

Selection of patients

Patients considered for tubal surgery need to be carefully selected, taking into consideration:

- patient's age
- site and extent of the tubal damage
- other factors that might influence fertility.

As with other treatments, age has an important effect on the outcome, and IVF may be better for older patients. Dis-tal tubal occlusion carries the worst prognosis, and surgery should be reserved only for cases in which damage is rela-tively minor. In women with minor damage, the live birth rate after surgery is around 40% over a period of 18 months. Women with a moderate to severe distal abnormality, and those with bipolar tubal disease (damage at more than one site on the same tube), have a very poor prognosis and IVF is more appropriate. However, with limited proximal dam-age, pregnancy rates of nearly 50% have been achieved after tubal surgery.

Techniques

Conventionally, tubal surgery has been performed by laparotomy, through a low transverse incision, with microsurgical techniques used to restore tubal patency. However, most tubal surgery is now performed laparoscop-ically. Even completely occluded tubes have been opened successfully laparoscopically using either a CO_2 laser or electrodiathermy. In skilled hands the results compare very favourably with conventional tubal surgery using an operat-ing microscope.

More recently, selective salpingography (passing a fine catheter through the uterus and along the fallopian tube under X-ray control) has been used successfully to treat some patients with proximal obstruction caused by a plug of amorphous debris.

Risks of tubal surgery

Patients who have undergone tubal surgery have a tenfold increased risk of having an ectopic pregnancy and should be advised to undergo an ultrasound scan at around 6 weeks' gestation to confirm the site of the pregnancy.

Endometriosis

Endometriosis is discussed in Chapter 16. There is no evidence that treating minimal peritoneal endometriosis with drugs improves fertility. Indeed, medical treatment of endometriosis involves creating anovulation for up to 6 months and this delays the patient from trying for a fam-ily. However, there is some limited evidence to suggest that surgery to ablate the endometriotic lesions and to divide adhesions that may have formed from endometriosis in-creases the chance of conception.

If the endometriosis involves the ovary or the fallopian tube, surgical treatment appears to be beneficial by cor-recting the anatomical defect. The results of surgery, even where the endometriosis is quite severe, appear to be quite encouraging. However, if pregnancy does not occur within 9–10 months, it is reasonable to consider IVF.

Male factor problems

Azoospermia and a raised serum FSH

Azoospermia and a raised serum FSH signify sperma-togenic failure (non-obstructive azoospermia). This can be confirmed by testicular biopsy. Occasionally, islands of spermatogenesis can be identified and sperm can be extracted from a testicular biopsy and used for intracy-toplasmic sperm injection (ICSI) as part of IVF treatment (see later). In most cases, however, the option likely to give the couple the best chance of a live birth is donor insemination.

Donor insemination (DI)

Men who donate sperm do so for altruistic reasons. Donors, to date, have been anonymous, although there are strong arguments for a change in practice to identified donors. All potential donors are carefully screened for a family history of medical conditions that could be passed to future chil-dren and for infection, particularly HIV. For the latter reason, semen is frozen in straws and quarantined for a minimum of 6 months. The donor is screened again for infection at the end of this period, and only if this second screen is negative is the sperm used for treatment. The need to freeze sperm reduces the pregnancy rates, as frozen sperm is not as ef-fective as fresh sperm.

Semen is inserted into the woman's cervix – or, if appro-priately prepared, into the uterus (see below) – at the time of ovulation. Ovulation is usually predicted by serial pelvic ultrasound scans or by the detection of the LH surge using a urinary assay. The chance of conception in the first cycle of treatment is 18.8%, falling rapidly to around 6% per cycle for the next 12 months.

Azoospermia and a normal FSH

Azoospermia in the presence of a normal FSH signifies a block of the vas deferens or epididymis. The most common group of men in this category are those who have had a vasectomy. Using microsurgical techniques the vas can be re-anastomosed (vasovasostomy) or attached to the epididymis (vasoepididymostomy), depending on the site of the obstruction. Although good anatomical results can be achieved, pregnancy rates are often disappointing, partly because the build-up of pressure distal to the obstruction may have damaged the delicate epididymis, and partly because antisperm antibodies may have formed. The time from the original vasectomy to the reversal procedure provides a useful guide to prognosis. Pregnancy rates are halved in the partners of men where the gap between the vasectomy and reversal is greater than 10 years (rates of 60% and 30%, respectively, with good surgical techniques).

Men in whom spermatogenesis is normal but surgery is not possible may be suitable for epididymal sperm aspiration in combination with IVF and ICSI. The sperm can be obtained under local anaesthesia by placing a needle percutaneously into the epididymis, or using more conventional microsurgical techniques under a general anaesthetic. As the sperm sample is usually of poor quality, direct ICSI into the oocytes is necessary (see below).

A significant proportion of men who have congenital absence of the vas (CAV) have been found to carry a variant of cystic fibrosis. They have compound heterogenicity, where each chromosome 7 carries a different mutation at the site of the transmembrane conductance regulator gene, which is responsible for cystic fibrosis. These couples therefore need careful screening for the common cystic fibrosis mutations. If his partner is found to be a carrier of one of the same mutations, there would be a 1:4 chance of their children having classical cystic fibrosis.

Hypogonadotrophic hypogonadism

Hypogonadotrophic hypogonadism can be treated successfully with exogenous gonadotrophins, FSH and hCG, or by using the LHRH infusion pump.

Idiopathic oligospermia

This is the most common diagnosis. A wide range of oral treatments have been employed: clomifene citrate or tamoxifen, mesterolone, kallikrein and even large doses of vitamin C. Although some studies have shown that the antioestrogens can increase the sperm count, there is no firm evidence that the use of any oral medication can improve conception rates. The mainstay of treatment, therefore, is IVF using sperm prepared in culture medium. In some men the sperm concentration is so low that standard IVF is not possible, and fertilization can only be achieved by ICSI (see below).

Varicocele

There is ultrasound evidence of a varicocele in 15% of the male population. Surgery to correct the defect is not justified in the absence of symptoms and with a normal semen analysis. If the sperm count is low, there is evidence that it can be improved with surgery; this is not, however, translated into a better conception rate.

Unexplained infertility

If no cause can be found and couples have been trying for less than 3 years, there is little evidence that medical intervention will improve their chances of conception. If infertility is longer than 3 years, the chance of spontaneous conception declines **(Fig. 8.4)** and evidence demonstrates that medical intervention can improve pregnancy rates. The simplest treatment used is oral clomifene citrate, which is generally given to the woman during days 2–6 of the menstrual cycle. Although it is commonly given for up to 6 months, a recent appropriately powered study showed clomifene to be of no benefit compared to a no-treatment arm.

Assisted conception

'Assisted conception' techniques are those in which gametes, either sperm or eggs, are manipulated to improve the chance of conception **(Table 8.4)**.

Intrauterine insemination (IUI)

IUI has been used to treat couples with unexplained infertility, a mild male factor, those with coital difficulties, and those with mild endometriosis. Sperm is prepared in culture medium, separating the seminal fluid, poorly motile sperm and other cellular debris in the ejaculate, and producing a clean sample of highly motile sperm. This is then placed directly into the uterine cavity via a fine plastic catheter. IUI is used alone, with the insemination timed to natural ovulation, or in conjunction with controlled ovarian stimulation. The latter involves ovulation-induction agents such as clomifene citrate or gonadotrophins, which are used to recruit up to three mature follicles. When the follicles reach an appropriate size, around 17 mm, ovulation is induced with hCG, and the prepared sperm is inserted into the uterine cavity. Randomized controlled trials indicate that results with IUI are little different whether no or mild stimulation is used.

Overall the live birth rates following IUI are around 8–9% per cycle. One complication of controlled ovarian stimulation is the unacceptably high rate of multiple pregnancy, which in some studies has been as high as 29%. For this reason it is a national recommendation that IUI should be used alone in patients with unexplained and mild male factor infertility. Recent studies, which have also contained a control

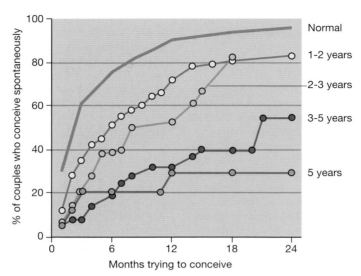

Fig. 8.4 Spontaneous pregnancy rates with increasing duration of unexplained infertility. (From Hull et al, British Medical Journal 1985, with permission.)

Table 8.4			
Assisted conception techniques			
Name	**Technique**	**Advantages**	**Disadvantages**
Superovulation with intrauterine insemination (IUI)	Mild ovarian stimulation Prepared sperm injected through the cervix	2.6-fold increase in pregnancy rate for those with unexplained infertility	Risk of multiple pregnancy
In-vitro fertilization (IVF)	Ovaries superovulated, eggs retrieved and mixed with sperm before transcervical transfer to the uterus	Effective for a number of indications, including 'unexplained' infertility	Risks of superovulation and multiple pregnancy Expensive
Gamete intrafallopian tube transfer (GIFT)	Similar stimulation to IVF, but gametes implanted laparoscopically into the fallopian tube	Effective for 'unexplained' infertility	More invasive than IVF; not suitable for tubal factor infertility (rarely used) Multiple pregnancy Expensive
Zygote intrafallopian tube transfer (ZIFT)	Similar to IVF, but fertilized zygotes transferred laparoscopically into the fallopian tube	Effective for a number of indications, including 'unexplained' infertility	More invasive than IVF; not suitable for tubal factor infertility (rarely used) Multiple pregnancy Expensive
Intracytoplasmic sperm injection (ICSI)	Stimulation and oocyte retrieval as for IVF, but sperm injected directly into the oocyte	Can be used to treat the majority of male factor infertility	Risks of superovulation and multiple pregnancy Some question marks over safety of offspring, increased proportion of children with chromosomal defects Expensive

'no-treatment arm', have shown that IUI with or without medication may not be any more effective than expectant management, questioning the value of IUI treatment.

In-vitro fertilization (IVF)

The term 'in-vitro fertilization' refers to the mixing of sperm and egg outside the body.

 History

The technique was pioneered in the 1970s by Patrick Steptoe and Professor Robert Edwards, initially in Oldham and then at Bourn Hall, Cambridge. The first pregnancy, an ectopic, was established in 1976, but it was not until 1978 that the first baby, Louise Brown, was born. Although this success was based

on the single oocyte developed during a normal ovulatory cycle, it soon became clear that a higher pregnancy rate could be achieved if a greater number of oocytes were obtained by superovulation.

Indications

IVF was originally developed for patients with tubal disease. However, the indications for IVF have expanded considerably and now include:

- male factor infertility
- severe endometriosis
- failed ovulation induction
- long history of 'unexplained' infertility
- preimplantation diagnosis for genetic disease
- surrogacy
- egg donation.

Technique
Hormonal regimen

The aim of the treatment is to recruit, or rescue, a cohort of antral stage follicles, and support their growth through to maturity. This is achieved by the administration of exogenous FSH, given by intramuscular or subcutaneous injection. Although there are two principal pituitary gonadotrophins involved in oocyte development – FSH and LH – only a relatively small background level of LH is needed. Most commercially available FSH-containing compounds are rich in FSH, with little or no LH component. They are manufactured either by extraction and purification from human postmenopausal urine, or by using recombinant DNA technology. In addition, most modern protocols use some form of pituitary suppression, either a gonadotrophin-releasing hormone (GnRH) agonist or an antagonist, principally to block an inappropriate LH surge. As the release of LH is blocked, hCG, which has a similar action, is used as a substitute, given approximately 36 hours before oocyte recovery.

Oocyte collection

During superovulation treatment, each ovary enlarges to the size of a tennis ball and they generally lie within 1 cm of the posterior fornix **(Fig. 8.5)**. This allows the oocytes to be collected using a needle passed through the vaginal vault, guided by a vaginal ultrasound probe, with the woman heavily sedated. The oocytes, with their cumulus cell mass, are identified easily **(Fig. 8.6)** and after removal are placed in an incubator.

Fertilization and incubation

On the morning of oocyte retrieval, the man collects a sperm sample by masturbation. After preparation in culture medium, the sperm are added to the test tubes containing the oocytes. The tubes are inspected 16 hours later for the characteristic signs of fertilization, the presence of a male and female pronucleus (see **Fig. 8.7**). The pronucleate embryos are returned to the incubator for a further 24 or 48 hours, with surplus embryos being frozen at this stage.

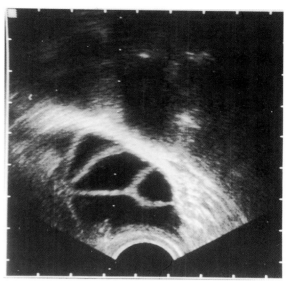

Fig. 8.5 Vaginal ultrasound illustrating superovulated ovary at egg collection.

Embryo transfer

Embryos can be transferred to the uterus at 48 or 72 hours after the oocyte collection, the 4- or 8-cell stage, respectively **(Fig. 8.8)**, or on day 5 at the blastocyst stage. Transferring at the blastocyst stage appears to provide the best chance of pregnancy. Although a maximum of two embryos can be transferred to the uterus in women under 40, there is a move in the UK to select out those women most at risk of a twin pregnancy, and electively transfer a single embryo (eSET). Analysis of the Human Fertilisation and Embryology Authority (HFEA) database demonstrates that 87% of all twins occur in those women under the age of 37 in their first cycle of treatment. An eSET policy is widely used in Europe and is associated with a significant reduction in the incidence of multiple pregnancies. In contrast, women over the age of 40, who are more likely to have aneuploid embryos, can have up to three embryos transferred.

Luteal support

As the pituitary gland has been desensitized, the luteal phase has to be supported with exogenous hCG or progesterone suppositories for 14 days, until the result of the pregnancy test is known.

Results

In the UK in the year 2005, 32,626 patients received 41,932 cycles of IVF and ICSI (43% ICSI). There were 9058 successful procedures, giving rise to 11,262 children.

Interpreting success rates

There is considerable variation in success rates from clinic to clinic, depending on the clinic's experience and the mixture of patients treated. In the UK, the Human Fertilisation and Embryology Authority (HFEA, see below), using the data

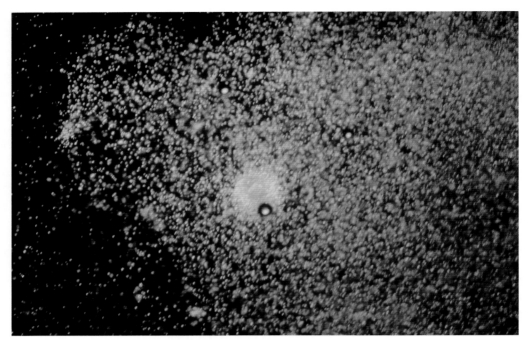

Fig. 8.6 Oocyte–cumulus cell complex identified at egg collection.

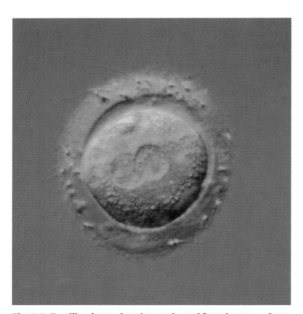

Fig. 8.7 Fertilized egg showing male and female pronucleus.

at their disposal, have produced a patient guide providing valuable information on outcomes in each clinic licensed for IVF. The most significant factor in determining an individual couple's chance of success is the woman's age, with a dramatic fall in pregnancy rates as age advances (**Fig. 8.9** and **Box 8.3**). Women over the age of 37 years appear to do less well, and by the age of 40 the 'take-home' baby rate

has fallen by 50% compared to women aged 30. Over age 45, the chance of pregnancy with a woman's own oocytes is only approximately 1%.

The live birth rates quoted represent the chance of success in a single cycle. The first cycle of treatment gives the patient the best chance of success, but the pregnancy rate in subsequent cycles is not dissimilar. The cumulative pregnancy rate in women under the age of 35 is 79% after six attempts. Interestingly, the cause of infertility does not appear to significantly affect the pregnancy rate after IVF.

Embryo freezing

Approximately 25% of patients have 'spare' embryos left over after the initial treatment. These can be frozen in liquid nitrogen and replaced during a subsequent natural or artificial cycle to give a further chance of a pregnancy. Only two-thirds of frozen embryos survive the thaw process. The live birth rate following frozen embryo transfer in 2005 was 18.0%.

Gamete intrafallopian tube transfer (GIFT)

This also involves the use of superovulation using the same protocols as described above for IVF, and oocyte collection by vaginal ultrasound. Thereafter the two techniques differ. With GIFT, the best three oocytes are selected and a laparoscopy is performed. The fallopian tube is cannulated and the selected oocytes, along with approximately 100,000 sperm, are returned to the tube. Fertilization then occurs in the fallopian tube.

Success rates of up to 36% per treatment cycle have been quoted, but GIFT is only applicable to those patients who have 'unexplained' infertility. As it involves a general anaesthetic and laparoscopy, it is more invasive than conventional IVF and very few centres now practise this technique. The only true indication is for those couples who cannot accept IVF on religious grounds.

Zygote intrafallopian tube transfer (ZIFT)

This is a combination of IVF and GIFT. The first part of the treatment is identical to IVF, but instead of replacing the embryos in the uterus, they are replaced, at laparoscopy, in the fallopian tube. Again, this treatment is more invasive

than conventional IVF and is generally only used if difficulties are encountered transferring the embryos through the cervix.

Intracytoplasmic sperm injection (ICSI)

This exciting technique, developed in Brussels by Professor Andre Van Steirteghem and colleagues, has revolutionized our ability to treat male infertility. The indications for ICSI are outlined in **Box 8.4**. If there are no sperm in the ejaculate and none in the epididymis, sperm can still be retrieved from testicular biopsies in a significant proportion (approximately 50%) of men. Sometimes multiple testicular biopsies are required to find areas of active spermatogenesis.

Technique

Oocytes are collected in the standard IVF fashion, and then prepared for ICSI by removing their surrounding cumulus cells. A smooth-ended glass pipette is used to hold the oocyte still, while a sharp ultrafine pipette pierces the egg and deposits one sperm along with a tiny amount of culture medium. Prior to injection the selected sperm needs to be immobilized to avoid damaging the delicate structure of the oocyte.

Results

The pregnancy outcome following ICSI is comparable to that of conventional IVF (live birth rate of 24.5% per cycle), although slightly lower pregnancy rates are reported in the more severe cases where testicular-derived sperm is required. ICSI is a more invasive procedure and some uncontrolled reports have suggested slightly increased rates of genetic and developmental defects in post-ICSI

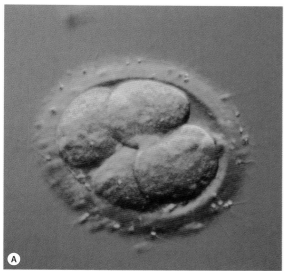

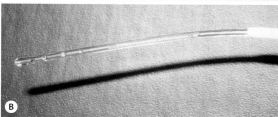

Fig. 8.8 Embryo transfer. (A) 4-cell embryo ready for transfer to the uterus. **(B)** Loaded embryo transfer catheter.

> ### Box 8.3
>
> #### Main factors affecting IVF outcome
>
> - Woman's age
> - Duration of infertility
> - Previous unsuccessful treatments
> - Previous pregnancies
> - Poor sperm quality

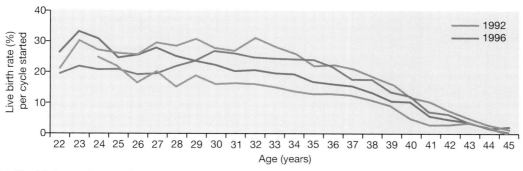

Fig. 8.9 Live birth rates by age of woman.

Box 8.4

Indications for ICSI

- Microepididymal sperm aspiration (MESA)
  - congenital absence of the vas deferens
  - obstructive azoospermia:
      post-infection:
      iatrogenic:
- <500,000 motile sperm in the ejaculate
- <5% morphologically normal sperm
- Repeated IVF failed fertilization

Box 8.5

Indications for egg donation

- Premature ovarian failure
- Gonadal dysgenesis
- Iatrogenic – surgery, radiation and chemotherapy
- Carriers of genetic disease
- Failed IVF – poor response, inaccessible ovaries, repeated failure to fertilize
- Recurrent miscarriage

pregnancies. Furthermore, there is clear evidence that a proportion of male infertility has a genetic basis, and by performing ICSI the abnormality may be passed on to the next generation. The true risk will only become evident in time as our understanding of the causes of impaired spermatogenesis become clearer, and the children born following ICSI are followed through to adulthood.

Egg donation

Patients with primary ovarian failure can only be treated by oocyte donation **(Box 8.5)**. This treatment is also increasingly being used for patients who appear to have an oocyte problem identified by repeated IVF failure. Another indication for egg donation (or for donor insemination) is genetic disease. Egg donors are in short supply and are generally women who, for altruistic reasons, wish to donate their eggs. Egg donation is much more complicated than sperm donation, as the donors have to undergo IVF treatment up to and including the stage of oocyte collection. Some centres offer an 'egg sharing' programme, whereby an infertility patient who cannot afford treatment agrees to go through an IVF cycle but donate half her eggs to a recipient who will fund both patients' treatment. This concept clearly raises ethical and moral concerns, although early research suggests that both parties benefit.

Results

This is a very successful treatment, with pregnancy rates generally higher than conventional IVF, and maintained even in women over the age of 40. This illustrates the fact that the quality of the oocyte is the most significant factor in the age-related decline of fertility.

Host surrogacy

Some women have functional ovaries but no uterus, due to either a congenital abnormality or previous hysterectomy. Such a patient could undergo IVF treatment, with the embryos then being transferred to another woman (a 'host surrogate') whose uterus has been suitably prepared by hormone treatment. The host will carry the pregnancy and then return the baby to the commissioning couple after delivery. According to English law the 'mother' is the woman who delivers the child. Therefore, the commissioning couple have to adopt the child, even though it is genetically theirs.

Preimplantation genetic diagnosis (PGD)

Couples who have a history of repeated pregnancy failure for genetic disease or who have had a child with a specific genetic abnormality may benefit from PGD. The couples undergo a conventional IVF treatment cycle, generally using ICSI as the means of fertilization. The embryos are left until day 3, by which stage they have divided to the 6- to 8-cell stage. Generally one and occasionally two blastomeres (embryonic cells) are removed and analysed for specific chromosomal abnormalities using fluorescent in situ hybridization (FISH) or a specific gene defect by polymerase chain reaction (PCR), or by identifying high-risk and low-risk haplotypes (based on a series of markers around the abnormal gene). Unaffected embryos are cultured through to the blastocyst stage, and single embryos are replaced in the usual manner. This allows the couple to potentially start a pregnancy knowing that the child is unaffected by the genetic condition generating the concern.

Results

The overall chance of success is slightly lower than for conventional IVF, but greater than 20% per treatment cycle.

Side-effects of assisted conception

Approximately 25% of all IVF pregnancies are twin pregnancies and there remain a few triplet pregnancies. The introduction of elective single embryo transfer, sanctioned by the HFEA, should reduce the multiple pregnancy rate to less than 10% within a period of 3 to 4 years.

Ovarian hyperstimulation syndrome (OHSS) is a condition where the ovaries over-respond to the gonadotrophin injections.

- More than 30 follicles may start to mature, resulting in ovarian enlargement and abdominal discomfort.
- Very high concentrations of oestradiol and progesterone make the patient feel nauseated.
- If the condition is severe, protein-rich ascites can accumulate, and more rarely pleural effusion may result. (This is akin to Meigs' syndrome.)

- The sudden shift in fluid can result in hypovolaemia, with resulting renal and thrombotic problems. The condition can be fatal.

The incidence of severe OHSS is low (<1%) and it only occurs if the hCG injection is given. Patients with polycystic ovaries are the most vulnerable and they have an increased risk of around 5%. Treatment is supportive with fluid replacement, generally with protein-rich fluids rather than simple crystalloid solutions. Serum electrolytes need careful monitoring because hyperkalaemia and/or hyponatraemia can develop. Hyperstimulation usually occurs in patients who conceive and can last throughout the early first trimester. If the patient fails to conceive, the condition is self-limiting and will resolve spontaneously.

Fetal abnormality

Out of a total of 7397 babies born following IVF/ICSI treatment in the UK in 1998, there were 95 babies with developmental defects and syndromes, 7 with chromosomal defects (predominantly Down syndrome), and 88 with congenital abnormalities, giving a congenital abnormality rate of 1.1% (IVF) and 1.6% (ICSI), respectively. This is almost identical to that in the general population.

The UK Human Fertilisation and Embryology Act

This Act, passed by the UK Parliament in 1990, brought about the formation of a regulatory body, known as the Human Fertilisation and Embryology Authority (HFEA). It regulates research on human embryos, the storage of gametes and embryos, and the use in infertility treatment of donated gametes and of embryos produced outside the body. The HFEA came into operation in August 1991, with the principal aim of ensuring that human embryos and gametes are used responsibly and that infertile patients are not exploited. Assisted conception treatment can only be performed in a centre licensed by the HFEA. This licence is renewed on an annual basis.

All patients who donate gametes (either sperm or eggs) or receive assisted conception treatment have to be registered with the HFEA. The outcome of treatment is also recorded. The HFEA also requires all patients considering assisted conception to be offered counselling by a trained counsellor. Paramount in the HFEA's philosophy is the welfare of the potential child.

Key points

- Infertility is defined as inability to conceive after 2 years of regular unprotected coitus. It affects approximately 1 in 6 couples.
- The commonest causes of infertility are ovulatory problems, semen abnormalities, and blockage of fallopian tubes. Other causes include coital difficulties and endometriosis.
- Investigation involves semen analysis, tests of ovulation (mid-luteal phase progesterone, or ultrasound monitoring) and tests for tubal patency (diagnostic laparoscopy or hysterosalpingography).
- Treatment of anovulation may include anti-oestrogens (particularly clomifene), pulsatile LHRH or exogenous gonadotrophins (which require careful monitoring).
- ICSI offers a treatment option to men with variable sperm counts.

Contraception and sterilization

Introduction

Over the last 70 years the global population has tripled from 2 billion to over 6 billion and it is estimated to reach 9 billion in the next 50 years **(Fig. 9.1)**. The current 'ecological footprint', the productive area of earth necessary to support the lifestyle of an individual, is approximately double the level that is sustainable long term. Currently, half the world's population does not have enough food to eat and this situation is likely to deteriorate. The number of people experiencing water shortages is likely to rise from the current level of around 500 million to 3 billion by 2050 and water tables under some cities in China, Latin America, and south Asia are falling by over a metre a year. Contraception is clearly important.

Contraception also has the potential to make a contribution to maternal and child survival. It has been estimated that family planning could save the lives of 3 million children a year by helping women to space births at least 2 years apart, and to bear children during their healthiest reproductive years. When women have the ability to space their births, they are better able to recover from nutritional depletion, blood loss and reproductive-system damage, allowing them to have healthier babies. Many women in the developing world would like to space or limit their births, but do not have access to family planning information or services.

Family planning programmes also help prevent the spread of HIV infection and other sexually transmitted diseases. Half of all new HIV infections in the developing world are among women and nearly 10% are among infants and children.

The provision of appropriate contraception is arguably one of the most important branches of medicine today. A wide variety of effective contraceptive methods are available, but there are no 'ideal' contraceptives and choice must be based on the balance of risks and benefits of each method for each individual. For most women the use of contraception is safe, but there are limited data on the use of contraception by women with certain medical conditions. In view of this, the World Health Organization (WHO) developed Medical Eligibility Criteria which provide evidence-based recommendations to facilitate the safe use of contraception without imposing unnecessary medical restrictions. A UK version is available (www.fsrh.org.uk) and the categories used to define risk are summarized in **Table 9.1**. For conditions given a UKMEC category 1, use of the method is unrestricted, whilst use of a method given a UKMEC category 4 poses an unacceptable health risk and should not be used. A UKMEC category 2 suggests the benefits generally outweigh the risks, while a UKMEC 3 suggests the risks may generally outweigh the benefits. Importantly, however, a method given a UKMEC category 3 may still be used, but this may require clinical judgement and/or referral to a specialist family planning provider.

Defining 'contraceptive failure' is not easy as it depends on the population studied: studies on a young population will suggest a higher failure rate than in an older group, as fertility is higher in younger people. Caution is therefore required in interpreting precise figures. The 'method' failure includes inherent risk of failure providing the method is used correctly. It is quantified in the units 'per 100 woman-years' – that is to say, the number of women who would become pregnant if 100 of them used that method of contraception for 1 year (or 50 women for 2 years etc). 'User' failure is said to occur when a given method is not used correctly. If used consistently and correctly, hormonal contraceptives (combined hormonal contraception, progestogen-only pills, injectable, implant and intrauterine system) and non-hormonal methods (copper intrauterine device, male and female sterilization) are more than 99% effective in preventing pregnancy. These methods, as well as emergency contraception, barrier methods and natural family planning methods, are covered in this chapter. Evidence-based guidance on all methods of contraception is available on the Faculty of Sexual and Reproductive Healthcare website (www.fsrh.org.uk).

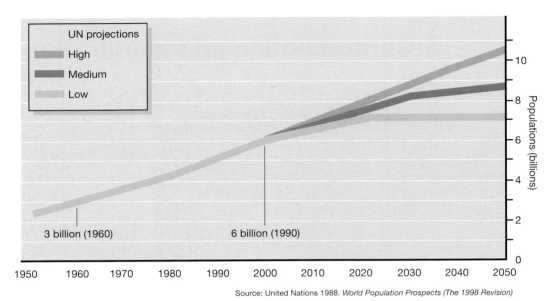

Source: United Nations 1988. *World Population Prospects (The 1998 Revision)*

Fig. 9.1 Global population growth, actual and projected.

Table 9.1	
UKMEC categories	
UKMEC category	**Definition**
UKMEC 1	A condition for which there is *no restriction* for the use of the contraceptive method
UKMEC 2	A condition for which the *advantages of using the method generally outweigh the theoretical or proven risks*
UKMEC 3	A condition where the *theoretical or proven risks usually outweigh the advantages* of using the method*
UKMEC 4	A condition which represents an *unacceptable health risk* if the contraceptive method is used

*The provision of a method to a woman with a condition given a UKMEc category 3 requires expert clinical judgement and/or referral to a specialist contraceptive provider since use of the method is not usually recommended unless other methods are not available or not acceptable.

Hormonal methods of contraception

Combined estrogen–progestogen methods (pills and patch)

Most data on the use and safety of combined hormonal contraception (CHC) relates specifically to the combined oral contraceptive pill (COC). The evidence is extrapolated to the transdermal patch as it also contains estrogen and progestogen. Information will be given here about the COC, with any additional information specific to the patch at the end of this section.

Combined oral contraceptive pills contain ethinylestradiol (EE) and a progestogen (a synthetic progesterone). The progestogens include *second generation* (levonorgestrel and norethisterone), *third generation* (desogestrel and gestodene) and *fourth generation* (drospirenone). Third-generation progestogens were introduced as they were thought to have fewer adverse effects on lipids than earlier preparations. Subsequent studies found that COCs containing these conferred a slightly higher risk of venous thromboembolism (VTE) than did those containing second-generation progestogens **(Table 9.2)**. The reason for this appears to be that third-generation progestogens are less effective at counteracting the thrombotic effects of EE than are older progestogens. Although the *relative risk* of VTE is increased three- to fivefold with combined hormonal contraceptive use–the *absolute risk* is very small **(Table 9.2)**.

While the COC works primarily by inhibiting ovulation, the cervical mucus is also less favourable to sperm penetration and the endometrium is more atrophic. Women considering the COC should be informed of the potential risks and benefits associated with use **(Table 9.3, Fig. 9.2)**. The COC is safe for the majority of women, and, indeed, a non-smoker may continue with COC use to age 50 years if she has no other contraindications for use. Deaths in COC users over 35 years of age are eight times more common in smokers than non-smokers. It is recommended that women who continue to smoke at the age of 35 years should use an alternative form of contraception (UKMEC category 3 if aged ≥35 years and smoking <15 cigarettes per day or UKMEC category 4 if smoking ≥15 cigarettes per day). The use of COC may pose an unacceptable health risk in women with cardiovascular disease (myocardial infarction, stroke, hypertension, venous thromboembolism), liver disease (severe cirrhosis, active

Table 9.2	
Risk of venous thromboembolism associated with COC use and non-use	
Absolute risk of VTE per 100,000 woman-years	**Circumstance**
5	For women not using COC and not pregnant
15	For women using a levonorgestrel- or norethisterone-containing COC (e.g. Microgynon 30, Loestrin 20, Loestrin 30)
25	For women using a desogestrel- or gestodene-containing COC (e.g. Marvelon, Mercilon, Femodene, Femodette)
60	In pregnancy

Table 9.3	
Risks and benefits associated with COC use	
Disease	**Relative risk with COC use in non-smokers**
Potential harms (risks)	
Coronary artery disease	Very small increase
Ischaemic stroke	Twofold increase
Venous thromboembolism	Threefold increase with levonorgestrel and norethisterone COCs (absolute risk small) Fivefold increase with desogestrel and gestodene COCs (absolute risk small)
Breast cancer	Any increased risk likely to be small and will vary with age No increased risk above background risk 10 years after stopping COC
Cervical cancer	Small increase after 5 years and a twofold increase after 10 years
Benefits	
Ovarian cancer	Halving of risk, lasting for >15 years
Endometrial cancer	Halving of risk, lasting for >15 years
Colorectal cancer	Reduction

viral hepatitis, tumours), or migraine *with aura* at any age or migraine *without aura* over the age of 35 years.

What is a suitable first-line method of COC?

A monophasic pill containing 30 to 35 μg of EE and a progestogen (either levonorgestrel or norethisterone) is recommended as a first-line COC. These pills are associated with the lowest risk of VTE. Gestodene- and desogestrel-containing pills can be used, if requested, after discussing the marginally higher VTE risk. A COC can be started up to and including day 5 of the menstrual cycle to provide immediate contraceptive protection. If started after this time, condoms or abstinence is advised for the next 7 days. Most COC packages contain 21 active tablets: one tablet is taken daily for 21 consecutive days, followed by a 7-day pill-free interval. A withdrawal bleed usually occurs in the pill-free interval due to the withdrawal of hormones which induces endometrial shedding. There are no proven benefits of a biphasic or triphasic COC over a monophasic pill. Women should be encouraged to take COCs daily at or around the same time every day. Current missed pill advice is summarized in **Figure 9.3.** In general, one pill can be missed at anytime in the packet without loss in efficacy or the need to use condoms.

Drug interactions

Liver enzyme-inducing drugs (including some antiepileptics, such as carbamazepine, some antiretrovirals, griseofulvin, rifampicin and St John's Wort) accelerate the hepatic breakdown of contraceptive steroids, thus potentially reducing the efficacy of the COC. The options for women using liver enzyme-inducing drugs long term who wish to continue with COC use is to increase the dose of EE to 50–60 μg per day (usually taking two pills per day), although this use is unlicensed. In addition, it is recommended to reduce the pill-free interval. Condoms should also be used, however, as there are no studies to identify the correct dose of COC required to maintain contraceptive efficacy in these situations. An alternative is obviously to use a method of contraception which is unaffected by liver enzyme-inducing medication (such as a progestogen-only injectable, the levonorgestrel-releasing intrauterine system [LNG-IUS] or a copper intrauterine device [Cu-IUD]).

The bacterial flora is involved in the breakdown of EE in the large bowel; this facilitates the secondary reabsorption of EE, the so-called enterohepatic circulation. Non-liver enzyme-inducing antibiotics alter this bowel flora, reducing the secondary reabsorption of EE. The effectiveness of COC must be assumed to be reduced when a non-liver enzyme-inducing antibiotic is used short term (<3 weeks) and for 7 days after the course is completed. Condoms should be used over the time the antibiotics are taken and for 7 days after the course is completed. If the pill-free interval falls within these 7 days, it should be omitted. If a non-liver enzyme-inducing antibiotic has been taken continuously for 3 weeks or more, the gut flora is restored and condoms are no longer required. The antibiotic rifampicin and the antifungal griseofulvin are potent liver enzyme inducers and advice is as for other liver enzyme-inducing drugs. Moreover, condoms are required for at least 4 weeks after cessation of these liver enzyme-inducing medications.

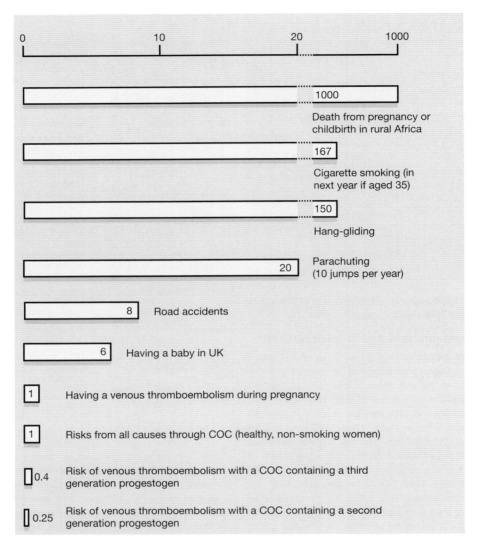

Fig. 9.2 Risks of the combined oral contraceptive pill compared to other risks in life.

Follow-up

A 12-month supply of COC can be given at the first visit, but for some women a follow-up at 3 months may be appropriate to assess any problems and provide re-instruction if necessary. Blood pressure should be assessed annually, but women should be encouraged to attend at any time if problems arise. The pill should be discontinued if any serious side-effects occur (e.g. chest pain, leg pain or swelling). Follow-up visits are also an opportunity to carry out other well woman screening (e.g. cervical cytology).

The COC should be stopped and an alternative method used at least 6 weeks before any planned major elective surgery where immobilization is expected.

Combined hormonal contraceptive patch

The risks and benefits associated with patch use are as described as for the COC **(Table 9.3)**. A patch can be applied to the abdomen, buttock or thigh on the same day each week for three consecutive weeks, followed by a patch-free week. The patch should be changed every 7 days, although a single patch will provide effective contraceptive protection for up to 9 days.

Progestogen-only contraception

Progestogen-only contraception (pills, injectables, implant and intrauterine system) avoid the potential side-effects attributed to estrogen. All progestogen-only methods can

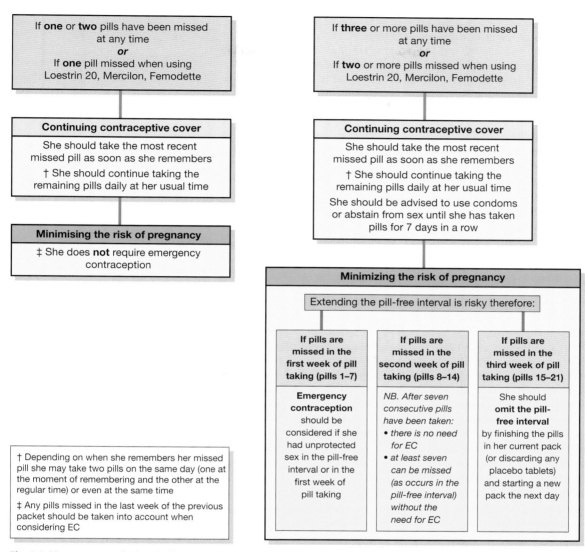

Fig. 9.3 Management of missed pills.

be associated with a disturbance in bleeding patterns and this is often the main reason for discontinuation of these otherwise very effective methods. Other side-effects have been reported (abdominal bloating, weight changes, acne, headaches and mood changes) but few have been directly related to progestogen use.

Drug interactions

The effect of liver enzyme-inducing drugs on the metabolism of progestogens is similar to that for estrogens. This reduces the efficacy of a progestogen-only pill or implant and this combination should not be used. The progestogen-only injectable depot medroxyprogesterone acetate (DMPA) and the levonorgestrel-releasing intrauterine system (LNG-IUS), however, are unaffected by liver enzyme inducing medication.

Progestogen is not reabsorbed from the large bowel and the efficacy of progestogen-only contraception is therefore *not* reduced by non-liver enzyme-inducing antibiotics.

Progestogen-only pills (POPs)

Traditional POPs (those containing levonorgestrel, norethisterone or etynodiol diacetate) and a newer POP (containing desogestrel) are currently available in the UK. Although POPs are suitable for most women, they are often used by women for whom a COC is contraindicated (e.g. when breastfeeding, with hypertension, for women over the age of 35 years who smoke or have migraine *without aura*, or for women of any age who have migraine *with aura*). All POPs thicken cervical mucus, thus preventing sperm penetration into the upper reproductive tract.

Traditional POPs inhibit ovulation in up to 60% of cycles, although the desogestrel-only pill inhibits ovulation in up to 97% of cycles and this is its main mode of action. A POP should be taken at or around the same time every day *without a pill-free interval*. A POP can be started up to and including day 5 of the menstrual cycle (within 7 days of a termination of pregnancy or up to day 21 postpartum) to provide immediate contraceptive protection. If started at other times, additional contraceptive protection, such as condoms, is required for the first 48 hours. A *traditional* POP is late if more than 27 hours have elapsed since the last pill was taken (i.e. more than 3 hours late). The desogestrel-only pill is late if more than 36 hours have elapsed between pill taking (i.e. more than 12 hours late).

Progestogen-only injectable contraception

The most widely used progestogen-only injectable in the UK is depot medroxyprogesterone acetate (DMPA) which is licensed to be given as an intramuscular injection every 12 weeks. Norethisterone enanthate (NET-EN) is licensed to be used short term only. The primary mode of action of progestogen-only injectables is inhibition of ovulation. Bleeding is common in the initial months of use but usually settles; indeed, up to 70% of women are amenorrhoeic at 1 year of use. Studies have suggested a *delay in return to fertility* following cessation of DMPA compared to other contraceptive methods, but *no reduction in fertility*. This is possibly due to the serum levels of MPA, which in some women can still be detected between 6 and 9 months after a single injection, and for some women in concentrations sufficient to inhibit ovulation.

It is recognized that there is a reversible loss in bone mineral density associated with DMPA use. There is no apparent increase in risk of fracture, and bone mineral density recovers after cessation of the method. There are few long-term data on the use of DMPA in women under the age of 18 years, who have yet to achieve peak bone density. Nevertheless, after counselling, women aged under 18 years can use DMPA (UKMEC 2, benefits outweigh risk). Moreover, women can use DMPA up to the age of 50 years, at which time an alternative method should be used. Women should be counselled about the risks and benefits of DMPA and lifestyle factors which may also be linked to bone loss (smoking, steroid use, etc) and this should be reassessed every 2 years if use is continuing. Weight gain can occur with DMPA use.

Progestogen-only subdermal implants

The only progestogen-only implant available in the UK is the single subdermal etonogestrel implant (Implanon; **Fig. 9.4**). It is made from a non-biodegradable polymer which contains an active slow-release progestogen formulation, and is about the size of a matchstick. The implant is licensed to provide contraception for up to 3 years. Changes in bleeding patterns are common and discontinuation due to bleeding is common (up to 43% within 3 years). Up to 20% of users will have no bleeding, but almost 50% will have

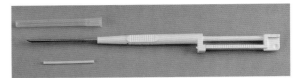

Fig. 9.4 Implanon. (Courtesy of Organon Laboratories Ltd.)

infrequent, frequent, or prolonged bleeding. These bleeding patterns may not settle with time. There is no evidence of a causal association between use of a progestogen-only implant and weight change, mood change, loss or libido, or headache. Health professionals who insert and remove progestogen-only implants should be appropriately trained.

Levonorgestrel-releasing intrauterine system (LNG-IUS)

The LNG-IUS offers a highly effective and reversible contraceptive method **(Fig.9.5A)**. It is licensed for 5 years' use as contraception or as a treatment for menorrhagia. It is licensed for up to 4 years' use as the progestogenic component of hormone replacement therapy. Failure rates for intrauterine contraception at 5 years use are low (1%). The LNG-IUS works primarily by its effect on the endometrium, preventing implantation. In addition, effects on cervical mucus reduce sperm penetration. Ovulation may be inhibited in up to 25% of women. Irregular bleeding is common in the first few months after insertion. Intermenstrual bleeding occurs frequently, but these problems often settle 5 or 6 months after insertion. Menstrual loss is reduced by an average of 90% at 12 months, and 20% of women experience complete amenorrhoea. Systemic side-effects due to absorption of levonorgestrel are often mild and usually settle with time. For women who have the device inserted after the age of 45 years, the LNG-IUS may be continued until the menopause is confirmed. The adverse effects and complications associated with insertion – including expulsion, perforation and infection – are as for a copper intrauterine device (outlined in the following section).

Non-hormonal contraception

Copper intrauterine devices (Cu-IUDs)

Copper is toxic to ova and sperm and a Cu-IUD works primarily by inhibiting fertilization. In addition, the endometrial inflammatory reaction has an anti-implantation effect and alterations in cervical mucus inhibit sperm penetration. Failure rates for intrauterine contraception at 5 years use are low (2% with a 380 mm² Cu-IUD). Banded Cu-IUDs which have 380 mm² of copper in the vertical stem and copper sleeves on the horizontal arms are the most effective intrauterine devices available and are recommended to be used as a first-line device **(Fig. 9.5B,C)**. Banded devices available in the UK can be used for up to 10 years. There

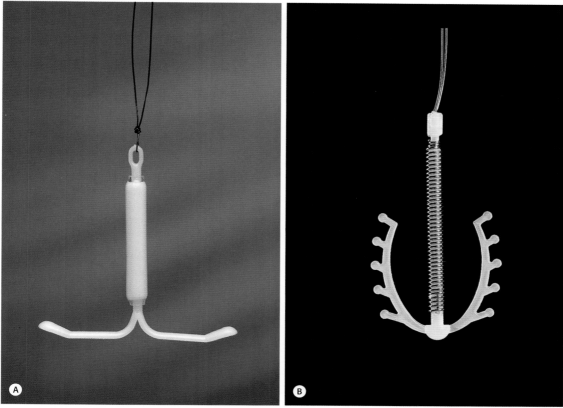

Fig. 9.5 Intrauterine contraceptive devices (IUDs). (A) Mirena; **(B)** Multiload 375.

is no delay in return to fertility after removal of intrauterine contraception. Spotting, light bleeding, or heavier or prolonged bleeding is common in the first 3 to 6 months of Cu-IUD use, but this may settle. There are few contraindications to use of intrauterine contraception **(Table 9.4)**. The management of common problems associated with Cu-IUD use are outlined in **Table 9.5**.

Insertion

Clinicians who insert intrauterine contraception should be appropriately trained, maintain competence and attend regular updates in dealing with emergencies. Discomfort during and/or after insertion of intrauterine contraception and the need for pain relief during insertion should be discussed with women in advance and administered when appropriate. Emergency equipment must be available in all settings where intrauterine contraception is being inserted, and local referral protocols must be in place for women who require further medical input.

Expulsion and perforation

The risk of expulsion with intrauterine contraception is around 1 in 20 and is most common in the first year of use, particularly within 3 months of insertion. The risk of uterine perforation associated with intrauterine contraception is up to 2 per 1000 insertions. Most perforations occur at the time of insertion, but a delayed 'migration' is recognized to occur. Immediate perforation may be detected because of acute pain or it may be detected later if pregnancy occurs. Most commonly, perforation is identified following the investigation of 'missing threads', although the most common reason for missed threads is that they have curled up and are intrauterine with a normally placed device. The management of suspected perforation and lost threads are outlined in **Table 9.5**. If the device is not in the uterine cavity, an abdominal X-ray will identify a Cu-IUD (or a LNG-IUS) if it is lying within the peritoneal cavity **(Fig. 9.6)**. Abdominally sited copper IUDs may cause dense adhesion formation and should be removed by laparoscopy or laparotomy.

Pelvic infection

There is an increased risk of pelvic infection in the 20 days following insertion of intrauterine contraception; after this, however, the risk is the same as for the non-IUD-using population. The risk of acquiring pelvic inflammatory disease is related to sexual activity and not the Cu-IUD. A clinical history (including sexual history) should be taken to identify those at higher risk of STIs (aged <25 years;

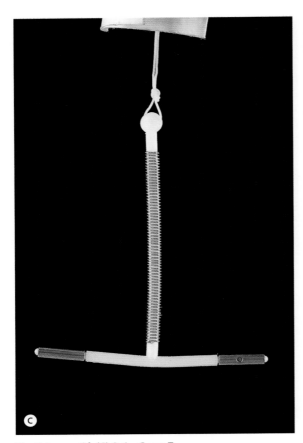

Fig. 9.5—cont'd (C) Ortho Gynae T.

these risks and should be carried out as soon as is practical, provided the threads are easily seen. If not, no attempt at retrieval should be made **(Table 9.5)**.

Barrier methods

Barrier methods of contraception aim to prevent sperm gaining access to the female upper reproductive tract. An extensive array of barriers has been used (male and female condoms, diaphragms and cervical caps). Barrier methods offer advantages in terms of safety and reversibility, but their efficacy is critically dependent upon quality of use. The failure rates can be low when they are used consistently and correctly by well-motivated couples. The contraceptive sponge (a delivery method for spermicide rather than a barrier method per se) is estimated to be between 80% and 90% effective at preventing pregnancy, but will not be mentioned further.

Male and female condoms

Used consistently and correctly, male condoms are up to 98% effective at preventing pregnancy and female condoms are up to 95% effective. In general, evidence supports the use of condoms to reduce the risk of STI transmission, but, even with correct and consistent use, transmission may occur. Men and women with latex sensitivity or allergy can use polyurethane or deproteinized latex condoms. An advance provision of emergency contraception should be offered to women using condoms as the sole method of contraception. Condom users should be made aware of the risk of pregnancy and STIs should a condom fail.

Male condoms are available in a variety of shapes and colours, and with or without spermicide. Condoms lubricated with non-spermicidal lubricant are recommended for use. Additional lubricant should be recommended for use of male condoms for anal sex to reduce the risk of breakage. Non-oil-based lubricants are recommended as they can be used safely with latex and non-latex condoms. Male condoms must be unrolled over the erect penis before there is any genital contact. Difficulties may occur when air is not excluded from the teat, or when trying to put them on inside out, or if snagging with fingernails occurs, and the condom should be held onto the penis during withdrawal from the vagina to avoid leakage of semen. The standard size available in a particular country may not meet the requirements of all men; a condom that is too large may roll off during intercourse.

The female condom is a polyurethane sheath, its open end attached to a flexible polyurethane ring which sits at the vaginal entrance, and comes in one size **(Fig. 9.8)**. It is marketed in the UK as the Femidom.

Female diaphragms and caps

These require a relatively high degree of user motivation, and failure rates are comparable to those seen with the male condom. They are divided into two groups: the diaphragm and those that cover the cervix (caps) **(Fig. 9.9)**.

or >25 years with a new sexual partner or more than one partner in the last year; or if their regular partner has other partners). Women who are at higher risk of STIs or who request swabs should be tested for *Chlamydia trachomatis* (as a minimum) and *Neisseria gonorrhoeae* (if deemed necessary from the history) in advance of insertion of intrauterine contraception. If results are unavailable before insertion, prophylactic antibiotics should be considered for this higher-risk group (at least to cover *C .trachomatis*). In asymptomatic women attending for insertion, there is no indication to test for or treat other lower genital tract organisms or delay insertion until results of tests are available.

Pregnancy

An IUD-failure pregnancy is rare, but if it occurs, the chance of having an ectopic pregnancy is higher than in those without a device **(Table 9.5)**. The overall risk of ectopic pregnancy is reduced with use of intrauterine contraception when compared to using no contraception, however. No particular device is associated with a lower rate of ectopic pregnancy. If the pregnancy is intrauterine, there is a considerable increase in the risk of spontaneous miscarriage and preterm labour **(Fig. 9.7)**. Removal of the IUD reduces

Table 9.4

UKMEC categories where risks may outweigh benefits or pose an unacceptable health risk for use of intrauterine contraception

UKMEC category 3 (risks outweigh benefits)	UKMEC category 4 (unacceptable risk)	Where Cu-IUD and LNG-IUS are given different UKMEC categories
<ul><li>Between 48 hours and <4 weeks postpartum</li><li>Current venous thromboembolism (on anticoagulants)</li><li>Initiation of method in women with ovarian cancer</li><li>Continuation of intrauterine methods in women with known pelvic tuberculosis</li></ul>	<ul><li>Pregnancy, puerperal sepsis, septic abortion</li><li>*Initiation* of the method in women with unexplained vaginal bleeding</li><li>Gestational trophoblastic neoplasia when serum hCG concentrations are abnormal</li><li>Initiation of the method in women with cervical cancer awaiting treatment or with endometrial cancer</li><li>Uterine fibroids or uterine anatomical abnormalities distorting the uterine cavity</li><li>Initiation of intrauterine methods in women with current pelvic inflammatory disease or purulent cervicitis</li><li>Initiation of intrauterine methods in women with known pelvic tuberculosis</li></ul>	**A UKMEC category 1 is given for a Cu-IUD and a category 3 is given for the LNG-IUS due to the progestogen content for the following medical conditions:** <ul><li>*Continuation* of LNG-IUS if a new diagnosis of ischaemic heart disease is made or if new symptoms of migraine with aura occur at any age</li><li>Past history of breast cancer with no recurrence in last 5 years*</li><li>Active viral hepatitis, severe decompensated cirrhosis or liver tumours (benign or malignant)</li></ul>**A UKMEC category 1 is given for a Cu-IUD and a category 4 is given for the LNG-IUS due to the progestogen content for the following medical conditions:** <ul><li>Current breast cancer*</li></ul>

*There is some evidence that the LNG-IUS has a protective effect on the endometrium against the stimulatory effects of tamoxifen. If other contraceptive methods are unacceptable the use of the LNG-IUS may be considered after counselling.
NOTES: Liver enzyme-inducing drugs are not thought to reduce the contraceptive efficacy of a Cu-IUD or the LNG-IUS. The UKMEC does not include Wilson's disease. No evidence was identified in the literature. It may be that in view of lack of evidence and potential toxic effect of copper the use of a Cu-IUD in a woman with Wilson's disease is not recommended.

The diaphragm consists of a soft dome, the edge of which contains a supporting metal spring to exert a slight pressure on the vaginal walls. It is inserted to lie diagonally across the vagina between the back of the symphysis pubis and the posterior fornix, but it does not form a complete barrier between the upper and lower vagina. Cervical and vault caps, and the vimule, depend on suction to hold the cap over the cervix or the vaginal vault. When used consistently and correctly, and with spermicide, diaphragms and cervical caps are estimated to be between 92% and 96% effective at preventing pregnancy.

There is limited evidence on the use of diaphragms, cervical caps or contraceptive sponge in reducing the risk of STIs. There may be some protection against cervical intraepithelial neoplasia (CIN) with diaphragms. Available evidence generally supports the use of female condoms to reduce the risk of STIs, but, even with consistent and correct use, transmission may occur. Women with sensitivity to latex proteins can use a silicone diaphragm or cervical cap, or a polyurethane female condom. The use of a diaphragm, cervical cap or contraceptive sponge by women who have or are at high risk of HIV or AIDS is not generally recommended. For women with a history of toxic shock syndrome the use of diaphragms, cervical caps and contraceptive sponge is also not generally recommended. Guidance on the correct use of diaphragms and caps is outlined in **Box 9.1**.

Spermicides

Spermicides are usually used with diaphragms and caps. The use of spermicide alone is not considered to provide effective contraception. Nonoxinol-9 (N-9) is the only spermicide commercially available in the UK. N-9 is a surfactant, which disrupts cell membranes. Epithelial disruption in the vagina and rectum has been identified in association with N-9 use in human and animal models. Repeated and high-dose use of N-9 is associated with an increased risk of genital lesions, which may increase the risk of HIV acquisition, and the WHO recommends that women at high risk of HIV infection should not use N-9. The risks of using a diaphragm or cervical cap (with N-9) in women with a high risk of HIV or those with HIV or AIDS generally outweigh the benefits (UKMEC 3; **Table 9.1**).

Natural family planning

Although the Billings' method is the most commonly used natural family planning method, it should be taught by an experienced teacher (history box). This technique requires the restriction of intercourse to those days of the menstrual cycle on which conception is least likely to occur.

Table 9.5

Managing common problems associated with intrauterine contraception

Problems associated with intrauterine contraception	Management
Suspected perforation at the time of insertion	The procedure should be stopped and vital signs (blood pressure and pulse rate) and level of discomfort monitored until stable. An ultrasound scan and /or plain abdominal X-ray to locate the device if it has been left in situ should be arranged as soon as possible.
'Lost threads'	Advise women to use another method (condoms or abstinence) until medical review. Consider the need for emergency hormonal contraception. If no threads are seen and uterine placement of the intrauterine method cannot be confirmed clinically, an ultrasound scan should be arranged to locate the device and alternative contraception recommended until this information is available. If an ultrasound scan cannot locate the intrauterine method and there is no definite evidence of expulsion, a plain abdominal X-ray should be arranged to identify an extrauterine device. If the intrauterine method is not confirmed on an ultrasound scan clinicians should not assume it has been expelled until a negative X-ray is obtained (unless the woman has witnessed expulsion). Hysteroscopy is not readily available in all settings but can be useful if the ultrasound scan is equivocal. Surgical retrieval of an extrauterine device is advised.
Abnormal bleeding	Gynaecological pathology and infections should be excluded if abnormal bleeding persists beyond the first 6 months following insertion of intrauterine contraception. Women using the LNG-IUS who present with a change in pattern of bleeding should be advised to return for further investigation to exclude infections, pregnancy and gynaecological pathology. For women using a Cu-IUD, non-steroidal anti-inflammatory drugs can be used to treat spotting, light bleeding, heavy or prolonged menstruation. In addition, antifibrinolytics (such as tranexamic acid) may be used for heavy or prolonged menstruation.
Pregnancy	Most pregnancies in women using intrauterine contraception will be intrauterine but an ectopic pregnancy must be excluded. Women who become pregnant with an intrauterine contraception in situ should be informed of the increased risks of second-trimester miscarriage, preterm delivery and infection if the intrauterine method is left in situ. Removal would reduce adverse outcomes but is associated with a small risk of miscarriage. If the threads are visible, or can easily be retrieved from the endocervical canal, the intrauterine contraceptive should be removed up to 12 weeks gestation. If there is no evidence that the intrauterine method was expelled prior to pregnancy, it should be sought at delivery or termination and, if not identified, a plain abdominal X-ray should be arranged to determine if the intrauterine method is extrauterine.
Suspected pelvic infection	For women using intrauterine contraception with symptoms and signs suggestive of pelvic infection, appropriate antibiotics should be started. There is no need to remove the intrauterine method unless symptoms fail to resolve within the following 72 hours or unless the woman wishes removal. All women with confirmed or suspected PID should be followed up to ensure: resolution of symptoms and signs, their partner has also been treated when appropriate, completion of the course of antibiotics, STI risk assessment, counselling regarding safer sex and partner notification.
Presence of *Actinomyces*-like organisms (ALOs)	Intrauterine contraceptive users with ALOs detected on a swab who have no symptoms should be advised there is no reason to remove the intrauterine method unless signs or symptoms of infection occur. There is no indication for follow-up screening. If symptoms of pelvic pain occur, women should be advised to seek medical advice. Other causes of infection (in particular, STIs) should be considered and it may be appropriate to remove the intrauterine method.

 History

John Billings (1918–2007), an Australian doctor who was described as a 'staunch Catholic', developed the method as a form of natural family planning in accordance with his religious faith. He was recognized with a Papal knighthood in life, and condolences for his death were given by the Pope. Billings strove to raise awareness of the significance of cervical mucus to fertility to all people, regardless of their religion.

Women assess cervical mucus changes throughout the cycle. Prior to ovulation (the fertile period) cervical mucus is clear, watery (i.e. of low viscosity) and is easily stretched into strands ('spinnbarkeit'). After ovulation (the non-fertile period) mucus is thick and sticky. This knowledge can be used to identify days where intercourse can occur with reduced likelihood of conception.

The lactational amenorrhoea method (LAM) provides a very effective technique (98%) if the woman is fully breastfeeding

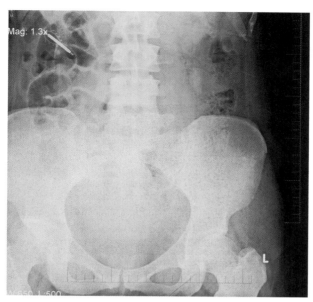

Fig. 9.6 The IUD has perforated the uterus and attached itself to the omentum.

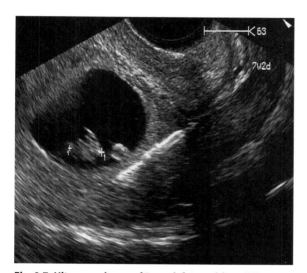

Fig. 9.7 Ultrasound scan of 7-week fetus with an IUD visible low in the uterine cavity.

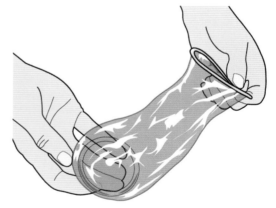

Fig. 9.8 Female condom.

- if combined pills are missed
- if progestogen-only pills are late.

Two methods are currently available: progestogen-only emergency contraception (POEC) and the Cu-IUD.

Progestogen-only emergency contraception (POEC)

The progestogen-only (levonorgestrel) method can be used up to 72 hours after unprotected intercourse. The pills inhibit or delay ovulation and prevent up to 84% of expected pregnancies. Levonorgestrel EC should be given as a single 1.5 mg dose as soon as possible after unprotected sex, and within 72 hours. Levonorgestrel EC may be considered between 73 and 120 hours after unprotected sex, but women should be informed of: the limited evidence of

day and night on demand with no supplementary feeds, she is less than 6 months postpartum, and she is amenorrhoeic. Another method of contraception should be introduced if menses occur (bleeding before 56 days can be ignored), or with the introduction of weaning, or after 6 months **(Fig. 9.10)**.

Emergency contraception

Emergency contraception (EC) can be used:

- after unprotected intercourse
- after 'accidents' with a barrier method (e.g. burst condom or diaphragm removed too early)

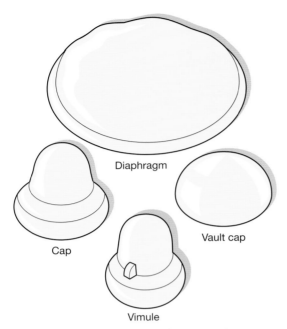

Diaphragm

Cap

Vault cap

Vimule

Fig. 9.9 Female barrier methods of contraception.

Box 9.1

Instructions for women using a diaphragm or cervical cap

- Initial assessment of diaphragm and cervical caps should be done by a suitably trained health professional
- All methods can be inserted anytime before intercourse
- The use of spermicide is recommended when using diaphragms and cervical caps
- If intercourse is repeated or occurs ≥3 hours after insertion, more spermicide is required and should be inserted with an applicator or as a pessary without removing the diaphragm or cervical cap
- The diaphragm or cervical cap must be left in situ for at least 6 hours after the last episode of intercourse. Sperm in the lower reproductive tract are unlikely to be alive after 6 hours
- Oil-based lubricants can damage latex, and women should be advised to avoid use when using latex diaphragms or cervical caps
- Women should be advised to check diaphragm or cervical cap regularly for tears, holes or cracks
- There is no evidence that a colour change or change in shape of the outer ring of a diaphragm reduces efficacy
- Women should be advised on the use of emergency contraception should female barrier methods be used incorrectly*
- Women should be advised to attend for a review of contraception if they have
  - any problems with the method
  - lost or gained more than 3 kg (7 lb)
  - had a pregnancy

*An advance provision of emergency hormonal contraception can be offered to women relying on female barrier methods for contraception.

efficacy; that such use is outside product licence; and the alternative of a Cu-IUD. Women who experience vomiting within 2 hours of administration of levonorgestrel EC should be advised to return as soon as possible for a repeat dose. Levonorgestrel EC does not provide contraceptive cover for the remainder of the cycle and effective contraception or abstinence must be advised. Women should be advised to have a pregnancy test if their expected menstruation is more than 7 days late, or lighter than usual.

A Cu-IUD

A Cu-IUD can be inserted up to 5 days after the first episode of unprotected sex or up to 5 days after the predicted date of ovulation (which may be more than 5 days after intercourse). Almost 99% of expected pregnancies can be prevented.

Sterilization

Female sterilization

Counselling and advice on sterilization procedures should be provided to women and men within the context of a service providing a full range of information and access to other long-term reversible methods of contraception. This should include information on the advantages and disadvantages and relative failures. Women should be informed that vasectomy carries a lower failure rate and that there is less risk related to the procedure. Women,

particularly those at increased risk from conditions such as previous abdominal surgery or obesity, should be informed of the risks of laparoscopy and the chances of laparotomy being necessary if difficulties are encountered at laparoscopy.

Women should be informed that tubal occlusion is associated with failure rates and that pregnancy can occur several years after the procedure. The lifetime risk of failure is estimated to be 1 in 200. The longest period of follow-up data available for the most common method used in the UK, the Filshie clip, suggests a failure rate after 10 years of 2–3 per 1000 procedures. The overall risk of ectopic pregnancy is not increased compared to women using no method of contraception; however, women should be informed that, if tubal occlusion fails, the resulting pregnancy may be ectopic.

Although women requesting sterilization should understand that the procedure is intended to be permanent, they should be given information about the success rates associated with reversal, should this procedure be necessary.

Women should be reassured that tubal occlusion is not associated with an increased risk of heavier or longer periods when performed after 30 years of age. There is an association with a subsequent increased hysterectomy rate, although there is no evidence that tubal occlusion leads to problems that require hysterectomy.

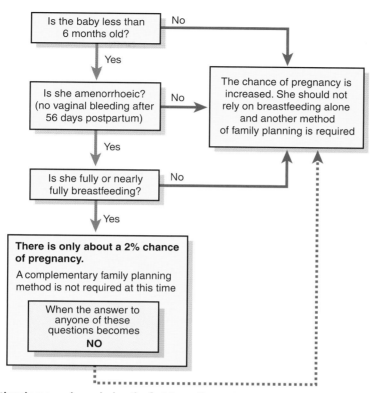

Fig. 9.10 Use of lactational amenorrhoea during the first 6 months postpartum.

Sterilization can be performed at the time of caesarean section if there has been appropriate pre-procedure counselling. Hysteroscopic methods of tubal occlusion are still under evaluation and should only be used within the present guidance system for new surgical interventions.

Vasectomy

Men should be informed that vasectomy has an associated failure rate of 1 in 2000 and that pregnancies can occur several years after vasectomy. Although men requesting vasectomy should understand that the procedure is intended to be permanent, they should be given information on the success rates associated with reversal, should this procedure be necessary. Men should be advised to use effective contraception until azoospermia has been confirmed. The way in which azoospermia is confirmed will depend on local protocols.

Men requesting vasectomy can be reassured that there is no increase in risk of testicular cancer or heart disease associated with the procedure. The association, in some reports, of an increased risk of being diagnosed with prostate cancer is at present considered to be non-causative. Men should be informed about the possibility of chronic testicular pain after vasectomy. Testosterone concentrations are unaffected.

Key *points*

- Worldwide, contraceptive provision is important but is affected by cultural, political and financial constraints.
- Medical eligibility criteria can be used to ensure the safe provision of contraception to women and men without imposing unnecessary medical restrictions.
- Efficacy of contraception is measured by failure rate expressed as pregnancies per 100 woman-years.
- Consistent and correct use of contraception is important to maintain efficacy. Methods which reduce the risk of user failure, such as long-acting methods (implant, injectable and intrauterine methods), are more effective than methods which rely on user input (pill taking or patch use).
- The combined hormonal methods (pill and patch) contain estrogen and a progestogen. These methods are contraindicated in some women, such as those with significant cardiovascular disease (e.g. myocardial infarction, stroke, hypertension, venous thromboembolism), those with thrombophilia, smokers aged ≥35 years, all women with migraine *with aura* and women aged ≥35 years with migraine *without aura*, and women with breast cancer.
- Progestogen-only contraception includes pills, injections, implants and the intrauterine system. These methods can be considered for use first line or by women who have contraindications to estrogen use.

- Barrier methods are less effective than other methods but can reduce the risk of sexually transmitted infections.
- 'Natural' contraception can provide effective contraception for well-instructed and motivated individuals.
- Emergency contraception comprises either a progestogen preparation which can be used up to 72 hours after unprotected intercourse, or a Cu-IUD, which may be used up to 5 days after the first episode of unprotected intercourse or up to 5 days after the expected date of ovulation.
- Male and female sterilization provide effective permanent contraception. Vasectomy has lower failure rates than female sterilization and can be performed without general anaesthesia. Progestogen-only implants are more effective than female sterilization but need to be changed every 3 years.

10 Miscarriage

Miscarriage is common, occurring in as many as 25% of all pregnancies. It is very upsetting for the parents and sensitivity is required at all gestations. Clinical management should be founded on two important principles:

1. Care must be taken not to advise uterine evacuation if there is any possibility of fetal viability. It should not be assumed that the pregnancy is non-viable simply because the gestation does not agree with the expected dates.
2. There should be a low threshold of suspicion for ectopic pregnancy. The absence of an ectopic pregnancy on ultrasound scanning does not mean that there is not an ectopic pregnancy.

Definition

Miscarriage can be defined according to the gestation or the weight of the fetus. The World Health Organization (WHO) definition is 'the expulsion from its mother of an embryo or fetus weighing 500 g or less' (500 g is approximately the 50th centile for 20 weeks' gestation). The term 'abortion' has connotations of induced abortion (Ch.11) and should not be used in connection with spontaneous pregnancy loss, where 'miscarriage' is appropriate.

In the UK any pregnancy loss before 24 weeks is regarded as a miscarriage, and any fetus born dead at or after 24 weeks of gestation is registered as a stillbirth. If a fetus shows signs of life after delivery at any gestation, however, the loss can be considered to be a live birth and subsequent neonatal death.

There is therefore a discrepancy between the legal definition used in the UK and the internationally accepted definition. Because of the rapid advances in neonatal intensive care and the survival of babies born at 23 weeks, most modern epidemiological studies follow the WHO guideline and confine the definition to losses occurring before 20 weeks.

Miscarriage has traditionally been classified in a clinical way, and much depends on skilled, carefully interpreted ultrasound scanning:

- *threatened:* vaginal bleeding and an ongoing pregnancy
- *inevitable:* the cervix to dilated
- *incomplete:* passage of some, but not all, of the products of conception
- *complete:* all products of conception have been expelled from the uterus
- *missed (silent):* where the fetus has died in utero before 20 weeks but has not been expelled; 'anembryonic pregnancy' is a type of 'missed' miscarriage in which embryonic development fails at a very early stage in the pregnancy
- *septic:* a complication of incomplete miscarriage or therapeutic (sometimes illegal) abortion, when intrauterine infection occurs
- *recurrent:* three or more consecutive miscarriages.

Incidence

The miscarriage ratio (the number of miscarriages divided by the total number of pregnancies in a population) lies between 10% and 25%. This risk is highest early in pregnancy and falls as the pregnancy advances. The quoted ratio, however, refers to clinically recognized pregnancies and it is possible for the embryo to die before any obvious signs of pregnancy have appeared. Evidence from studies of chorionic gonadotrophin (hCG) assays in very early pregnancy and from assisted conception units suggests that rates of such very early miscarriage may be as high as 50–60%.

The incidence of miscarriage has been shown to increase with maternal age, rising by a factor of 10 after the age of 40 years compared to before 35 years. Overall, however, when the fetus is found to be viable on ultrasound scan, the chance of a successful outcome is high (4% risk of miscarriage if heartbeat present at 6 weeks, 2% risk of miscarriage if heartbeat present at 8 weeks).

Recurrence risk

This knowledge is important for parental counselling. While a few women have a specific recurring cause (such as uterine abnormality) which excludes them from general risk estimation, it is reasonable to reassure the couple that the outlook for future pregnancies is good. A woman experiencing a first miscarriage does not have a materially increased risk of miscarriage in her next pregnancy.

Aetiology

There are a number of conditions recognized as causing sporadic and/or recurrent miscarriage.

Fetal chromosomal abnormalities

About half of all clinically recognized first-trimester losses are chromosomally abnormal, with 50% of these being autosomal trisomy, 20% 45XO monosomy, 20% polyploidy, and 10% with various other abnormalities.

In second-trimester miscarriage, the incidence of chromosomal abnormality is lower at about 20% overall. Attempts to confirm the presence of chromosomal abnormality in a particular instance are often unsuccessful owing to failure of culture.

Endocrine factors

Women with polycystic ovary syndrome have an increased incidence of both sporadic and recurrent miscarriage and, although this has been attributed to high circulating levels of luteinizing hormone in the follicular phase of the cycle, there is no evidence of any effective therapy. Inadequate luteal function has been reported in association with recurrent miscarriage in 20–60% of cases, but there is no convincing evidence to support the use of artificial progestogens.

In women with diabetes mellitus who have poor control around the time of conception, the incidence of miscarriage is high at around 45%. Women whose control is good are no more likely to have a miscarriage than those who do not have diabetes. There is no clear association between thyroid dysfunction and miscarriage.

Immunological causes

Recent advances in reproductive immunology have revealed both autoimmune and alloimmune associations with miscarriage.

Autoimmune disease

Approximately 15% of women who are investigated for recurrent miscarriage (three or more consecutive pregnancy losses) are found to be positive for lupus anticoagulant, antiphospholipid antibodies, or both. Untreated, they have a subsequent rate of fetal loss approaching 90%. Effective treatment can be provided with low-dose aspirin and low-molecular-weight heparin. These antibodies are also associated with arterial and venous thrombosis, fetal growth restriction, pre-eclampsia and thrombocytopenia, and this should be borne in mind for later pregnancy management. The lupus anticoagulant is not synonymous with systemic lupus erythematosus (SLE), being present in only 5–15% of patients with SLE.

Alloimmune disease

Immunological tolerance of pregnancy is partly related to the special properties of the fetomaternal interface:

- the lack of classic major histocompatibility antigen from the trophoblastic cells of chorionic villi
- the presence of antigens, encoded by paternal genes, which are thought to stimulate production of 'blocking' antibodies.

This process is complex and it has been suggested that some miscarriages may result from maternal immunological rejection of fetal trophoblast cells. Attempts to immunize women against paternally derived antigens have been unsuccessful.

Uterine anomalies

Structural uterine anomalies, such as bicornuate or septate uteri, may cause miscarriage in a few instances, particularly if the loss has occurred in the second trimester. Uterine fibroids may also interfere with early pregnancy growth, but the extent to which they cause miscarriage is difficult to determine because of other associated factors such as age, hormonal dysfunction and subfertility.

Infections

Any serious maternal infection causing high fever at any time in pregnancy may adversely affect the fetus and lead to pregnancy loss. There are also a number of specific maternal infections, however, which may precipitate miscarriage. Viruses, such as rubella and cytomegalovirus, have the ability to cross the placenta and affect the placenta and fetus. Such congenital infection in early pregnancy may lead to miscarriage, as well as to later fetal abnormality and neonatal illness (p. 274). Malaria, trypanosomiasis, *Chlamydia trachomatis*, mycoplasma, *Listeria monocytogenes* and syphilis have also all been implicated in early pregnancy loss.

Environmental pollutants

Cigarette smoking, both active and passive, and high alcohol consumption are associated with higher rates of sporadic and recurrent miscarriage.

Unexplained

At least 50% of miscarriages, either sporadic or recurrent, have no identifiable cause.

Clinical presentation and management

Presentation

There is usually a history of bleeding per vaginam (p.v.) and lower abdominal pain. The passage of tissue is sometimes reported **(Fig.10.1)**. The bleeding can vary from being life-threateningly severe, requiring urgent and aggressive resuscitation to the smallest brown spotting.

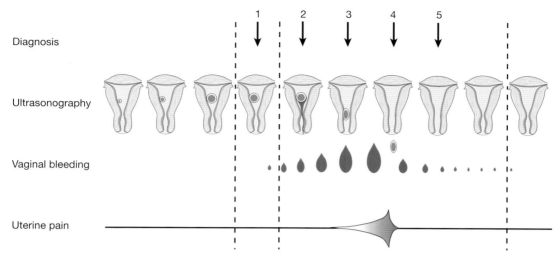

Fig. 10.1 Clinical and ultrasound features of a miscarriage. 1. Ultrasound may show fetal heart activity, or the pregnancy may appear non-viable. 2. Vaginal bleeding and pain begin. 3. The cervical os is open – an inevitable miscarriage. 4. The gestational sac is extruded. 5. Pain and bleeding usually settle rapidly.

Occasionally there may be no symptoms at all and an empty gestational sac, or fetal pole with absent fetal heartbeat, may be found at a routine booking scan. It is seldom possible to make consistently reliable diagnoses based on clinical examination alone, and management is largely based on ultrasound scan (USS) findings. This management relies on an understanding of the ultrasound findings in a normally developing pregnancy **(Table 10.1)**. Ultrasound is usually commenced transabdominally, but the transvaginal approach provides superior images and is widely employed.

Viable intrauterine pregnancy

The prognosis is good and the parents can be offered reasonable reassurance **(Fig. 10.2)**.

Empty gestational sac

If there is an empty gestational sac greater than 25 mm in maximum diameter, the pregnancy is very likely to be non-viable **(Fig. 10.3)**. If a pregnancy test was positive more than 3 weeks previously, the gestation is likely to be at least 6+ weeks and a fetal pole would always be expected on transvaginal (TV) ultrasound scanning. If the first positive pregnancy test was less than 3 weeks previously, however, conservative management is most appropriate, with a repeat scan in at least 10 days. Although this will add anxious waiting time for the mother, it is preferable to arranging a uterine evacuation on a potentially viable pregnancy.

A true gestational sac should be differentiated from a 'pseudosac' **(Fig.10.4)**. This is caused by fluid secreted under the hCG stimulation of an ectopic pregnancy, and it

Table 10.1			
The first nine weeks			
Days	**Weeks**	**Clinical features**	**Scan features**
0	0	Menses	
7	1		
14	2	Conception	
21	3		
28	4	Pregnancy test positive [menses due]	Empty uterus
	5		Gestational sac (hCG >2000 IU)
	6	Nausea Breast tenderness	Yolk sac, Fetal heartbeat on transvaginal scan Fetal pole 4 mm
	7		Fetal pole 10 mm
	8		Fetal heartbeat on transabdominal scan Fetal pole 14 mm
	9		Fetal pole 22 mm

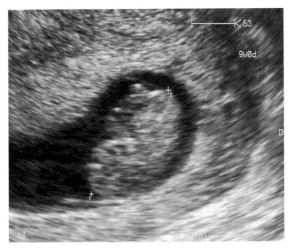

Fig. 10.2 An intrauterine 22 mm fetal pole, consistent with 9 weeks' gestation. Fetal heart activity was seen.

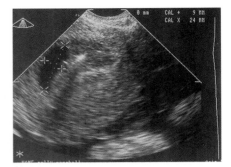

Fig. 10.4 A pseudosac and intrauterine contraceptive device in the presence of an ectopic pregnancy.

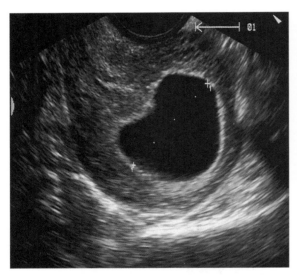

Fig. 10.3 An empty gestational sac at 8 weeks' gestation. This pregnancy was an anembryonic, sometimes referred to as a 'silent', miscarriage.

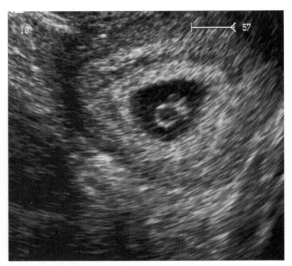

Fig. 10.5 Intrauterine gestational scan containing a 6 mm fetal pole with a yolk sac. There was no fetal heart activity on transvaginal scan. Note the double decidual ring consistent with intrauterine pregnancy.

lacks the 'double decidual ring' outline seen with a true sac (Figs 10.3 and 10.5).

Fetal pole with no fetal heartbeat

A fetal heartbeat is usually seen on a TV scan if the fetal pole is more than 2–3 mm, but will always be seen by 6 mm **(Fig.10.5)** if present (15 mm is appropriate for a transabdominal scan). If there is any doubt, re-scanning should be arranged in 7–10 days.

Empty uterus

Either there has been a complete miscarriage (tissue may have been passed), or the pregnancy is very early (e.g. <5 weeks), or there is an ectopic pregnancy. Ectopic pregnancy

must be excluded. An intrauterine sac will usually be seen on TV scan if the hCG is >1000 IU, and its absence raises the possibility of an ectopic pregnancy. Serum levels of hCG should rise by more than 66% in 48 hours if the pregnancy is viable and intrauterine; a smaller rise suggests an ectopic pregnancy (see fig 15.2). If the level doubles and the woman remains well, the ultrasound scan should be repeated in 1 week to ensure that the pregnancy is ongoing. If less than doubling, steady, or only slightly reduced, a laparoscopy should be considered to exclude ectopic pregnancy.

Gestational Trophoblastic disease

See page 211.

Management of early pregnancy loss

Once a diagnosis has been established and explained to the woman and her partner, providing there is no ongoing heavy vaginal bleeding, the options for subsequent management can be discussed. Surgical uterine evacuation and medical uterine evacuation with mifepristone and a synthetic prostaglandin are technically analogous to the methods employed in the therapeutic termination of pregnancy (Ch. 11). Conservative management with no scheduled medical or surgical intervention may be appropriate, but the woman needs to be warned that the onset, duration and magnitude of the inevitable vaginal bleeding are unpredictable. If the diameter of retained products is small on ultrasound examination (e.g. less than 40 mm) and the woman wishes conservative management, she may be reviewed in 2 weeks and re-scanned, at which time about 20% of women will still have retained products. This small number of women may then be offered surgical or medical management as outlined.

Rhesus isoimmunization

Rhesus isoimmunization may occur in rhesus-negative women who have lost a rhesus-positive fetus (p. 313). As there is no practical way of determining fetal blood group in miscarriage, all rhesus-negative women should be offered anti-D immunoglobulin as appropriate:

- *Confirmed miscarriage:* anti-D should be given to all non-sensitized rhesus-negative women who miscarry after 12 weeks, whether complete or incomplete, and to those who miscarry below 12 weeks when the uterus is evacuated (either surgically or medically).
- *Threatened miscarriage:* anti-D should be given to all non-sensitized rhesus-negative women with threatened miscarriage after 12 weeks. Routine administration of anti-D is not required below 12 weeks when the fetus is viable, unless the bleeding is heavy or associated with abdominal pain. If there is clinical doubt, then anti-D should be given.

After the miscarriage

There has been a bereavement; the emotional trauma experienced will vary from one couple to the next, but the negative impact of a miscarriage should not be underestimated. There may be some medical benefits in waiting before trying again, but this has to be weighed against the loss of fertility opportunities; contraception may be offered. Support groups, such as The Miscarriage Association, are available.

Septic abortion

Fortunately, this is rare unless after illegal terminations with inadequate asepsis and therefore is more commonly encountered in countries where termination of pregnancy is not legal. There is usually pyrexia, tachycardia, malaise, abdominal pain, marked tenderness and a purulent vaginal loss. Endotoxic shock may develop and there is a significant maternal mortality. The responsible organisms include Gram-negative bacteria, streptococci (haemolytic and anaerobic) and other anaerobes (e.g. *Bacteroides*).

Recurrent spontaneous miscarriage

This is the consecutive loss of three or more fetuses weighing <500 g. The incidence of 1% is greater than would be expected by chance alone, which is estimated at 0.34%. Only a proportion of women will therefore have an underlying cause for their recurrent losses.

Investigation is based on the principles discussed above and includes:

- *Karyotype* from both parents. The incidence of chromosomal abnormality in this group, usually a balanced translocation, is around 3–5%. The finding of such an abnormality should prompt genetic referral since it has implications for future pregnancies.
- Maternal blood for *lupus anticoagulant* and *anticardiolipin antibodies*. The antiphospholipid syndrome can be diagnosed in this context if the assays are positive on more than one occasion at least 6 weeks apart. Treatment in a subsequent pregnancy with low-dose aspirin is associated with a 40% likelihood of successful outcome, but a 70% success can be obtained with low-dose aspirin and low-molecular-weight heparin.
- *Thrombophilia screen.* Retrospective studies have indicated an increased incidence of thrombophilic defects in those with recurrent miscarriage (activated protein C resistance, antithrombin III deficiency, protein C deficiency, and protein S deficiency, and possibly hyperhomocystinaemia). Evidence for effective treatment in this group is lacking.
- *Pelvic ultrasound scan* (uterus and ovaries) to look for uterine abnormalities. Three-dimensional transvaginal ultrasound is particularly informative. However, it is very difficult to estimate the significance of anatomical abnormalities and caution is required before undertaking significant surgical procedures to correct uterine anomalies.

Amongst women with mid-trimester loss, the possibility of cervical incompetence should be considered. Cervical incompetence indicates that the internal os of the cervix is unable to retain the pregnancy within the uterus. The diagnosis is supported by a history of relatively painless cervical dilatation, and there may be a background history of prior surgery to the cervix. There is no single diagnostic test of cervical incompetence, which makes reliable diagnosis impossible. Inserting a cervical suture (cervical cerclage) may be of benefit, but at the risk of infection developing after insertion **(Fig.10.6)**. Transabdominal cerclage is also used where a vaginal approach either has been technically not possible due to the short length of the cervix or a vaginally placed suture has failed.

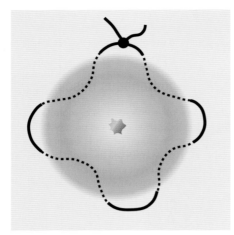

Fig. 10.6 A cervical suture.

Where no specific abnormalities are found, counselling and reassurance are the mainstays of successful management: 60–75% of women who have suffered three consecutive miscarriages and who have no apparent underlying cause will have a successful pregnancy at their next attempt. The use of unproven treatments should be resisted.

Conclusion

For most miscarriages, whether sporadic or recurrent, no specific cause can be found. Competent management of the acute episode and timely investigation of women with recurrent miscarriage are the mainstays of treatment.

Key points

- Miscarriage is the loss of a pregnancy before 24 weeks' gestation.
- There are few successful interventions for preventing miscarriage and management is centred on accurate diagnosis, counselling, and minimizing complications.
- Care must be taken not to advise uterine evacuation if there is any possibility of viability. It should not be assumed that the pregnancy is non-viable simply because the gestation does not agree with the expected dates.
- There should be a low threshold of suspicion for ectopic pregnancy.
- Ultrasound services provided by early pregnancy assessment units represent the most relevant initial investigation and appropriate care setting for the vast majority of women experiencing bleeding and/or pain in early pregnancy.

11

Therapeutic abortion

Introduction

Termination of pregnancy, or therapeutic abortion, has been carried out for thousands of years. The provision of abortion in a legal, medically supervised, and safe framework is one of the most contentious issues in modern-day medicine. Many people have strongly held and often divergent opinions about abortion. Those who are pro-abortion maintain that they are 'pro-choice' and support the right of individuals to make their own decisions. They are sensitive to the difficulties of bringing an unwanted baby into the world, and are aware of the impact on both the woman concerned and society more broadly. Those who are anti-abortion, or 'pro-life', argue that the fetus is more than just part of the mother; it is a life in itself and should be protected, even if that means limiting the mother's choices regarding her body.

There are many factors leading to unplanned pregnancy: contraception may have failed, or perhaps was not used at all; occasionally, intercourse without the woman's consent has resulted in pregnancy. Of course, a woman may have an unplanned pregnancy but be pleased to be pregnant and continue the pregnancy. Another may have planned to be pregnant but then her circumstances may change and she feels unable to continue. Amongst women attending antenatal clinics, research demonstrates that only two-thirds of women had an intended pregnancy, with the rest either ambivalent or having an unplanned pregnancy. Although abortion should not be considered as a method of contraception, contraceptive failures do occur, and access to abortion allows women complete fertility regulation.

Abortion care forms a large part of the gynaecology workload in the UK, and therapeutic abortion is one of the commonest gynaecological procedures. Although doctors may have differing degrees of involvement in abortion services, most will come into contact with women who are seeking abortion at some point in their career, so need to be familiar with the legal framework and options open to the women.

Worldwide perspectives

There are over 100 million acts of sexual intercourse every day across the world, resulting in over 900,000 pregnancies. It is estimated that about 50% of these pregnancies are unplanned, and about 25% actually unwanted. Many women with an unwanted pregnancy will seek an abortion, and, as a result, about 150,000 pregnancies are terminated by induced abortion every day. There are over 50 million abortions worldwide every year and around one-third of these abortions are carried out in unsafe conditions. Illegal abortions are often performed in unclean conditions by unqualified people, causing considerable morbidity and mortality. Between 100,000 and 200,000 women die each year from unsafe abortion. In contrast, abortion performed in appropriate conditions with trained staff is an extremely safe procedure, with extremely low morbidity and mortality.

UK perspectives

The Abortion Act was passed in 1967, and after this, there was a rapid rise in the number of abortions carried out in England, Wales and Scotland. Currently, over 185,000 abortions are carried out each year in England and Wales, with a further 12,500 in Scotland. Women of all reproductive ages have abortions, although the highest rate is amongst women aged 18–24 years. About three-quarters of women having abortions are unmarried, although many of these will have a regular partner. Almost half of women have already had a child and one-third have had an abortion previously. Most terminations (60%) are carried out before 9 weeks of pregnancy, and a smaller number (13%) are carried out in the second trimester.

Legal and ethical aspects

Abortion is not available 'on demand' in the UK, and can only be carried out if certain criteria are met. The 1967 Abortion Act, as amended in 1991, states that abortion can be performed if two doctors agree that the pregnancy should be terminated on one or more grounds **(Box 11.1)**.

Most abortions (95%) are carried out under Clause C of the Abortion Act, where two doctors agree that continuing the pregnancy would carry greater risk to the physical or mental health of the woman than abortion. A smaller number of abortions (3%) are carried out to protect the health of existing children. Clauses C and D carry an upper gestational limit of 24 weeks. The 1967 Abortion Act does not apply to Northern Ireland, where abortion is only legal under exceptional circumstances, e.g. to save the life of the mother.

Current methods of inducing abortion are now so safe that it is safer for the woman to have an early abortion than to continue to term and have a delivery. Of course, that does not mean that abortion should be recommended, but a clinician may consider a request for abortion when a woman feels that her health (or that of her children) will be adversely affected by continuing the pregnancy.

Although uncommonly used, the Abortion Act also allows abortion to be performed in an emergency situation upon the single signature of the doctor performing the abortion. Such an emergency abortion can be carried out either to save the life of the pregnant woman, or to prevent grave permanent injury to the physical or mental health of the pregnant woman.

Recent opinion polls have shown that most of the public support the right to abortion, with 65% agreeing that if a woman wants an abortion she should not have to continue with her pregnancy. Women requesting abortion need the agreement of two doctors, and will often rely on the support of their general practitioner for referral. Over 80% of British general practitioners described themselves as 'broadly pro-choice', and 18% as 'broadly anti-abortion'. No doctor has to be involved in referring women for abortion, but British Medical Association guidance advises that if a doctor is unable to make a referral for termination, then a timely referral of the woman to a colleague who does not hold similar views is obligatory; every doctor has an obligation to treat in an emergency situation.

Counselling before abortion

When a woman is considering abortion, it is important that she is able to weigh up the practical and emotional aspects of her decision, to ensure that the best choice is made in the circumstances. She will require sympathetic but non-directional support so that she is able to explore her own feelings and to make her own informed decision. Many women with an unplanned pregnancy will make their decision within a few days of knowing that they are pregnant. Other women may remain undecided for some time. It is important that the decision to abort is made freely by the woman, and that she is not coerced by another party, for example a parent or partner. For this reason, it may be important to speak to the woman alone at some point during the consultation.

Psychological problems and rates of depression are not increased after abortion when compared with background population risk, but some women may experience coping problems and distress. The counselling process can help to identify these women, and ensure that appropriate support is offered both before and after the abortion. **Box 11.2** outlines risk factors for emotional problems.

Women who blame themselves for the pregnancy and subsequent abortion can struggle to come to terms with their decision. It can help to identify what went wrong that led to the pregnancy. Jointly agreeing a contraceptive plan with the woman can return a sense of control to her, and give her something positive for the future to take from the experience.

We are used to taking a structured gynaecological history, collecting factual information, such as date of last menstrual period, but we can help the woman to express her emotional needs by using some basic counselling techniques:

- Ask open-ended questions, e.g. 'How did you feel about the pregnancy?', rather than 'Were you upset when you found out?'
- Listen to the patient, e.g. show interest in her views, and show understanding.

Circumstances in which an abortion may be carried out under the Abortion Act 1967 (amended 1991)

A. The continuance of the pregnancy would involve risk to the life of the pregnant woman greater than if the pregnancy were terminated
B. The termination is necessary to prevent grave permanent injury to the physical or mental health of the pregnant woman
C. The pregnancy has *not* exceeded its 24th week and continuance of the pregnancy would involve risk, greater than if the pregnancy were terminated, of injury to the physical or mental health of the pregnant woman
D. The pregnancy has *not* exceeded its 24th week and continuance of the pregnancy would involve risk, greater than if the pregnancy were terminated, of injury to the physical or mental health of the existing child(ren) of the family of the pregnant woman
E. There is a substantial risk that if the child were born it would suffer from such physical or mental abnormalities as to be seriously handicapped

---

Factors associated with coping problems and distress after abortion

- Women with a history of mental health problems
- Younger women
- Women from cultural or religious group who do not believe in abortion
- Women with low self-esteem
- Women without a close supportive person to talk to
- Women undergoing later abortions
- Women in whom the pregnancy was initially planned
- Women who feel there is no choice, e.g. due to financial pressures

- Reassure her that her feelings are normal, e.g. saying 'I understand that you are finding this difficult to talk about'.
- Encourage questions, e.g. say 'What would you like to ask me about your choices?' rather than 'Any questions?'

Some women need practical information to make their choice, such as details about maternity leave, housing rights etc., or information about adoption. Timely referral to a social worker should be available.

Pre-abortion investigations

Once the woman has decided to proceed to abortion, there are a number of investigations which are usually performed, to ensure that the abortion is as safe as possible:

- *Blood tests:* haemoglobin is measured, and a sample is sent for ABO and rhesus blood grouping. Women who are rhesus negative will require anti-D immunoglobulin after the abortion (250 IU if less than 20 weeks, and 500 IU if over 20 weeks). HIV, haemoglobinopathy and other tests can be performed if indicated.
- *Estimation of gestation:* this can be performed by either clinical examination or ultrasound. Most abortion clinics in the UK now use ultrasound to confirm gestation before abortion. Ultrasound is essential if there is a possibility of ectopic pregnancy, or where gestation is unclear. Some women will not make the decision until they know the gestation of the pregnancy, i.e. they may decide to abort an early pregnancy, but would not wish to undergo a later abortion. Occasionally, women may request a copy of the scan, as a memento of the pregnancy. Ultrasound will sometimes reveal a silent miscarriage (missed miscarriage).
- *Prevention of infection:* infection can occur in about 10% of women after abortion, but can be reduced with the use of antibiotics. Some clinics treat everyone having an abortion with prophylactic antibiotics (commonly metronidazole and azithromycin), whereas others screen women for sexually transmitted infections, including chlamydia, and treat positive women and their partners.
- *Cervical cytology:* if a woman is due cervical cytology, then this can be offered at the time of the clinic visit.
- *Provision of information:* information given verbally should be supported with written information for the woman to take away. This should include information about the types of abortion available, the risks and complications of abortion, and who to contact if there are any problems after the procedure.

Methods of abortion

Historically, a wide range of surgical and medical techniques have been used to cause therapeutic abortion. In the past two decades, advances in abortion techniques mean that safe and effective methods are now available at all stages of gestation. Medical methods have been increasing in frequency since the licensing of mifepristone in 1991. Both medical and surgical abortion can be offered up to 24 weeks, but availability varies in different geographical areas. The most appropriate method depends on gestation, parity, medical history and the woman's preference **(Box 11.3)**.

Medical abortion

Mifepristone is a synthetic steroid which blocks the biological action of progesterone by binding to its receptor in the uterus and other organs. It is given orally under supervision of a doctor or nurse, in a premises licensed to carry out abortion. The woman is then allowed home. She returns to the unit 24–72 hours later (usually 48 hours) and is admitted for administration of a prostaglandin, usually administered vaginally. Bleeding usually starts within a few hours, followed by uterine contractions which expel the fetus and placenta. The woman normally goes home later the same day. Most women experience period-like pains but there is much variation, with some women needing no pain relief while others (about 10–20%) require opiates. Bleeding usually continues for about 10 days after medical abortion.

Box 11.3

Abortion options depend on gestation. Providing a choice of abortion method increases satisfaction with method chosen.

Medical abortion

- 'Early' medical abortion
  - under 9 weeks
  - mifepristone plus single dose misoprostol
- 'Late' first-trimester medical abortion
  - between 9 and 12 weeks
  - mifepristone plus misoprostol (more than one dose of misoprostol may be required)
- Mid-trimester medical abortion
  - 13–24 weeks
  - mifepristone plus repeated doses of misoprostol (need to perform feticide intervention if over 22 weeks)

Surgical abortion

- Manual vacuum aspiration
  - below 7 weeks
  - under local anaesthesia
  - higher failure rate
  - careful follow-up required
- Suction abortion
  - between 7 and 14 weeks
  - cervical preparation recommended
  - usually general anaesthesia
- Dilatation and evacuation
  - between 14 and 24 weeks
  - requires specially trained surgeon
  - not available in all areas

Early medical abortion (up to 9 weeks' gestation)

When a woman is less than 7 weeks' pregnant, medical abortion is the most effective type of termination, with a lower failure rate than early surgical abortion. It is also a good choice between 7 and 9 weeks' (63 days') gestation.

The normal regimen is:

Mifepristone 200 mg orally, followed by misoprostol 800 μg vaginally 24–72 hours later.

Medical abortion in the late first trimester (9–13 weeks)

In the past, surgical termination alone has been offered to women in the late first trimester. However, it is now recommended that medical abortion can be offered as an alternative to surgical termination in the late first trimester.

The normal regimen is:

Mifepristone 200 mg orally, followed by misoprostol 800 μg vaginally 36–48 hours later. Up to a further four doses of misoprostol 400 μg, either vaginally or orally, can be given until abortion occurs.

Medical abortion in the second trimester (13–24 weeks)

Traditionally, mid-trimester medical abortion was carried out using prostaglandin alone, or in combination with an oxytocin infusion. Not uncommonly, it would take several days for the abortion to be completed. Giving mifepristone prior to prostaglandin has been shown to reduce the length of time taken for the abortion to occur.

The normal regimen is:

Mifepristone 200 mg orally, followed by misoprostol 800 μg vaginally 36–48 hours later. Up to a further four doses of misoprostol 400 μg orally, can be given until abortion occurs.

Surgical abortion

Surgical abortion below 7 weeks' gestation

Surgical abortion below 7 weeks' gestation has a higher failure rate than later surgical procedures and medical abortion at this gestation. For these reasons, surgical abortion is usually delayed until 7 weeks. However, a few centres offer manual aspiration abortion at very early gestation. This is performed using a narrow suction curette of 4 or 5 mm diameter, inserted into the uterus under local paracervical block. The early pregnancy is aspirated using a 50 ml syringe. It is very important to ensure that the abortion is complete, either by identifying the products of conception or by hCG follow-up.

Surgical abortion at 7–14 weeks

Surgical abortion at this gestation is performed by suction or vacuum aspiration, using a flexible suction curette, and a mechanical or electrical pump. The suction curette is inserted into the uterine cavity, after cervical dilatation, and the contents aspirated **(Figs 11.1 and 11.2)**. The procedure is usually carried out under general anaesthesia, but local anaesthesia or conscious sedation can also be used.

Complications increase with advancing gestation, and some doctors do not offer surgical termination beyond 12 weeks. Cervical treatment with prostaglandin before surgical abortion reduces the risk of cervical trauma and uterine perforation, and should certainly be used when the woman is under 18 years of age, or gestation is above 10 weeks. Many clinics give all women prostaglandin before surgical abortion.

The recommended regimen is:

Misoprostol 400 μg vaginally, 3 hours prior to surgery.

Late surgical abortion (15–24 weeks)

Cervical preparation followed by dilatation and evacuation (D&E) can be offered in the second trimester. It is the method of choice in the USA, but in the UK is offered by a

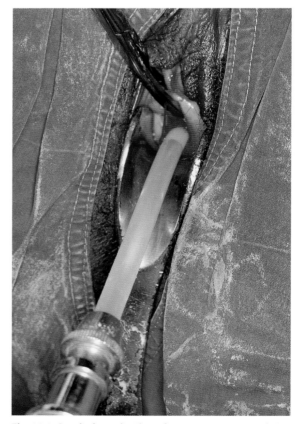

Fig. 11.1 Surgical termination of pregnancy at 10 weeks' gestation.

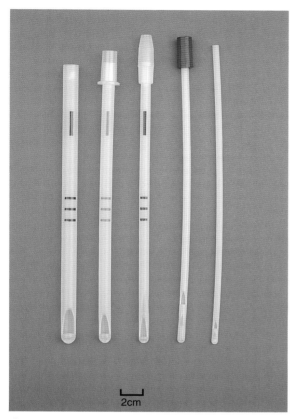

2cm

Fig. 11.2 A selection of suction curettes for surgical pregnancy termination.

limited number of doctors experienced in the technique. It may be necessary to dilate the cervix up to a diameter of 20 mm before the fetal parts can be extracted using special instruments. D&E has the advantage that the woman is unaware of the procedure. There is evidence from the USA that women prefer D&E to medical methods, although many nurses and doctors find the procedure disturbing.

Complications of abortion

Women should be advised that the risk of complications is low. Indeed, a termination is safer than continuing the pregnancy to term. Complications do occasionally occur, however, and women should be given information about where to seek help if there are problems.

Retained products of conception

This is the commonest complication following abortion, occurring in up to 5% of women. It is more common after medical abortion, and when surgical abortion is carried out at either very early or late gestations. Some women with retained products will require (further) surgical evacuation of the uterus, particularly if there is heavy or prolonged

bleeding. Many women will pass the retained tissue spontaneously. Antibiotics can be given to reduce the risk of secondary infection until the tissue is passed.

Failure of abortion

Ongoing pregnancy after an abortion procedure is unusual, but occurs in 2.3 per 1000 women undergoing surgical abortion, and between 1 and 14 per 1000 women having medical termination. Women should be advised of the importance of returning for follow-up, particularly if there was any doubt over completeness at the time of termination, or there are continuing symptoms of pregnancy.

Post-abortion infection

Pelvic infection can occur in up to 10% of women after termination, but this can be halved with pre-abortion STI screening and use of antibiotics at the time of termination. Women should be advised about signs of infection such as pyrexia, pelvic pain and offensive vaginal discharge, and should return if concerned.

Haemorrhage

Significant haemorrhage at the time of termination occurs in around 1 in 1000 cases, and is more common when abortion is carried out at later gestation.

Trauma to the genital tract

Perforation of the uterus happens in about 1 in 1000 surgical cases, and is more common with later-gestation abortions. Cervical trauma is also uncommon (less than 1 in 100) and is reduced by cervical preparation with prostaglandin. Uterine rupture has been described very occasionally with mid-trimester medical abortion.

Future fertility

Women often ask about the chance of an abortion affecting their future fertility. There is no established positive association between previous termination of pregnancy and future infertility, ectopic pregnancy or placenta praevia. There may be a slight increase in risk of subsequent miscarriage and preterm delivery with later abortion, although the evidence is unclear.

Psychological sequelae

There is no evidence of lasting psychological harm to women undergoing abortion. Some women may be at higher risk of distress after the abortion, and can be identified at the time of pre-abortion counselling and offered greater support.

Abortion aftercare

A follow-up visit at about 2 weeks can be offered to all women after abortion, to check there have been no complications, and to encourage use of contraception. Follow-up can be with the general practitioner, family planning clinic or abortion service.

Post-abortion contraception

About a third of terminations are carried out on women who have had a termination in the past, and ensuring that there is adequate contraception available can help to reduce the chance of a further abortion. All methods of hormonal contraception (combined pill, progestogen pill, implant, injection) can be started on the day of surgical abortion, or on the prostaglandin treatment day of medical abortion, with immediate contraceptive cover. Intrauterine contraception can be fitted immediately following termination. This can be done at the end of the surgical procedure, or following expulsion of the pregnancy with medical termination. Condoms can be used immediately after termination. Women are usually advised not to use a diaphragm within 6 weeks of mid-trimester abortion, in case refitting is required. Decisions about sterilization are better delayed until at least 6 weeks after termination, as there is a higher failure rate and later regret when sterilization is performed immediately after abortion.

Conclusion

Almost 200,000 women undergo therapeutic abortion each year in the UK. Women need to be well informed about pregnancy and abortion options, and supported with counselling to make an informed choice. A choice between medical and surgical abortion can often be offered. A range of contraceptive options should be made available to women at the time of termination.

Key *points*

- Unsafe abortion is a great threat to women's health worldwide, and causes many maternal mortalities.
- Therapeutic abortion is a common, safe and effective procedure in the UK, and is carried out under the terms of the Abortion Act.
- Women considering termination need information about options to inform their choice, and non-directive counselling to ensure they reach the most appropriate decision.
- A choice between medical and surgical abortion can often be offered.
- A contraceptive plan should be agreed and in place immediately after the abortion.

12

Sexual problems

Introduction

It is important for any doctor to be able to take a sexual history and to have some idea of how sexual problems are managed. Understanding the physiology of the normal sexual response will allow the doctor to help many of the simpler sexual problems. This is still true even in our age of apparent openness about sex.

Scientific investigation of the normal sexual response is necessary to our understanding, but, because of society's disapproval, few scientists have chosen to work in this area until recently. Early workers were:

- Sigmund Freud (1856–1939), an Austrian doctor, was the founder of psychoanalysis and the first to recognize the importance of childhood influences on sexuality. His studies were on patients rather than normal subjects.
- Havelock Ellis (1859–1939) studied medicine at St Thomas's Hospital, London. His seven-volume *Studies in the Psychology of Sex* (1897–1928) caused controversy but was the first detached treatment of the subject.
- Alfred Kinsey (1894–1956), an American zoologist, became director of Indiana University's Institute for Sex Research in 1942. To investigate 'normal' sexual experience, 18,500 Americans were interviewed. *Sexual Behaviour in the Human Male* was published in 1948, and *Sexual Behaviour in the Human Female* in 1953.
- Masters and Johnson: William Masters (b. 1915), a doctor, and Virginia Johnson (b. 1925), a psychologist, working at Washington University, St Louis, carried out the first direct observations on sexual activity under laboratory conditions. *Human Sexual Response* appeared in 1966, and *Human Sexual Inadequacy* in 1970.

Normal sexual response

The normal human sexual response can be regarded as having five phases: desire, arousal, orgasm, resolution, and the refractory phase **(Fig. 12.1)**.

Desire

Sexual desire refers to the general level of interest in sexuality. It is modulated by hormones – hence the change in sexual interest at puberty. The main modulator in both sexes is testosterone.

Arousal

This phase has three components: central arousal, genital response, and peripheral arousal.

Central arousal

This refers to the response to sexual stimuli, which may be visual or tactile or may result from internal imagery or from a relationship. These stimuli act through the cerebral cortex **(Fig. 12.2)**. The areas of the brain involved in sexual arousal are thought to be in the limbic system. There are thought to be excitatory centres with endorphins as the neurotransmitter, and inhibitory centres, linked to the centres for pain and fear.

Genital response

The spinal pathways leading to the genitalia are not precisely known but appear to be near the spinothalamic pathways for pain and temperature. Genital responses are due to vasocongestion and neuromuscular changes. Arteriolar

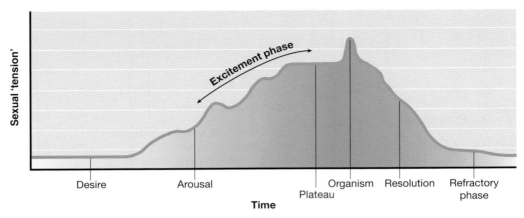

Fig. 12.1 The normal sexual response.

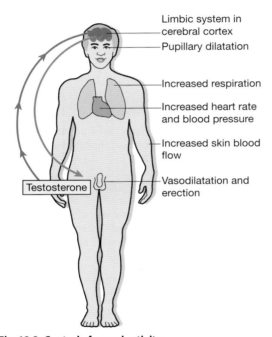

Fig. 12.2 Control of sexual activity.

dilatation is probably controlled by the parasympathetic sacral outflow at S2, 3 and 4 via the nervi erigentes. Thoracic sympathetic outflow also plays a part. The local neurotransmitters involved include vasoactive intestinal polypeptide (VIP), a potent vasodilator found in the penis and vagina.

In the male, engorgement of the corpora cavernosa is due mainly to arteriolar dilatation and probably a reduction in the venous outflow **(Fig. 12.3)**. The scrotum tightens due to contraction of the dartos muscle and the testes are elevated due to contraction of the cremaster muscle.

In the female, there is engorgement of the venous plexus surrounding the lower part of the vagina, and of the erectile bulbs of the vestibule on either side of the introitus **(Fig. 12.4)**. There is reddening and pouting of the labia minora. The clitoris becomes erect and later is said to retract against the symphysis pubis.

The vagina becomes lubricated by a transudate as the blood supply to the vaginal wall increases. This fluid is not the product of mucous glands: beads of fluid appear all over the vaginal wall. Mucus secretion from the cervix makes relatively little contribution to vaginal lubrication (which is therefore usually unaffected by hysterectomy). Secretion from Bartholin's glands, formerly thought to be mainly responsible for lubrication, is only moderate in amount and occurs relatively late during arousal.

Relaxation of the woman's pelvic floor muscles occurs after vaginal lubrication has started. In the later stages of arousal the uterus becomes engorged, increases in size, and rises in the pelvis. The upper part of the vagina 'balloons' and there may be slow irregular contractions of the lower third of the vagina.

In both sexes, but particularly in the male, the genital response interacts with the central response, so that arousal becomes self-amplifying.

Peripheral arousal

Sexual arousal causes:

- a rise in systolic and diastolic blood pressure (which may only be transient)
- general flushing of the skin
- change in heart rate (either an increase or a decrease)
- respiratory changes
- pupillary dilatation.

Plateau phase

When arousal is complete, there may be a 'plateau' phase during which the couple prolong the pleasure of intercourse before orgasm. If this continues too long, however, coitus may become painful for one or both partners.

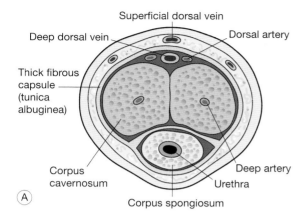

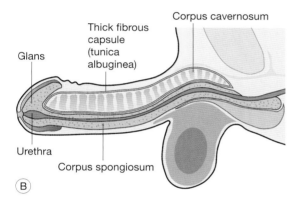

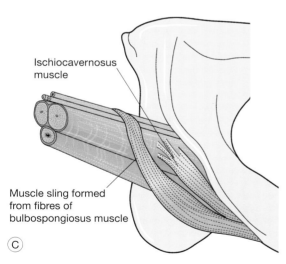

Fig. 12.3 The penis. (A) Cross-section showing erectile spaces and principal blood vessels. **(B)** Erectile tissues. Each crus of the corpora cavernosa is inserted into the pubic bone. **(C)** Muscles.

Orgasm

Orgasm involves genital, muscular and sensory changes, as well as cardiovascular and respiratory responses.

In the male

First there is smooth muscle contraction of the epididymis, vas deferens, seminal vesicle, prostate and ampulla, propelling seminal and prostatic fluid into the urethral bulb. Then the male becomes aware that orgasm is imminent and ejaculation usually follows within a few seconds. The internal bladder sphincter remains shut but the external sphincter relaxes and semen is propelled along the urethra by rhythmic contractions of the bulbospongiosus and ischiocavernosus muscles.

In the female

A few seconds after the onset of the subjective experience of orgasm there is a spasm of the muscles surrounding the lower third of the vagina (the 'orgasmic platform') followed by a series of rhythmic contractions, usually five to eight in number. These do not expel fluid from the vagina. Uterine contractions may also occur.

In both sexes

There is contraction of rectus abdominis, pelvic thrusting, contraction of the anal sphincter and sometimes carpopedal spasm. Systolic and diastolic blood pressure rises by at least 25 mmHg, and hyperventilation occurs. There is a feeling of intense pleasure and an alteration of consciousness to a variable degree.

Resolution

The events of arousal are gradually reversed. In men there is a moderate immediate loss of erection, followed by a slower complete reversal. In women, if no orgasm has occurred, pelvic congestion may take hours to resolve and may be uncomfortable. In both sexes there is a subjective feeling of relaxation, though its duration may differ between the man and the woman.

Refractory phase

There follows an interval during which further stimulation does not produce a response. In men this varies from minutes in young men to many hours in older men. Some women do not experience a refractory period, but only a minority of women (14% according to Kinsey) can have multiple orgasms.

The effect of age

Normal sexual behaviour differs from couple to couple. It also alters with age and with the evolution of a sexual relationship. Patients may present with problems due to

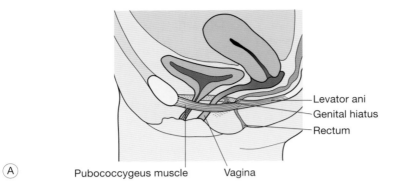

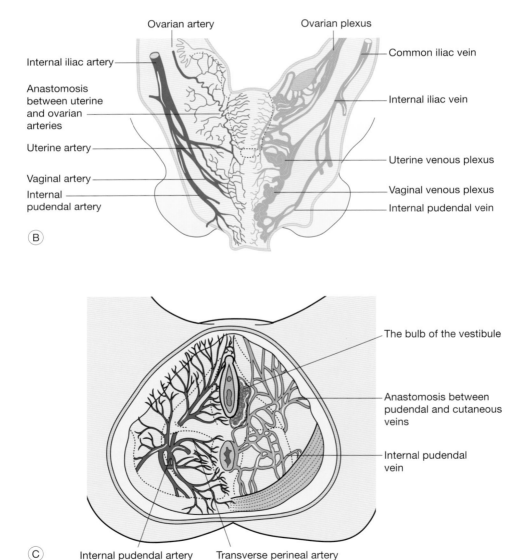

Fig. 12.4 Female reproductive organs. (A) The muscular supports of the vagina. This shows the sling of muscle fibres that surround the urethra, vagina and rectum, running from the pubic bone to the coccyx. The levator plate formed by these fibres supports the rectum and vagina in its non-aroused horizontal position. **(B)** Arteries and veins supplying the female reproductive organs. **(C)** Blood vessels of the pelvic floor, showing the rich arterial and venous networks surrounding the vaginal opening.

difficulties in adjusting to the change from one phase to the next phase of a relationship.

Adolescence

An adolescent usually has a high capacity for sexual arousal and a need to find out whether he or she is sexually attractive. Alongside the need to learn about sexual behaviour there is emotional vulnerability. Unsatisfactory sexual experience at this time can set the scene for continuing problems later. Young women in their late teens are at high risk of unwanted pregnancy due to uncertainty about contraceptive needs.

The couple

The early months of a relationship may be characterized by frequent sex, but a couple need to learn quickly how to establish good communication and to adjust their sexual behaviour to each other's needs. Otherwise, dysfunctional patterns may develop; for example, of premature ejaculation, or of the man continually making inappropriate sexual advances and being rebuffed.

Early parenthood

The time taken for sexual interest to return after childbirth is variable and in some women can be a year or more. Problems may be due to a painful episiotomy or postnatal depression but more commonly are due to tiredness and the difficulty of coping with the demands of the new baby.

Middle age

When the novelty of a sexual relationship has worn off, sexual activity becomes less frequent and this may cause anxieties. Couples may feel they 'ought' to be having sex more often. Stresses at work for both partners may combine with social commitments to make it difficult to relax together. In the years before the menopause women often have menstrual problems. After the menopause there may be a reduction in sexual interest or a problem with vaginal dryness; these can usually be corrected by hormone replacement therapy. One partner may no longer find the other physically attractive, or may be increasingly put off by what he or she considers irritating characteristics.

Old age

Loss of erectile capacity increases with age and may also be due to physical disease **(Fig. 12.5)**. Couples used to an active sex life may find these changes difficult to accept and men may seek treatment to restore their youthful abilities.

The functions of sex

It is important to remember how much people differ from one another and how wide the range of normality may be.

Reproduction

Now that the average number of children per family is around two, reproductive sex is often limited to a short interval in a couple's relationship. Couples who have had a problem with infertility may find that it causes difficulty with their sex life, or conversely may find that after they achieve pregnancy it is difficult to have sex for pleasure only.

Pleasure

Though sex is readily associated in people's minds with pleasure, the many taboos that surround it make purely 'recreational' sex more often a fantasy than a reality.

Pair-bonding

Enjoying sex means lowering one's defences, and sharing this experience strengthens the bond between the partners. People who have had to build particularly strong

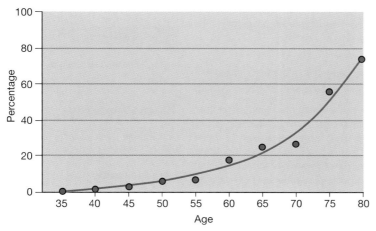

Fig. 12.5 Impotence increases with age. (From Bancroft 1989, with permission. Data from Kinsey et al 1948.)

defences – for example, after emotional abuse in childhood – may have difficulty in relinquishing them.

Asserting masculinity or femininity

People may use sexual activity to reassure themselves about their sexuality. This is normal in adolescence, but for some people the pattern continues or recurs at times of stress.

Bolstering self-esteem

Satisfactory sex improves a person's self-esteem and unsatisfactory sex has the opposite effect. People who have had an unsatisfactory sexual relationship may hurry straight into another one to try to re-establish their confidence, often with the opposite result.

Achieving power

Some people see the sexual relationship in terms of dominance and submission. This can apply to coitus itself, or to the power to allow or deny access to sex.

Expressing hostility

For many people anger is incompatible with sexual arousal but for some people anger enhances arousal and aggressive sex may be used to express anger. Rape or sexual assault may have more to do with aggression than with sex.

Reducing anxiety or tension

The use of orgasm to relieve tension applies particularly to people who habitually masturbate. They may do so more often at times of stress. A person who has got used to relieving sexual tension by masturbation may have difficulty adjusting to a shared sex life after marriage.

Risk-taking

The risks of sexual activity range from fear of discovery to contracting HIV infection. For some people, an element of risk adds to their pleasure.

Material gain

Prostitution is the most obvious form of sex for gain, and is often the result of poverty. Marriage, even nowadays, may also be a way of using sex to buy security.

History-taking

Some sexual problems may present disguised as another symptom such as pelvic pain, or are discovered apparently fortuitously, for example when a routine enquiry is made about contraception. It is inappropriate to take a detailed sexual history from every patient whatever their complaint, but it is reasonable, particularly in a gynaecological clinic, to ask one or two questions about sex as a matter for routine; for example, 'Do you have any trouble with intercourse?' or, if appropriate, 'Is this symptom worse after intercourse?' For some patients this will not be necessary, but for others

it will be a chance to mention a sex problem. An evasive reply may suggest that all is not well. Obtaining accurate information requires skill and practice.

Elucidating a sexual problem relies mainly on the history, though useful information may be obtained from examination or investigation. The interviewer must be comfortable with the subject as the patient is likely to be embarrassed by talking about a sexual problem. A sympathetic but matter-of-fact approach may help to reduce this embarrassment. The vocabulary used must also be appropriate, using words that avoid, on the one hand, being too technical and, on the other hand, appearing too crude.

It is usually helpful to see both partners, but not necessarily together on the first occasion. A patient may be more frank if interviewed alone, but the partner may give quite a different version of the history. When treatment is planned, however, both partners should ideally be involved.

The history needs to be thorough, but, if too intrusive, it may be off-putting. If a topic seems painful, the subject can be changed and then returned to later. Sometimes more than one interview is necessary, with sensitive topics being explored on the second occasion after a rapport has been built up. A detailed account of a specific instance may be more helpful than asking general questions. For example, if the patient is asked 'How often do you have intercourse?' the reply is likely to be a vague guess which depends partly on what the patient thinks is expected (e.g. 'About twice a week'). It may be better to ask 'When did you last have intercourse?', and then, if the couple's last attempt was unsatisfactory, to ask in detail about what went wrong. Open-ended questions should also be used; for example, 'How did you feel when that happened?'

Many patients, especially if talking about their sexual problem for the first time, find it difficult to put their feelings into words. It may be helpful to offer the occasional summing-up: 'What I think you're saying is that …'. The patient will usually give a clearly positive response if the doctor has summed up the situation correctly. If the patient's response is more guarded, the doctor should be cautious about the conclusions drawn.

Sex problems

Problems with sex include sexual variations and sexual dysfunction.

Sexual variations

Only a minority of patients requesting treatment are homosexual or have problems of deviant sexuality.

Homosexuality

Homosexual behaviour has been tolerated or approved of in many primitive societies but widely rejected in western societies. Male homosexual acts were illegal in England until 1967 and the ban on lesbians and gay men in the armed forces was lifted only in the year 2000. Kinsey reported that 30% of men had experienced orgasm during a homosexual encounter at least once, but only about 3% were exclusively homosexual, with another 3% having extensive homosexual experience. The incidence of female homosexuality is much lower, with 6% of women having at least one homosexual experience, 2% having significant experience and 1% being exclusively homosexual.

Problems encountered by homosexual people are of two types: (1) sexual dysfunction or (2) dissatisfaction with their sexual orientation. Fear of an unsympathetic response may inhibit them from seeking treatment for dysfunction. Prejudice by their family or by society often adds to their problems.

Transsexuality

A transsexual is a man or woman who believes himself or herself to be of the opposite gender in spite of his or her anatomy. Transsexuals are likely to seek medical help to alter their bodies to be consistent with their psychological gender. There are a number of 'gender identity clinics' in various parts of the world, which provide specialist services for transsexuals, using the combined expertise of psychologists, psychiatrists, endocrinologists and surgeons.

Transvestism

A transvestite is someone who enjoys dressing in the clothes of the opposite gender. This group includes transsexuals and some homosexuals but also people (mainly men) who enjoy cross-dressing without the wish to change sex, and men who obtain sexual gratification from wearing women's clothes. A high proportion of the latter groups are married and parents: they may be referred to a specialist clinic because of the strain that their behaviour is putting on their relationship.

Sadomasochism

Moderate pain inflicted during sexual arousal (e.g. as a 'love bite') was enjoyed by 50% of subjects in Kinsey's study. Ritualized dominance and submission are enjoyed by a small number of people, almost entirely male, most of whom can switch between dominant and submissive roles. Submission may be a way of avoiding responsibility if sex is associated with guilt. Such people rarely request treatment.

Fetishism

Particular parts of the body, articles of clothing (e.g. shoes) or materials (e.g. nowadays, rubber or plastic) can become objects of sexual gratification. Fetishism hardly ever occurs in women. These men rarely request treatment.

Sexual dysfunction

Sexual dysfunction may be due to psychological or relationship problems or may have a medical or surgical cause. It is so common as to be almost physiological. Not everyone with sexual dysfunction considers that they have a problem. In one survey of married couples, nearly 66% of the women reported some degree of difficulty with arousal and 40% of the men reported problems, mainly premature ejaculation. In another study, only one-third of anorgasmic women considered themselves to have a problem.

The incidence of dysfunction varies with age. Kinsey reported that 50% of women had not experienced orgasm by their late teens: by the age of around 35 the proportion was 10%. Permanent erectile impotence becomes more common with age **(Fig. 12.5)**, the incidence rising from about 2% at age 40 to about 25% at 70 and 75% at 80, according to Kinsey's survey. This does not necessarily cause a problem if the woman's interest in sex has also decreased with age.

The common disorders of sexual function can be classified according to the physiological stages described early in this chapter:

- impaired desire (diminished libido in both sexes)
- disorders of arousal (erectile dysfunction in men, vaginismus in women)
- disorders of orgasm (premature ejaculation in men, anorgasmia, usually in women)
- dyspareunia (mainly in women).

The causes of sexual dysfunction can be classified into pathological or psychological factors but it is unhelpful to make a sharp distinction between the two as they often coexist. For example, painful intercourse due to a physical cause such as a herpetic lesion may lead to secondary anxiety in both partners. On the other hand, anxiety due to sexual abuse in childhood may lead to pelvic congestion or spasm of the pelvic floor muscles. Treatment often needs to be directed towards physical and psychological causes at the same time.

A list of pathological causes of sexual dysfunction is given in **Box 12.1**. These causes are more common in older people. More usually, however, the cause of sexual dysfunction is due to psychological factors. These can be classified as in **Box 12.2**.

Female sexual dysfunction

Impaired desire

This is the commonest symptom presenting to specialist sexual medicine clinics, although it is not such a frequent symptom in routine gynaecology clinics. The woman complains that she is just not interested in sex. Such 'loss of libido' may be primary or secondary. The unhelpful and offensive term 'frigidity' is no longer used.

Primary

Some women have never felt interested in sex and in these cases there is usually impairment of arousal and orgasm as well. The underlying cause is often in an upbringing in

---

Box 12.1

Pathological causes of sexual dysfunction

Medical disorders

- Acute and chronic illness
- Psychiatric illness
- Cancer – especially gynaecological
- Neurological problems, e.g. spinal cord injuries, multiple sclerosis, neuropathy
- Endocrine, e.g. diabetes
- Cardiovascular, e.g. myocardial infarction
- Respiratory
- Arthritic
- Renal, e.g. dialysis
- Gynaecological, e.g. vaginitis

Surgical procedures

- Mastectomy
- Colostomy
- Gynaecological – oophorectomy, episiotomy, vaginal repair
- Amputation

Drug effects

- Anticholinergics
- Anticonvulsants
- Antihypertensives
- Anti-inflammatories
- Hormones
- Hypnotics and sedatives
- Major tranquillizers
- Alcohol
- Opiates

Box 12.2

Psychological factors in sexual dysfunction

Remote

- Repressed family attitudes to sex
- Poor sex education
- Sexual or physical trauma

Precipitant

- Psychiatric illness
- Childbirth
- Infidelity
- Partner's dysfunction
- Relationship problem – may be cause or effect

Maintaining

- Anxiety
- Poor communication
- Lack of foreplay
- Depression
- Poor information

---

which sex was regarded as dirty. The woman may choose a partner who also has an apparently low sex drive.

Secondary

More commonly, loss of libido follows an interval of apparently normal sex drive, during the woman's teens or early 20s, or early in the relationship with her partner. Loss of interest in sex may occur after childbirth, when both parents (particularly the woman) devote all their attention to the baby, often nowadays combining motherhood with a return to the woman's paid employment. If there has been postnatal depression, this will exacerbate the problem.

Other causes include:

- depression
- bereavement
- the menopause
- gynaecological investigation, e.g. for an abnormal cervical smear; hysterectomy causes loss of libido in only a few instances, and more commonly improves a woman's sex life
- loss of self-esteem (e.g. problems at work).

Sometimes, the secondary loss of libido has no obvious specific cause. A woman who has suffered sexual or physical abuse in childhood, or who has had a sexually repressed upbringing, may go through a phase of normal or increased sexual activity in her teens and 20s and then present with loss of libido due to the long-term effects of her childhood experiences.

Often, the man reacts to the woman's loss of interest by making persistent sexual demands and then, after some years, giving up approaching her for sex. Loss of desire is often due to a problem with the relationship, and counselling will be directed towards improving communication between the partners. A specific cause, such as childhood abuse, may require specialist referral, e.g. for psychotherapeutic counselling. Hormone therapy is appropriate for postmenopausal women but not for those who still have a normal menstrual cycle.

Orgasmic dysfunction

Inability to achieve orgasm is usually associated with lack of interest in sex, but sometimes can be an isolated symptom in a woman who has an otherwise satisfactory sex drive and is able to experience normal arousal.

Primary

As noted above, Kinsey reported that 10% of women had never achieved orgasm by the age of 35, and other studies indicate that up to a third of women are dissatisfied in some way with their orgasmic ability. Only a small proportion of these will seek medical treatment.

Inability to achieve orgasm despite adequate arousal may be due to inexperience of the woman or her partner, or unrealistic expectations, e.g. reading erotic fiction may have led the couple to believe that orgasm occurs automatically on penetration. Sometimes, the cause is more deep-seated; because of childhood repression the woman is unable to let go her defences. Psychological counselling may be helpful.

Secondary

Secondary orgasmic dysfunction follows an interval of adequate sexual functioning. It is usually associated with reduced desire or arousal, as discussed in the previous section.

Situational orgasmic dysfunction

Some women can achieve orgasm through masturbation but not coitus, or with one partner but not with another.

Vaginismus

Vaginismus is involuntary spasm of the pelvic floor muscles and perineal muscles, provoked by attempted penetration. It is also provoked by vaginal examination or by attempts to insert a tampon or the woman's own finger into the vagina. When severe, the conditioned reflex includes spasm of the adductor muscles of the thighs.

Primary

In most cases the problem is primary vaginismus and is discovered during the first attempt at intercourse. It may be due to apprehension that intercourse will be painful or due simply to failure to control the pelvic musculature. Persistent attempts at penetration cause more pain and a 'vicious circle' is set up, reinforcing the vaginismus.

Primary vaginismus may also be due to more deepseated psychological problems, such as an unwillingness to accept sexual maturity, or sexual repression in childhood.

Secondary

Vaginismus may also follow a physically painful experience, such as a sexual assault, an obstetric problem at delivery or an insensitive vaginal examination.

Management of vaginismus

The vulva and vagina should be examined for any painful lesion, though in most cases no such cause will be found. In a few cases examination will reveal a firm intact hymen and this may require dilatation under anaesthesia. This is necessary in only a small minority of cases.

Most cases of primary and secondary vaginismus respond well to simple treatment, involving training in relaxation and the use of vaginal dilators. The woman should be helped to relax completely: she should let her head rest on the pillow and vaginal examination should not be attempted until the adductor muscles of the thighs have fully relaxed. The woman is then taught to insert a small vaginal dilator: such patients need a combination of gentleness and encouragement to overcome their apprehension. Once she is comfortable about inserting the small dilator regularly, she can progress to gradually larger sizes. During treatment she is also taught pelvic floor exercises, which help her to gain control of the muscles. It may take several weeks or months before full control is achieved.

Attempts at intercourse should be discouraged until she is able to insert the larger-sized vaginal dilators. In some cases it then becomes apparent that the husband has a problem with erectile dysfunction, but in most instances satisfactory intercourse follows. An alternative to vaginal dilators is for the woman to use her own finger and then for the partner to insert one and then two fingers into the vagina. In most instances that present to the clinic, however, the couple are reluctant to do this and prefer the dilators. If primary vaginismus is due to more deep-seated problems, treatment may take many months and the prognosis is less good. Psychotherapy may be appropriate in these cases.

Dyspareunia

Pain on intercourse is the commonest sexual problem presenting to the routine gynaecology clinic. It is usually classified into superficial and deep dyspareunia, but it is not always possible to make a clear distinction between the two **(Box 12.3)**. With superficial dyspareunia, there is a pain at the vaginal introitus on attempted penetration, often making full intercourse impossible. In deep dyspareunia there is pain in the pelvis on deep penetration. Bimanual examination may reveal a specific area of tenderness, e.g. on moving the cervix or on palpating the posterior fornix, the rectum, or one or other lateral fornix. Sometimes, however, the tenderness is more general and a specific site cannot be identified.

Examination of the vulva may reveal the inflammatory appearance of candidal infection, the lesions of herpes, or the presence of atrophy or dystrophy. Careful examination may be necessary to reveal the localized inflammation of vestibulitis. Vulval and vaginal swabs should be taken for microbiological examination and treatment given if appropriate. If no cause is found for what appears to be superficial dyspareunia, it may be necessary to consider the causes of deep dyspareunia.

Deep dyspareunia is often associated with other symptoms such as dysmenorrhoea or persistent pelvic pain. The history should include questions about bowel habit. Bowel dysfunction is not uncommon and can be treated with a high-fibre diet. The timing of the pain in relation to the cycle should also be noted – it may occur just before ovulation or menstruation. Bimanual examination may reveal a pelvic mass.

The finding of a retroverted uterus is unlikely to be significant, as uterine retroversion is common. Occasionally, however, a sharply retroverted uterus can be the only site of tenderness. High vaginal and cervical swabs should be taken if there is any suspicion of pelvic infection. In most

---

Box 12.3

Causes of dyspareunia

Superficial dyspareunia

- Infection, e.g. candida, herpes
- Atrophic change, particularly after the menopause
- Vulval dystrophy
- Vaginismus

Deep dyspareunia

- Endometriosis
- Pelvic inflammatory disease
- Bowel dysfunction
- Pelvic mass
- 'Unexplained' pelvic pain

cases laparoscopy is necessary to diagnose or exclude endometriosis or pelvic inflammatory disease.

When a specific cause is identified, the appropriate treatment is given. If laparoscopy is negative, a high-fibre diet may help even in the absence of obvious bowel symptoms. If no cause is found and the deep dyspareunia is not associated with other symptoms, the problem may be due to too little foreplay, leading to inadequate arousal and insufficient relaxation of the upper vagina. The couple should try allowing more time for arousal, and may be advised to avoid positions (such as the woman sitting on top of the man) in which penetration is particularly deep.

If deep dyspareunia is associated with 'unexplained pelvic pain', treatment can be difficult and may require a combination of endocrine manipulation and psychological support.

Male sexual dysfunction

Male sexual dysfunction can be classified as impairment of desire, erection or ejaculation. There is considerable overlap between these disorders.

Impaired desire

In the male, libido is dependent on normal testosterone levels, and serum testosterone should be checked in men complaining of lack of libido. If the level is normal, testosterone supplements are unlikely to help.

As noted above, male libido diminishes with age. This is not simply due to falling testosterone levels. Older men may seek treatment because they are unwilling to accept this physiological change.

There is an assumption among many men that the male should always be ready for sex. There is also a widespread expectation that medications exist which can increase libido. Male patients are often unwilling or unable to change a busy lifestyle which leaves little time for sex.

Erectile dysfunction

Inability to achieve or maintain a satisfactory erection ('impotence') is the commonest sex problem among men. It may be associated with impaired desire, but desire usually is normal. Indeed, the anxiety provoked by the erectile dysfunction may increase his awareness of sexual stimuli.

Erectile dysfunction is usually due to psychological factors but it is important to investigate possible physical causes. If a physical cause is found, it may indicate a general disease and it may be treatable. The patient may not accept a diagnosis of a psychological cause until possible physical causes have been excluded **(Box 12.4)**.

In addition to a full sexual history, the man should be asked about the duration of the problem, whether it is primary or secondary, and whether it is situational (i.e. does he get 'early morning' erections, or can he get an erection by masturbation but not with his partner). Enquiry should

---

> **Box 12.4**
>
> ### Physical causes of erectile failure
>
> **Endocrine disorders**
> - Disorders causing reduced plasma testosterone may cause erectile failure, but these usually cause loss of libido as well.
> - Diabetes may cause impotence. The incidence of erectile failure at age 50 is 40% among diabetic men, and only 5% among non-diabetic men. The mechanism may be either diabetic neuropathy or vascular disease.
>
> **Neurological disorders**
> - Multiple sclerosis may cause erectile failure.
> - Spinal injury causes erectile failure but, after the initial phase of 'spinal shock', reflex erectile ability may return if the sacral segments of the spinal cord are intact.
>
> **Vascular disorders**
> - There is a decline in sexual activity after myocardial infarction and, interestingly, before a heart attack.
> - Hypertension, when untreated, is also associated with erectile dysfunction.
>
> **Drugs**
> - Antihypertensives, particularly methyldopa, may cause erectile failure. Beta-blockers are less likely to cause erectile failure, though it can occur idiosyncratically.
>
> **Psychiatric illness**
> - Severe depression causes loss of sexual interest in over 60% of cases.
>
> **Surgery**
> - Prostatectomy need not cause impotence, particularly if it is by the transurethral or retropubic route. Perineal prostatectomy for cancer is a more radical operation and usually causes erectile failure.
>
> **Physiological**
> - Ageing reduces the frequency of erections. Some men may also fail to understand the refractory period, and may have unrealistic expectations of how soon erection can recur after orgasm.

---

be made about symptoms of general disease, including those listed above; for example, does exercise bring on claudication?

Clinical examination should include a check for signs of systemic disease. The genitalia should be examined for abnormalities of the penis (such as hypospadias) or abnormally small testes. Serum testosterone should be checked as a matter of routine, and, if it is low, serum sent for follicle-stimulating hormone (FSH) and prolactin assay.

Drug treatment is now often used in addition to, or instead of, psychosexual counselling. Therapeutic options include:

- Phosphodiesterase inhibitors, e.g. sildenafil (Viagra). Penile erection is due to relaxation of the smooth muscle around the cavernosal vascular spaces, allowing them to fill with blood. This is under the control of the autonomic nervous system, mediated by cyclic guanosine monophosphate (cGMP). These drugs are taken orally and enhance erection by blocking breakdown of cGMP. Alternatives to sildenafil are vardenafil (Levitra), which acts more quickly, and tadalafil (Cialis), which has a longer duration of action. They work best in psychogenic erectile failure and milder organic problems, in which the success rate is ≈ 85%. Side-effects are mild and transient and include flushing, dyspepsia, headache and disturbance to colour vision. These drugs must not be used by men who use nitrates or have severe cardiac disease, as they may lead to a life-threatening profound drop in blood pressure.

- Alprostadil (PGE_1). This drug also relaxes cavernosal smooth muscle but has to be injected directly into the corpora cavernosa. It is more effective than sildenafil in erectile failure due to more severe organic problems. It is also available as a urethral pellet (MUSE) but this is much less effective.
- Other treatments used include vacuum devices **(Fig. 12.6)** and penile implants, the latter only where no other treatment has been effective.

Ejaculatory dysfunction

The most common type of ejaculatory dysfunction is premature ejaculation. Retarded ejaculation is much less common and may be associated with other psychological problems. Painful ejaculation is relatively rare.

Premature ejaculation is normal in early sexual experiences. It is difficult to define, and the best guide is if the man feels he has insufficient control to satisfy himself and his partner. Sometimes, ejaculation occurs before penetration or within a few seconds of penetration. The cause of premature ejaculation is usually psychological, with anxiety increasing each time the problem occurs.

Treatment requires the cooperation of the partner and it is difficult to help a man who presents for treatment without his partner's knowledge. If the couple have a good relationship, they can be instructed in the 'stop–start' technique, in which the partner manually stimulates the penis until orgasm is near, when he signals her to stop. Practice with this technique helps to build a feeling of control. The 'squeeze' technique – firm pressure at the level of the frenulum – may also help to retard ejaculation.

Treatment of sexual problems

The treatment of sexual problems can be divided into two categories:

- counselling, which should be within the scope of a general practitioner
- sex therapy, which requires specialist training.

Counselling

Some problems can be helped by a single consultation or a few consultations. Simple counselling may include the following.

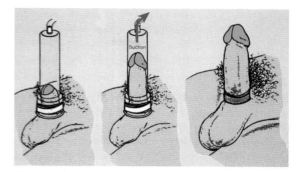

Fig. 12.6 The use of a vacuum device to manage impotence.

Permission-giving

A patient may become very anxious about some activity, such as masturbation, and may be helped to know that it is normal. Simply talking about sexual matters in a matter-of-fact way is helpful to many patients who feel they are unique in experiencing difficulties.

Limited information

An explanation of normal anatomy or physiology may also be helpful. He or she may be reassured by an examination, which shows that the genitalia are normal. The clinician may also recommend a book which explains sexual matters.

Advice

Commonsense advice on sexual technique may be helpful. In spite of the apparent openness about sexual matters in many countries, many people do not seem to understand the importance of foreplay, the pleasures of non-penetrative sex, or the fact that the positions adopted during intercourse can be varied. Many couples, with both partners leading busy lives, seem to expect to be able to 'switch on' sexual activity during the brief interlude when it is convenient, and sensible advice about making time for each other may be helpful.

Sex therapy

Some problems are resistant to simple counselling and require specialist referral. Specialist treatment usually involves an average of about 12 sessions. About two-thirds of couples benefit from specialist therapy; vaginismus and premature ejaculation respond particularly well, but results are less good for reduced desire. The components of therapy are a graduated behavioural programme and counselling.

Graduated behavioural programme

This involves first banning attempts at intercourse or touching the breasts or genitalia. 'Sensate focus' then follows, in which the partners make time to touch each other's bodies, tell each other what feels enjoyable, and relax without feeling pressure to have sex. The third stage is to touch the genital areas, though the ban on intercourse remains. After that stage, the couple progress to 'vaginal containment', which means penetration without movement, and then to intercourse including movement within the vagina.

Counselling

The graduated behavioural programme usually takes several months, and while the couple are proceeding through it they attend regularly for counselling. The counsellor may help the couple to reconsider their attitudes to sexual matters, and may discuss the feelings they have for sex and for each other. Counselling also involves permission-giving, education, reassurance, summing up feelings that the couple may not have recognized, and reinforcing positive aspects of the relationship.

Conclusion

Sexual problems cause much unhappiness and may present to any clinician. Some can be treated easily with simple advice; others need more prolonged specialist treatment. A few never respond to treatment. The main aim for a young doctor is to be able to discuss the subject comfortably. This is not easy, particularly when the patient is older than the doctor but still expects advice because the doctor has a medical degree. With sexual problems, more than with many aspects of medicine, the learning curve is long.

When treatment is successful, however, patients are very grateful and it can be very gratifying to be able to help so much, merely by listening and talking to them.

Key *points*

- Sexual problems are important and history-taking requires considerable skill. The problems may present directly or in the guise of another condition or may be discovered coincidentally.
- Normal sexual response has five phases: desire (general sexual interest), arousal (which involves central and genital responses), orgasm, resolution, and a refractory phase during which further arousal does not occur.
- Sexual response varies with age and with different phases of a relationship.
- Sex has several functions in addition to reproduction, e.g. the strengthening of the pair bond.
- Commonest male problems include erectile failure and premature ejaculation.
- Commonest female problems include loss of libido, orgasmic dysfunction and vaginismus.
- Causes of sexual dysfunction may be physical, medical or psychological. Psychological factors include predisposing factors (e.g. poor sex education or childhood abuse). Dysfunction is also more likely after childbirth, or if there has been infidelity, anxiety or poor communication.
- Treatment involves counselling and education, hormonal therapy, and relaxation exercises. Sometimes, couple, group or psychotherapy is required.

13

Female genital infections

Introduction

Genital infections in females can be caused by sexually transmitted infections (STIs) such as *Chlamydia trachomatis* or human papillomavirus (HPV), or by infections such as bacterial vaginosis and *Candida albicans* which are not sexually transmitted. The World Health Organization (WHO) in 2002 identified unsafe sex as the second most important cause (after being underweight) of ill-health in the world, causing 17% of all economic losses through ill-health in the developing countries. It estimates that there are over 340 million cases of the four major curable STIs (syphilis, gonorrhoea, chlamydia and trichomoniasis) in adults aged 15–49 throughout the world each year, 90% in developing countries. The Joint United Nations Programme on HIV/AIDS (UNAIDS) estimated that in 2007, 33 million adults and children were living with HIV/AIDS worldwide. The incidence of new HIV infections peaked in the late 1990s at around 3 million per year. Currently around 70% of the 2.5 million new HIV infections each year occur in sub-Saharan Africa, where three women are newly infected to every two men. African women aged 15–24 carry an even more disproportionate burden of infection, with a ratio of three women to every one man infected.

There have been dramatic changes in the pattern of infections over the past 50 years. In the UK there was a decline in syphilis following the end of the Second World War, and in gonorrhoea from the 1970s, until the 1990s. However, during this time there was an increase in chlamydia, herpes, wart virus and HIV infections. From the mid-1990s the downward trend in the bacterial STIs then reversed, and viral STIs continued to increase. The number of new diagnoses of HIV in the UK doubled between 2000 and 2004, stabilizing at around 7800 new cases per year. Between 1997 and 2006, cases of chlamydial infection increased year on year by a total of 294%. In contrast, gonorrhoea rates rose steadily to a peak in 2002 and then declined. A dramatic rise in cases of syphilis between 2000 and 2006 is largely attributable to cases in men, particularly men-who-have-sex-with-men, although there has also been a 438% rise in cases in women. Rises in STIs in women have been greatest in those aged 15–19 years, and have continued despite advances in diagnosis and treatment. Among the factors believed responsible for the increases are changes in sexual behaviour, particularly the use of non-barrier contraceptives, the emergence of drug-resistant strains, symptomless carriers, a highly mobile population, lack of public education, and the reluctance of some patients to seek treatment.

STIs including *Chlamydia trachomatis,* syphilis and genital herpes can cause long-term morbidity. In women, untreated infections can lead to chronic pain or infertility and may significantly increase susceptibility to sexual transmission of HIV. During pregnancy they may cause miscarriage, premature birth, or infection of the newborn. Certain features increase the likelihood of someone having an STI. These are: age under 25 years; lack of barrier contraception use; being single, separated or divorced; and having an occupation involving staying away from home. Also, women undergoing termination of pregnancy and those with an infection such as genital warts are at increased risk of STIs. In reality these factors are surrogate markers of sexual activity and rates of partner change, which are what mainly determine the risk of transmission and acquisition of an STI. For many women, particularly in developing countries, it is the social and demographic risk factors affecting the community from which she chooses a regular partner, rather than her own individual risk factors, that determine STI risk.

Principles of STI management

Most STIs are asymptomatic and only a small proportion of women who present with symptoms such as vaginal discharge have an STI. Confining STI testing to those who present with symptoms has little or no effect on prevalence. Many of the more serious infections may cause no symptoms in women until complications arise, so prompt diagnosis and appropriate management is crucial in reducing adverse outcomes. About 70% of women with chlamydia, 50% with gonorrhoea, 65% with pelvic inflammatory disease (PID), 30% with genital warts, and 50% with genital herpes have no symptoms. Programmes of vaccination, opportunistic testing and epidemiological treatment, based on population or subpopulation risk factors in women attending for other routine healthcare are an important factor in control. Opt-out testing for HIV and syphilis infection are routine parts of antenatal care in the UK, and screening for chlamydia in women and men under 25 is becoming widespread. In clinical practice, the only way to detect these infections is by examining and testing for them in both symptomatic and asymptomatic women. The clinician must be alert to the presence of risk factors in the clinical history: women under 25 seeking contraception, for example, should always be offered testing for chlamydia.

Partner notification (contact tracing) is an essential part of the management of curable bacterial STIs to prevent re-infection and to avoid further onward transmission. Partner notification strategies include: patient referral, where the patient informs recent partner(s); provider referral, where details are passed to a healthcare professional who then contacts the partners; and conditional referral, where provider referral is initiated if patient referral has not occurred after an agreed period in as elapsed. In provider referral it is usual to protect the identity of the index patient. Enhanced partner notification strategies such as providing the patient with antibiotic treatment for the partner, or with a pharmacy voucher for treatment, are also used. Patients should abstain from sex until they and their partner(s) have completed treatment. A follow-up consultation (in person or by phone) may be performed after treatment to check that medication has been completed, that there has been sexual abstinence, and that the partner(s) has been treated.

The need to accurately assess risk factors and to sensitively and appropriately identify current and previous partners makes good sexual history-taking a critical factor in STI management.

Sexual history

A woman who is complaining of genital symptoms expects to be asked questions related to this, but may or may not have considered the possibility of an STI. Asymptomatic women attending for other reasons, such as termination of pregnancy, may also be unaware of STI risk. Time, sensitivity and privacy must be ensured: interviews should take place in a soundproof setting. Accurate answers to a risk assessment may not be possible with a partner or relative present. Questioning should be sensitive, inclusive and appropriate, but direct, and avoid euphemisms. As with all history-taking, choice of words, and appropriate facial expressions and body language in the questioner are important. Use open language to avoid conveying any impression of being judgmental; examples are the use of inclusive words such as 'partner' rather than 'boyfriend'. Permission-giving might involve providing a selection of possible answers to a question that includes those which might be judged socially or morally unacceptable, such as non-use of condoms, or anal intercourse. Carefully introducing subjects or words that the patient might find difficult, the words 'consent' and 'rape' for example, can help with disclosure.

The history-taking should start by asking about the presenting complaint. An open question followed by more open questions is usually the best approach. A small number of direct closed questions will often clarify details of vaginal discharge, dysuria, vulval lumps or ulcers, or lower abdominal pain. Supplementary questions about these symptoms are given below. The patient should then be asked about her gynaecological history. The final part should be the sexual history, in order to assess the risk of STIs. Asking 'Do you have a (sexual) partner?' can be a gentler introduction if the woman is not expecting questions about sexual contacts. This can lead to questions about the woman's most recent sexual exposure:

- How long ago was it?
- Was this with a regular or casual partner?
- If a regular partner, how long has the relationship been?
- Was it a man or a woman?
- What kind of contraception/protection was used?
- If condoms were used, were they used consistently and properly, and have there been any recent breakages?
- Has the sexual partner got any genital symptoms?

Other sexual partners Asking about 'previous' sexual partners immediately conveys an expectation of serial monogamy, making it even harder for a woman to disclose a concurrent partner. Around 9% of sexually active women in the UK report a concurrent sexual partnership in the previous year.

- When did she last have sex with a different partner? If within the past few months, the same details as above need to be obtained.
- How many different partners have there been over the past few months?

Assessment of HIV risk Supplementary questions about risk of exposure to HIV infection should also be asked:

- Has the woman ever injected drugs?
- Are any male partners known to be bisexual, injecting drug users, or from areas of the world with high HIV levels such as sub-Saharan Africa and Asia?

Examination for genital infections

Clinical symptoms are not helpful at indicating the site of infection and are of limited use in determining which infection is likely to be present. Examination and microbiological testing should therefore be performed. It is again important to consider the setting in which an examination is performed. It should be in a private room and the woman should be provided with a gown to cover the areas not being examined. All women should be offered a chaperone for both the history and examination regardless of the practitioner's gender. It is essential that all males have a chaperone when examining a woman's genital tract. The procedure should be explained to the woman prior to the examination. Simple considerations, such as making sure the patient is in a comfortable position and warming the speculum, will usually result in a more cooperative patient. This will allow a thorough examination with properly taken swabs. The woman should be in the lithotomy position, and there should be a good light source behind the examiner. The following genital examination should be performed:

- Inspect the pubic hair and surrounding skin for pubic lice and any skin rashes.
- Palpate the inguinal region for lymphadenopathy.
- Inspect the labia majora and minora, clitoris, introitus, perineum and perianal area for warts, ulcers, erythema or excoriation.
- Inspect the urethral meatus and Skene's (history box) and Bartholin's glands for any discharge or swelling.
- Insert a bivalve speculum into the vagina.
- Inspect the vaginal walls for erythema, discharge, warts, ulcers.
- Inspect the cervix for discharge, erythema, contact bleeding, ulcers or raised lesions. Mucopurulent discharge from the cervix is not a reliable indicator of infection.
- Perform a bimanual pelvic examination to assess size and any tenderness of the uterus, cervical motion tenderness (cervical excitation) and adnexal tenderness or masses.

 History

Alexander Johnston Chalmers Skene (1837–1900) was a Scottish gynaecologist who described the lesser vestibular, periurethral glands, also known as the Skene's glands.

Taking swabs for genital infections

It is important that swabs are performed adequately and that the specimen is placed in the appropriate culture or transport medium. For urethral and endocervical specimens, cellular material needs to be obtained. To take a urethral specimen, a fine swab should be gently inserted into the urethral opening rotated and then placed in the medium. For an endocervical sample, the swab should be inserted about 1 cm into the endocervical canal and it should be rotated for several seconds and placed in the medium. Nucleic acid amplification testing (NAAT) is increasingly available for chlamydia, gonorrhoea, herpes simplex, and, less commonly, syphilis and trichomoniasis.

The swabs required will depend on the laboratory facilities available locally and the symptoms, but assessment may include the following:

- A urethral swab for culture for gonorrhoea placed in Amies, Stuart's or similar transport medium.
- A first-pass urine sample for chlamydia DNA amplification testing (if genital examination is not possible).
- Observe the vaginal discharge to see if it has the homogeneous, white appearance typical of bacterial vaginosis.
- Swab the lateral vaginal walls and the pool of discharge in the posterior fornix. Smear some of the discharge onto a glass slide and allow to air dry (for Gram staining by the laboratory for clue cells, pseudohyphae and spores). Place the swab in Amies, Stuart's or similar transport medium for *Candida* and *Trichomonas vaginalis* culture.
- Test the pH of the vaginal discharge either by touching the swab used to take the vaginal specimen onto narrow-range pH paper, or the paper can be pressed against the lateral vaginal walls with sponge holders. It is important that cervical secretions are avoided for this, as cervical mucus has a pH of 7 and any contamination will give a falsely high reading.
- Any vaginal secretions should be wiped from the cervix.
- An endocervical swab for identification of gonorrhoea (for culture placed in Amies, Stuart's or similar transport medium with the urethral swab, or into a commercial medium for gonococcal DNA amplification testing).
- An endocervical sample for chlamydia DNA amplification testing.
- A blood sample for syphilis serology.
- A blood sample for hepatitis B testing if the woman or any of her sexual partners are from areas of high hepatitis B prevalence (e.g. sub-Saharan Africa or Asia), followed by hepatitis B immunization if the test is negative.
- A blood sample for hepatitis B and C testing if the woman or any of her sexual partners have ever injected drugs, followed by hepatitis B immunization if the test is negative.
- A blood sample for HIV testing if the patient gives informed consent.
- If vesicles, ulcers or fissures are seen, a sample for herpes culture should be taken from the base of the lesion and sent to the laboratory in viral transport medium.

Symptoms associated with genital infections

None

Many infections are completely asymptomatic, so testing should be considered on the basis of risk factors.

Vaginal discharge

An increase in vaginal discharge may be due to a number of infective and non-infective conditions **(Table 13.1)**. Even in areas of high STI prevalence, the great majority of women presenting with vaginal discharge will not have an STI. Physiological discharge can only be diagnosed after negative swabs have excluded the infective causes.

Questions that help discriminate between the various causes are:

- Does the discharge have an offensive odour?
- Is there any vulval itching or soreness?
- Are there any other symptoms such as dysuria, intermenstrual or postcoital bleeding, or abdominal pain?

Dysuria

Dysuria is usually due to acute bacterial cystitis, urethritis or vulvitis **(Table 13.2)**. External dysuria, particularly in the absence of frequency or abdominal pain, indicates irritation at the urethral meatus.

Questions that help distinguish between the causes are:

- Is the dysuria external, i.e. is it as the urine comes into contact with the vulval mucosa?
- Is there any urinary frequency, nocturia or haematuria?
- Is there any vaginal discharge, postcoital or intermenstrual bleeding, or abdominal pain?
- Are there any vulval sores or itching?

Vulval lumps

Raised lesions on the vulva can be due to infections, or anatomical variants. Genital warts are by far the most common cause of vulval lumps **(Table 13.3)**.

Questions that help distinguish between the causes are:

- Are the lumps painful?
- How many are there?
- How long have they been present?
- Are there any other symptoms such as dysuria, intermenstrual or postcoital bleeding, or abdominal pain?

Vulval ulcers

Infective lesions are the most common cause of vulval ulcers, with genital herpes being the main infection in the UK **(Table 13.4)**.

Table 13.1	
Causes of vaginal discharge	
Vaginal infections	Bacterial vaginosis *Candida albicans* *Trichomonas vaginalis*
Cervical infections	*Chlamydia trachomatis* *Neisseria gonorrhoeae*
Physiological discharge	Cervical ectopy
Other causes	Retained tampon Retained products of conception

Table 13.2	
Causes of dysuria	
Acute bacterial cystitis	Coliform bacteria *Staphylococcus saprophyticus*
Urethritis	*Chlamydia trachomatis* *Neisseria gonorrhoeae*
Vulvitis	Genital herpes Candidal infection *Trichomonas vaginalis* Vulval dermatological conditions

Table 13.3	
Causes of vulval lumps	
Viral infections	Genital warts Molluscum contagiosum Vulval intraepithelial neoplasia and vulval cancer
Bacterial infections	Syphilitic condylomata lata Skene's or Bartholin's gland abscesses due to *Chlamydia trachomatis* or *Neisseria gonorrhoeae*
Anatomical variants	Sebaceous glands Vulval papillae
Other	Sebaceous cysts

Table 13.4	
Vulval ulcers – types	
Infective	Genital herpes Syphilis
Non-infective	Aphthous ulcers Behçet's syndrome (history box)

Behçet's disease is named after Hulusi Behçet (1889–1948), a Turkish dermatologist and scientist who first recognized the syndrome in one of his patients in 1924.

Questions that help distinguish between the causes are:

- Are the ulcers painful?
- How many are there?
- How long have they been present?
- Are there any other symptoms such as dysuria, inter-menstrual or postcoital bleeding, or abdominal pain?

Lower abdominal pain

Lower abdominal pain can be caused by a number of differing conditions **(Table 13.5)**. Infective causes are particularly common in young (under 25 years) sexually active women.

Questions that help distinguish between the causes are:

- Is there any vaginal discharge, postcoital or intermenstrual bleeding, or deep dyspareunia?
- When was her last menstrual period (LMP), what contraception has she been using, and is there any possibility of her being pregnant?
- Has she any dysuria, urinary frequency, nocturia or haematuria?
- Has she any nausea, vomiting, diarrhoea or constipation?

Specific infections

Bacterial vaginosis (BV)

Background information

BV is the most common cause of vaginal discharge in women of reproductive age, found in around 9% of women in general practice, 12% of pregnant women, and 30% of women undergoing termination of pregnancy. BV is due to an overgrowth of anaerobic bacteria, genital mycoplasmas and *Gardnerella vaginalis* (all of which can be present in small numbers in the vagina). It is not sexually acquired, so sexual partners do not need to be treated.

Symptoms and signs

- About 50% of women with BV are asymptomatic.
- If symptoms are present, they are mainly increased vaginal discharge and fishy odour, usually without any itch or irritation. The odour is often worse after sexual intercourse and during menstruation.

Table 13.5

Causes of lower abdominal pain

Uterus	Endometritis due to *Chlamydia trachomatis*, *Neisseria gonorrhoeae* or bacterial vaginosis Endometriosis
Fallopian tubes	Salpingitis due to *C. trachomatis* and/or *N. gonorrhoeae* Ectopic pregnancy
Ovary	Torsion of, or haemorrhage into, an ovarian cyst
Urinary tract	Cystitis
Bowel	Acute appendicitis Irritable bowel syndrome

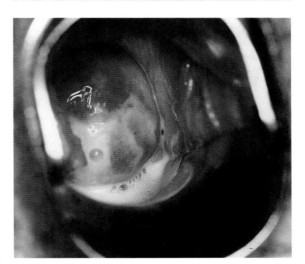

Fig. 13.1 Bacterial vaginosis. BV is due to an overgrowth of anaerobic bacteria, genital mycoplasmas and *Gardnerella vaginalis*. The discharge is milky white, adherent to the vaginal walls, and may be frothy.

- On examination, the discharge is milky white and adherent to the vaginal walls, and may be frothy **(Fig. 13.1)**. There is no inflammation of the vulva or vagina.

Diagnosis

A Gram-stained vaginal smear showing a depletion of normal lactobacilli and the presence of mixed organisms is the preferred method of diagnosis. BV can also be diagnosed clinically. Amsel's criteria require that three of the following should be present: the typical thin homogeneous discharge on examination; vaginal pH greater than 4.5; amine odour after adding 10% potassium hydroxide to the vaginal fluid (the whiff test); clue cells on microscopy (at least 20% of all epithelial cells). The latter are epithelial cells covered with bacteria that are 'clues' to the diagnosis. Where microscopy is unavailable, a combination of typical symptoms and a raised pH may be used to make a presumptive diagnosis. Menses, semen, and infection with *T. vaginalis* can also give a raised pH and positive amine test. Culture of vaginal secretions has no place in the diagnosis of BV. 30–50% of women are colonized with *G. vaginalis*, anaerobes and mycoplasmas, as part of their normal vaginal flora.

Treatment and management

Treatment is recommended in all women with symptoms and those undergoing gynaecological surgery (including termination of pregnancy), and recommended treatments are:

- metronidazole 400 mg orally twice daily for 5–7 days
- metronidazole 2 g orally single dose
- metronidazole 0.75% vaginal gel, 5 g daily for 5 days
- clindamycin 2% vaginal cream, 5 g daily for 7 days.

Complications

BV increases vaginal vault infection following hysterectomy, postpartum endometritis following caesarean section, and post-abortal pelvic inflammatory disease (PID) after surgical termination of pregnancy. In pregnancy it may increase the risk of late miscarriage and preterm birth.

It increases a woman's risk of acquiring HIV infection two- to threefold.

Candidal infections

Background information

75% of all women experience at least one episode of symptomatic candida in their lifetime. About 20% of asymptomatic women have vaginal colonization with candida. Increased rates of colonization (30–40%) are found in pregnancy and uncontrolled diabetes. Recognized predisposing factors that are associated with symptomatic candida are pregnancy, diabetes, immunosuppression, antimicrobial therapy, and vulval irritation/trauma. It is not sexually acquired, so sexual partners do not need to be treated.

Symptoms and signs

- Vulval itching, present in nearly all symptomatic women. Thick, white vaginal discharge, vulval burning, external dysuria, and superficial dyspareunia may also be present.
- On examination, vulval erythema, sometimes with satellite lesions, fissuring, excoriation and oedema may be present. There may be the typical white plaques on the vaginal walls **(Fig. 13.2)**, but the discharge may be minimal.

Diagnosis

Microscopy and culture is the most sensitive method of diagnosis. Clinical diagnosis is insensitive, but sensitivity increases with the number of symptoms and signs present. Up to half of women who self-diagnose candidal infection have another condition.

Treatment and management

There are a number of effective intravaginal and oral antifungal agents available, such as:

- Topical treatments:
  - clotrimazole pessaries for 1, 3, or 6 nights
  - econazole pessaries for 1 or 3 nights
  - miconazole pessaries for 1 or 14 nights.
- Oral treatments (should not be used during pregnancy):
  - fluconazole 150 mg single dose
  - itraconazole 200 mg twice daily for 1 day.

Complications

There are no known long-term complications from candidal infections.

Chlamydia trachomatis

Background information

C. trachomatis is the most frequently seen bacterial STI, affecting at least 3–5% of sexually active women in the UK, and as many as 14% of those aged under 20 years. The natural history of infection is not fully understood and in around 50% of cases the infection resolves spontaneously without complications. However, it can cause pelvic inflammatory disease, chronic pain and infertility, so is considered to be a serious public health issue. Screening for, and treating, asymptomatic chlamydia reduces the rate of pelvic inflammatory disease, and some countries have instituted population screening programmes.

Symptoms and signs

- The cervix is the primary site of infection, but the urethra is also infected in about 50%.
- Approximately 70% of women with chlamydia are asymptomatic.
- If symptoms are present, they are usually non-specific, such as increased vaginal discharge and dysuria.
- Lower abdominal pain and intermenstrual bleeding may be present if the infection has spread beyond the cervix.
- On examination there may be mucopurulent cervicitis **(Fig. 13.3)** and/or contact bleeding **(Fig. 13.4)**, but the cervix may also look normal.

Diagnosis

The widely used method of choice is a nucleic acid amplification test such as PCR, with a sensitivity of over 90%. Cervical or vulvovaginal swab samples are suitable for PCR testing, and first voided urine samples are also satisfactory. Self-taken vulval swabs perform as well, or better than, physician-taken cervical swabs and may be used for home-based testing. Enzyme immunoassay (EIA) tests have sensitivity of only 60–70% and are outdated.

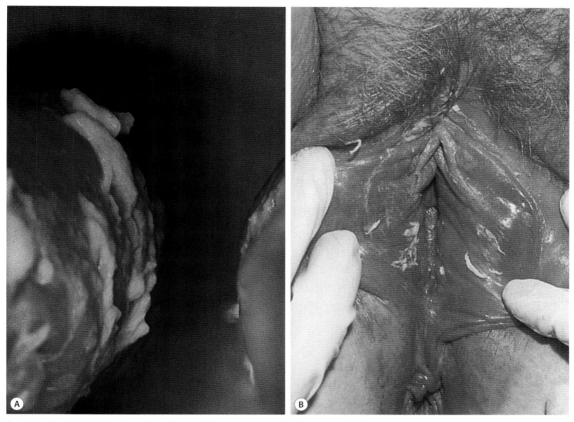

Fig. 13.2 Candidal infection. Although candida may present with these 'typical' white plaques, the discharge is sometimes minimal. (*A*, From McMillan A, Young H, Ogilvie MM, Scott GR (eds), *Clinical Practice in Sexually Transmissible Infections*, Saunders 2003. *B*, From Clutterbuck D, *Specialist Training in Sexually Transmitted Infections and HIV*, Mosby 2005.)

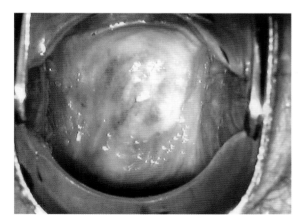

Fig. 13.3 Mucopurulent cervicitis. This may be a feature of infection with *C. trachomatis*. The cervix, however, can look normal.

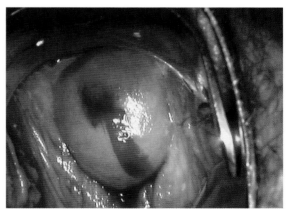

Fig. 13.4 Contact bleeding. This can occur for a number of reasons, one of which is *C. trachomatis* infection.

Treatment and management

Uncomplicated chlamydial infection can be treated with:

- azithromycin 1 g single dose
- doxycycline 100 mg twice daily for 1 week.

Pregnant and lactating women can be treated with:

- erythromycin 500 mg twice daily for 14 days.

Patients should abstain from sex until they and their partner(s) have completed treatment. A test of cure is not necessary, unless erythromycin has been prescribed (as it has a lower cure rate). However, reinfection rates are 10–30%, so retesting after 6–12 months is indicated.

Complications

C. trachomatis can spread beyond the lower genital tract, causing Skene's and Bartholin's gland abscesses, endometritis, salpingitis and perihepatitis. Around 3–10% of women with chlamydia develop symptomatic ascending infection (pelvic inflammatory disease; PID), which may lead to tubal damage, predisposing to tubal pregnancies and tubal infertility as well as causing chronic pain. Although asymptomatic upper genital tract infection also leads to tubal damage, the proportion of women who develop infertility following asymptomatic chlamydial infection is thought to be low (<1%). Chlamydial infection during pregnancy can cause miscarriage, preterm birth, postpartum infection and neonatal infection. In genetically susceptible people, a sexually acquired reactive arthritis (SARA) can occur (Reiter's syndrome – history box). Chlamydial infection increases a woman's risk of acquiring HIV infection three- to fourfold.

History

Hans Conrad Julius Reiter was a German bacteriologist and hygienist (1881–1969) who described the syndrome which in its full-blown picture consists of urethritis, arthritis and conjunctivitis.

Neisseria gonorrhoeae

Background information

Gonococcal infection rates are around 10-fold lower than those of chlamydia in the UK. There has been a steady fall in the number of infections in the UK since 2002. Rates are highest in women aged 15–19 years, in urban areas and in some black ethnic minority populations. *N. gonorrhoeae* is a highly adaptive organism and antibiotic resistance requires intensive and continuing surveillance.

Symptoms and signs

- The cervix is the primary site of infection, but the urethra is also infected in 70–90%.
- About 50% of women with gonorrhoea have no symptoms.
- The most common symptoms are increased vaginal discharge, dysuria, and postcoital bleeding.
- Lower abdominal pain and intermenstrual bleeding may also be present if the infection has spread beyond the cervix.
- On examination there may be a purulent **(Fig. 13.5)** or mucopurulent cervicitis and/or contact bleeding, but again the cervix may look normal.

Diagnosis

Nucleic acid amplification tests (NAAT) for *N. gonorrhoeae* are increasingly used and offer increased sensitivity but lower specificity than culture. Confirmation of NAAT positive results by culture is recommended and has the advantage of allowing antibiotic sensitivity testing.

Treatment and management

Uncomplicated gonorrhoea in all women, including pregnant and lactating women, can be treated with:

- cefixime 400 mg orally single dose
- ceftriaxone 250 mg i.m. single dose.

About 40% of females with gonorrhoea also have *C. trachomatis* infection, so they should be tested and treated for chlamydia. Patients should abstain from sex until they and their partner(s) have completed treatment.

Complications

N. gonorrhoeae can spread locally beyond the lower genital tract, causing Skene's and Bartholin's gland abscesses, endometritis, salpingitis and perihepatitis. About 10–20% of women with acute gonococcal infection will develop salpingitis, the resulting damage predisposing to tubal pregnancies and tubal infertility. Infection in pregnancy can cause miscarriage, preterm birth, postpartum infection and neonatal infection. Rarely, gonococcal septicaemia can occur and present as an acute arthritis/dermatitis syndrome (disseminated gonococcal infection). Gonorrhoea increases a woman's risk of acquiring HIV infection four- to fivefold.

Pelvic inflammatory disease (PID)

Background information

PID results when infections ascend from the cervix or vagina into the upper genital tract. It includes endometritis, salpingitis, tubo-ovarian abscess and pelvic peritonitis. The

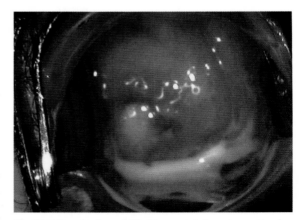

Fig. 13.5 Purulent cervicitis. The cervix is the primary site of infection in 90% of cases of gonococcal infection, and a purulent discharge may be seen.

main causes are *C. trachomatis* and *N. gonorrhoeae*, but *Mycoplasma hominis* and anaerobes are frequently also found. Sometimes in women with laparoscopically proven PID no bacterial cause is found. The true incidence of PID is unknown because about two-thirds of cases are asymptomatic.

Symptoms and signs

- Clinical symptoms and signs vary from none to very severe.
- The onset of symptoms often occurs in the first part of the menstrual cycle.
- Women with chlamydial PID usually have clinically milder disease than women with gonococcal PID.
- Lower abdominal pain is the most common symptom, with increased vaginal discharge, irregular bleeding, postcoital bleeding and deep dyspareunia also present in some women.
- The cervix may have a mucopurulent discharge with contact bleeding, indicative of cervicitis.
- Adnexal and cervical motion tenderness on bimanual examination is the most common sign, but pyrexia and a palpable adnexal mass may also be present.

Diagnosis

No specific symptoms, signs or laboratory tests are diagnostic of PID and the diagnosis is often made on clinical findings (presence of lower abdominal pain, increased vaginal discharge, cervical motion tenderness and adnexal tenderness on bimanual examination), which together have a specificity of 65–70% compared to laparoscopy. Non-specific tests of inflammation such as the ESR, white cell count and C-reactive protein may be raised, and swabs taken only from the lower genital tract showing sexually transmitted pathogens are supportive evidence. Negative results do not exclude the diagnosis. The absence of pus cells on a slide taken from the cervix or vaginal wall is a sensitive marker of the absence of PID. Differential diagnoses, including appendicitis and, ectopic pregnancy should be considered and a pregnancy test should be performed. Laparoscopy, with microbiological specimens from the upper and lower genital tract, is considered the 'gold standard' for diagnosis, but this is not always available or appropriate, particularly for those with mild symptoms. Clinical symptoms and signs do not accurately predict the extent of tubal disease found at laparoscopy.

Treatment and management

Treatment should not be delayed while waiting for bacteriological test results, as early antibiotic therapy improves outcomes. Outpatient therapy with oral antibiotics is appropriate for clinically mild to moderate disease, but hospitalization is required if there is diagnostic uncertainty, severe symptoms or signs, or failure to respond to oral therapy. Intravenous therapy for the first few days is recommended in women with severe clinical disease.

Recommended regimens are:

- cefoxitin 2 g i.v. three times daily plus doxycycline 100 mg (i.v. or oral) twice daily plus metronidazole 400 mg (i.v. or oral) twice daily for 14 days
- ofloxacin 400 mg (i.v. or oral) twice daily plus metronidazole 400 mg (i.v. or oral) twice daily for 14 days
- ceftriaxone 250 mg i.m. single dose, or cefoxitin 2 g i.m. single dose with probenecid 1 g orally single dose, plus doxycycline 100 mg (i.v. or oral) twice daily plus metronidazole 400 mg (i.v. or oral) twice daily for 14 days.

Appropriate analgesia should be given. Patients should abstain from sex until they and their partner(s) (where an STI is diagnosed) have completed treatment. Women with moderate or severe clinical findings should be reviewed after 2–3 days to ensure they are improving. Lack of response to treatment requires further investigation, intravenous therapy and/or surgical intervention. All patients should be seen after treatment to check their clinical response, and that medication has been completed. Repeat testing of initially positive swabs is recommended.

Complications

The main complications from PID are due to tubal damage, with the risk of all complications increasing with severity of infection. Tubal infertility occurs in 10–12% of women after one episode of symptomatic PID, 20–30% after two episodes, and 50–60% after three or more episodes. The risk of ectopic pregnancy is increased 6- to 10-fold, with higher rates in women with several episodes. Abdominal or pelvic pain for longer than 6 months occurs in 18% of women. Women with a past history of PID are 5 to 10 times more likely to need hospital admission and undergo hysterectomy.

About a third of women have repeated infections. This may be due to relapse of infection because of inadequate treatment, reinfection from an untreated partner, post-infection tubal damage, or further acquisition of STIs. In 5–15% of women with salpingitis, the infection spreads from the pelvis to the liver capsule, causing perihepatitis (Fitz-Hugh–Curtis syndrome – history box).

h | *History*

Fitz-Hugh–Curtis syndrome is named after the two American physicians Thomas Fitz-Hugh Jr (1894–1963) and Arthur Hale Curtis (1881–1955) who first reported this condition, in 1934 and 1930, respectively.

Trichomonas vaginalis (TV)

Background information

TV is uncommon in the UK – less than 6000 diagnoses per year – but in other parts of the world, e.g. Africa and Asia, it remains a major cause of vaginal discharge. It is sexually transmitted and only infects the urogenital tract. Unlike bacterial vaginosis, TV causes significant inflammation.

Symptoms and signs

- It may be asymptomatic in 10–50% of women.
- The most common symptom is vaginal discharge, with a malodour. There may also be vulval pruritus, external dysuria and dyspareunia.
- On examination there may be vulval erythema and excoriation, and the purulent discharge may be visible on the vulva. The vaginal mucosa is often inflamed, with a yellow or grey discharge.

Diagnosis

Culture is the most sensitive method of diagnosis. Microscopy of a wet-mount preparation, in which motile trichomonads can be seen, is about 70% sensitive compared to culture.

Treatment and management

The recommended treatment is:

- metronidazole 2 g single oral dose, or
- metronidazole 400 mg orally twice daily for 5–7 days.

30% of women with TV have gonorrhoea and/or chlamydia, so they should be tested for other STIs. Patients should abstain from sex until they and their partner(s) have completed treatment.

Complications

TV increases a woman's risk of acquiring HIV infection and in pregnancy is associated with low birth weight and preterm delivery.

Genital warts

Background information

Genital warts are the commonest viral STI in the UK. The prevalence of infection with human papillomavirus (HPV) types 6 and 11 in women aged 19–23 years in one UK vaccine study was 23%, and the incidence of clinical genital warts is around 0.8% per annum. HPV is highly infectious: two-thirds of sexual partners will develop warts, and HPV infection is also seen in adolescents who have had only non-penetrative sexual contact. Infection causes painless, benign, epithelial tumours caused by HPV types 6 and 11. The incubation period of months to years means that warts may appear some time into an exclusively monogamous relationship. The immunosuppression of pregnancy may cause warts to appear or recur. Vaccines against oncogenic HPV types (16 and 18) are available. Some of these also protect against HPV 6 and 11.

Symptoms and signs

- Genital warts are painless, so in women they may be asymptomatic.
- If symptomatic, it is usual that the woman has felt the vulval lumps.

- On examination the flesh-coloured papules can be seen around the introital opening. They can spread onto the labia, perineum, and perianal area. They may be single but are usually multiple **(Fig. 13.6)**.
- On the mucous membranes they are usually soft and cauliflower-like (condylomata acuminata).
- On the drier surfaces they are harder and keratinized.

Diagnosis

They are diagnosed by their clinical appearances. Atypical lesions should be biopsied, particularly in older women, as premalignant and malignant lesions can look similar.

Treatment and management

Warts may resolve spontaneously. No one treatment modality has been shown to be effective in all cases. Fewer (less than 5) or keratinized warts can be treated with ablative therapy such as cryotherapy, trichloroacetic acid, curettage or electrocautery. All of these can be used in pregnancy and a single treatment may be effective. Multiple, soft warts (condylomata acuminata) can be treated with podophyllotoxin solution or cream. It is a cytotoxic agent, so is contraindicated in pregnancy. Imiquimod cream works by stimulating local cell-mediated immunity, resulting in clearance of the warts. It can be used on both soft and keratinized warts, but should also not be used in pregnancy. All treatments can have recurrence rates of up to 25%, because of residual subclinical viral infection. Treatment failure should be followed by change of treatment, and management algorithms improve outcomes. Women with genital warts should be tested for chlamydia, and, depending on risk assessment, may require testing for other STIs. There is evidence that condoms reduce the spread of HPV, so patients should be advised to use condoms with new partners.

Complications

Genital warts are mainly a cosmetic problem. Psychological morbidity may arise because of their appearance, fears about cervical cancer, or concerns about fidelity if they appear in a regular relationship. Physical complications are rare; HPV 6 and 11 are not associated with cervical cancer and vertical transmission is rare.

Genital herpes

Background information

Genital herpes can be caused by herpes simplex virus (HSV) type 1 or 2. Over 50% of first-episode genital herpes in the UK is due to HSV type 1. Cases rose 32% between 1995 and 2006, following a sixfold rise since the 1970s. HSV-2 antibodies are found in 7.6% of blood donors, but less than 50% of donors give a clinical history of herpes, suggesting that many people have subclinical infection.

It is initially an acute vesicular/ulcerating eruption, frequently followed by recurring lesions.

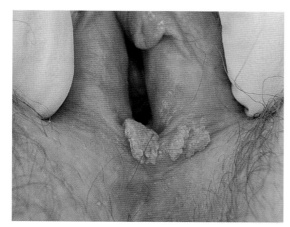

Fig. 13.6 Flesh-coloured papules characteristic of warts.
They may be single, but are usually multiple, and can spread
onto the labia, perineum, and perianal area. (From Clutterbuck D,
Specialist Training in Sexually Transmitted Infections and HIV, Mosby
2005.)

HSV ascends the peripheral sensory nerves into the
dorsal root ganglion, where latent infection develops. This
can reactivate, giving recurrent lesions. These are not
always noticeable; asymptomatic, subclinical, viral shedding occurs up to 20% of the time in HSV-2 infection. All
of these reactivated episodes are potentially infectious and
around 75% of first-episode infections are acquired from
an asymptomatic partner.

Symptoms and signs

Symptoms range from mild irritation and soreness to severe
systemic illness with extensive, confluent anogenital ulceration. Genital lesions classically pass through erythematous, vesicular and ulcerative stages before resolution.

Primary infection

- This is the first-ever exposure to either HSV-1 or -2. It
  can cause vulval soreness and external dysuria, but it
  can also be asymptomatic. As the symptoms are non-
  specific it may be misdiagnosed as either a urinary tract
  infection or candida.
- On examination there are multiple painful superficial
  ulcers **(Fig. 13.7)**. Tender inguinal lymphadenopathy is
  also usually present.

Non-primary, first-episode genital herpes

This occurs in people with previous orolabial HSV-1 who
then acquire genital HSV-2 infection. There is some cross-
protection from this prior infection, resulting in a milder illness
than in primary infection. These non-primary infections are
more likely to be asymptomatic than are primary infections.

Recurrent herpes

- These episodes may be asymptomatic (subclinical shedding). If symptoms are present they are usually milder

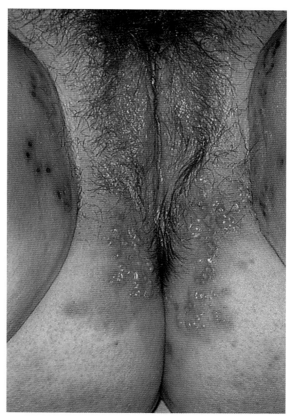

Fig. 13.7 Primary herpes. Multiple painful superficial ulcers
are present. (From Clutterbuck D, *Specialist Training in Sexually
Transmitted Infections and HIV*, Mosby 2005.)

than in first infections. They may be preceded by a prodrome of tingling, itching or pain in the area.
- On examination there are usually just a few ulcers confined to a small area.
- 90% of people with HSV-2 infection and 60% with
  HSV-1 will develop recurrences within the first year. The
  median number of recurrences in year 1 is one in HSV-1
  infection and five in HSV-2. Long-term studies show that
  symptomatic recurrences gradually decrease with time.

Diagnosis

Nucleic acid testing (NAAT) of swabs from the lesions for
HSV-1 and -2 DNA is the most sensitive method of diagnosis. Viral culture for HSV may be used. Type-specific
serological tests for HSV-1 and -2 are available and may be
useful in assessing the susceptibility of a partner to primary
infection (e.g. during pregnancy).

Treatment and management
Primary and first-episode genital herpes

Antiviral drugs reduce the severity and duration of the
symptoms. They do not prevent latency, so have no effect
on future recurrences.

Recommended regimens are:

- aciclovir 200 mg five times daily for 5 days
- famciclovir 250 mg three times daily for 5 days
- valaciclovir 500 mg twice daily for 5 days.

Aciclovir can be used in pregnancy and breastfeeding.

Analgesia and saline bathing are recommended. Patients can be advised to pass urine in a bath or under a shower spray of warm water, to ease external dysuria. Testing for other STIs should be performed, but this can wait until the vulval ulcers have healed, when it will be more comfortable to insert a vaginal speculum. The natural history of HSV infection should be explained, covering recurrences, sub-clinical viral shedding, the potential for sexual transmission, and treatments that are available.

Recurrent genital herpes

Recurrences are self-limiting and can often be managed with supportive therapy. Infrequent but severe recurrences can be treated with episodic antiviral therapy. If started early, therapy will reduce the severity and sometimes the duration of an attack, but will not reduce the number of recurrences. The patient should initiate treatment at home as soon as a recurrence is noticed.

Episodic treatment regimens are:

- aciclovir 200 mg five times a day for 5 days
- famciclovir 125 mg twice daily for 5 days
- valaciclovir 500 mg twice daily for 5 days.

For frequent recurrences (more than six recurrences in a year) suppressive therapy may be considered. In around 80% of cases, recurrences are stopped altogether. Therapy does not modify the natural history of infection, but after 12 months of treatment about 20% of patients will have fewer recurrences due to the natural decay in episode frequency. It may be restarted if frequent recurrences persist.

Suppressive treatment regimens are:

- aciclovir 400 mg twice daily
- famciclovir 250 mg twice daily
- valaciclovir 500 mg once daily.

Patients should be advised to avoid sexual contact during the prodrome and recurrence, as this is when the risk of transmission is highest. It should be explained that there is a low risk of transmission even when they have no obvious recurrence, because of subclinical viral shedding. Condoms reduce this risk and suppressive therapy has an additional effect.

Complications

Women who acquire primary genital herpes during pregnancy, particularly in the third trimester, may transmit the infection to the baby at the time of delivery. The risk of perinatal transmission with recurrent HSV is low. Genital herpes increases the acquisition and transmission of HIV two- to threefold and may be a highly significant cofactor in the worldwide HIV epidemic. Many people with recurrent HSV infection develop psychological problems and fear rejection by sexual partners. Aseptic meningitis and autonomic neuropathy can occasionally occur with primary infection, even leading to urinary retention. Rarely, the infection can disseminate, causing a life-threatening condition. This is more likely in the immunocompromised and in pregnancy.

Syphilis

Background information

Syphilis is caused by the spirochaete *Treponema pallidum*. Before the mid-1990s, cases of infectious syphilis in women were so rare in the UK that the value of antenatal screening for syphilis was being questioned. A dramatic resurgence of the disease since 2000 has confirmed the need for continued vigilance. Fifteen cases of congenital syphilis were seen in UK GUM clinics in 2006.

Symptoms and signs

Syphilis can be asymptomatic, and identified on screening serology such as in antenatal testing.

There are several stages of symptomatic syphilis infection.

- *Primary syphilis.* About 3 weeks after exposure, a chancre appears. This is usually a single, painless ulcer with rolled indurated edges, which usually goes unnoticed in women. Even without treatment, it heals spontaneously. Syphilis serology may still be negative at this stage of infection.
- *Secondary syphilis.* After several weeks, a generalized illness develops, with fever, malaise, and skin and mucosal rashes. The rash is present on the trunk, limbs, palms and soles. Wart-like moist papules occur on the vulva (condylomata lata). Even if untreated, these symptoms and signs resolve after 3–12 weeks. Syphilis serology is strongly positive at this stage of infection.
- *Late syphilis.* Up to 40% of untreated patients will develop symptomatic late syphilis, with neurosyphilis, cardiovascular syphilis or gummata.

Diagnosis

Syphilis can be diagnosed by serological testing. The initial test is likely to be an enzyme immunoassay (EIA), but, if positive, the Venereal Disease Research Laboratory (VDRL) test or rapid plasma reagin (RPR) test, and the *Treponema pallidum* haemagglutination (TPHA) test and fluorescent treponemal antibody absorption (FTA-abs) test should be performed.

Treatment and management

The treatment of all stages of syphilis requires long courses of antibiotics, and long-term follow-up. Penicillins remain the treatment of choice. Management should be undertaken by a department of genitourinary medicine.

Complications

Without adequate treatment, complications of late syphilis can occur. Syphilis in pregnancy can cause miscarriage and stillbirth, and can be transmitted to the infant, causing congenital syphilis.

HIV infection

Background information

HIV infection can be transmitted by contact with body fluids (either sexually, or through needles or blood transfusion) and by vertical transmission from mother to baby. It was estimated that 73,000 people were living with HIV in the UK in 2000, but that 30% were unaware of their infection. Antiretroviral therapy with three or more drugs has dramatically improved morbidity and mortality from HIV. There are now less than 500 deaths from AIDS each year in the UK. Late diagnosis remains a problem: 40% of these deaths occur in people diagnosed too late for effective therapy.

Symptoms and signs

- Most people with HIV infection have no symptoms in the first few years of infection.
- There may be a mild systemic illness with fever, malaise and rash at the time of seroconversion 6–12 weeks after infection. This is rarely recognized as being HIV-related.

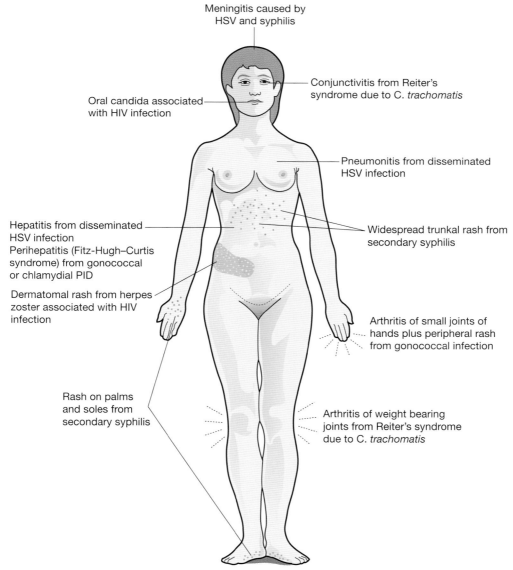

Fig. 13.8 Systemic presentations of sexually transmitted infections.

■ As the immune function is starting to deteriorate, infections such as oral candida and herpes zoster may occur.

■ Women with HIV infection get more frequent episodes of vaginal candida and HSV recurrences.

■ Opportunistic infections and HIV-related malignancies can present in many different ways.

Diagnosis

Serology for evidence of antibodies to HIV is the method of diagnosis. HIV testing should be offered as a routine part of STI screening and requires informed consent but not specialist counselling.

Treatment and management

Patients should have their CD4 count (this measures cell-mediated immune function) and HIV viral load (this measures the level of viral replication) performed about every 3 months. Antiretroviral therapy with three or more drugs should be started when the CD4 count drops to $350–400 \times 10^9/l$.

Complications

Without treatment, there is increasing damage to the cell-mediated immunity, leading to susceptibility to opportunistic infections and eventually death, a median of 9–12 years after infection. Treating the pregnant woman with triple antiretroviral therapy and avoiding breastfeeding can reduce vertical transmission. Rates of transmission are now as low as 1%. Delivery by caesarian section reduces vertical transmission in women who are not taking antiretroviral therapy, but is not thought to offer additional benefit in those on effective treatment.

Systemic presentations of sexually transmitted infections

STIs do not always present with genital symptoms or signs. Many can cause systemic infections, which produce symptoms and signs in other systems of the body. HIV almost always presents in this way. It is not within the scope of this chapter to cover all the presentations of HIV-related opportunistic infections and malignancies, but the common early presentations are shown in **Figure 13.8**.

Key *points*

- STIs in females are often asymptomatic. Detection depends on risk assessment and testing in all women presenting for care.
- If symptoms and signs are present, they are usually non-specific. Most women with vaginal discharge do not have an STI.
- High rates of STIs are found in sexually active women aged less than 20 years.
- STIs often coexist; screen for other infections if one is diagnosed.
- The management of STIs, but particularly chlamydia, gonorrhoea and PID, includes treatment of the sexual partner(s) and advice about abstinence from sex until the patient and partner(s) have completed treatment, in order to prevent reinfection.

14 Heavy menstrual bleeding and dysmenorrhoea

Heavy menstrual bleeding

Heavy menstrual bleeding (HMB) is defined, for clinical purposes, as bleeding that has an adverse impact on the quality of life of a woman; it may occur alone or with other symptoms. Menstrual blood loss can be measured, but this is usually only performed for research purposes. HMB is often called 'menorrhagia' and is the commonest cause of iron-deficiency anaemia in women in the affluent world.

Menstrual problems are becoming more prevalent since women experience more periods in their lifetime than did their predecessors 100 years ago (approximately 400 periods vs. 40). This is because women have fewer children and breast-feed less (lactational amenorrhoea). Only 50% of women who complain of excessive heavy bleeding, however, actually suffer from loss that falls outside the normal range for a population of women not complaining of any menstrual abnormality (>80 ml per month).

The medical and surgical treatment of HMB is also an appreciable burden to health-service resources. HMB is a common indication for hysterectomy, although the numbers have fallen in the last 10 years with the introduction of alternative, effective treatments. Although a commonly performed operation, hysterectomy is a major surgical procedure and its use needs to be balanced against the potential associated mortality and morbidity. Satisfaction rates with hysterectomy are, however, very high.

Causes of HMB

The causes are summarized in **Table 14.1**.

Uterine pathology

HMB is associated with both benign pathology (e.g. uterine fibroids, endometrial polyps, adenomyosis, pelvic infection) and, extremely rarely, malignant pathology (e.g. endometrial cancer). Over half of those women with an excessively heavy loss of >200 ml will have fibroids.

Endometrial polyps are common benign localized overgrowths of the endometrium. They consist of a fibrous tissue core covered by columnar epithelium, and it is believed that they arise as a result of disordered cycles of apoptosis and regrowth of endometrium. Although it is uncertain that they cause HMB, it is likely that intrauterine endometrial polyps do increase the likelihood of irregular bleeding **(Fig. 14.1)**. It is unlikely, however, that small endocervical polyps detected at the time of a routine cervical smear cause the same effect. Malignant change of such a polyp is rare.

Uterine fibroids (leiomyomas) are benign tumours of the myometrium which are present in approximately 20% of women of reproductive age. They are well-circumscribed whorls of smooth muscle cells with collagen and may be single or multiple **(Fig. 14.2)**. Size varies from microscopic growths to tumours that weigh as much as 40 kg and they are more common in women of Afro-Caribbean origin. Submucous fibroids project into the uterine cavity, intramural fibroids are contained within the wall of the uterus, and subserosal fibroids project from the surface of the uterus; cervical fibroids arise from the cervix.

Many are asymptomatic, but when symptoms do occur, they are often related to the site and size of the fibroid. Presenting symptoms include menstrual dysfunction, infertility, miscarriage, dyspareunia and pelvic discomfort. The mechanism by which fibroids adversely affect reproduction is unclear, but may be related in part to distortion of the uterine cavity affecting implantation or due to fibroids causing disturbance of uterine blood flow. Fibroids may also present because of pressure effects on surrounding organs, such as frequency of micturition as a result of pressure on the bladder, or even hydronephrosis due to ureteric compression. Growth of fibroids is mediated by sex steroids, particularly oestrogen, and they therefore grow during pregnancy and shrink after the menopause. Occasionally during pregnancy, necrosis of the fibroid ('red degeneration') leads to acute abdominal pain. The incidence of malignant change (leiomyosarcoma) in fibroids is considered to be extremely low (0.1%).

Dysfunctional uterine bleeding (DUB)

DUB is said to be the cause for HMB in the absence of recognizable pelvic pathology or systemic disease. It is thus a diagnosis of exclusion and is the commonest 'diagnosis' reached after investigating women with HMB. Some clinicians further classify DUB as 'anovulatory DUB' or 'ovulatory DUB', although clinically this is not an important distinction as treatment is the same in both cases. The underlying cause of DUB is likely to reside at the level of the

Table 14.1		
The main causes of menorrhagia		
1	Uterine pathology	Common
2	Dysfunctional uterine bleeding (DUB)	Very common
3	Medical disorders, including clotting defects	Very rare

endometrium, although the precise nature of the vascular and endocrine abnormality remains elusive.

Medical disorders and clotting defects

Very rarely, HMB is associated with such medical problems as thyroid disease (both hypo- and hyperthyroidism), hepatic disease, and renal disease (although the majority of those with end-stage renal failure are amenorrhoeic). Other symptoms of the disorder are likely to be present.

Certain coagulation abnormalities (e.g. von Willebrand's disease) and platelet defects (e.g. thrombocytopenia) are associated with an increased incidence of HMB.

Assessment of HMB

History

The number of sanitary towels used, duration of bleeding, or passage of clots seems to have little correlation with the actual volume of blood lost. However, complaints of 'flooding' (leakage of heavy blood loss onto clothing) and having to use 'double sanitary protection' (pad and tampon) to prevent leakage of blood onto clothes are indicative of HMB and are likely to have a negative impact upon the woman's quality of life. It is important, therefore, to ask about the degree of inconvenience experienced, such as time lost from work, or becoming housebound during menses owing to fear of social embarrassment from an episode of flooding in public.

A history of irregular bleeding, dyspareunia, pelvic pain, or intermenstrual or postcoital bleeding may raise the suspicion of underlying pathology and often require additional investigation. They can be termed 'red light' symptoms.

The woman should also be questioned about symptoms suggestive of anaemia, such as fatigue and light-headedness. A history suggestive of systemic disease such as a thyroid disorder or a clotting abnormality would signal that further investigation for such causes would be required. The woman should also be questioned about risk factors for endometrial cancer, such as use of unopposed oestrogen, tamoxifen use, polycystic ovary syndrome, and family history of endometrial or colon cancer. It is also important to establish if she has a history of thromboembolism, as many medical treatments for HMB are hormonal and thus their use may be relatively or absolutely contraindicated.

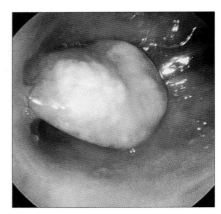

Fig. 14.1 Hysteroscopic view of intrauterine polyp.
(Courtesy of Karl Storz Endoscopy (UK) Ltd.)

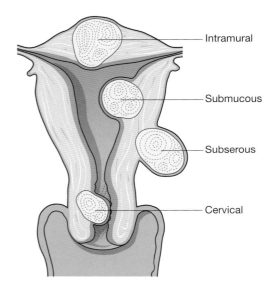

Fig. 14.2 Sites of fibroids throughout the uterus.

Examination

The woman should be examined for signs of anaemia. An abdominal, bimanual and speculum examination should be considered. An enlarged, 'bulky' uterus suggests uterine fibroids, and tenderness suggests endometriosis, pelvic inflammatory disease or adenomyosis.

Investigations

Laboratory tests A full blood count should be carried out in all women, to diagnose/exclude anaemia. Thyroid function tests and tests of coagulation should be performed only if there are features suggestive of this in the history. No other endocrine tests are routinely indicated.

Ultrasound A pelvic ultrasound scan should be performed if history or examination suggests structural uterine pathology, or if it is not possible to assess the uterus clinically because of obesity. The site and size of abnormalities such

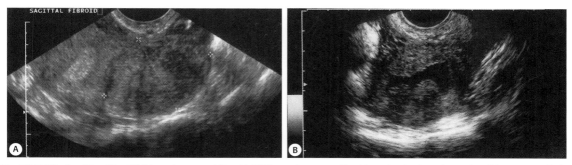

Fig. 14.3 Uterine fibroids. (A) A large intramural fibroid. **(B)** Two submucous fibroids projecting into the cavity of the uterus, which contains a small amount of fluid (saline infusion ultrasound scan).

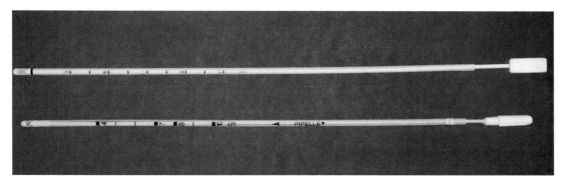

Fig. 14.4 Two varieties of endometrial samplers.

as fibroids can be determined, together with assessment of the ovaries **(Fig. 14.3)**.

Endometrial assessment This should be performed in all women aged >45 years, and in younger women with persistent HMB in spite of medical treatment, 'red light' symptoms such as irregular bleeding, or for whom there are risk factors for endometrial cancer. This can take the form of an endometrial biopsy or a hysteroscopy, both of which can be carried out either as an outpatient or inpatient **(Fig. 14.4** and p. 193).

Cervical cytology This should be performed if it is due, or if the cervix looks suspicious.

Treatment of causes of HMB

Focal uterine pathology

Benign intrauterine polyps will usually be removed by polypectomy using hysteroscopic techniques. If malignant pathology is detected, then this should be treated as appropriate.

Fibroids may be treated medically or surgically.

Medical

Unfortunately, the symptoms caused by fibroids respond poorly to medical treatments such as those used in the treatment of DUB (see below). Since growth of fibroids is hormone dependent, gonadotrophin-releasing hormone (GnRH) analogues (which result in hypo-oestrogenism) may be used to cause fibroid shrinkage. GnRH analogues are derivatives of natural GnRH, but peptide substitutions give the agonists greater potency and longer activity. Depot injection of the GnRH analogue, however, leads to pituitary downregulation with hypo-oestrogenism. Fibroids shrink by approximately 50% over 3 months of treatment, but regrowth occurs on cessation of treatment. During treatment, hypo-oestrogenism can result in symptoms such as hot flushes and also bone loss. In view of concern about osteoporosis, use of GnRH analogues is limited to short-term use (<6 months). 'Add-back' hormone replacement therapy (HRT) is required to minimize the risk of osteoporosis and side-effects.

Surgical

Hysteroscopic resection of small submucous fibroids is often possible, which can lead to improved fertility and relief of menstrual problems. Ablation of small submucous fibroids can be achieved by microwave endometrial ablation (MEA, see below).

If a woman wishes to conserve her fertility, myomectomy is an option. This involves incision of the pseudocapsule of the fibroid, enucleation of the bulk of the tumour, and closure of the resulting defect. The operation is usually performed as an open abdominal procedure, although laparoscopic techniques are sometimes employed. Myomectomy is associated with a similar degree of morbidity to that of hysterectomy. There is a risk of haemorrhage (due to the vascularity of fibroids) and the small possibility that an emergency hysterectomy may need to be performed during surgery, to arrest uncontrollable bleeding. Furthermore, there is a risk of adhesion formation, which could compromise fertility (as a result of tubal obstruction), and the possibility that residual seedling fibroids may grow and lead to recurrence of fibroids. GnRH analogues are often used preoperatively to shrink the fibroids, with associated decreased intraoperative blood loss. Pregnancies after myomectomy are frequently delivered by planned caesarean section because of concern regarding uterine rupture in labour.

Uterine artery embolization (UAE), performed by interventional radiologists, is an effective and safe technique. It involves interruption of the blood supply to the fibroid by blocking the uterine arteries with coils or foam delivered through a catheter placed in the femoral artery. The healthy myometrium revascularizes immediately, owing to the development of collateral circulations from vaginal and ovarian vessels. Fibroids, however, do not appear to revascularize, and shrink by about 50%, a reduction which appears to be sustained. Pain following occlusion of the vessels is often severe and usually requires opiate analgesia. Potential complications include infection, fibroid expulsion, and the effects of exposure of the ovaries to ionizing radiation. The incidence of these is low and immediate morbidity is less than following hysterectomy, although pain and fever from post-embolization syndrome is not uncommon and deaths, though rare, have occurred. There are now several reported series of pregnancies following UAE; this treatment is therefore an option, after careful counselling, for women wishing to maintain their fertility.

If childbearing is complete and the woman is experiencing severe symptoms as a result of her fibroids, then hysterectomy may be considered (see below).

Dysfunctional uterine bleeding (DUB)

In the majority of cases of HMB, no specific cause is found and the diagnosis is DUB. Sometimes a woman is seeking reassurance that there is no pathology and does not necessarily wish treatment. For most women, however, treatment is requested. The following treatments may be considered.

Medical treatment

Intrauterine progestogens The levonorgestrel intrauterine system (LNG-IUS) delivers progestogen directly to the uterus **(Fig. 14.5)**. and is a first-line treatment for HMB, being particularly suitable for women requiring contraception: it is a highly effective reversible method of contraception and can stay in place for up to 5 years. After 12 months, menstrual blood loss is reduced by around 95% and many women are amenorrhoeic. The main problems with the LNG-IUS are the high incidence of irregular bleeding, particularly within the first 3–6 months after insertion, and an expulsion rate of 5%.

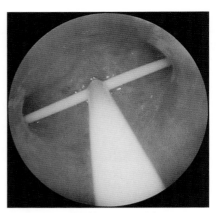

Fig. 14.5 An intrauterine progestogen-releasing system in the uterus. (Courtesy of Karl Storz Endoscopy (UK) Ltd.)

Prostaglandin synthesis inhibitors Non-steroidal anti-inflammatory drugs (NSAIDs) taken during menstruation reduce menstrual blood loss by around 25%, by reducing endometrial prostaglandin concentrations. The NSAID most commonly used for treatment of HMB is mefenamic acid, although other NSAIDs have not dissimilar efficacies. Side-effects include gastrointestinal complaints, dizziness and headache. These drugs are also of benefit for treating dysmenorrhoea.

Antifibrinolytics Antifibrinolytics, such as tranexamic acid, work by inhibiting plasminogen activator, thereby reducing the fibrinolytic activity in the endometrium. This increases clot formation in the spiral arterioles and reduces menstrual loss. Tranexamic acid taken during menstruation reduces blood loss by around 50%. Gastrointestinal side-effects, nausea and tinnitus can occur. The drug should not be taken by women who are predisposed to thromboembolism.

The NSAIDs and antifibrinolytics are the best options for women wishing to conceive, since they are only taken during menstruation and do not suppress ovulation

Combined oral contraceptive pill This reduces blood loss by approximately 50%. Its mechanism for doing so is thought to be due to suppressive effects on the endometrium. There is no age restriction on use of the combined oral contraceptive in women at low risk (see p. 84).

Systemic progestogens Oral progestogens are widely prescribed for HMB but overviews of well-designed trials of this therapy do not demonstrate a meaningful reduction in menstrual loss. Taken in a cyclical fashion, however, oral progestogens are often useful in regulating otherwise irregular cycles. If the depot injectable progestogen (medroxyprogesterone acetate) is administered for long enough, amenorrhoea frequently results. During initial months of use, however, bleeding can be unpredictable and heavy. Side-effects of progestogens include nausea, bloating, headache, breast tenderness, weight gain and acne.

GnRH analogues Amenorrhoea occurs as a result of pituitary downregulation and thus inhibition of ovarian activity. Women may experience problems, however, associated with the resultant hypo-oestrogenism – particularly, hot flushes and vaginal dryness. GnRH analogues are usually reserved for short-term use only (up to 6 months) and add-back HRT is usually prescribed to relieve symptoms of hypo-oestrogenism.

Danazol This is a synthetic androgen with anti-oestrogenic and anti-progestogenic activity which reduces menstrual blood loss but is no longer recommended because of its poor side-effect profile which includes irreversible virilization.

Surgical treatment

Endometrial ablation Using a number of different techniques it is possible to destroy most or all of the endometrium, thereby lessening or stopping menstrual loss altogether. Since endometrium regenerates from the basal layer it is essential to ablate to the endo–myometrial border. Endometrial ablation offers a safer method of symptom control, much shorter hospital stay, and shorter recovery period than hysterectomy. Early techniques involved a hysteroscopic procedure under general anaesthesia during which the endometrium was treated, under direct visualization, with either laser or diathermy or by resection. Newer, non-hysteroscopic procedures include ablation with a heated balloon (e.g. Thermachoice, Cavaterm), bipolar radiofrequency impedance-controlled endometrial ablation (e.g. NovaSure), and microwave endometrial ablation (MEA) **Fig. 14.6**. These newer procedures carry fewer risks than the hysteroscopic resections and some can be performed under local anaesthesia.

The success rates of the different ablative techniques are broadly similar. All three are associated with a 70–80% overall satisfaction rate, and an amenorrhoea rate of 20% for balloon treatment and around 50% for impedance-controlled ablation and MEA. Complications are rare but include uterine perforation, hyponatraemia and infection. Pregnancy is contraindicated after an ablation procedure and women are urged to use a reliable, if not permanent, form of contraception.

Hysterectomy This is the only treatment that guarantees amenorrhoea and as a consequence it is associated with a high level of satisfaction. Hysterectomy is performed by the abdominal or vaginal route, the latter with or without laparoscopic assistance (laparoscopically assisted vaginal hysterectomy or LAVH). Abdominal hysterectomy involves a laparotomy incision, which is usually transverse; a vaginal hysterectomy involves an incision through the vaginal wall. The choice between the two procedures depends on the size of the uterus, the degree of uterine descent, the wish to remove the ovaries (difficult by the vaginal route), and the skills and preferences of the surgeon **(Table 14.2)**. Complications of hysterectomy include haemorrhage, bowel trauma, damage to the urinary tract, infection, postoperative thromboembolism, and risk of vaginal prolapse in later years. Complications are significantly greater in those with

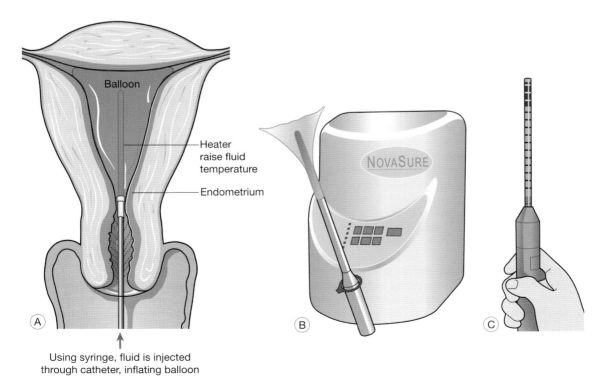

Balloon

Heater raise fluid temperature

Endometrium

Using syringe, fluid is injected through catheter, inflating balloon

(A)   (B)   (C)

Fig. 14.6 Conservative surgical treatments for menorrhagia. (A) A thermal balloon; **(B)** impedance-controlled ablation; **(C)** microwave endometrial ablation.

Table 14.2

Pros and cons of different hysterectomy methods

	Pros	Cons
Total abdominal hysterectomy (TAH)	Cervix is removed, therefore no further smears or risk of cervical malignancy (thus particularly suitable for those with a history of abnormal cytology) Good access to ovaries	Increased surgical morbidity
Subtotal abdominal hysterectomy	Fewer complications than TAH (↓bleeding, ↓infection, ↓bladder injury, ↓ureteric damage) Good access to ovaries	Risk of cervical cancer remains as before
Vaginal hysterectomy	May be lower incidence of bladder and bowel injury in straightforward cases (compared to abdominal hysterectomy) No painful abdominal wound	There is only limited ovarian access Is contraindicated with: • large uterus • restricted uterine mobility • limited vaginal space • adnexal pathology • cervix flush with vagina

uterine fibroids. Women undergoing a vaginal procedure recover more quickly from the operation than do those undergoing an abdominal hysterectomy, but the incidence of major complications, whilst low, is slightly higher with the vaginal route.

For women with DUB who are undergoing an abdominal hysterectomy and who have a history of normal cervical cytology, there is the choice of having a 'subtotal' hysterectomy. This involves removing the body of the uterus but leaving the cervix behind. The advantages of a subtotal compared to a 'total' hysterectomy are that the operation is quicker, with less risk of damage to structures surrounding the cervix (bowel and urinary tract) **(Fig. 14.7)**. There are also reported, but unproven, advantages of less disruption to the bowel, bladder and sexual functioning postoperatively. If the cervix is left, the surgeon must be careful to remove any residual endometrium in the cervical canal at the time of surgery. This is to minimize the small risk that menses would continue from the endometrium in the cervical canal. The disadvantages of a subtotal hysterectomy are that the woman must continue in the cervical cytology screening programme. The risk of cervical cancer arising in the stump of cervix is extremely small (<0.1%) provided that cervical cytology was normal prior to the operation.

Whether to remove the ovaries at the time of abdominal hysterectomy depends on several factors, including the woman's preferences, her age, her family history of breast or ovarian carcinoma, and her attitude towards HRT. In someone who is 50 years old, it is unlikely that there will be much further ovarian function (average age of menopause 51), and bilateral salpingo-oophorectomy will significantly reduce the incidence of later ovarian carcinoma and surgery for benign ovarian tumours. Residual ovaries (ovaries not removed at time of hysterectomy) may also occasionally cause chronic pain or dyspareunia if adherent to the vagina or side wall of the pelvis. In a woman who is 40, however, a further 10 years of ovarian oestrogen

secretion may be expected and many women will not wish to take HRT for such duration. It may therefore be appropriate to discuss 'routine' oophorectomy in women over 45 and ovarian conservation in women under 45. The decision must remain, however, a very individualized consideration.

Medical disorders and clotting defects

Referral should be made to the appropriate physician/haematologist to institute further investigation and treatment of the underlying condition.

Dysmenorrhoea

Excessive menstrual pain (dysmenorrhoea) is a significant clinical problem. It is characteristically a cramping lower abdominal pain, which may radiate to the lower back and legs and may be associated with gastrointestinal symptoms or malaise. It has been estimated that dysmenorrhoea affects 30–50% of menstruating women. It is also one of the most frequent causes of absenteeism from school and of days off work. As with heavy menstrual bleeding, dysmenorrhoea may be idiopathic (primary dysmenorrhoea) or due to pelvic pathology (secondary dysmenorrhoea).

Primary dysmenorrhoea

This generally begins with the onset of ovulatory cycles, typically within the first 2 years of the menarche. Pain is usually most severe on the day of menstruation or the day preceding this. There is good evidence that prostaglandins are involved in the aetiology, with higher concentrations of PGE_2 and $PGF_{2\alpha}$ in the menstrual fluid of women who suffer from dysmenorrhoea. $PGF_{2\alpha}$ increases the contractility of the myometrium and can lead to the dysmenorrhoea pain.

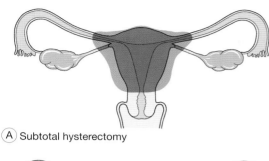

(A) Subtotal hysterectomy

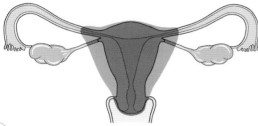

(B) Total hysterectomy

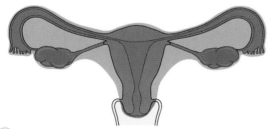

(C) Total hysterectomy with bilateral salpingo-oophorectomy

Fig. 14.7 Types of Abdominal Hysterectomy (A) Sub-total abdominal hysterectomy; **(B)** Total abdominal hysterectomy; **(C)** Total abdominal hysterectomy with bilateral salpingo-oophorectomy.

Management of primary dysmenorrhoea

Pelvic examination may not be helpful in primary dysmenorrhoea and not appropriate when dealing with an adolescent. A transabdominal ultrasound scan will reveal normal pelvic organs and provide considerable reassurance to a young woman and her family. Discussion and reassurance are an essential part of the management. If dysmenorrhoea is unresponsive to standard medical therapy (see below), then consideration should be given to the possibility of underlying pathology and appropriate investigation instituted.

Treatment of primary dysmenorrhoea

Prostaglandin synthesis inhibitors NSAIDs reduce the uterine production of $PGF_{2\alpha}$ and thus dysmenorrhoea. Most NSAIDs have been shown to be effective treatments, but mefenamic acid and ibuprofen are preferred in view of their favourable efficacy and safety profiles.

Combined oral contraceptive pill Suppression of ovulation with the combined contraceptive pill is highly effective in reducing the severity of dysmenorrhoea.
Depot progestogens The injectable progestogen-only contraceptive suppresses ovulation and thus may be a useful treatment in alleviating dysmenorrhoea.
Levonorgestrel intrauterine system (LNG-IUS) In addition to reducing menstrual blood loss, the LNG-IUS is effective at reducing dysmenorrhoea. Insertion of the device may, however, be difficult in those who have not been pregnant.

Secondary dysmenorrhoea

This is, by definition, associated with pelvic pathology. It usually has its onset many years after the menarche. Common associated pathologies are endometriosis, adenomyosis, pelvic infection and fibroids. It may also be associated with the presence of an intrauterine contraceptive device. In contrast, however, the LNG-IUS is associated with reduced dysmenorrhoea.

Management of secondary dysmenorrhoea

Women who have no other complaints but dysmenorrhoea and who have no abnormalities on abdominal, pelvic or speculum examination, may be safely treated without further investigation. Swabs from the genital tract, however, are helpful to exclude active pelvic infection, particularly *Chlamydia trachomatis*. If pelvic masses such as fibroids are suspected, a pelvic ultrasound may be helpful. A laparoscopy is indicated if endometriosis or pelvic inflammatory disease is suspected, or for those women in whom standard medical therapy has been ineffective.

Treatment of secondary dysmenorrhoea

Treatment is dependent on the underlying pathology.

Key *points*

- HMB (heavy menstrual bleeding) can be classified as being related to structural uterine pathology (e.g. fibroids) or as dysfunctional uterine bleeding (DUB), i.e. no identifiable structural cause. Very rarely, HMB may be secondary to some specific medical disorders, including clotting defects.
- Medical treatment for DUB includes prostaglandin synthesis inhibitors, antifibrinolytics, the combined contraceptive pill, systemic progestogens, intrauterine progestogens, GnRH analogues and danazol. Endometrial ablation and hysterectomy are the two surgical options.
- Dysmenorrhoea may be idiopathic (primary dysmenorrhoea) or due to pelvic pathology (secondary dysmenorrhoea). Treatment is with prostaglandin synthesis inhibitors, the combined contraceptive pill, or depot or intrauterine progestogens.

15

Pelvic pain and ectopic pregnancy

Introduction

Physiological pelvic pain with menstruation or childbirth is almost universal, but many women will present with pelvic pain for other reasons. This is most commonly acute pelvic pain – for example with appendicitis, a miscarriage or an ectopic pregnancy – but the pain may also be chronic, lasting for many months or years.

With acute pain there is usually a well-defined pathological cause which either resolves spontaneously or can be effectively treated. Chronic pelvic pain (CPP) is a symptom, not a diagnosis. CPP presents in primary care as frequently as does migraine or low back pain. Aiming for accurate diagnosis and effective management from the first presentation may help to reduce the disruption of the woman's life and may avoid a seemingly endless succession of referrals, investigations and operations.

Pelvic pain is considered under the two headings of 'acute' and 'chronic', although it is important to note that there is significant overlap. Although focusing on the gynaecological causes of pelvic pain, the non-gynaecological causes are also important and it is for this reason that a multidisciplinary approach, particularly for those women with CPP, is important.

Pain

Pain is a subjective phenomenon. Many of the factors affecting pain are centrally mediated, such that pelvic pain is often made worse by psychological, psychiatric or social distress. Unlike external organs such as the skin, which contains pain sensors, the organs within the peritoneal cavity (the viscera) are sensitive to inflammation, chemicals, and stretching or distortion caused by specific stimuli, for example adhesions or gaseous distension. The sensitivity of different organs to varying stimuli is an important factor influencing pelvic pain: the cervix and uterus are relatively insensitive, for example, whereas the fallopian tubes are exquisitely sensitive. Crushing of the bowel is associated with minimal discomfort, whereas stretching and distension cause severe pain. Unlike cutaneous painful stimuli, localization of visceral pain is often very difficult.

History

The history is arguably the most important factor in determining how quickly the diagnosis is reached and appropriate treatment instigated. Particular attention should be given to the time of onset of the pain, the characteristics, radiation, duration, severity, exacerbating and relieving factors, cyclicity, and analgesic requirements. Associated symptoms of gastrointestinal, urological or musculoskeletal origin should be sought. It is also important to take a detailed menstrual history, in particular the frequency and character of vaginal bleeding, any intermenstrual bleeding or vaginal discharge, and their relationship to the pain. Ectopic pregnancy can occur without recognizable amenorrhoea.

A sexual history may be of help, particularly details of any superficial or deep dyspareunia, contraception and sexually transmitted infections (STIs). There may be a family history of gynaecological disorders, for example endometriosis. A cervical cytology history should be recorded.

With chronic pain, there is often value in detailing a family and social history, including marital or relationship problems, pressure at work, financial worries, and childhood or adolescent problems such as sexual abuse. Listening is a centrally important facet of the history-taking which may in itself be therapeutic for some women. It is useful to ask some open-ended questions such as: 'What do you think the cause of your pain might be?' and 'How is the pain affecting your life?' to give the woman an opportunity to tell you about aspects of the problem which might not be apparent from a more systematic history.

If the history suggests there is a non-gynaecological component to the pain, referral to the relevant healthcare professional, such as gastroenterologist, urologist, genitourinary medicine physician, physiotherapist, psychologist or psychosexual counsellor, should be considered.

Examination

The examination is most usefully undertaken when there is time to explore the woman's fears and anxieties. The examiner should be prepared for new information to be revealed at this point. Observation of the woman's general demeanour is important when assessing the severity of pain. Eye-witness accounts from other health professionals and friends or family may also be helpful. The temperature, pulse and blood pressure should be recorded.

Abdominal examination should include inspection for distension or masses, palpation for tenderness, rebound and guarding, and abdominal auscultation if gastrointestinal obstruction or ileus is suspected. Inspection of the vulva and vagina at speculum examination may reveal abnormal discharge (suggestive of infection) or bleeding. Permission should then be sought to perform a vaginal and rectal examination.

A bimanual examination may reveal uterine or adnexal enlargement suggestive of a pelvic mass, fibroids or an ovarian cyst. Cervical excitation (pain associated with digital displacement of the cervix) is associated with ectopic pregnancy and pelvic infection. Tenderness or pain elicited by bimanual palpation of the pelvic organs themselves is suggestive of an ongoing inflammatory process which may be infective (e.g. chlamydia) or non-infective (e.g. endometriosis). A fixed immobile uterus suggests multiple adhesions from whatever cause, and nodularity within the uterosacral ligaments (sometimes palpable only by combined rectovaginal examination) can be a feature of endometriosis.

Acute pelvic pain

There are many causes of acute pelvic pain, but the most important gynaecological conditions are ectopic pregnancy, miscarriage, pelvic inflammatory disease, and torsion or rupture of ovarian cysts **(Box 15.1).** If the urine pregnancy test (UPT) is negative, a high vaginal swab, endocervical swab and full blood count should be performed for evidence of infection. All sexually active women below the age of 25 years who are being examined should be offered opportunistic screening for chlamydia. An ultrasound scan is helpful in identifying ovarian cysts, but non-gynaecological causes of pain should not be forgotten.

Whilst the results of investigations are awaited, it is important to continue monitoring the vital signs and to provide analgesia. If the diagnosis is unclear and the pain is not resolving, a diagnostic laparoscopy may be warranted.

The management of miscarriage, pelvic inflammatory disease and ovarian cysts is discussed in the appropriate chapters. An innocent cause of pain is that experienced mid-cycle with ovulation – so-called 'mittelschmerz'. This pain is usually sudden in onset, can be quite severe, and, if persistent in each cycle, will respond to ovulation suppression with the combined oral contraceptive.

Ectopic pregnancy

Although non-intrauterine pregnancies can be ovarian, cervical or intra-abdominal, the majority are tubal **(Fig. 15.1).** The incidence of ectopic pregnancy is 1 in 200 and it remains one of the major causes of maternal mortality.

The history and examination should particularly include the date of the last menstrual period, the date of any pregnancy tests, and symptoms suggesting pelvic infections. Pelvic examination should be gentle to avoid tubal

---

Box 15.1

Causes of acute pelvic pain

■ *Gynaecological:* ectopic pregnancy, miscarriage, acute pelvic infection, ovarian cysts
■ *Gastrointestinal:* appendicitis, constipation, diverticular disease, irritable bowel syndrome
■ *Urinary tract:* urinary tract infection, calculus
■ *Other causes:* musculoskeletal

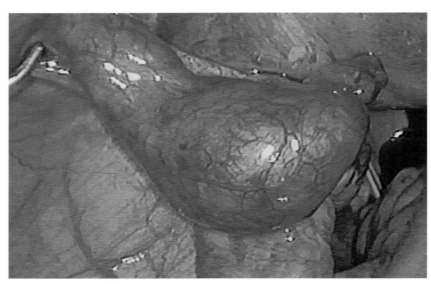

Fig. 15.1 An ectopic pregnancy in the ampulla of the fallopian tube.

rupture. If the pregnancy test is positive and the woman is not shocked, an ultrasound scan (often transvaginal) will be helpful to distinguish between ectopic pregnancy, miscarriage and continuing intrauterine pregnancy. A pseudosac (fluid in the thickened endometrium) can be confused with an intrauterine gestation sac in 20% of ectopic pregnancies. A serum beta human chorionic gonadotrophin (hCG) level which does not increase by over 66% in 48 hours increases the likelihood of ectopic pregnancy.

Management depends on the overall clinical picture, the scan result and the serum level of hCG. Tubal pregnancy can be managed by laparotomy, operative laparoscopy, medically, or occasionally by observation alone. Management must be tailored to the clinical condition and future fertility preferences of the woman. **(Fig. 15.2)**.

- If the woman is shocked on admission, an immediate pregnancy test should be performed to exclude ectopic pregnancy, with consideration given to an urgent laparotomy if the result is positive. Resuscitation and sometimes blood transfusion will be required.
- If the UPT is positive with clinical signs of ectopic pregnancy (pelvic tenderness and/or cervical excitation and/or shoulder tip pain due to diaphragmatic irritation from haemoperitoneum) and an empty uterus on ultrasound, a diagnostic laparoscopy should be carried out. In the presence of an ectopic pregnancy, laparoscopic salpingectomy or salpingotomy is appropriate. In a haemodynamically stable woman, a laparoscopic approach to the surgical management of tubal pregnancy is preferable to an open approach. In the presence of a healthy contralateral tube, there is no clear evidence that salpingotomy should be preferred to salpingectomy. Postoperative tracking of serum hCG is necessary following salpingotomy, to identify the small number of cases complicated by persistent trophoblast.
- In a well woman with a positive UPT and an empty uterus on transvaginal ultrasound, a serum hCG level is performed. If the level is over 1500 IU/l, a laparoscopy should be considered, as an intrauterine sac is usually seen above this level. Otherwise, hCG should be rechecked in 48 hours. If levels are not doubled, steady or only slightly reduced, a laparoscopy should be considered.
- Medical therapy with methotrexate, either as a single- or multiple-dose regimen, is an option for women with ectopic pregnancy who have minimal symptoms, are clinically stable and have a serum hCG level of less than 3000 IU/l. If medical therapy is offered, women should be given verbal and written information about the possible need for further treatment and adverse effects following treatment. Women should be able to return easily for assessment at any time during follow-up.
- Expectant management is an option for clinically stable asymptomatic women with an ultrasound diagnosis of ectopic pregnancy and a decreasing serum hCG, initially less than 1000 IU/l.

When serum hCG levels are below the discriminatory zone (<1000 IU/l) and there is no pregnancy (intra- or extrauterine) visible on transvaginal ultrasound scan, the pregnancy can be described as being of unknown location (pregnancy of unknown location or PUL). Using an initial upper level of serum hCG of 1000–1500 IU/l to diagnose PUL, women with minimal or no symptoms but at risk of ectopic pregnancy should be managed expectantly with 48-hour follow-up and should be considered for active intervention if symptoms of ectopic pregnancy occur, serum hCG levels rise above the discriminatory level (1500 IU/l) or levels start to plateau. Intervention has been shown to be required in 20–30% of cases of PUL. If women are managed expectantly, serial serum hCG measurements should be performed until hCG levels are less than 15 IU/l. In addition, women selected for expectant management of PUL should be given clear information about the importance of compliance with follow-up and should be within easy access of the unit treating them.

Non-sensitized women who are rhesus negative with a confirmed or suspected ectopic pregnancy should receive anti-D immunoglobulin.

Chronic pelvic pain (CPP)

Healthcare costs associated with CPP are very considerable and do not take into consideration the disability and suffering of the woman and loss of earnings to both the individual and employer. CPP can lead to loss of employment, family and marital discord, divorce, medical misadventures and litigation. Amongst high-quality studies, the rate of dysmenorrhoea was 16.8% to 81%, that of dyspareunia was 8% to 21.8%, and that of non-cyclical pain was 2.1% to 24% worldwide.

The definitions of CPP are numerous but one suitable definition is 'intermittent or constant pain in the lower abdomen or pelvis of at least 6 months duration, not occurring exclusively with menstruation or intercourse and not associated with pregnancy'. A comparison between acute and chronic pelvic pain is shown in **Table 15.1**.

The management of CPP is particularly challenging as there are so many possible causes and contributory factors **(Box 15.2)**. An association with dysmenorrhoea, dyspareunia, irregular menstruation, abnormal vaginal discharge, cyclical pain and infertility may all be helpful in suggesting an underlying gynaecological problem. Altered bowel habit, excess flatulence or flatus, constipation or diarrhoea, on the other hand, point to a gastrointestinal problem, particularly irritable bowel syndrome. Psychiatric, urological and musculoskeletal causes of chronic pain are further possibilities.

Physical and sexual abuse, as well as pelvic pathology such as endometriosis, adhesions and pelvic varices, predispose women to CPP. It is believed that adhesions may be a cause of pain, particularly on organ distension or stretching. Dense vascular adhesions are likely to be a cause of

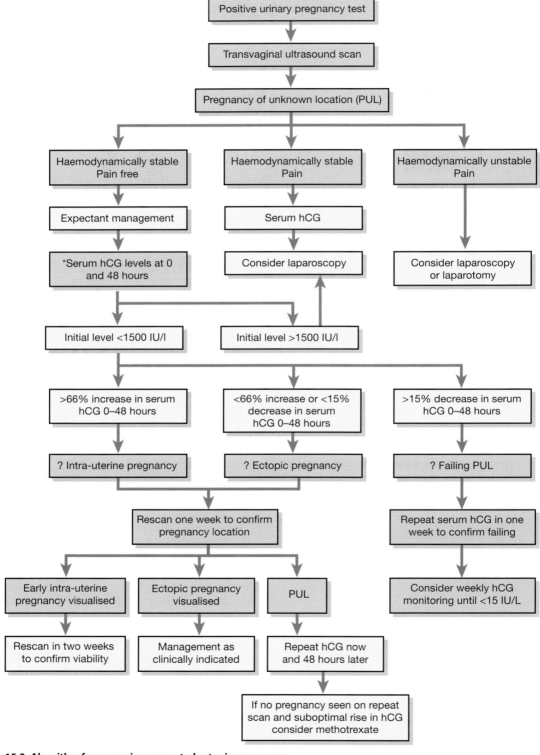

Fig. 15.2 Algorithm for managing suspected ectopic pregnancy.

Table 15.1	
Comparison of acute and chronic pelvic pain	
Acute	**Chronic**
Well-defined onset	Ill-defined onset
Short duration	Unpredictable duration
Rest often helpful	Rest usually not helpful
Variable intensity	Persistent
Anxiety common	Depression common
Disease symptom	May not be possible to identify an underlying disease process

---

Box 15.2

Differential diagnoses for women with chronic pelvic pain

- *Gynaecological:* endometriosis, adhesions (chronic pelvic infection), adenomyosis, leiomyoma, pelvic congestion syndrome, ovarian cysts
- *Gastrointestinal:* adhesions, appendicitis, constipation, diverticular disease, irritable bowel syndrome
- *Urinary tract:* urinary tract infection, calculus, interstitial cystitis
- *Skeletal:* degenerative joint disease, scoliosis, spondylolisthesis, osteitis pubis
- *Myofascial:* fascitis, nerve entrapment syndrome, hernia
- *Psychological:* somatization, psychosexual dysfunction, depression
- *Neuropathic:* pudendal nerve entrapment, spinal cord neuropathies

---

CPP, as dividing them appears to relieve pain. Symptoms suggestive of irritable bowel syndrome or interstitial cystitis are often present in women with CPP. These conditions may be a primary cause or a component of CPP.

Up to 40% of women with CPP, however, do not have an identifiable biological cause despite extensive investigations. It is therefore important to plan which investigations are necessary, carry them out, and then call a halt to any further investigations if no pathology is identified. In gynaecology, such investigation often involves a diagnostic laparoscopy. Further management then depends on whether a pathological cause has been identified or not, and this is considered below. Again, there is some overlap between the two groups **(Fig. 15.3)**.

Endometriosis

See Chapter 16.

Pelvic infection

Chronic pelvic infection is associated with a high incidence of tubal damage, and consequently an increased incidence of ectopic pregnancy, infertility or CPP. It may be due to

relapse of infection because of inadequate treatment, re-infection from an untreated partner, post-infection tubal damage, or further acquisition of STIs. The severity of the problem is related to the number of episodes of pelvic inflammatory disease and the extent of pelvic adhesions.

Ovarian cysts

The majority of ovarian cysts are benign, particularly those presenting with acute pain. Pain may occur because of torsion, cyst rupture, or bleeding occurring into a cyst. Management depends on the presenting clinical situation, but suspected torsion necessitates surgical removal.

Other causes

If investigations are negative and there remains significant diagnostic doubt about whether a pain is gynaecological or not, it may be worth considering a 3-month trial of ovarian suppression with a GnRH analogue. A dramatic reduction of symptoms following suppression with recurrence after treatment suggests a true gynaecological cause, including the possibility of adenomyosis, and there is evidence that hysterectomy will lead to long-term improvement in around three-quarters of this responding group. Many, however, may not wish or be suitable for such radical surgery, and others will be no better despite the suppression.

No identifiable pathological cause for the pain

Treating a woman with CPP without a specific diagnosis is particularly difficult because of the uncertainty for both the clinician and woman, and the problems that this then causes in choosing an appropriate therapeutic intervention. The first step has to be that both the clinician and woman accept 'chronic pelvic pain syndrome' as a disease entity in its own right and then devise strategies to relieve the physical, psychological and social distress that this causes.

Management options range from psychosocial therapy, analgesia management including use of anticonvulsants like gabapentin, hormonal treatments, antidepressants (like amitriptyline) and complementary therapies, to surgery, including surgical excision of nerves (uterine nerve ablation) and pelvic clearance. Communication with the woman should include sharing of information, honest and realistic discussion of the pros and cons of various investigation and treatment options and the likelihood of there being a beneficial outcome. It may also be helpful to involve the woman's partner or friend in the decision-making process.

Encouragement to lead as normal a life as possible whilst investigation and treatment are instigated is acknowledged to be very important in the likelihood of making a full recovery. This would include encouraging return to work, exercise, maintaining a healthy diet, avoiding the inappropriate use of analgesia, and looking for alternatives to analgesia

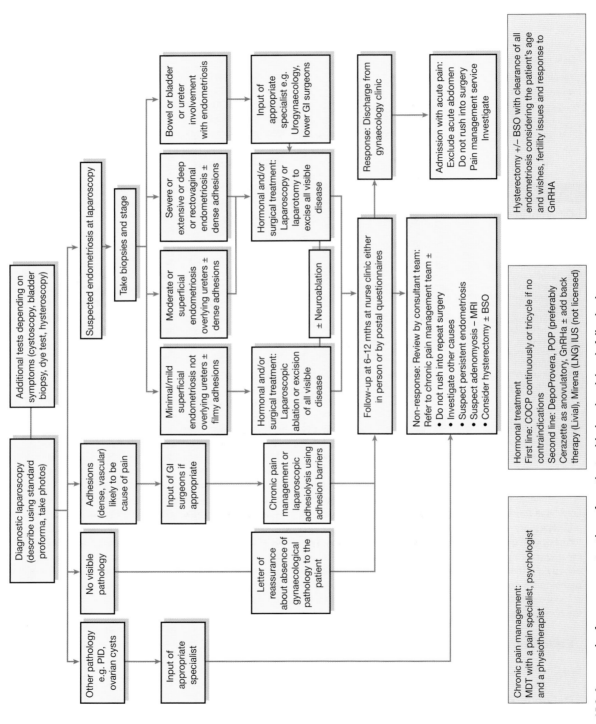

Fig 15.3 An example of a management pathway for patients with chronic pelvic pain following laparoscopy.

where possible. Complementary therapies such as reflexology, homeopathy and acupuncture may be helpful.

The risks of medical misadventure associated with CPP can be minimized by adopting a sympathetic and caring multidisciplinary approach, or by referral to healthcare professionals with a special interest and expertise in managing this condition. A multidisciplinary team approach should ideally include expertise in gastroenterology, neurology, pain management, psychiatry and psychology. Specific psychological approaches to the management of CPP, with input from psychologists and liaison psychiatrists, may be helpful to many women. These approaches include behavioural therapy, cognitive behavioural therapy, group therapy and pharmacological therapy. Pharmacological therapy (e.g. antidepressants and anxiolytics) may be particularly valuable for those individuals who have become secondarily depressed as a consequence of their chronic pain.

Key points

- Acute and chronic pelvic pain have numerous, occasionally overlapping, causes (**Boxes 15.1** and **15.2**).
- Many women present because they want an explanation for their pain. Often, they already have a theory or a concern about the origin of the pain. These ideas should preferably be discussed in the initial consultation.
- The multifactorial nature of chronic pelvic pain should be discussed and explored from the start. The aim should be to develop a partnership between clinician and patient to plan a management programme.
- Diagnostic laparoscopy has been regarded in the past as the 'gold standard' in the diagnosis of chronic pelvic pain. It may be better seen as a second line of investigation if other therapeutic interventions fail. Transvaginal scanning and MRI are useful tests to diagnose adenomyosis.
- Women with cyclical pain should be offered a therapeutic trial using the combined oral contraceptive pill or a GnRH agonist for a period of 3–6 months before having a diagnostic laparoscopy.
- Women with symptoms suggestive of irritable bowel syndrome should be offered a trial of antispasmodics and try amending their diet to control symptoms.
- Women should be offered appropriate analgesia to control their pain, even if no other therapeutic manoeuvres are yet to be initiated. If pain is not adequately controlled, consideration should be given to referral to a pain management team or a specialist pelvic pain clinic.
- While the commonest causes of chronic pelvic pain are endometriosis and chronic pelvic infection, over a third will have no identifiable pathology. It is important to call a halt to unnecessary investigations: accept the 'chronic pelvic pain syndrome' as a disease entity in its own right.

16

Endometriosis

Introduction

Although endometriosis is a common condition, our knowledge about it is incomplete. Debate remains about its origins, pathological features, diagnosis, prognosis and treatment.

The term 'endometriosis' refers to tissue resembling the endometrium which is lying outside of the endometrial cavity. It usually lies within the peritoneal cavity and predominantly in the pelvis, commonly on the uterosacral ligaments behind the uterus **(Fig. 16.1)**. Rarely, it can also be found in distant sites such as the umbilicus, abdominal scars, perineal scars, and even the pleural cavity and nasal mucosa. Like the true endometrium it responds to cyclical hormonal changes and it bleeds at menstruation. Such bleeding may cause problems.

Adenomyosis occurs when there is endometrial tissue within the myometrium of the uterus. The uterus is enlarged and feels 'boggy'. There is painful and heavy menstruation. Adenomyosis is difficult to diagnose clinically and is usually only apparent retrospectively, with histological examination of the uterus after hysterectomy. It is commonly considered to be a separate entity from endometriosis, occurring in a different population and having a different aetiology.

Incidence

Endometriosis occurs in approximately 1–2% of women of reproductive age, but among infertile women the incidence may be 20 times greater. As it is oestrogen dependent, it is rarely diagnosed postmenopausally, but recurrence has been associated with the use of hormone replacement therapy.

Aetiology

The precise aetiology of endometriosis remains unclear, with no single explanation reliably explaining all its features. Sampson's 'implantation' theory (history box) postulates that endometrial fragments flow in a retrograde manner along the fallopian tube during menstruation, 'seeding' themselves on the pelvic peritoneum. In support of this theory is the fact that it is sometimes possible to see blood flowing from the fimbrial end of the fallopian tube if a laparoscopy is carried out during menstruation. Seeding is also observed onto scars such as after hysterectomy or caesarean section, or on perineal scars after delivery, and there is some animal research in which endometrial tissue has been surgically implanted directly onto the peritoneum.

h History

John Albertson Sampson (1873–1946), from Massachusetts, was a prolific writer, publishing 17 papers while still a resident. He proposed that endometriosis is a process produced by the retrograde escape of endometrial tissue, which leads to secondary reactions of inflammation, repair and scar formation.

This theory, however, cannot be the only mechanism of endometriosis formation, as endometriosis has been reported in women with congenitally obstructed fallopian tubes. Meyer's 'coelomic metaplasia' theory (history box) proposes that cells of the original coelomic membrane transform to endometrial cells by metaplasia, possibly as a result of hormonal stimulation or inflammatory irritation. This could explain the presence of endometriosis in nearly all the distant sites, although it is also possible that spread from the uterus to these distant sites occurs by venous or lymphatic microembolism.

h History

Robert Meyer (1864–1947), a German-born gynaecologist and pathologist, proposed that endometriosis is the result of peritoneal metaplasia. It is acknowledged that retrograde menstruation may be a stimulus for the metaplasia.

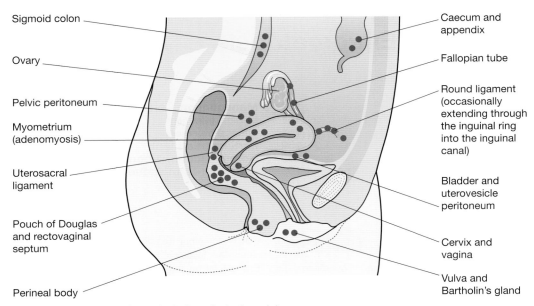

Sigmoid colon

Ovary

Pelvic peritoneum

Myometrium
(adenomyosis)

Uterosacral
ligament

Pouch of Douglas
and rectovaginal
septum

Perineal body

Caecum and
appendix

Fallopian tube

Round ligament
(occasionally
extending through
the inguinal ring
into the inguinal
canal)

Bladder and
uterovesicle
peritoneum

Cervix and
vagina

Vulva and
Bartholin's gland

Fig. 16.1 Common sites for endometriotic deposits in the pelvis.

In some instances, the presence of endometriosis may be explained by neoplasia. This is particularly so in the ovary, where a solitary ovarian endometrioma is sometimes included in the classification of ovarian neoplasia as the benign counterpart of endometrioid carcinoma.

The question remains as to why endometriosis becomes established in some, but not all, women and it is possible that there is some genetic or immunological predisposition to account for such wide variation.

Clinical presentation

In most instances, clinical presentation occurs because of pelvic disease. Endometriosis is the commonest cause of secondary dysmenorrhoea. There is usually a continuous, non-spasmodic pain, which is worse immediately before and throughout menstruation, and colicky dysmenorrhoea may also occur in association with heavy menstrual loss and the passage of clots. In addition, there may be dyspareunia, which may relate to endometriotic deposits in the pouch of Douglas or to ovarian endometriomas. Typically this pain settles when the period ends, but some women also describe a continuous, lower abdominal pain that is not specifically related to their cycle or to sexual activity.

One of the puzzles regarding endometriosis is the lack of correlation between the severity of these symptoms and the extent of the disease. Extensive deposits leading to the obliteration of the pouch of Douglas and involving the ovaries, fallopian tubes and other pelvic organs may be completely asymptomatic; conversely, women with lesions only a few millimetres across may be debilitated by pain.

Menstrual disturbances may be associated with endometriosis, and in particular with adenomyosis. Where there is also significant ovarian involvement, the menstrual cycle may become erratic. Rarely, postcoital bleeding is experienced in the presence of endometriosis involving the ectocervix, or where deposits in the pouch of Douglas penetrate into the posterior fornix.

Endometriosis in distant sites is rare but may generate local symptoms, such as cyclical epistaxes with nasal deposits, or catamenial pneumothoraces with pleural deposits. Monthly rectal bleeding may occur if the bowel mucosa is affected.

Examination

The clinical diagnosis of endometriosis is aided by findings of:

- thickened pelvic ligaments, particularly the uterosacral ligaments, which may be nodular; on speculum examination, blue nodules may be seen in the posterior vaginal fornix.
- a fixed (immobile) retroverted uterus
- uterine or ovarian enlargement if these organs are involved.

There may also be tenderness in the lateral and posterior fornices and with applied pressure on the uterosacral ligaments. Attempts to move the uterus may also provoke pain. This pain often resembles the presenting symptom, particularly when this was dyspareunia.

With the exception of visualizing endometriotic nodules, none of these features is diagnostic of endometriosis and

Table 16.1	
Possible mechanisms by which endometriosis may reduce fertility	
System	**Mechanism**
Coital function	Dyspareunia, leading to reduced frequency of coitus
Sperm function	Inactivation of spermatozoa by antibodies Phagocytosis of spermatozoa by macrophages
Tubal function	Fimbrial damage Reduced tubal motility with prostaglandins
Ovarian function	Anovulation LUF syndrome (see text) Luteolysis caused by prostaglandin $F_{2\alpha}$ Altered release of gonadotrophins

Box 16.1
Laparoscopic and histological appearances
■ Haemosiderin deposits covered with peritoneum resemble the classical appearance of endometriosis, but may arise from local haemorrhage of any origin. The typical chocolate-coloured cysts contained within the ovary, for example, need not be caused by endometriosis, and histological examination often shows that these have arisen from haemorrhage into a follicular or corpus luteum cyst. ■ A wide range of subtle peritoneal changes, such as clear 'sago' blisters, glandular papillae, white opacified patches, red flame-like lesions and circular peritoneal defects, may prove on biopsy to be a result of endometriosis **(Fig. 16.2)**. ■ Even more perplexing is the finding that normal peritoneum, when biopsied and studied with scanning electron microscopy, may contain cells of endometrial type. These may be more common in patients with proven disease elsewhere, but can also be found in apparently normal women. ■ As many as 52% of patients with pelvic pain but no visible peritoneal deposits of endometriosis have been found on histological examination to harbour lesions deep in the uterosacral ligaments.

conversely their absence does not exclude the disease. There are many other causes of pelvic pain, including irritable bowel syndrome and recurrent urinary infection, which can confuse the differential diagnosis. In particular, chronic conditions such as pelvic inflammatory disease and pelvic venous congestion mimic many features of endometriosis. Laparoscopy is therefore usually necessary to make the diagnosis.

Endometriosis and infertility

Endometriosis is commonly diagnosed in women who are undergoing laparoscopic investigations for infertility but who do not have specific symptoms. Although endometriosis and infertility are associated more commonly than can be explained by chance, the exact mechanism of their interrelationship is uncertain **(Table 16.1)**.

While it is recognized that severe disease can cause infertility by forming periovarian and peritubular adhesions and by destroying ovarian tissue, the association between mild endometriosis and infertility is less clear. Theoretically, high prostaglandin production from endometriotic tissue could impede tubal motility, or the spermatozoa may be affected by adverse immunological factors.

Another possibility is that infertility caused by some unrelated factor may predispose to endometriosis simply because, in the absence of pregnancy and lactational amenorrhoea, there will have been more periods. Other theories suggest that both endometriosis and infertility are manifestations of a third, unidentified problem. An association with the luteinized unruptured follicle (LUF) syndrome, in which follicular development proceeds along apparently normal lines but oocyte release does not occur, provides another explanation. As endometriosis is more common in this condition, it has been proposed that failure to release follicular fluid mid-cycle may result in a preferential environment for endometriosis to become established.

Investigation

Transvaginal ultrasound can detect gross endometriosis involving the ovaries (endometriomas or chocolate cysts) and MRI can delineate the extent of active endometriosis lesions greater than 1 cm in diameter in deep tissues, e.g. rectovaginal septum. Laparoscopy remains the traditional standard diagnostic method. Active endometriotic lesions are classically described as red, puckered and inflamed, or 'burnt match heads' (cigarette burns). Inactive lesions look like scars. The degree to which laparoscopic visualization alone may be adequate, however, has been questioned (see **Box 16.1**).

Little is known about the rate of progression of low-grade endometriosis, but a proportion of untreated patients may deteriorate over as little as 6 months. The prompt return of symptoms after treatment, seen in many patients, may represent re-extension of uneradicated residual disease.

It is impossible to guarantee a cure after treatment. Routine repeat laparoscopy after completion of treatment, therefore, has limited prognostic value and is probably best reserved for those patients with recurrent symptoms.

Management

Medical treatment with non-steroidal anti-inflammatory drugs and/or simple analgesics is widely employed and many women will be self-prescribing prior to diagnosis. Medical treatment with ovulation suppression is most useful for symptomatic relief, but is of no value for the treatment of endometriosis in patients wishing to conceive. Treatment is usually limited to between 3 and 6 months.

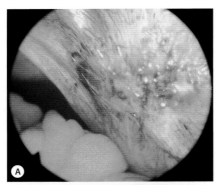

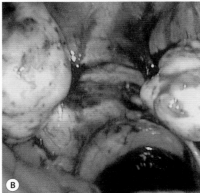

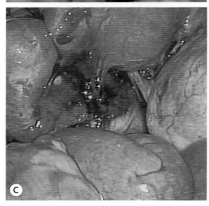

Fig. 16.2 Peritoneal appearances of endometriosis.
Laparoscopic views show **(A)** clear blisters ('sago' granules), 'blood blisters', yellow-brown patches, 'powder burns', atypical vascularity and telangiectasia; **(B)** bilateral endometriomas; **(C)** severe endometriosis with adhesions. (Parts **(B)** and **(C)** courtesy of Karl Storz Endoscopy (UK) Ltd.)

Surgical treatment may be conservative, with laser or diathermy ablation, or radical, involving hysterectomy and oophorectomy.

Medical treatment

Ovulation suppression limits the likelihood of conception, but nonetheless it is still advisable for women to use barrier methods of contraception (unless using the combined oral contraceptive as their treatment method). To avoid inadvertent administration during pregnancy, all therapies should be initiated within the first 3 days of the start of a menstrual period. Medical treatment is founded upon the observation that endometriosis improves during both pregnancy and the menopause; so, creating a 'pseudo-pregnancy' with progestogens or combined oral contraceptives and a 'pseudo-menopause' with gonadotrophin-releasing hormone (GnRH) analogues is appropriate and frequently effective.

For symptomatic endometriosis, continuous progestogen therapy (e.g. medroxyprogesterone acetate 10 mg three times daily for 90 days) is most cost-effective, has fewer side-effects and is more suitable for long-term use compared with more expensive alternatives. Progestogens have a direct action on the endometrial target tissue by binding to progestogen receptors. This produces decidualization of the endometrial tissue, which then leads to subsequent necrosis. The combined oral contraceptive pill is also an appropriate alternative whereby it is taken continuously in order to induce amenorrhoea. The usual risk factors for the suitability or otherwise for using the combined pill should be evaluated, but if appropriate and symptoms are alleviated, it can be continued for several years or even longer.

Second-line drugs are the GnRH analogues (which can be administered by nasal spray, implants or injection), and the orally administered androgen danazol. GnRH analogues bind to GnRH receptors in the pituitary, initially stimulating gonadotrophin release but rapidly desensitizing the pituitary to GnRH stimulation, thereby in turn suppressing gonadotrophin release and hence ovarian steroid secretion. The profound hypo-oestrogenic state produced not only affects endometrial tissue but also causes side-effects mimicking the climacteric. Therapy is limited to 4–6 months and it is routine to prescribe 'add-back' hormone replacement therapy to alleviate the predictable menopausal side-effects and negative effects upon bone density. Danazol combines androgenic activity with anti-oestrogenic and anti-progestogenic activity, and it inhibits pituitary gonadotrophins. It has a relatively high incidence of androgenic and perimenopausal side-effects, making it an infrequent treatment choice.

Medical treatment can also be used as a diagnostic tool. By achieving amenorrhoea and symptom relief, then it is extremely likely that the symptoms were due to endometriosis. If symptoms persist, a review of the diagnosis is necessary and other causes of pelvic pain considered.

Surgical treatment

When continued fertility is required, conservative surgery is appropriate. This is usually carried out laparoscopically and includes diathermy destruction, laser vaporization or excision of endometriosis deposits. It may bring about symptom relief and has a role in subfertile women (see below). Recurrence risks following conservative surgery are as high as 30%.

Hysterectomy with bilateral oophorectomy for women who have completed their childbearing is usually curative. Hormone replacement will be needed; although this may activate residual disease, the possibility may be minimized by using some form of combined preparation rather than an oestrogen-only form.

Fertility treatment

There is no evidence that medical treatment of endometriosis is of any value in the management of subfertility. Surgical ablation or excision of minimal and mild endometriosis does improve fertility, but whether surgery has a role in moderate and severe endometriosis is less clear. Surgical treatment of large ovarian endometriotic cysts probably enhances spontaneous pregnancy rates and will improve transvaginal access if in vitro fertilization (IVF) is considered. In cases of moderate and severe endometriosis, assisted reproduction techniques should be considered as an alternative to surgery, or following unsuccessful surgery.

Complications, prognosis and long-term sequelae

Depending upon the severity of the disease, adhesions and fibrosis may distort bowel, bladder, ureters and other neighbouring viscera, leading to chronic problems with these systems. The physical and psychological morbidity from long-term pain can be considerable.

Key points

- Endometriosis is caused by endometrium-like tissue outside the uterine cavity. Endometrium-like tissue growing within the uterine wall is referred to as adenomyosis, and may be a different pathological entity.
- Endometriosis may be caused by the seeding of endometrial cells when menstrual fluid spills retrogradely along the fallopian tubes. Other possible aetiological mechanisms are coelomic metaplasia and venous or lymphatic spread.
- Clinical endometriosis affects 1–2% of women, but the incidence is higher among women with subfertility. Symptoms include secondary dysmenorrhoea, dyspareunia, lower abdominal pain and menorrhagia. There may be ovarian enlargement, thickening of uterosacral ligaments, fixed retroversion of the uterus and tenderness on pelvic examination.
- Diagnosis usually requires laparoscopy.
- Medical management is by progestogens, the combined oral contraceptive pill, danazol or GnRH analogues. Surgical management may involve laparoscopic ablation or excision of deposits, open surgery with local resection, or hysterectomy with or without bilateral oophorectomy.

17

Premenstrual syndrome

Introduction

Premenstrual syndrome (PMS) can usefully be defined as 'a condition manifesting with physical, behavioural and psychological symptoms in the absence of organic or psychiatric disease, which regularly occurs during the luteal phase of each ovarian cycle and which disappears or significantly regresses by the end of menstruation'. PMS is considered severe if it impairs work, relationships or usual activities. Some observers note that as many as 95% of women suffer mild symptoms, and between 5% and 10% of women have symptoms severe enough to disrupt their lives, principally in the 2 weeks leading up to the start of menstruation.

Over 150 symptoms have been attributed to PMS, but particularly:

- mood changes/irritability
- abdominal bloatedness
- breast tenderness (cyclical mastalgia)
- headaches
- oedema.

Aetiology

The aetiology of PMS remains largely unknown. Ovulatory cycles are generally considered to be a necessary pre-requisite. Many hypotheses have considered whether there might be abnormal levels of specific hormones, and research has focused on progesterone, oestrogen, adreno-corticotrophic hormone, vasopressin, luteinizing hormone, prolactin and thyroid-stimulating hormone. There is no consistent evidence that any of these are abnormal in PMS, but there are suggestions that it is the changing patterns of hormone levels, rather than the absolute levels, which is important. There may be an abnormality in levels of neurotransmitter function, particularly serotonin, and this is discussed further under 'Management' below.

Clinical presentation

As there are no specific biochemical tests for PMS, the diagnosis is dependent on a prospective charting of symptoms to confirm that there is a true exacerbation in the luteal phase when compared to the follicular phase of the cycle **(Fig.17.1)**. A simple calendar record of the presence or absence of a woman's three principal symptoms and days of menstruation is appropriate. There are numerous specific criteria, many of them research tools which are not necessarily always applied strictly to clinical practice. An example of one of these is shown in **Box 17.1**.

Differential diagnosis

Symptoms that are worse other than premenstrually are not attributable to PMS. Other conditions such as endometritis, migraine headaches, depression and anxiety disorders are exacerbated premenstrually, but again should not be confused with the more specific diagnosis of PMS. Perimenopausal mood changes are usually non-cyclical and consideration may be given to checking a serum follicle-stimulating hormone (FSH) level. A normal FSH level does not exclude the menopause, but the investigation may be of particular value in those who have had a hysterectomy with ovarian conservation (since there is no menstruation).

The breast pain of PMS is usually cyclical, bilateral and poorly localized, and 'lumpiness' is common. By contrast, non-cyclical breast pain is precisely localized and rarely bilateral.

In those with abdominal swelling, it is important to consider intra-abdominal pathology such as ovarian cysts or ascites. The abdominal bloating of PMS is rapidly relieved by the onset of menstruation, perhaps owing to the relaxing effect of prostaglandins on smooth muscle or to comparative stasis of the gut in response to morphine-like endorphins. Hypothyroidism and anaemia should be considered

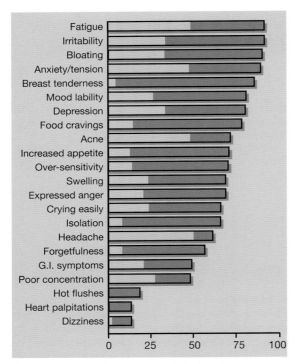

Fig. 17.1 Incidence (percent of cycles) with which individual symptoms were reported in the follicular phase of the cycle (open bars) and luteal phase of the cycle (entire bars) in 170 women. GI, gastrointestinal.

Box 17.1

Example of a set of diagnostic criteria for PMS

1. The presence, by self-report, of at least one of the following somatic and affective symptoms during the 5 days before menses in each of the three previous cycles:

Affective symptoms:	Somatic symptoms:
Depression	Breast tenderness
Angry outbursts	Abdominal bloating
Irritability	Headache
Anxiety	Swelling
Confusion	
Social withdrawal	

2. Relief of the above symptoms within 4 days of the onset of the menses, without recurrence until day 12
3. Presence of the symptoms in the absence of any pharmacological therapy, hormone ingestion, drug or alcohol misuse
4. Reproducible occurrence of symptoms during two cycles of prospective recording
5. Identifiable dysfunction in social or economic performance by one of the following criteria:

   ■ Discord in relationship confirmed by partner
   ■ Difficulties in parenting
   ■ Poor work or school performance
   ■ Increased social isolation
   ■ Legal difficulties
   ■ Suicidal ideation
   ■ Medical attention sought for somatic symptoms

From Mortola et al 1990, Obstet Gynecol 76:302

---

in those complaining predominantly of fatigue. The characteristics of endogenous depression are different to those of the mood changes and irritability commonly observed in PMS, but, since both conditions are relatively common, it is not unusual to encounter both in the same woman.

Management

Women with mild PMS do not usually need medical treatment and may be helped by reassurance and counselling. General health measures such as improved diet, increased exercise, self-relaxation, and reducing smoking and drinking might be helpful. Some women find self-help groups supportive, while others choose yoga or hypnosis. Treatment can be aimed at the symptoms, or at a hypothesized underlying cause.

Symptomatic treatment

A number of symptomatic treatments are in use, although the evidence supporting their effectiveness is limited. Those with premenstrual bloatedness can be treated in the same way as those with irritable bowel syndrome, and those with oedema may respond to a diuretic. Breast tenderness can also be treated with diuretics, as well as with bromocriptine or low-dose danazol. Mood changes are considered in more detail below.

Treatment aimed at the hypothesized underlying cause

A wide variety of medical treatments have been considered, many of which are still in current use. Close scrutiny, however, reveals that only a limited number of these are of proven value, and the treatment modalities are classified this way in **Box 17.2**. The 'probably effective' group consists of treatments demonstrated to be effective by good-sized trials, usually randomized placebo-controlled trials. The use of a placebo arm is particularly important in PMS research, as most placebo treatments demonstrate symptom improvements of around 30%. Treatments classified as 'probably not effective' have also been examined in well-conducted studies, and no significant benefit has been demonstrated over placebo. The 'may be effective' group include therapies in which studies have been inconclusive, often because of small patient numbers. The three groups will be considered in more detail below.

Probably not effective
Progesterone or progestogens

The rationale for the use of progesterone or progestogens in the management of PMS is based on the unsubstantiated premise that there is a progesterone deficiency. Although initial data suggest there to be abnormal concentrations of metabolites of progesterone (pregnenolone and allopregnenolone),

Box 17.2

Possible treatments for PMS

Probably effective

- SSRIs
- Suppression of ovulation
- Oophorectomy

May be effective

- Diet
- Exercise
- Psychological approaches
- Vitamin B6
- Complementary therapy

Probably not effective

- Progesterone
- Evening primrose oil
- Vitamin E

there is no consistent evidence that low concentrations of progesterone are found in women with PMS; overviews of randomized trials do not suggest any useful clinical benefit. Intramuscular depot progestogen may be helpful (see later).

Evening primrose oil

The hypothesis is that there is a deficiency in essential fatty acids, particularly gamolenic acid, leading to low levels of prostaglandin E1 and therefore premenstrual symptoms. Evening primrose oil contains essential fatty acids, including gamolenic acid, and is available in many countries without a prescription. It is heavily promoted as an effective treatment for a range of conditions, including PMS, and it appears to have minimal side-effects. Trials demonstrate marginal, if any, clinical improvement, principally in the relief of mastalgia.

Vitamin B$_6$ (pyridoxine)

It has been suggested that treatment with pyridoxine, the active form of which is a coenzyme in amino acid metabolism, may act by correcting some deficiency within the hypothalamus. Pyridoxine is involved particularly in the metabolism of dopamine and serotonin, low levels of which lead to high levels of prolactin and aldosterone, possibly explaining the fluid retention experienced in PMS. It may also account for some of the psychological symptoms attributable to alterations in neurotransmitter levels.

Vitamin B$_6$ is taken daily, and this can be on a continuous basis or during the second half of the menstrual cycle. Placebo-controlled randomized trials do not demonstrate any meaningful benefit of B$_6$ in PMS. There are safety concerns with its use since doses greater than 200 mg per day are associated with peripheral neuropathy.

May be effective

Diet

The usual recommendations are for a reduction in salt, sugar, alcohol and caffeine, and an increase in carbohydrates. It is suggested that the increased carbohydrate intake increases serotonergic activity, which in turn improves symptoms.

Exercise

Aerobic activity leads to increased endorphin levels, which are recognized to improve mood, and several studies suggest there may be some benefit in the treatment of PMS.

Psychological approach

Techniques aimed at reducing stress may be beneficial. Cognitive behavioural therapy, which encourages relaxation, and the use of 'coping skills' may also be helpful. A clinical psychology service should ideally be made available to women with severe disease.

Complementary therapy

Studies have explored the use of homeopathy, dietary supplementation, relaxation, massage, reflexology, chiropractic therapy and biofeedback. While there were some positive findings, there is no compelling evidence to support any of these therapies. Agnus Castus may be of benefit, but there is no standard quality-controlled preparation available. St John's Wort has the potential for significant interaction with conventional medicines, including SSRIs.

Probably effective

Selective serotonin reuptake inhibitors (SSRIs)

PMS often presents with symptoms similar to those of anxiety and depression and this association has resulted in treatment with a variety of antidepressants. Reduced platelet uptake of serotonin and reduced levels in the blood of women with PMS during the luteal phase have been used to imply a role for SSRIs in PMS treatment. Meta-analysis shows that SSRIs are effective, with around 60% of those with severe PMS reporting a reduction in physical and behavioural symptoms compared to around 30% of controls. This effectiveness is often apparent after only one or two cycles. Side-effects include insomnia, gastrointestinal disturbances, fatigue and loss of libido, but may be acceptable at the recommended low dose. Intermittent use in the luteal phase may be as effective as continuous daily dosing. A gradual rather than abrupt withdrawal of SSRIs is appropriate if the SSRI has been taken on a continuous basis, in order to avoid symptoms of withdrawal.

Ovarian suppression

Since the majority of PMS symptoms can be attributed to cyclical ovarian hormone production, the suppression of ovulation is a logical treatment option. The effectiveness of the combined oral contraceptive (COC) pill for the treatment of PMS is uncertain; some research suggests an improvement in symptoms, whereas other research suggests symptom exacerbation. Limited evidence supports the use of a recent-generation COC containing drospirenone as the progestogen. It is logical to consider taking the COC continuously. Depot medroxyprogesterone, a long-acting injectable progestogen, may also be helpful.

The synthetic androgen danazol suppresses ovulation and a relatively low dose of 200 mg twice daily is effective in improving the symptoms of mastalgia. Use of danazol is limited by its potential for irreversible virilization, and effective contraception should be used to avoid virilization of a female fetus.

Transdermal oestrogen (100 µg/day), by way of patches designed for hormone replacement therapy (HRT), is associated with an improvement in PMS symptoms. If the woman has not had a hysterectomy, a progestogen is required to avoid endometrial stimulation, hyperplasia and possible malignant transformation. The lowest dose of progestogen is appropriate; the levonorgestrel intrauterine system is particularly suitable since the serum level of progestogen is very low, thus minimizing the risk of progestogenic side-effects (which may mimic/exacerbate PMS).

Gonadotrophin-releasing hormone (GnRH) analogues are a highly effective way of suppressing ovarian function, and are therefore a highly effective treatment for severe refractory PMS. As oestrogen is suppressed to postmenopausal levels, however, the PMS symptoms may be replaced by menopausal ones, including hot flushes. These in turn can be minimized with the use of continuous combined 'add-back' HRT. A therapeutic trial of GnRH analogues with add-back HRT is often beneficial in clarifying the diagnosis and establishing that the woman can tolerate an HRT preparation should oophorectomy become appropriate (see below). Treatment with GnRH analogues cannot be continued long term, however, because of the risks of osteoporosis and other side-effects associated with a premature menopause. GnRH analogues are licensed for use over 6 months only and are not specifically licensed for use in PMS.

Bilateral oophorectomy

This is an effective treatment for PMS. It is, however, a surgical procedure and therefore not without significant short-term surgical risks. There are also the longer-term risks of premature menopause as with the GnRH analogues, particularly if compliance with subsequent HRT is poor. This surgical option is therefore only suitable for those very likely to benefit from it, as suggested by a definite response to a GnRH analogue, and only in those who have completed their family. It is also reasonable not to opt for this procedure if the natural menopause is likely to be occurring in the near future.

Individual management strategy

Given the large number of treatments advocated, it can be difficult to find a practical way through them. As PMS is usually a chronic condition, it is important to consider the side-effect profile of treatments that may be used over many years. Once the diagnosis is established by prospective symptom diary-keeping, it seems sensible to try those treatments with fewest significant side-effects, initially diet, regular aerobic exercise, and techniques aimed at stress reduction. A significant proportion of women will benefit from these three tried together, and drug therapy can then be considered for those who do not improve sufficiently.

An SSRI is the most appropriate first-line drug, used initially for the second half of the cycle and then throughout the cycle if there is no improvement over the first two or three cycles. The next stage is ovarian suppression with a GnRH analogue. Successful symptom improvement, however, leaves a dilemma, as continuous treatment is not appropriate. Long-term suppression with medroxyprogesterone acetate 3-monthly i.m. (which may be associated with significant side-effects) and surgical oophorectomy are the main subsequent options to be considered.

Key *points*

- Premenstrual syndrome (PMS) can be defined as a regular pattern of symptoms occurring in the time before menstruation, with a lessening of symptoms soon after the start of bleeding.
- The aetiology of the condition is poorly understood, and diagnosis is dependent on prospectively charting the symptoms to confirm that there is a true cyclical variation.
- Only a limited number of treatments are of greater value than placebo and these are listed in **Box 17.2**. Initial treatment should include dietary advice, regular aerobic exercise, and techniques aimed at stress reduction. An SSRI is the most appropriate first-line drug; if unsuccessful, it may be appropriate to institute a trial of ovarian suppression. Long-term suppression with medroxyprogesterone acetate or surgical oophorectomy may be considered.

18

The menopause

Introduction

Human female fertility terminates relatively abruptly in middle age. This seems to be rather a puzzle as, in evolutionary terms, those genes that 'favour' giving birth to as many offspring as possible would be expected to proliferate. In other words, the genes of mothers who continued giving birth to children for as many years as they could would be expected to be successful. Human children, however, remain dependent on their mothers for many years after birth and, if mothers continued to reproduce until the end of their lives, they would be less able to support the later children to independent maturity. The incidence of congenital abnormality also increases with maternal age. This would be a waste of personal resources without genetic benefit, and would also limit the support such a mother could offer to her grandchildren, in whom she has a quarter-part genetic investment.

The flaw in this otherwise reasonable teleological argument, however, is that the vast majority of women previously died long before reaching the current average age of menopause, thus diluting the role of longevity in the evolutionary process. The true reasons behind this process of ovarian failure, the menopause, are therefore not yet fully elucidated.

Menopause literally means 'last menstrual period' but the word is often used to cover the physiological changes that occur around this time. The fluctuating levels of oestrogen resulting from declining ovarian function lead to changes in a number of systems, and may give rise to significant symptoms. Although physiological, the menopause has important adverse long-term effects on health **(Table 18.1)** which can, in part, be offset by the use of hormone replacement therapy (HRT). The pros and cons of this treatment will be discussed in more detail and need to be carefully considered on an individual basis before treatment is started.

Physiology

The perimenopause (or climacteric) may begin months or years before the last menstrual period, and symptoms may continue for years afterwards. The median age at menopause in the UK is 50.8 years and it occurs when the supply of oocytes becomes exhausted. A newborn girl has over half a million oocytes in her ovaries: one-third of these disappear before puberty and most of the remainder are lost during reproductive life. In each menstrual cycle, some 20 or 30 primordial follicles begin to develop and most become atretic. As only about 400 cycles occur during an average woman's lifetime, most oocytes are lost spontaneously through ageing rather than through ovulation.

In premenopausal women, oestradiol is produced by the granulosa cells of the developing follicle, but, as the menopause approaches, this production becomes very variable. The proportion of anovulatory menstrual cycles increases and progesterone production declines. Pituitary production of follicle-stimulating hormone (FSH) and luteinizing hormone (LH) rises because of diminishing negative feedback from oestrogen and other ovarian hormones such as inhibin, but other pituitary hormones are not affected. Serum levels of FSH over 30 IU/l can be used clinically to clarify the diagnosis of menopause (see below), although levels begin to rise significantly around the age of 38 even in normally cycling women. Anti-Müllerian hormone is a better marker of follicular reserve than FSH and is now used in medical practice.

Circulating androstenedione, mainly of adrenal origin, is converted by fat cells into oestrone, a less potent form of oestrogen than oestradiol. After the menopause, this is the predominant circulating oestrogen rather than ovarian oestrogens.

Table 18.1

The consequences of oestrogen deficiency

Short-term problems	Vasomotor (85% of women)	• Headaches • Hot flushes • Night sweats • Palpitations • Insomnia
	Psychological	• Irritability • Poor concentration • Poor short-term memory • Depression • Lethargy • Loss of libido/self-confidence • Generalized aches
Intermediate problems	Urogenital	• Urethral symptoms • Uterine prolapse • Stress/urge incontinence • Dyspareunia • Atrophic vaginitis/vulvitis
	Cutaneous/connective tissue	• Vaginal dryness • Dry skin • Dry hair • Brittle nails
Long-term problems (>50% of women)	Arterial	• Cardiovascular disease • Cerebrovascular disease
	Skeletal	• Osteoporosis

Reproduced with permission from: National Osteoporosis Society, 1994 and Oldenhave A et al, *Am J Obstet Gynecol* 1993; 168: 772–80.

Signs and symptoms (Table 18.1)

Vaginal bleeding

Irregular periods before the menopause are usually the result of anovulatory menstrual cycles, and, if irregular bleeding persists, endometrial assessment may be required to exclude the possibility of endometrial carcinoma. The menopause itself can be recognized only in retrospect after an arbitrary length of amenorrhoea, usually taken as 6 months or a year. Further vaginal bleeding after this is 'postmenopausal' and endometrial assessment may again be required. Approximately 10% of those with postmenopausal bleeding have a gynaecological malignancy.

Hot flushes

A 'hot flush' is an uncomfortable subjective feeling of warmth in the upper part of the body, usually lasting around 3 minutes. Approximately 50–85% of menopausal women experience such vasomotor symptoms, although only 10–20% seek medical advice. Flushes are sometimes accompanied by nausea, palpitations and sweating, and may be particularly troublesome at night. They are thought to be of hypothalamic origin and may in some way be related to LH

release. It is thought that a fall in oestrogen levels affects central alpha-adrenergic systems which in turn affect central thermoregulatory centres and LH-releasing neurons.

About 20% of women begin experiencing flushes while still menstruating regularly. Flushes slowly improve as the body adjusts to the new low oestrogen concentrations, but in approximately 25% of women they continue for more than 5 years. Exogenous oestrogen administration, in the form of HRT, is effective in relieving these symptoms in about 90% of cases.

Genitourinary atrophy

The genital system, urethra and bladder trigone are oestrogen-dependent and undergo gradual atrophy after the menopause. Thinning of the vaginal skin may cause dyspareunia and bleeding, and loss of vaginal glycogen causes a rise in pH which can predispose to local infection. Urgency of micturition may result from atrophic change in the trigone. Unlike flushes, these atrophic symptoms may appear years after the menopause and do not improve spontaneously, although they respond well to a short course of local or systemic oestrogen.

Other symptoms

Some studies have suggested that many symptoms, including irritability and lethargy, can be improved by hormone therapy more effectively than by placebo. Most investigators, however, feel that the symptom of depression is not due directly to oestrogen withdrawal, although it has been reported that oestrogen treatment can improve the symptoms of depression. It is possible that this effect may be related to the indirect relief of specific symptoms, such as insomnia caused by night sweats.

Long-term effects

The menopause alters a woman's susceptibility to breast cancer, cardiovascular disease and osteoporosis.

Breast cancer

Although the risk of breast cancer increases with increasing age, the rate of increase slows after the menopause. The risk of breast cancer is decreased if the menopause is premature and increased if it occurs late, such that a woman who has had a menopause in her late 50s has double the risk of breast cancer when compared to a woman who has had a menopause in her early 40s.

Cardiovascular disease

A premenopausal woman's risk of developing coronary artery disease is less than one-fifth of that of a man of the same age, a sex difference that has disappeared by the age of 85 years. This has been assumed to indicate that oestrogens protect against vascular disease, but the phenomenon may be due to other risk factors affecting the male and to the fact that high-risk men die before they reach old age.

Studies looking at the effect of postmenopausal oestrogen therapy on cardiovascular disease suggest that unopposed oestrogen treatment may reduce the risk of ischaemic heart disease. More recent studies, however, looking at the incidence of subsequent myocardial infarction, have found no protective effect. Starting combined HRT at the time of the natural menopause (i.e. around 50 years) does not seem to be associated with an increased incidence of cardiovascular events, although there may be an adverse impact in women over 60 years of age at initiation of HRT.

Osteoporosis

Bone resorption by osteoclasts is accelerated by the menopause **(Fig. 18.1)**. Oestrogen receptors have been demonstrated on bone cells, and oestrogens have been shown to stimulate osteoblasts directly. Calcitonin and prostaglandins may also be involved as intermediate factors in the link between oestrogen and bone metabolism.

In the first 4 years after the menopause there is an annual loss of 1–3% of bone mass, falling to 0.6% per year thereafter. This leads to an increased rate of fractures, particularly of the distal radius, the vertebral body and the upper femur, and one or more of these fractures will affect 40% of women over 65 years. Wedge compression fractures of the spine, leading to the so-called 'dowager's hump' affect 25% of white women over 60 years **Fig. 18.2**, and fractures of the hip have occurred in 20% of women by the age of 90 years. Women who are underweight have a higher risk of osteoporosis because of reduced peripheral conversion of androgens to oestrogen. Women of Afro-Caribbean origin have a smaller risk of osteoporosis than white or Asian women, as they have a greater initial bone mass.

Osteoporosis has important consequences for women and for health services. In the UK, over 35,000 postmenopausal women suffer femoral fractures every year and 17% of them die in hospital. HRT has a very significant benefit in reducing the incidence of osteoporosis and osteoporotic fractures.

Administration of oestrogen decreases fracture risk; however, it is not recommended as a first-line treatment, as the long-term risks (particularly stroke) are considered to outweigh the benefits.

Diagnosis

The menopause may be confused with premenstrual syndrome (PMS), depression, thyroid dysfunction, pregnancy, and, rarely, phaeochromocytoma or carcinoid syndrome. Vasomotor symptoms may be caused by calcium antagonists and by antidepressive therapy, especially tricyclics.

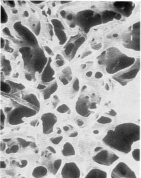
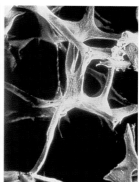

Fig. 18.1 Normal (left) and osteoporotic (right) bone. (Reproduced with permission from Dempster D et al, *American Journal of Bone and Mineral Research* 1: 15–21.)

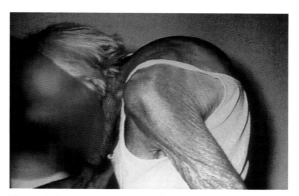

Fig. 18.2 Severe osteoporosis of the spine. (Reproduced with permission from slide set *A woman's guide to osteoporosis*, produced by Wyeth Laboratories.)

The diagnosis of menopause is usually clinical and can only be made in retrospect after 6–12 months of amenorrhoea. If there is clinical confusion, there may be some value in checking the serum FSH level, which should be >30 IU/l postmenopausally. Perimenopausally, the level may be normal, and it should be noted that FSH levels peak physiologically in mid-cycle, making it worth rechecking apparently high levels a second time. If there is diagnostic doubt about whether a woman is perimenopausal, especially over 45 years of age, a therapeutic trial of HRT may be considered. Absence of a satisfactory response suggests that symptoms are unrelated to low levels of oestrogen.

Hormonal therapy

Oestrogen supplementation is the basis of replacement therapy. Although progestogens may have a small role in relieving vasomotor symptoms, they are added to oestrogen to protect the endometrium and reduce the hyperplasia that would otherwise result. The oestrogens may be systemically administered as daily oral tablets, twice-weekly or weekly transdermal patches, or subcutaneous implants administered every 6–8 months. Daily nasal sprays, skin creams and 3-monthly vaginal rings are also used.

Whatever the route of administration, women who have not undergone hysterectomy should be placed on a regimen which includes a progestogen to minimize the risk of endometrial cancer associated with unopposed oestrogen therapy as mentioned above. This advice applies also to women who have undergone endometrial resection. Women who have had a hysterectomy do not require a progestogen.

Oral preparations

The oral route may have a more beneficial effect than parenteral therapy on lipid profiles, leading to higher HDL and lower LDL levels, but it is potentially more thrombotic. Tablets may be given as an oestrogen-only preparation for those who have had a hysterectomy, or as a combined oestrogen–progestogen preparation for those who have not. The combined form may be administered cyclically or continuously.

Cyclical preparations, which usually lead to monthly withdrawal bleeds, are used perimenopausally, and the continuous combined preparations, the so called 'no-period' HRT, are an option from more than 2 years after the last menstrual period. This continuous combined therapy is more convenient for the 80+% who do not suffer unscheduled bleeding, but erratic bleeding beyond the first 6 months of treatment warrants further investigation.

Alternatives to these oestrogen–progesterone preparations are tibolone and raloxifene. Tibolone is a synthetic steroid with weak oestrogenic, progestogenic and androgenic effects, which may be started 2 years after periods have ceased in a similar way to the continuous combined preparations. Raloxifene, a synthetic selective oestrogen-receptor modulator (SERM), has oestrogenic effects on bone and lipid metabolism but has a minimal effect on uterine and breast tissue. It is therefore ineffective for controlling perimenopausal symptoms but it has a useful role in protecting against osteoporosis and it does not cause vaginal bleeding.

Transcutaneous administration

Transdermal patches are available as an unopposed oestrogen form, or as cyclical or continuous oestrogen–progestogen combinations. Skin reactions, ranging from hyperaemia to blisters, affect only a very small percentage of users.

The clinical advantage of transcutaneous administration is that it should avoid gastrointestinal side-effects, and minimize the effects on hepatic production of both lipoproteins and coagulation factors. Patches are usually applied to the buttock, and each patch lasts for between 3 and 7 days, depending on the formulation. This method appears to be as effective as oral preparations in treating symptomatic women and for the prevention of osteoporosis.

Percutaneous oestrogen gels are also available. A measured dose is rubbed into the skin and avoids the prolonged skin contact of patches. The same contraindications apply as for other unopposed oestrogens.

Subcutaneous implants

Estradiol may be implanted in subcutaneous fat, usually in the lower abdomen, at intervals of no less than 5 or 6 months. The oestradiol level does not always fall away to baseline before symptoms recur and there is a risk of tachyphylaxis (persistent symptoms despite ever-increasing oestradiol levels) unless strict dose control is observed. Providing that pre-implant oestradiol levels are monitored, however, the risk of tachyphylaxis is minimized. Testosterone implants can be used where there is low libido.

Vaginal preparations

These include estradiol tablets, low-dose estradiol-releasing Silastic ring pessaries, and estriol vaginal pessaries and vaginal cream. They are all useful in the treatment of atrophic vaginitis.

Risks and side-effects of hormone treatment

General

Nausea and breast tenderness occur in about 5–10% of patients. Uterine bleeding is less common with low-dose regimens and, in general, the lowest dose that controls symptoms should be used. Irregular bleeding should be investigated as appropriate. There is a slight risk of cholelithiasis, and there is a theoretical chance of glucose tolerance impairment.

Endometrial carcinoma

Unopposed therapy (i.e. oestrogen only) increases the incidence of endometrial cancer fourfold, and it should therefore be used only for those who have had a hysterectomy. The incidence is reduced to a relative risk of less than 1.0 with opposed therapy (i.e. with the addition of progesterone for at least 10 days per cycle). The levonorgestrel-releasing intrauterine system (Mirena) protects the endometrium effectively when used in conjunction with oestrogen-only HRT in postmenopausal women.

Breast cancer

A link between oestrogen treatment and breast cancer is biologically plausible because of the connection between late menopause and breast cancer as noted above. There is a small increase in likelihood of having breast cancer with combined HRT after 5 years of use, although oestrogen alone in hysterectomized women does not have this adverse effect. There is no increased risk in those who stopped taking HRT more than 5 years previously. It may be that breast cancer diagnosed while on HRT is more curable.

Other cancers

The evidence of any adverse effect on other cancers, such as ovarian, is equivocal and any effect is likely to be very small.

Venous thromboembolic disease

There is an increased risk of venous thromboembolic disease in the first year of HRT treatment, with a relative risk of approximately 4.0 in the first 6 months and 3.0 in the second 6 months (baseline risk 1.3/1000/year). There is apparently no increased risk in those taking it beyond 1 year. Routine pretreatment screening for thrombophilia is not recommended, but it should be carried out in those with a personal or family history of venous thromboembolic disease.

Stroke

There is a significant increase in the likelihood of stroke in all age groups, although the impact is small in younger menopausal women as the baseline risk of stroke is so low.

Contraindications to hormone treatment

Pregnancy, thromboembolic disease and a history of recurrent venous thromboembolism are recognized contraindications to HRT, as are liver disease and undiagnosed vaginal bleeding. Treated hypertension and other cardiovascular risk factors are probably not contraindications.

Use of oestrogen-containing HRT is widely considered to be contraindicated following breast carcinoma (including intraductal carcinoma) and following advanced endometrial carcinoma. There are also theoretical reasons why it should be avoided in those who have had ovarian cancer.

Duration of HRT

When oestrogens are given for vasomotor symptoms, they are generally continued for 2 or 3 years and then stopped. Whether to continue therapy beyond this time depends on whether symptoms recur and on a weighing up of the risks of osteoporosis against the potential side-effects of breast cancer and venous thromboembolic disease for that particular individual.

Non-hormonal treatment

Drugs

Vasomotor symptoms may be reduced by clonidine, which acts directly on the hypothalamus, but in practice it is of limited value. The selective serotonin reuptake inhibitors (SSRIs) have also been shown to be effective. Palpitations and tachycardia may be improved by beta-blockers. Sedatives, hypnotics and antidepressants may be helpful in the treatment of non-vasomotor symptoms.

The first-line treatment for osteoporosis is now a bisphosphonate, and oestrogen is used only for those where this is inappropriate. In elderly women, supplementation with calcium, calcitonin and vitamin D reduces the risk of hip fractures. Moderate exercise may slow the rate of bone loss, though compliance with exercise programmes is often poor.

Psychological support

Some women with menopausal symptoms need only reassurance. Others may have particular stresses at this time of life, such as children leaving home, which may accentuate their perimenopausal symptoms. The marked placebo benefits in various studies show the importance of psychological support and a sympathetic ear.

> ### Key points
>
> - The average age of women experiencing spontaneous menopause is 51.
> - The menopause is caused by ovarian failure as the supply of oocytes is depleted. FSH rises as oestrogen production falls, and an FSH of >30IU/l is suggestive of postmenopausal status.
> - Cessation of periods is often preceded by irregular bleeding. A vaginal bleed more than a year after menopause probably warrants investigation.
> - Vasomotor symptoms such as hot flushes affect around two-thirds of women and may continue for more than 5 years after the menopause. Other symptoms include genitourinary atrophy and, possibly, some psychological symptoms.
> - Long-term health risks of the post menopause include cardiovascular disease and osteoporosis. Fractures of the radius, vertebral body or femoral neck affect 40% of women over the age of 65 years.
> - HRT is offered to treat menopausal symptoms and to reduce long term hypo-oestrogenic side-effects. If the woman still has a uterus, opposed HRT (oestrogen and progesterone) is necessary to avoid the risk of endometrial carcinoma. Oral, transcutaneous and vaginal preparations are available, as well as subcutaneous implants.
> - Side-effects of HRT include an increased incidence of breast carcinoma and venous thromboembolic disease.

19

Genital prolapse

Introduction

Uterovaginal prolapse is described as the descent of some of the pelvic organs (urethra, bladder, uterus, small bowel and rectum) into the vagina. The structures lying immediately above the vagina are in close proximity to each other and, if the integrity of pelvic fascia is disrupted, descent of a single organ seldom occurs in isolation. This becomes important when considering different modalities of treatment and how best to relieve symptoms.

Aetiology

The aetiology of genital prolapse is multifactorial and the main predisposing factors are listed in **Box 19.1**. In addition, obesity, chronic cough and constipation, which all raise intra-abdominal pressure, can aggravate the condition.

Childbirth

Childbirth results in trauma to the pelvic floor and loss of tissue support to the female pelvic organs. Vaginal delivery, and in particular multiparity, may disrupt the fascia and cause ligament weakening. A prolonged labour, in particular a prolonged second stage, a large baby, and perineal trauma have all been implicated in causing direct damage to the fascia and neuromuscular tissue of the pelvic floor.

Menopause

The menopausal state, characterized by oestrogen deficiency and loss of connective tissue strength, is a causative factor in the development of prolapse. This may be because oestrogen influences collagen formation.

Congenital

Congenital weakness and neurological deficiency of the tissues account for prolapse in a small proportion of women. Rarely, children may be born with prolapse or they may develop significant prolapse during childhood. There may also be anatomical variants that may make certain women more susceptible to prolapse in later life.

Gynaecological surgery

Although surgery is often used to treat prolapse, it may be responsible for a small number of cases. Suprapubic surgical procedures for urinary incontinence (e.g. Burch colposuspension – history box) alter the anatomy such that the bladder neck is approximated behind the symphysis pubis. This increases gravitational effects on the pouch of Douglas, prolapse of which leads to enterocele. Prolapse of the vaginal vault is a not uncommon long-term consequence of a hysterectomy.

b | *History*

John Burch (1900–1977), from Nashville, followed his father into gynaecology and developed the Burch colposuspension per-operatively when he was unable to suspend the bladder neck from the retropubic periosteum (the usual operation of the time).

Genetic

Genetic factors have been implicated in the development of prolapse. It is uncommon, for example, in the African population, possibly related in some way to the different collagen content of tissues.

Classification

The classification of prolapse, and the main symptoms, are summarized in **Table 19.1**.

Urethrocele/cystocele

A urethrocele is descent of the part of the anterior vaginal wall which is fused to the urethra. This is approximately the first 3–4 cm of the anterior wall superior to the urethral meatus. Any descent of this tissue may alter the urethrovesical angle and disrupt the continence mechanism, predisposing to stress urinary incontinence (SUI).

The bladder base lies immediately above this. Descent of this area is termed a cystocele **(Fig. 19.1)**. Urethroceles and cystoceles are often considered together, and when both are present the term cystourethrocele is used.

Uterus and cervix

The cervix occupies the upper third of the vagina and descends when there is uterine prolapse. Uterine prolapse may be described as first, second or third degree **(Fig. 19.2)**:

- First degree – there is descent of the uterus and cervix within the vagina but the cervix does not reach the introitus.
- Second degree – descent of the cervix to the level of the introitus.
- Third degree – the cervix and uterus protrude out of the vagina.

Procidentia is a term used when the cervix, uterus and vaginal wall have completely prolapsed through the introitus. Exposure of the cervix and vagina outside the introitus may lead to ulceration of the cervix and thickening of the vaginal mucosa.

Rectocele

Weakening of the tissue that lies between the vagina and rectum (rectovaginal fascia) allows the rectum to protrude into the lower posterior vaginal wall, causing a rectocele **(Fig. 19.3)**. Laxity of the perineum may also be present which gives a gaping appearance to the fourchette (the posterior margin of the introitus).

Table 19.1

Types of genital prolapse

Original position of organs	Prolapse	Symptoms[*]
Anterior	Urethrocele and cystocele	Urinary symptoms (stress incontinence, urinary frequency)
Central	Cervix /uterus (1st, 2nd, 3rd degree and procidentia)	Bleeding and/or discharge from ulceration in association with procidentia
Posterior	Rectocele and enterocele	Bowel symptoms, particularly the feeling of incomplete evacuation and something having to press the posterior wall backwards to pass stool

*In addition to the general symptoms of discomfort, dragging, the feeling of a 'lump', and, rarely, coital problems.

Enterocele

An enterocele is the only type of vaginal prolapse which is truly a hernia **(Fig. 19.4)**. It has a sac, neck and contents. The sac is a protrusion of the peritoneum of the pouch of Douglas and may contain small bowel, or omentum.

Symptoms

Prolapse may be asymptomatic and it may only be detected when women present for cervical cytology. If symptoms are present, they are usually non-specific but there may be features that are related to a specific type of prolapse **(Table 19.1)**.

Non-specific symptoms may be attributable to the 'stretch effect' on tissues. Women may describe an uncomfortable dragging feeling or backache that characteristically improves when lying down. Women may also describe 'something coming down'. Coital difficulties are an uncommon presenting symptom.

Anterior wall prolapse may cause urinary symptoms because it involves bladder and urethra. Over 50% of women with SUI have a significant cystourethrocele. Other urinary symptoms such as frequency and urgency may also be present. A large cystocele can cause problems of incomplete emptying of the bladder, and retained urine then predisposes to recurrent urinary tract infections.

Uterine prolapse does not usually present until the woman feels a 'lump'. If there is a procidentia, then there may be bleeding or discharge from ulceration of the cervix or vaginal wall.

Bowel symptoms related to a rectocele involve a feeling of incomplete evacuation of the bowel contents. When straining occurs with defecation, the rectocele balloons forward and some women need to digitally reduce the rectocele to pass stool. Enteroceles usually present as a

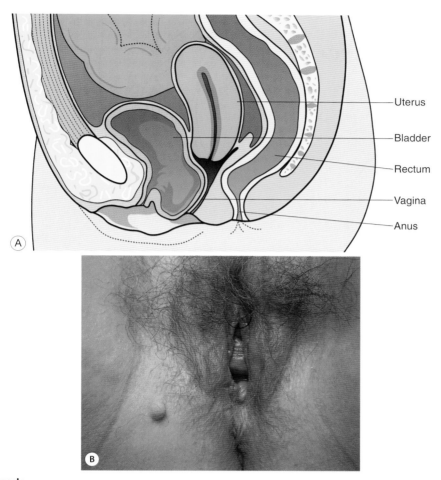

A

Uterus

Bladder

Rectum

Vagina

Anus

B

Fig. 19.1 Cystocele.

lump but may be also associated with non-specific lower abdominal discomfort.

Signs

Examination for prolapse forms part of the general gynaecological examination. Abdominal examination focuses on the possibility of a pelvic mass which may be pushing the pelvic organs downwards.

Pelvic examination is then performed, initially with the patient supine. On inspection of the vulva, one may note atrophic changes (scanty hair, thinning of the labia). The woman is asked to abduct her legs and strain. By gently parting the labia majora with the thumb and index finger of the left hand, prolapse may be seen appearing at the introitus. Urinary leakage may also be apparent and an assessment of the perineum can also be made. A bimanual examination may then be performed, and may give a useful indication of uterine descent.

Examination in the left lateral position can also be helpful. This allows a systematic examination of the entire vagina, exerting gentle traction with the speculum on the posterior vaginal wall. Sponge forceps are occasionally used during this examination to reduce a large prolapse or to enable the examiner to distinguish the anatomy. The speculum can then be slowly withdrawn along the posterior wall of the vagina and the full extent of any rectocele will come into view. If a prolapse is not apparent with the woman lying down, it may sometimes be necessary to examine her in the standing position.

Management

If a prolapse is not causing symptoms and the woman is unaware of it, then one must question whether any treatment is necessary. Simply because a doctor notices laxity within the vagina does not mean that surgery should be performed.

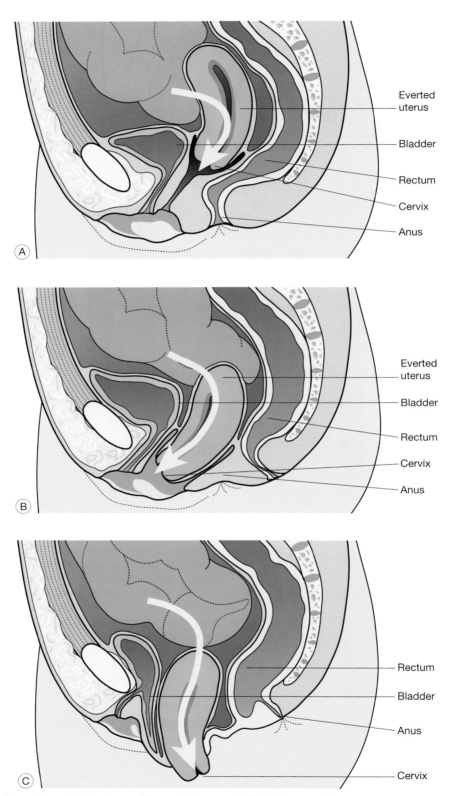

Everted uterus

Bladder

Rectum

Cervix

Anus

Everted uterus

Bladder

Rectum

Cervix

Anus

Rectum

Bladder

Anus

Cervix

Fig. 19.2 Uterine prolapse. (A) First-degree, **(B)** second-degree, and **(C)** third-degree prolapse.

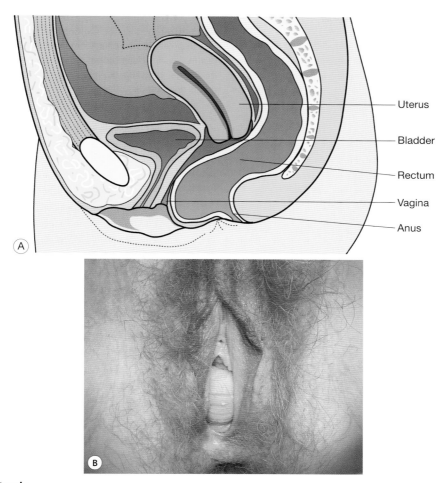

Uterus

Bladder

Rectum

Vagina

Anus

Fig. 19.3 Rectocele.

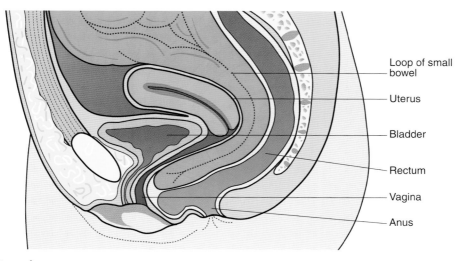

Loop of small bowel

Uterus

Bladder

Rectum

Vagina

Anus

Fig. 19.4 Enterocele.

Conservative

Conservative treatment may be considered if a woman does not want, or is not fit enough for, surgery. Conservative measures may also be used for temporary relief before surgery and even as a therapeutic test to see if reduction of the prolapse improves specific symptoms.

Pelvic floor exercises are not effective when prolapse is well established. They do have a role in the treatment of associated urinary incontinence, but their main value may be as a prophylactic intervention, particularly postpartum and postoperatively.

Pessaries are commonly used. A ring pessary is an inert plastic ring which is placed in the vagina so that one edge of the ring is behind the symphysis pubis and the other is in the posterior fornix **(Figs 19.5 and 19.6)**. The ring tends to support the uterus and vault of the vagina. It may also help reduce cystocele but it will not reduce a rectocele. Once a ring is fitted, arrangements are usually made to change

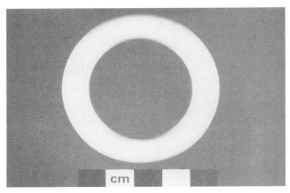

Fig. 19.5 Ring pessary (50 mm diameter).

it every 4–6 months. At this examination, the vagina is inspected thoroughly for atrophic changes and ulceration due to pressure necrosis. Complications from the ring may include urinary symptoms (frequency, infection), vaginal discharge, bleeding or, very rarely, fistula formation (if the ring is neglected). Other types of ring pessary are available, particularly the 'shelf' pessary which has a useful role in procidentia.

If atrophy of the lower genital tract is noted in association with prolapse, a course of oestrogen therapy (commonly administered topically as a cream) may improve vaginal tissue thickness. This may improve some symptoms and it facilitates any planned vaginal surgery.

Surgery

Most procedures for the treatment of genital prolapse are performed through the vagina, with only a few requiring an abdominal approach. When considering a surgical technique, particular attention should be given to preserving the calibre of the vagina if the woman wishes to remain sexually active. This aspect should always be discussed before operation.

Anterior vaginal wall – anterior repair (anterior colporrhaphy)

Anterior vaginal wall prolapse may be associated with stress urinary incontinence which may need to be investigated prior to surgery. The principle of an anterior repair is to make a midline incision through the vaginal skin and to reflect the underlying bladder off the vaginal mucosa. Once this is achieved, lateral supporting sutures are placed into fascia in order to elevate the bladder and bladder neck. The remaining redundant vaginal skin that has been 'ballooning' down is excised, and the vaginal skin is then sutured closed.

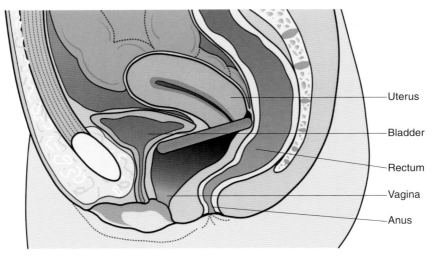

Uterus

Bladder

Rectum

Vagina

Anus

Fig. 19.6 Ring pessary in situ. Note that the anterior vaginal wall is elevated to reduce the cystocele and the uterine prolapse has been corrected.

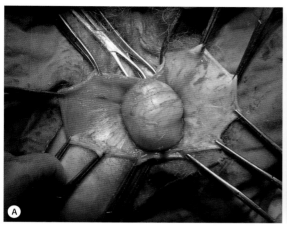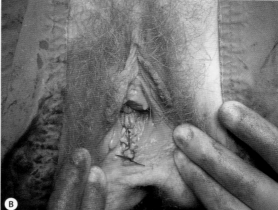

Fig. 19.7 Posterior colporrhaphy. (A) The posterior wall is opened in the midline to expose the rectum. **(B)** The posterior wall is closed after reducing the prolapse.

Uterine descent – vaginal hysterectomy or Manchester repair

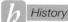 *History*

William Fothergill (1865–1926) was born in Southampton to a Quaker family. He proposed suturing the stumps of cardinal ligaments to the cervical stump to provide uterine support.

Vaginal hysterectomy is commonly performed for uterine prolapse. However, one must not presume that just because the uterus is prolapsing, it can be removed vaginally, as it may be too large to remove because of, for example, associated fibroids. One should also consider whether the uterus is being pushed down from a mass above (e.g. advanced ovarian cancer with gross ascites), or whether bowel is likely to be adherent to the uterus (e.g. after previous abdominopelvic surgery, endometriosis or severe infection). Once the uterus is removed, it is important that the supporting ligaments are approximated so as to prevent further prolapse of the vaginal vault.

Manchester repair (also called 'Fothergill repair' – history box) has a role in treating uterine prolapse, but is less commonly performed than vaginal hysterectomy. The uterosacral ligaments are divided and shortened, the cervix is amputated, and the shortened ligaments are approximated anterior to the cervical stump. The body of the uterus is not removed.

Posterior vaginal wall – posterior repair (posterior colpo-perineorrhaphy)

The principles of a posterior repair are similar to those of an anterior repair. An incision is made in the vaginal wall and the rectum is separated from the vagina **(Fig. 19.7)**. Supporting sutures are placed laterally to reduce the prolapse. The lax vaginal skin is then excised and the incision closed. This operation can be combined with a repair of the perineal

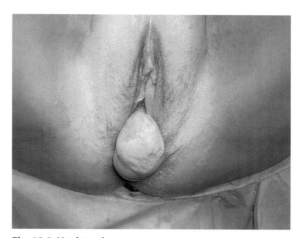

Fig. 19.8 Vault prolapse.

body to support the perineum. Again, particular care must be taken not to narrow the vagina and create dyspareunia.

As the procedure reaches the apex of the rectocele, the surgeon must identify whether or not there is an enterocele present. If one is present, the peritoneum must be opened (avoiding bowel injury). The hernial sac must be transfixed and excised, and supporting lateral tissue approximated in order to prevent recurrence.

Total vault prolapse (after hysterectomy)

This condition refers to the complete eversion of the vagina following a hysterectomy **(Fig. 19.8)**. It is effectively a procidentia without the uterus, not unlike a sock that has been turned inside out. Surgical options are sacrocolpopexy, sacrospinous fixation and vaginal mesh insertion.

Sacrocolpopexy

Sacrocolpopexy involves suturing the vaginal vault to the body of the sacrum, either directly, or indirectly by using a graft (porcine dermis, Gore-Tex, Marlex) interposed

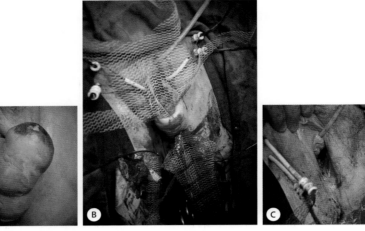

Fig. 19.9 Repair of complete vault prolapse.

between the two structures. The procedure is performed through an abdominal incision but can be carried out laparoscopically.

Sacrospinous fixation

Sacrospinous fixation requires the surgeon to suture the top of the vaginal vault to the sacrospinous ligament. The procedure is performed through the vagina. Complications of the procedure include damage to the sciatic nerve and pudendal vessels.

Vaginal mesh repairs

Recurrence of prolapse after surgical correction is common, with up to 30% of women requiring a second operation within 5 years. The recurrence may be due to the fact that the repaired tissues were weak even before the original operation; consequently, there is increased interest in mesh-augmented pelvic floor repair. Meshes are used with the aim of improving tissue strength and support. Types of mesh used are synthetic biocompatible meshes (e.g. polypropylene) and biological meshes (e.g. porcine dermis or bovine pericardium), and these can also be either absorbable or non-absorbable.

Currently, mesh is most popularly provided as 'mesh repair kits'. They use monofilament, low-weight, macroporous polypropylene meshes to reinforce the pubocervical and rectovaginal fascia. The operation involves the blind insertion of trocars into the obturator foramen, ischiorectal fossa, ileococcygeus muscle and sacrospinous ligament. Most meshes have three parts, which are placed between the bladder and vagina, through each obturator foramen and between the rectum and vagina (**Fig. 19.9**).

Meshes have been associated with an increased risk of complications, however, partly from the risks of insertion and partly because they are foreign bodies. Operative complications include bladder injuries, rectal injuries and vascular damage (cystoscopy is recommended to exclude bladder damage). Long-term complications include dyspareunia, erosion or rejection of the mesh, and mesh-related infections. Infection after use of a vaginal polypropylene mesh has been reported in around 8% of cases, with erosions occurring in about 12%. Necrotizing fasciitis is also a possibility.

Although mesh repair kits are associated with low recurrence and low morbidity rates, some of the uncommon complications are serious and potentially life-threatening, and it is suggested that these repairs should be carried out only by specialists.

Key *points*

- Genital prolapse describes the descent of the pelvic organs (urethra, bladder, uterus, small bowel and rectum) into the vagina.
- It is more common after childbirth and in obese women, postmenopausal women and those with conditions which raises intra-abdominal pressure, such as chronic cough or constipation.
- Prolapse may be classified as: anterior compartment defects (urethrocele or cystocele – urethra or bladder, respectively); a central compartment deficit leading to the prolapse of the uterus (first-, second- or third-degree prolapse); or a posterior compartment deficit (prolapse of the rectum or small bowel – rectocele and enterocele, respectively).
- Women with prolapse may present with a 'something coming down', discomfort, or urinary or bowel symptoms. Asymptomatic prolapse does not usually need to be treated.
- Treatment may be conservative (ring pessaries, pelvic floor exercises) or surgical repair, i.e. repairing the vaginal wall defect or performing vaginal hysterectomy for uterine prolapse.

20

Urinary incontinence

Introduction

Urinary incontinence is defined as the condition in which there is involuntary loss of urine which can be objectively demonstrated and which is a social or hygienic problem. It should be noted that the volume of urine lost is not a feature of the definition, but the ability of an independent person to confirm that there is urine loss is essential.

Urinary incontinence is an important condition because it causes significant distress. It is generally accepted that between 10% and 20% of the adult female population are incontinent of urine on one or more occasion per month. The prevalence changes little with age until over the age of 75 years, when it affects between 25% and 50% of women. Certain conditions predispose to urinary incontinence, including faecal impaction, decreased mobility, confusional states, and the presence of certain drugs, including diuretics and hypnotics. There is contradictory evidence on any relationship between incontinence and previous hysterectomy; retrospective studies suggest that there is a causal relationship, but prospective studies suggest that there is not.

Types of urinary incontinence

The commonest types of urinary incontinence in women are:

- stress urinary incontinence (SUI)
- overactive bladder (OAB)
- retention with overflow
- fistula.

Stress urinary incontinence (SUI) is the commonest cause of urinary incontinence in adult women, accounting for between 60% and 70% of cases. SUI is a sign or a symptom, but if this is proven at urodynamic testing, then it is called urodynamic stress incontinence (USI). This has replaced the old term 'genuine stress incontinence'. SUI is leakage that occurs when there is a rise in intra-abdominal pressure without a detrusor contraction; women therefore notice leakage on coughing, laughing, sneezing etc. and, in severe cases, even on walking or on rising from sitting.

An overactive bladder (OAB; previously called detrusor instability, detrusor overactivity or detrusor hyperreflexia) occurs when a woman is incontinent in response to an involuntary detrusor contraction. This accounts for about 30% of cases of incontinence in adult women. The woman will experience urgency, and if she cannot reach the toilet and the bladder contraction persists, she will be incontinent. As the problem tends to happen both day and night, she will usually also complain of urinary frequency and nocturia, and, in severe cases, enuresis (bed wetting).

Retention with overflow is only common in elderly female patients or in those with a neurological problem. The denervated bladder continues to fill until it simply spills over, resulting in leakage.

A fistula is an abnormal communication between two epithelial surfaces and, in the UK, usually results as a complication of surgery. In less affluent countries, obstructed labour is a much common cause. Any communication between the lower urinary tract (ureter, bladder or urethra) and the genital tract (uterus and vagina) will result in continuous dribbling incontinence. Fistulae account for only 1 in 1000 cases of incontinence in the female in the UK.

It is important to be aware that any incontinent woman may have more than one type of coexisting incontinence. An overactive bladder often coexists with both stress incontinence and, somewhat confusingly, with voiding difficulty or retention.

The mechanism of continence

The mechanism of continence must be understood if the pathophysiology of incontinence is to be understood. In the normal woman, continence is maintained at the level of the bladder neck. If, for instance, a radio-opaque medium were to be placed in the bladder of a normal, continent woman and that woman was asked to stand, an X-ray would demonstrate that urine does not flow into the urethra. The concept therefore arose of a so-called proximal urethral sphincter, a mechanism present in the region of the bladder neck and proximal urethra which maintains continence. It was originally considered that this was an arrangement of smooth muscle in the proximal urethra. However, no such sphincter mechanism based upon muscle exists. There is smooth muscle in the proximal urethra but it generally runs in a longitudinal rather than a circular direction and as such could not maintain continence.

It is now considered that the so-called proximal urethral sphincter mechanism is a water-tight seal which maintains the pressure in the urethra greater than the pressure in the bladder. The anatomical basis of that seal is considered to be a series of arteriovenous anastomoses within the wall of the proximal urethra. These can be demonstrated on histological examination. They allow some degree of turgor pressure to be exerted circumferentially around the urethra, which results in the formation of a hermetic seal by keeping the urethra occluded. The effect of any pressure exerted around the periphery of a hollow tube is to occlude that tube. If the pressure is exerted in numerous places around the circumference of the tube, then the tube will simply close. Such is the proximal urethral sphincter.

The situation becomes more complex in that if a pressure study is performed to compare the pressure in the urethra with the pressure within the bladder, then whilst the pressure in the proximal urethra exceeds that in the bladder, the greatest pressure difference exists at the mid-urethra. This is the so-called distal urethral sphincter mechanism. This does have an anatomical basis in muscle in that striated muscle, innervated by spinal roots S2–4, is found within the wall of the mid-urethra.

There are further features which aid the maintenance of continence, particularly the supporting tissues around the urethra which maintain the proximal urethra in an intra-abdominal position. The importance of this position is that if the proximal urethra is intra-abdominal, then any pressure rise within the abdomen will be transmitted equally to the bladder and the proximal urethra; the pressure difference will not change and continence will therefore be maintained. Weakness or damage to the supporting tissues may predispose to genuine stress incontinence. The supporting tissues are characterized anatomically as the pubourethral ligaments, derived from the fascia of the pelvic floor, and, to a lesser degree, the pelvic floor musculature, namely levator ani. It has been demonstrated that vaginal delivery may denervate both the pubourethral ligaments and levator ani, the nerve damage being manifest within the pudendal nerve. Thus, vaginal delivery may predispose towards SUI. Secondly, there is the concept of bladder stability. The bladder muscle, the detrusor, should only contract during micturition, whereas it should relax during bladder filling. Such a situation is described as a 'stable' bladder. In women who have an overactive bladder, the detrusor initially relaxes during filling but then contracts involuntarily. Such a situation is termed an overactive bladder (OAB). If the contraction is modest, then the woman will appreciate the contraction as urinary urgency, but if the contraction is strong enough to elevate the pressure in the bladder above that in the urethra, then there will be the symptom of urge incontinence.

Aetiology

Stress urinary incontinence

SUI clearly requires some degree of weakness of both the proximal and distal urethral sphincter mechanisms. Whilst no single aetiological factor exists in all women with SUI, there are a series of predisposing factors which often explain the condition. These include:

- pregnancy
- prolapse
- menopause
- collagen disorder
- obesity.

Pregnancy

Vaginal delivery may cause denervation of the pudendal nerve and hence damage to the supporting tissues of the urethra. Moreover, the pudendal nerve in part supplies innervation to the distal urethral sphincter. The first vaginal delivery is more likely than a subsequent vaginal delivery to cause SUI, and this incontinence may be preventable by elective caesarean section. There is also a transient form of SUI which occurs during pregnancy but is not present outside of pregnancy. The mechanism of this incontinence is a combination of the raised intra-abdominal pressure related to uterine contents together with the smooth-muscle-relaxant effect of progesterone. Thus, some women will describe SUI during pregnancy but not at other times.

Prolapse

Prolapse is not a cause of SUI per se but the same pathophysiological abnormality which causes the incontinence may cause prolapse, namely a deficiency of supporting tissues. Anterior vaginal wall prolapse is therefore often a surrogate indicator of a predisposition to SUI.

Menopause

Many women date the onset of their symptoms from the menopause. There is evidence that the withdrawal of oestrogen reduces the so-called maximal urethral closure pressure; hence the pressure in the urethra is not as great as it used to be. The effect of this pressure reduction is that a smaller rise in intra-abdominal pressure will result in SUI.

Pathophysiology of overactive bladder

- Idiopathic
- Neurogenic
- Psychogenic

Possible agents involved include: glutamate, ATP, nerve growth factor, nitric oxide, brain-derived neurotropic factor Receptors under investigation: vanilloid, purinergic and neurokinin receptors

Collagen disorder

Collagen is a major component of the pubourethral ligaments. There are several different types of collagen within the body and there is evidence that there are different types of collagen in varying proportions in the pubourethral ligaments of women who become incontinent compared with the pubourethral ligaments of those who do not.

Overactive bladder

The aetiology of OAB is summarized in **Box 20.1**. In the majority of women the aetiology is unknown.

Voiding difficulty

The aetiology of voiding difficulty in the female is the opposite of that in the male. In women it is due to an underactive detrusor (hypotonia) in 90% of cases, and in only 10% of cases does it reflect anatomical obstruction. The aetiology of the detrusor hypotonia is usually simply ageing, with the natural reduction in muscle fibres and muscle strength being enough to bring about a clinical problem. There is some evidence that young women who put off voiding during their adult life ('infrequent voiders') are more prone to this problem. Women with neurological disease can have voiding difficulty due to either detrusor hypotonia or obstruction, in the latter case secondary to inappropriate contraction of the urethral sphincter.

Clinical presentation

Stand-alone symptoms are uncommon and so urinary incontinence usually presents as part of a symptom complex comprising stress incontinence, frequency, urgency and nocturia. Urge incontinence will usually be present if the patient is suffering from an overactive bladder. One must also enquire about voiding problems, and the symptoms in women are the same as in men with prostatic enlargement: hesitancy, poor stream, intermittent stream, straining to void, feeling of incomplete emptying, and post-micturition dribbling. Symptoms of haematuria or recurrent urinary tract infections are concerning and merit urological assessment of upper and lower urinary tracts.

Prolapse will coexist with stress incontinence in up to 50% of cases, so an enquiry about symptoms is essential.

Likewise, although the symptoms are often unvoiced, anal incontinence is often present in association with urinary incontinence and must be sought. A full medical history and drug history will allow assessment of whether these problems are contributory to the patient's incontinence.

Urinary incontinence is a major quality-of-life issue and it is essential to assess to what degree the woman's symptoms are impacting on her lifestyle. Incontinence can prevent a woman from socializing and following her pastimes and in severe cases have a significant detrimental effect on personality. It is not unheard of for incontinence to render someone incapable of leaving the house. It can likewise have a significant negative impact upon a woman's sex life, and incontinence during intercourse is a common but usually unvoiced problem. Nocturia is a significant problem, leaving the sufferer lacking sleep and often having difficulty with concentration and even working. Nocturia in the elderly also carries the risk of falls, with fractured neck of femur the common outcome. It should be noted that in the elderly, urinary incontinence is the second commonest reason for a patient being unable to return to independent living.

Diagnostic evaluation

Clinical examination

All women should undergo an abdominal and pelvic examination. This should be done after she has emptied her bladder. Abdominal examination may reveal a palpable bladder suggesting urinary retention, and infrequently an otherwise unsuspected pelvic mass may be palpable. Pelvic examination may reveal pelvic organ prolapse or vaginal atrophy. Coexisting symptomatic prolapse will suggest a surgical solution for the incontinence, whilst atrophic changes require treatment with vaginal oestrogens. Stress urinary incontinence may be demonstrable; the woman should be asked to give a single sharp cough. A brief neurological assessment of the S2,3,4 dermatomes should be performed, and if symptoms of anal incontinence are present the anal sphincter tone should be determined by digital examination.

Further assessment

Urinalysis

Every woman presenting with lower urinary tract symptoms should have a urinalysis performed. The presence of leucocytes and nitrites suggests a urinary tract infection and this may be causing or worsening the patient's symptoms. Treatment with a broad-spectrum antibiotic should be started and an MSSU sent if there is no response. The presence of haematuria should prompt cystoscopy, and ultrasound of the upper renal tracts. The presence of glycosuria may suggest diabetes, which can predispose to recurrent urinary tract infections and urinary frequency.

Table 20.1			
Bladder diary (frequency/volume chart)			
Patient A	**Patient B**	**Patient C**	**Patient D**
0800 500 ml	0800 400 ml	0800 450 ml	0800 150 ml
1200 300 ml	1000 200 ml	1000 400 ml	1000 150 ml
1600 200 ml	1030 50 ml	1300 350 ml	1200 150 ml
1900 350 ml	1100 50 ml	1430 400 ml	1400 150 ml
2300 200 ml	1400 250 ml	1600 500 ml	1600 150 ml
	1700 250 ml	1900 350 ml	1800 150 ml
0400 250 ml	1900 75 ml	2100 400 ml	2000 150 ml
	1930 50 ml	2300 400 ml	2200 150 ml
	2230 300 ml		
			0000 150 ml
	0300 100 ml		0200 150 ml
	0400 50 ml		0400 150 ml

Frequency–volume chart

This simple non-invasive assessment (sometimes also called a bladder chart or bladder diary) can be extremely useful in determining the cause of a woman's symptoms; she keeps a note of how often she voids and how much she passes each time. Preferably 2–3 days should be monitored. **Table 20.1** shows an example from four patients. Patient A is normal. Patient B has a normal bladder capacity (400 ml) but is emptying her bladder with as little as 50 ml in it, and this is typical of an overactive bladder. Patient C is over-drinking and this is giving her urinary frequency and high urinary output. Patient D has a pathologically small bladder – probably inflammatory in nature. As the woman responds to treatment, her frequency–volume chart will improve, acting as a simple form of biofeedback.

Cystoscopy

Cystoscopy is required only for the assessment of haematuria or recurrent urinary tract infections. It is not required for those suffering purely from an overactive bladder.

Ultrasound measurement of post-void residual

This is a simple non-invasive test that should be performed in the presence of symptoms of voiding difficulty or in an elderly patient with incontinence.

Quality-of-life questionnaires

Much more emphasis is being placed upon quality of life and a woman's subjective assessment of her problem and response to treatment than has previously been the case. With this in mind, several quality-of-life questionnaires have been developed and validated for women suffering from lower urinary tract symptoms. This should be a part of the assessment of every woman both before

Box 20.2
Indications for urodynamic studies
■ In patients with symptoms of voiding difficulty
■ In patients with neurological disease
■ When conservative treatment has been tried and failed
■ Prior to surgery
■ When surgery has failed

and after treatment, along with an impression of what she expects from treatment; shared goals will improve patient satisfaction.

Urodynamic studies

These tests are a dynamic assessment of the lower urinary tract and offer objective information about bladder and urethral function. They are, however, invasive, embarrassing, expensive and time-consuming. Furthermore, they are not foolproof in providing a diagnosis. All of these facts have led to a trend in putting less emphasis on the result of urodynamic studies and more on the patient's perspective of her symptoms. The aim of urodynamics is to achieve a diagnosis, and differentiating between SUI and OAB in a woman with a mixture of symptoms is arguably the most useful information these tests provide. They can also predict the success of surgery and, too, the complications of surgery. The indications for urodynamic studies are listed in **Box 20.2**.

Treatment

Treatment options for urinary incontinence comprise:

■ conservative treatment (lifestyle interventions and bladder retraining)
■ physiotherapy
■ drug therapy
■ surgery.

Treatment should start with conservative treatment and this usually includes two distinct approaches: lifestyle interventions and bladder retraining. The GP or practice nurse can provide these; however, in reality, the time and experience these require mean it is probably better to involve a trained continence advisor or clinical nurse specialist.

Lifestyle interventions

Appropriate lifestyle changes are shown in **Box 20.3**. These changes are often difficult to achieve, but that is no reason for not educating the patient about what she can do to improve things herself. Indeed, it is imperative that we do, as often more invasive therapies are not without significant potential side-effects.

Box 20.3

Lifestyle interventions

- Normalize fluid intake. Many women drink too much, worsening frequency and incontinence, though many people with OAB over-restrict the amount of fluid they drink, increasing the risk of bladder irritation. 1.5 litres per day is the aim
- Cut down alcohol and restrict caffeine. These drinks should constitute no more than a third of the total daily fluid intake
- Lose weight if BMI >30
- Stop smoking
- Avoid carbonated drinks
- Treat chronic constipation and chronic cough

Bladder retraining

This physical therapy is another common non-pharmacological intervention, the objective of which is to re-establish cortical control over voiding. The patient emptying her bladder to a strict time schedule, usually hourly to begin with, achieves this. The time interval between voids is then increased to achieve a normal micturition pattern. The best results are achieved when done under the supervision of a continence nurse or specialist physiotherapist. To aid bladder retraining the following techniques are usually taught:

- distraction techniques, or doing something that requires concentration
- sitting on a hard seat or across a tightly rolled towel
- pelvic floor squeezes.

Physiotherapy

Physiotherapy is the first-line treatment for incontinence caused by pelvic floor dysfunction, but is also of some benefit to those with OAB. Treatment involves muscle training using pelvic floor exercises, which are regular voluntary contractions and relaxations of the pelvic floor muscles. It aims to both improve urethral resistance and pelvic visceral support by increasing the strength of the voluntary pelvic floor muscle contraction, and teach voluntary contraction of the muscles before increases in abdominal pressure. It may take 6 months to train muscles effectively, and women should be advised of this.

Biofeedback can be used as an adjunct to physiotherapy. It allows the patient to recognize the strength of an appropriate pelvic floor muscle contraction by verbal feedback during digital palpation, or electromyogenic feedback using vaginal electrodes.

Cones can be inserted vaginally for short periods to produce contractions in an attempt to retain them. Patients exercise daily with increasing weights, retaining the cone for 10–20 minutes each time. Cure or improvement rates after physiotherapy as high as 60% have been noted. Programmes cannot be successful in women who cannot locate and properly contract their pelvic floor muscles.

An instructor followed-up training programme is more effective than home exercise. It appears that the most benefit occurs in women with mild or moderate incontinence, although improvement can still be seen in those with severe symptoms.

Drug therapy

Conservative measures and physiotherapy can help up to three out of four women and are the only available interventions with no side-effects. If these fail, medical therapy should be prescribed. The mainstays of medical treatment for the overactive bladder are the antimuscarinics. Seven anticholinergic or antimuscarinic agents are currently licensed for treatment of OAB in the UK:

- oxybutynin (Lyrinal XL, Ditropan, Kentera)
- darifenacin (Emselex)
- solifenacin (Vesicare)
- tolterodine (Detrusitol and Detrusitol XL)
- trospium (Regurin)
- propiverine (Detrunorm).

The best estimate of the effectiveness of antimuscarinics is that on average about 50% of women will have up to 50% improvement. Side-effects – including dry mouth, dizziness, nausea and constipation – remain problematic; however, given that if drug therapy fails, further treatments for OAB are either very serious or unlikely to be effective, one must ensure that several if not all of the above drugs have been tried before abandoning medical treatment.

Medical therapy for SUI comprises oestrogens or duloxetine. Vaginal oestrogens should be prescribed to all women with urinary incontinence who are postmenopausal and who are not taking a systemic HRT preparation. Duloxetine is a combined serotonin and noradrenaline reuptake inhibitor licensed for use in moderate to severe SUI. Blockade of serotonin and noradrenaline reuptake in the spinal cord stimulates pudendal motor neurons, increasing stimulation of urethral striated muscles in the sphincter, and enhancing contraction. Duloxetine improves SUI by increasing urethral closure pressure and electrical activity of the sphincter. Adverse effects are related to increases in noradrenaline and serotonin, and include gastrointestinal disturbances, dry mouth, headache and, rarely, suicidal ideology.

Surgery

Surgical treatment of SUI and OAB are entirely different, with the former condition usually responding to minimally invasive procedures. OAB, however, requires major surgery with significant complications, and here, surgery is very much a last resort.

Surgery for SUI

Historically, there are several different surgical methods of treating SUI.

Anterior colporrhaphy This was used for decades to correct both incontinence and anterior vaginal wall prolapse. The bladder neck is elevated and supported by deep sutures placed on either side of it. These stitches are inserted into paraurethral tissue and the anterior portion of pubococcygeus. Continence 5 years following this procedure is approximately 50%.

Open (Burch) colposuspension The bladder neck and base are elevated by suturing the upper lateral vaginal walls to the iliopectineal ligaments. This procedure is highly effective and appears to remain so with time. Throughout the 1970s and 1980s this was the surgery of choice, with a success rate of 85% after 5 years. Complications following surgery are voiding disorder, detrusor overactivity and genitourinary prolapse.

Laparoscopic colposuspension The open procedure has been reproduced laparoscopically, but can only be performed by skilled minimal access surgeons. Cure rates are equivalent to those of the open procedure, but the technique has by and large been superseded by vaginal tape (sling) surgery.

Conventional sling surgery Sling procedures using autologous or synthetic material have high efficacy rates that are sustained with time. When using autologous material, strips of rectus fascia are placed in a sling under the bladder neck and cause urethral closure when the sling is stretched.

The procedures mentioned above have largely been replaced by the newer procedures described below.

Tension-free vaginal tape (transvaginal tape; TVT) sling This procedure was first introduced in the mid-1990s. The tape is inserted vaginally, provides mid-urethral support and exits suprapubically, being left under no tension **(Fig. 20.1)**. Cure rates of 94% are reported. Complications include vascular and bladder injuries which are related to

penetration of the retropubic space. Urinary tract infection rates postoperatively are around 5%, as is the rate of voiding difficulty and overactive bladder. At least in the short term, TVT is as effective as colposuspension for the treatment of primary stress incontinence.

Trans-obturator tape (TOT) sling This procedure was described in 2002. Here, the tape is suspended under the urethra through the obturator and puborectalis muscles **(Fig. 20.2)**. The success rates with this procedure are equivalent to those with the TVT procedure. TOT has the advantage over TVT of avoiding blind entry into the retropubic space, therefore reducing the risk of damage to the internal organs. The incidence of overactive bladder and voiding difficulty are similar to with the TVT and both procedures have a 1–2% incidence of vaginal tape erosion requiring oversewing of the vagina or removal. A TVT or TOT procedure may be combined with a prolapse repair.

Surgery for OAB

If medical treatment fails, then all of the following treatments have a place. All are specialized procedures and are typically the domain of the urologist.

- sacral nerve root stimulation (neuro-modulation)
- botulinum toxin A injections
- detrusor myectomy
- augmentation cystoplasty.

Treatment of voiding disorders

The treatment of voiding difficulty is first and foremost clean intermittent self-catheterization (CISC). This puts the woman in control of her voiding function and carries less

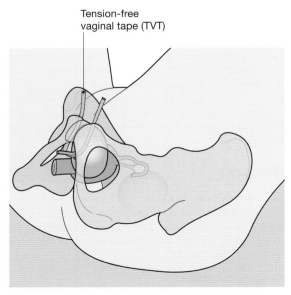

Tension-free
vaginal tape (TVT)

Fig. 20.1 Tension-free vaginal tape (TVT). © 2004 Gynecare, Worldwide, division of Ethicon Inc.

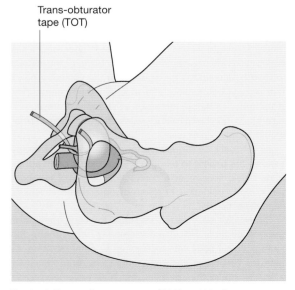

Trans-obturator
tape (TOT)

Fig. 20.2 Trans-obturator tape (TOT). © 2004 Gynecare, Worldwide, division of Ethicon Inc.

risk of infection than does an indwelling catheter. If she does not have the mental agility or physical ability to perform CISC, an indwelling catheter (urethral or suprapubic) may be required.

Treatment of genitourinary fistulae

If a period of indwelling catheterization fails to close the fistula, surgical correction will be required.

Key *points*

- Urinary incontinence is a major quality-of-life issue.
- Urinary incontinence is present in between 10% and 20% of adult females.
- Many will also suffer from anal incontinence, but this will usually not be voiced.
- Lifestyle advice is an essential starting point in the management of incontinence.
- Tape surgery is successful in up to 90% of cases of stress urinary incontinence.

21

Ovarian neoplasms

Introduction

Ovarian cancer is the most common of the gynaecological malignancies in most affluent countries, and the incidence is rising. In the UK there are around 5000 newly diagnosed cases each year and approximately 3700 women annually die of the disease. The overall 5-year survival is around 25%.

Ovarian cancer occurs predominantly in the fifth, sixth and seventh decades of life, with the peak age being around 75 years.

Natural history

Unlike cervical cancer, there is no clearly defined preinvasive ovarian lesion. Benign, borderline and invasive tumours are recognized but these are distinct pathological entities and there is little evidence of progression from one to the other **(Fig. 21.1)**. Indeed, there is even controversy about whether malignant epithelial tumours, which are the most common, arise from the ovary and then metastasize or arise as multicentric disease de novo. The multicentric theory is supported by the fact that ovarian-like tumours can arise in the peritoneum of women who have previously had both ovaries removed. Cancer in this case is called primary peritoneal cancer.

Aetiology

It is entirely possible that the different types of ovarian neoplasm have differing aetiologies, particularly as germ cell tumours, which account for 25% of ovarian neoplasms, occur in much younger women than do the epithelial tumours.

Reproductive history

Reproductive history is an important determinant of epithelial ovarian cancer risk. Nulliparous women have a higher risk than parous women and the risk is inversely correlated with parity **(Fig. 21.2)**. It is thought that the number of ovulation events in a woman's reproductive life is the main risk factor.

Exogenous oestrogens

Oral contraceptives

Overwhelming evidence now exists that women who have used the combined oral contraceptive pill at some stage in the past have a reduced risk of developing ovarian cancer. The longer the use, the lower the risk. This is again thought to be through the reduction in the number of ovulation events.

Hormone replacement therapy (HRT)

In postmenopausal women the effect of oestrogen replacement therapy has been investigated because of a reported increased risk in women who received diethylstilbestrol (a non-steroidal oestrogen) early in life. The balance of evidence, however, suggests that HRT has no significant effect on ovarian cancer risk.

Repeated (incessant) ovulation

It has been suggested that the more often a woman ovulates, the greater the risk of ovarian carcinoma. The apparently protective effects of both pregnancy and the combined oral contraceptive pill further support this theory. The mechanism is uncertain, but it may be that repeated monthly repair of the ovarian epithelium after ovulation predisposes to

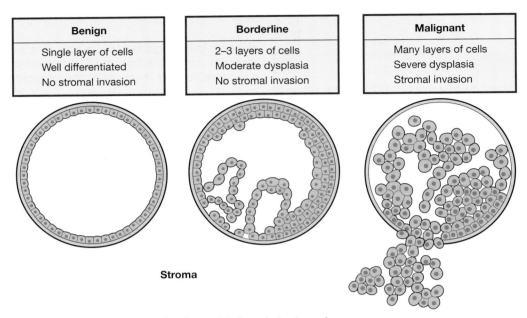

Benign	Borderline	Malignant
Single layer of cells Well differentiated No stromal invasion	2–3 layers of cells Moderate dysplasia No stromal invasion	Many layers of cells Severe dysplasia Stromal invasion

Stroma

Fig. 21.1 Morphology and behaviour of surface-epithelium-derived neoplasms.

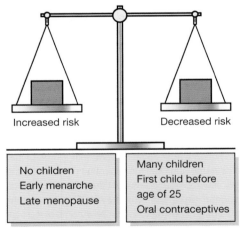

Increased risk	Decreased risk
No children Early menarche Late menopause	Many children First child before age of 25 Oral contraceptives

Fig. 21.2 Risk factors in ovarian cancer.

malignant change. Despite this plausible theory, however, it is likely that ovarian carcinogenesis is multifactorial.

Genetic factors

It is now accepted that a genetic predisposition exists in at least a proportion of ovarian cancer cases. Although overall there is a slightly increased risk of ovarian cancer in those with a family history, the risk is small for most categories except for those of early onset, and those with more than one affected first-degree relative. If one affected primary relative has ovarian cancer and the cancer was diagnosed when she was less than 50 years old, a woman's risk of developing ovarian cancer is around 5%. If there are two primary relatives under the age of 50 years with the disease, the risk is approximately 25%.

Only 5–10% of cases of ovarian carcinoma, however, have a direct genetic association. Of particular significance in this small group are the breast–ovarian cancer tumour suppressor genes *BRCA1* and *BRCA2*, as these are associated with a 10–50% lifetime risk of developing ovarian carcinoma. Mismatch repair genes associated with cancer of the colorectum, endometrium, stomach, urinary tract and small bowel are also responsible for a small proportion of this hereditary group. Women with such a history may warrant regular screening, and it is reasonable to consider bilateral oophorectomy after completion of their family. Such an operation will substantially reduce the risk but will not prevent primary peritoneal carcinoma.

Other factors

There has been controversy about the possible role of asbestos and talcum powder in the aetiology of ovarian cancer. Insufficient evidence in the form of case-controlled studies exists to completely dismiss reported associations. Similar problems beset the assessment of smoking, diet and alcohol consumption.

Pathology

Neoplasms can arise from any of the elements that comprise a mature ovary, including its surface serosal or mesothelial elements **(Fig. 21.3)**. A number of simpler themes can be drawn from a wide diversity of tumour types, namely: epithelial tumours, which are by far the most common (70% of primary ovarian tumours); sex cord/stromal tumours; germ cell tumours; and metastatic tumours **(Table 21.1)**. Most of the epithelial tumour types can be further broadly classified as benign, borderline or malignant.

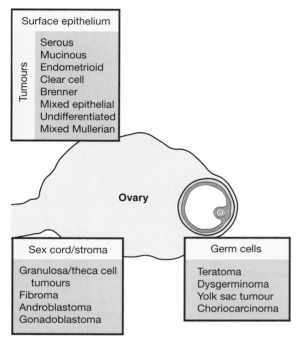

Fig. 21.3 Ovarian neoplasms arise from three basic tissue components.

Borderline tumours

The term 'borderline' is reserved for tumours which display the characteristics of malignant tumours but show no evidence of invasion. Women with borderline ovarian tumours have a much better prognosis than those with frankly malignant tumours. Nevertheless, long-term survival is by no means as high as might be expected and late recurrence up to 20 years after removal of the primary does occur. Despite lacking the features of invasion, these tumours may present at an advanced stage, raising the possibility of multicentric origin. The treatment of these is predominantly surgical as they tend to be resistant to chemotherapy.

Epithelial tumours

Serous tumours

Serous tumours are the most common ovarian neoplasm, accounting for almost 50% of ovarian cancers. They also account for 20% of all benign ovarian tumours, and these cases occur primarily in women of reproductive age. Serous cystadenomas (benign) are usually unilocular cysts, filled with straw-coloured fluid and of variable size **(Fig. 21.4)**. They are bilateral in 20% of cases. Serous cystadenocarcinomas involve both ovaries in over 50% of cases and may have both cystic and solid components. Psammoma bodies, concentrically laminated calcified concretions, are a frequent histological finding.

Mucinous tumours

These comprise 20% of all ovarian tumours and less than 10% are malignant. Benign tumours are usually unilateral and only 20% of malignant tumours are bilateral.

Table 21.1			
Pathology of ovarian tumours			
Borderline		Common	Separate clinical entity; do not invade
Epithelial	Serous	Common	Benign and malignant
	Mucinous	Common	Benign and malignant; associated with pseudomyxoma peritonei
	Endometrioid	Uncommon	Usually malignant
	Clear cell	Uncommon	Usually malignant
	Urothelial-like (Brenner)	Uncommon	Rarely malignant
Sex cord/stromal	Granulosa cell	Rare	Low grade; often secrete sex hormones
	Thecoma/fibroma	Rare	Rarely malignant; may secrete sex hormones; Meigs' syndrome
	Sertoli/Leydig	Rare	May secrete sex hormones
Germ cell tumours	No differentiation	Rare	Dysgerminoma; may secrete hCG
	Extra-embryonic differentiation	Rare	Yolk sac tumours (endodermal sinus tumours), malignant ovarian choriocarcinoma
	Embryonic differentiation (teratoma)	Common	Mature teratomas (benign) may contain epithelium, hair, teeth and greasy white sebum; immature (malignant) are rare
Metastases		Common	Especially endometrial, gastrointestinal tract and breast

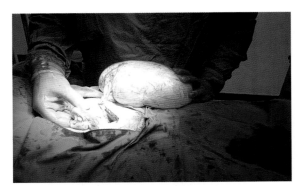

Fig. 21.4 A unilateral benign cystadenoma.

Mucinous tumours are usually multiloculated and contain mucinous fluid of variable viscosity. They are generally the largest of the common epithelial tumours. In less than 5% of cases, concomitant pseudomyxoma peritonei may be present. There is characteristic gelatinous tumour within the peritoneal cavity. It is unclear to what extent pseudomyxoma peritonei truly arises from the ovary rather than from a primary mucinous tumour of the appendix.

Endometrioid tumours

Endometrioid tumours are usually malignant and closely mimic endometrial cancer in histological appearance. In around 30% of cases there is a coexistent second primary in the endometrium.

Clear cell tumours

These are virtually all malignant and may be a variant of endometrioid tumours. They are the most frequent epithelial tumour found in association with ovarian endometriosis.

Urothelial-like tumours

Urothelial-like or Brenner tumours (history box) are uncommon, usually unilateral and rarely malignant. They in part comprise epithelium of urothelial type but their main component is ovarian stroma. A rare aggressive variant is the urothelial or transitional cell carcinoma.

 History

Fritz Brenner (1877–1969), a German-born physician who later emigrated to South Africa, first characterized the tumour in 1907; the term Brenner tumour was first used by Robert Meyer, in 1932.

Sex cord/stromal tumours

Rare neoplasms, they comprise 5% of all ovarian tumours.

Granulosa cell tumours

These are functional low-grade cancers and account for around 5% of ovarian malignancies. Three-quarters secrete sex hormones, most commonly oestrogen, which in turn may lead to precocious pseudopuberty, irregular menstrual bleeding or postmenopausal bleeding, depending on the age of presentation. They tend to recur late but can be monitored with serum oestradiol measurements. Characteristically they contain cells with 'coffee bean' nuclei and 'gland-like' spaces called Call–Exner bodies (history box), which are pathognomonic.

 History

Call–Exner bodies are granulosa cells arranged haphazardly around a space containing eosinophilic fluid. They are named after Friedrich von Call (1844–1917), an Austrian physician, and Sigmund Exner (1846–1926), an Austrian physiologist.

Thecoma/fibroma

These tumours are usually unilateral and rarely malignant. They contain cells ranging from theca cells to fibroblastic-type cells. Tumours containing the former are oestrogenic although they are less common than granulosa cell tumours. Rarely, ovarian fibromas may present with non-malignant ascites and pleural effusion, which resolve after removal of the tumour (Meigs' syndrome – history box).

 History

Meigs' syndrome is the triad of ascites, pleural effusion and benign ovarian tumor, named after Joe Vincent Meigs (1892–1963), an American obstetrician and gynaecologist. For reasons unknown, the pleural effusion is classically on the right side.

Sertoli/Leydig cell tumours

These are among the rarest ovarian tumours, accounting for <1% of such. They occur in young women, the mean age being in the mid-20s. They are almost invariably unilateral and are commonly androgenic, though many are non-functional and only a few are oestrogenic. They contain either Sertoli cells or Leydig cells (history boxes) and in the case of the latter may be accompanied by stroma-derived fibroblasts.

 History

Enrico Sertoli (1842–1910) was an Italian physiologist who discovered Sertoli cells in 1865 while studying medicine at the University of Pavia, Italy.

History

Leydig cells are found adjacent to the seminiferous tubules and were named by Franz von Leydig (1821-1908), a German zoologist and comparative anatomist.

Germ cell tumours

This heterogeneous group of tumours affects mainly children and young women and comprises 20–25% of all ovarian tumours. Around 4% are malignant. They represent the majority of ovarian tumours in children, where around one-third are malignant.

Dysgerminoma

Dysgerminoma is the most common malignant germ cell tumour, comprising at least 50% of this group. Nevertheless, it is relatively uncommon and represents only 3% of all ovarian cancers. 75% occur in females aged 10–30 years, the median being 22 years, and it is the most frequently encountered ovarian malignancy in pregnancy. It is also the malignancy most likely to be associated with gonadoblastoma in gonadal dysgenesis. At least 10% are bilateral and there may be a raised serum human chorionic gonadotrophin (hCG) level.

Endodermal sinus or yolk sac tumour

This is the second most common malignant germ cell tumour of the ovary but comprises only 1% of all ovarian cancers. It rarely affects women over 40, the median age being 19 years. Presentation is commonly with a sudden onset of pelvic symptoms and a pelvic mass. Elevated serum levels of alpha-fetoprotein are found with normal hCG levels. Co-existent teratomas are found in 20% of patients.

Choriocarcinoma

These secrete hCG and may present with precocious pseudopuberty. They have a poor prognosis and do not respond well to chemotherapy (unlike uterine trophoblastic disease).

Teratoma

Teratomas are colloquially known as ovarian dermoid cysts, and these are usually benign. They characteristically contain elements from all three embryonic germ cell layers and are thought to occur via parthenogenesis, a form of reproduction in which the ovum develops without fertilization. Mature teratomas may contain epithelium, hair, teeth and greasy white sebum, and constitute 20% of all ovarian neoplasms. They are commonest in women in their 20s but account for 50% of ovarian neoplasms in females under 20 years. Malignant change, usually squamous cell, is rare (<1%) and usually occurs in postmenopausal women.

Immature teratomas are rare, characteristically occurring in children under 15 years of age. Specialized tissue derivatives from a single germ layer are found in 3% of teratomas, notably among those with predominantly thyroid tissue (struma ovarii) and carcinoid tumours.

Metastatic tumours

Secondary tumours in the ovaries are surprisingly common. Cervical cancer only rarely metastasizes to the ovaries, but spread from endometrial cancer is far more frequent. Breast cancer may also metastasize to the ovaries, and patients presenting with single or bilateral ovarian masses should be examined carefully to exclude a breast lesion.

Cancers of the gastrointestinal tract also metastasize to the ovary and in the case of gastric cancer give rise to the so-called Krukenberg tumour (history box). This contains mucin-producing 'signet ring' adenocarcinoma cells. Such tumours may elicit a stromal response in the ovary which may cause hormone production; as a result, virilization may be a presenting complaint. In such cases, confusion with sex cord/stromal tumours is possible, although these, unlike Krukenberg tumours, are usually unilateral.

b *History*

A Krukenberg tumor refers to a secondary ovarian malignancy whose primary site arises in the gastrointestinal tract. It was named by Friedrich Ernst Krukenberg (1871–1946), a German physician, who first described them as 'fibrosarcoma ovarii mucocellulare carcinomatodes'.

Spread

Ovarian cancer spreads trans-coelomically whereby tumour is 'seeded' onto the surfaces of the intraperitoneal structures and organs. Those who die usually do so from intestinal obstruction and cachexia as a consequence of widespread intraperitoneal disease. Intrahepatic metastases and malignant pleural effusions are seen, and para-aortic lymph node metastases are found in up to 18% of cases where the disease appears otherwise to be confined to the ovary.

Presentation

As a rule, ovarian cancer tends to present at a late stage. Occasionally, ovarian cancers are diagnosed incidentally during pelvic or abdominal palpation for another reason. This mode of presentation, however, is the exception rather than the rule. In general the symptoms are diverse and non-specific. As a result, patients often do not recognize the sinister nature of their symptoms, and the disease progresses insidiously until they develop gastrointestinal complications or bowel obstruction secondary to widespread intraperitoneal malignancy.

The varied nature of these symptoms results in many cases being referred to inappropriate specialties for investigation. The most frequent complaint is abdominal distension due either to ascites or masses **(Table 21.2)**.

Table 21.2

Symptoms in ovarian cancer

Symptom	% of patients
Pain	50–60
Abdominal swelling	50–65
Anorexia	20
Nausea and vomiting	20
Weight loss	15
Abnormal vaginal bleeding	15
Frequency	10
Malaise	5
Change in bowel habit	5
Virilization	Rare
Precocious puberty	Rare

Table 21.3

Signs in ovarian cancer

Sign	% of patients
Pelvic mass	70–80
Abdominal mass	60–70
Ascites	30–40
Pleural effusion	10–15
Hepatomegaly	<5
Cervical lymphadenopathy	<5

Table 21.4

Staging of ovarian cancer

Stage	Definition	5-year survival
I_A	One ovary	
I_B	Both ovaries	60–70% but can be 95% for IA
I_C	I_A or I_B with ruptured capsule, tumour on the surface of the capsule, positive peritoneal washings or malignant ascites	
II_A	Extension to uterus and tubes	
II_B	Extension to other pelvic tissues, e.g. pelvic nodes, pouch of Douglas	30%
II_C	II_A or II_B with ruptured capsule, positive peritoneal washings or malignant ascites	
III_A	Pelvic tumour with micro-scopic peritoneal spread	
III_B	Pelvic tumour with peritoneal spread <2 cm	10%
III_C	Abdominal implants >2 cm ± positive retroperitoneal or inguinal nodes (Fig. 21.5)	
IV	Liver parenchymal disease. Distant metastases. If pleural effusion, must have malignant cells	10%

The most common clinical signs are an abdominal or pelvic mass and ascites **(Table 21.3)**.

Investigation and staging

If there is a low index of suspicion, investigation is often with ultrasound and tumour markers. The risk of malignancy index (RMI) aids in the differentiation of benign from malignant lesions (RMI = ultrasound score × menopausal score × CA125). If the index of suspicion is high, then CT or MRI can be used in addition to the tumour markers to examine the pelvis, and to look for peritoneal spread, ascites, liver metastases and ureteric obstruction. An X-ray or CT scan of the chest is important to look for pleural effusions or macroscopic chest disease.

Ovarian cancer is staged surgically according to the FIGO system **(Table 21.4)**.

Tumour markers

Around 80% of epithelial ovarian cancers are associated with elevated levels of a tumour marker (blood test) called CA125. This marker is of value in the assessment of patients presenting with pelvic masses, as well as in sequentially monitoring the response to treatment and to help identify presymptomatic relapse during follow-up. However, CA125 may also be elevated in the serum of women with benign conditions, such as endometriosis, or where peritoneal trauma has taken place. A positive result, therefore, while suggestive of ovarian cancer, is not diagnostic. Conversely, a negative result for tumour markers does not exclude a diagnosis of ovarian cancer, as 50% of stage 1 (confined to the ovary) ovarian cancers will have a normal CA125.

About 65% of ovarian germ cell tumours produce elevated serum levels of hCG, alpha-fetoprotein or both. These markers can again, if elevated, be very useful in monitoring response to therapy and in detecting tumour recurrence after completion of therapy.

Treatment

Benign tumours

Benign tumours require either excision or possibly drainage under laparoscopic control. There may be difficulties in deciding whether a cyst is benign or malignant. In general, ovarian cysts in young women tend to be benign and the risk

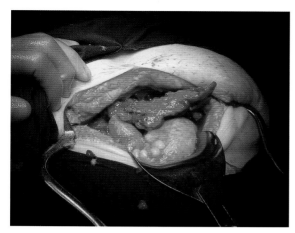

Fig. 21.5 The omentum in this stage III$_C$ cystadenocarcinoma is almost completely replaced with tumour. Optimal debulking was not achieved.

of malignancy increases with age. A cyst is often assumed at surgery to be benign if it is unilateral and unilocular with smooth external and internal surfaces and no solid elements **(Fig. 21.4)**. Although not conforming to this rule, teratomas are benign and the diagnosis is usually obvious when they are opened after removal.

Epithelial cancers

Most patients with epithelial ovarian cancer present late and the overall survival is poor **(Fig. 21.5)**. Because of this and because of new developments, particularly with chemotherapeutic agents, the modern approach to treatment is to consider ovarian cancer as a chronic disease. This means that the tumour is primarily treated with the aim of achieving remission but accepting that the tumour will probably become active again in the future. When this occurs, further treatment to achieve control will be given. In this way, whilst most patients will not be cured in the conventional sense, many patients will have a prolonged period of good-quality life.

Treatment is usually a combination of surgery and chemotherapy. Traditionally this has been in the form of aggressive surgery attempting to remove all areas of tumour and including removal of both ovaries, uterus and omentum. Complete removal of tumour is often unrealistic though, and the concept of surgical debulking has arisen. This is where the tumour deposits are removed as far as possible, aiming to reduce the size of deposits to below 1 or 2 cm in dimension. Chemotherapy will almost certainly be used as well. In this setting it is called 'adjuvant chemotherapy'. There are many active chemotherapeutic agents that can be used in ovarian cancer. In the first-line setting the current standard is platinum based. This is usually carboplatin, which will usually be combined with a taxane. This chemotherapy is given over six cycles and usually in the outpatient setting.

Recently, in many cancer centres, a different approach has been adopted for the most advanced cases of ovarian cancer. These patients are frequently unfit and with the advent of CT imaging it is easier to identify patients in whom surgery will achieve little. In these cases, after histological confirmation with guided needle biopsy, chemotherapy is used first of all rather than surgery. Surgery will usually be considered midway through the chemotherapy treatment. The effect of this is more rapid control of the cancer and a reduction in the surgical related morbidity. This approach of neoadjuvant chemotherapy followed by surgery is currently being evaluated by randomized trial.

Most patients with advanced ovarian cancer will relapse at some point after primary treatment. In this situation, further chemotherapy will usually be considered. The specific type of chemotherapy will depend upon the chemotherapy that has been used in the past, as well as the interval since chemotherapy was last used. In the case of the first relapse, if the interval since treatment is significant, then further challenge with carboplatin will frequently be tried. Other drugs include the taxanes, topotecan and Caelyx. Ideally, patients should be considered for entry into clinical trials, as the evidence suggests that patients who are entered into trials tend to have better outcomes. Many patients will have several lines of chemotherapy over a number of years before eventually dying of their disease. As most patients will eventually die of their disease progression it is important to consider formal palliative care when appropriate.

In young women who wish fertility to be preserved and in whom the disease appears confined to one ovary, it is reasonable to consider conservative surgery. The other ovary and omentum, a common site for metastases, should be biopsied and a thorough inspection made of all peritoneal surfaces.

Non-epithelial tumours

These tumours frequently occur in young women where preservation of fertility is an important consideration. It is also clear that many of these tumours, especially those of germ cell origin, are exquisitely sensitive to chemotherapy, and radical surgery is therefore inappropriate. Extremely good survival can be achieved with limited surgery and subsequent combination chemotherapy.

Survival

Overall 5-year survival (all stages) is in the order of 25% **(Table 21.4)**, a figure which has remained unaltered for many years. A better prognosis can be expected for women with malignant germ cell tumours, where the reported 5-year survival from most studies is in excess of 75%.

The only real prospect for improving survival in epithelial cancers is either detection at an early stage or development of better chemotherapy. Screening is still the subject of research, with trials involving the combination of tumour markers (such as CA125) and ultrasound. At present it seems unlikely that screening and early detection of low-risk groups is going to be a useful proposition.

Key *points*

- Ovarian cancer is the commonest gynaecological cancer. The incidence is increasing, with around 5000 newly diagnosed cases each year in the UK. The 5-year survival is about 25%.
- Unlike cervical cancer, there is no recognised pre-malignant stage and most new cases present with advanced disease (stage III or IV).
- Genetic factors have been identified (e.g. the *BRCA1* and *BRCA2* tumour suppressor genes) which identify a small proportion of women at risk. Other risk factors include low parity. Use of the oral contraceptive pill protects against ovarian cancer.
- Presentation is usually with pelvic mass, malaise and weight loss. Treatment is primarily surgical, although advances have been seen recently in chemotherapy, particularly with platinum-based drugs and the taxanes.
- Management strategies are directed towards earlier diagnosis and improved chemotherapies. Currently available tests do not fulfil the criteria for a screening programme aimed at low-risk women.

22 Uterine neoplasia

Introduction

The uterus consists of both the cervix and the body (or 'corpus' of the uterus). For many reasons, however, including their causative factors and their treatment, tumours arising from the corpus and the cervix are usually regarded as originating from two separate organs. This chapter will consider cancers arising from the uterine body; cancers arising from the cervix are discussed in Chapter 24.

The majority of malignancies arising from the uterine body arise from the endometrium. The endometrium consists of both glandular and supporting (or 'stromal') elements and it is possible for either to undergo malignant change. The majority of uterine malignancies are adenocarcinomas arising from the endometrial glands **(Figs 22.1, 22.2A)**. Sarcomas of the muscle of the uterus, the myometrium or the stromal tissues of the endometrium are much rarer **(Fig. 22.2B)**.

Incidence

Endometrial cancer is the second most common gynaecological malignancy in the UK, after cancer of the ovary, and there are approximately 4000 new cases per year diagnosed in England and Wales. Its incidence is low in women under 40 years of age (less than 2 per 100,000) but rises rapidly between the ages of 40 and 55 years, levelling off after the menopause to around 44 per 100,000.

Approximately 5% of endometrial carcinomas will develop in women under the age of 40 and 20–25% will be diagnosed before the menopause. There is evidence that the incidence is rising in developed countries.

Aetiology

The majority of endometrial cancers are associated with conditions in which there are relatively, rather than absolutely, high levels of oestrogen production and it is therefore postulated that oestrogen has a role in the development of the disease **(Box 22.1)**.

High levels of oestrogen may be physiological, as with obesity (due to the aromatization in body fat of peripheral androgens to oestrogens), nulliparity (due to anovulation) and late menopause. The relationship between diabetes/hypertension and endometrial cancer is a result of the increased incidence of obesity in these groups of women. Non-physiological causes of increased oestrogen include unopposed oestrogen hormone replacement therapy (HRT), which increases the risk fourfold. This risk is reduced to a relative risk of less than 1.0 with opposed HRT (i.e. with the addition of progestogen for at least 10 days per cycle). Oestrogen-secreting tumours, which are rare, also increase the risk of endometrial carcinoma.

Endometrial cancer is also seen less frequently in women who have used the combined oral contraceptive pill, probably because it administers progestogens throughout the cycle. Women who smoke, and are therefore likely to reach an earlier menopause, also have a lower than expected incidence of the disease.

The more common and oestrogen-dependent type of endometrial cancer is sometimes called type I disease and is seen in women around the time of the menopause or soon after. It is generally diagnosed at an earlier stage and as a result has a better prognosis. There may be premalignant change (see 'Endometrial hyperplasia' below) and the tumour cells of type I disease usually have oestrogen and progesterone receptors. This form of the cancer has characteristic growth factor alterations which distinguish it from normal endometrium.

Type II endometrial cancer is probably not related to oestrogen production. It is seen in older women, progresses more rapidly, and is not associated with a hyperplastic or in situ phase. The chances of surviving 5 years with this type of cancer are considerably lower than for the type I form, even with early-stage disease.

Clinical features and diagnosis

Abnormal uterine bleeding is the cardinal symptom of endometrial carcinoma. The bleeding is most commonly postmenopausal, and women with this symptom should be regarded as having malignancy until proven otherwise.

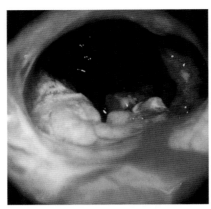

Fig. 22.1 A hysteroscopic view of an endometrial carcinoma arising from the posterior uterine wall. (Courtesy of Karl Storz Endoscopy (UK) Ltd.)

Box 22.1

Risk factors for endometrial carcinoma

Increase risk

- Obesity, especially upper body obesity
- Nulliparity
- Late menopause
- Unopposed oestrogen therapy, including tamoxifen
- Oestrogen-secreting tumours (granulosa/theca cell ovarian tumours)
- Carbohydrate intolerance
- Polycystic ovary syndrome
- Personal history of breast or colon cancer
- Family history of breast, colon or endometrial cancer

Decrease risk

- The combined oral contraceptive pill
- Progestogens

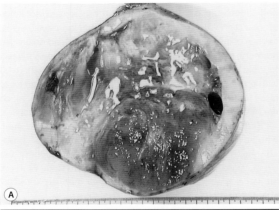

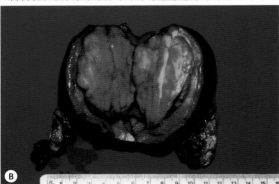

Fig. 22.2 Macroscopic picture of (A) endometrial carcinoma and (B) endometrial sarcoma. (Courtesy of Dr N Wilkinson, Department of Pathology, Leeds.)

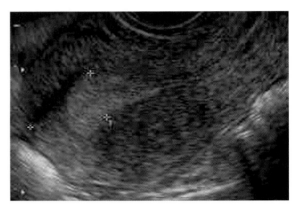

Fig. 22.3 Transvaginal ultrasound image demonstrating thickened endometrium. (Courtesy of Dr C Hardwick, Glasgow.)

A less common mode of presentation in the postmenopausal group is that of vaginal discharge – either blood stained, watery or purulent. Pain is rarely associated with early disease and usually indicates late spread to involve bone or nerve roots. Endometrial carcinoma can also present with abnormal cells on a smear consistent with endometrial origin.

Mode of spread is principally direct through the fallopian tubes and myometrium. Lymphatic and haematogenous spread may also occur.

There are four main methods of investigation as listed below. The method chosen depends on the patient's risk factors and the local facilities.

Ultrasound

Transvaginal scanning can be used to measure the endometrial thickness in postmenopausal women **(Fig. 22.3)**. If the thickness is less than 4 mm, endometrial

Around 5–10% of women with postmenopausal bleeding will have a primary or secondary malignancy, most commonly endometrial cancer (80%), cervical cancer, or (rarely) an ovarian tumour. As the condition can occur in premenopausal women, any irregular uterine bleeding in those over 40 years of age should also be investigated.

cancer is very unlikely. Fluid in the endometrial cavity on ultrasound in these women is associated with malignancy in 25% of cases.

Endometrial biopsy

An outpatient biopsy can be obtained using one of a number of samplers, for example the Pipelle **(Fig. 22.4)**, or the Vabra aspirator. These are both 3 mm in diameter, the Pipelle being a thin plastic tube and the Vabra a stainless steel device attached to an electrical suction pump. The Pipelle is the most convenient, best tolerated and least expensive, but samples only around 4% of the endometrial surface and will miss around a third of tumours. The Vabra samples around 40% of the endometrial surface and picks up more tumours, but is more painful and more expensive. In view of the relatively high false negative rates, endometrial biopsy alone is appropriate only for those at relatively low risk of carcinoma.

Dilatation and curettage

This is usually carried out under general anaesthesia. The cervix is dilated sufficiently to allow the introduction of a sharp curette, which is used to sample the endometrium. Used alone, this will miss around 10% of endometrial cancers.

Hysteroscopy

The inside of the uterine cavity can be visualized directly using a hysteroscope, which can be introduced with or without anaesthesia, depending on the instrument and the local facilities **(Fig. 22.1)**. Biopsy or curettage (see above) can also be performed at the same time. Hysteroscopy with biopsy is considered to be the 'gold standard' investigation.

Pathology

Endometrial pathology can be divided into hyperplasia, carcinoma or sarcoma.

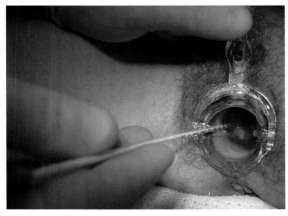

Fig. 22.4 Pipelle endometrial biopsy.

Endometrial hyperplasia

Endometrial hyperplasia is a potentially premalignant condition which is thought to result from persistent and prolonged oestrogenic stimulation of the endometrium. The nomenclature of this condition is confusing and the terms simple hyperplasia, glandular hyperplasia, cystic glandular hyperplasia and endometrial hyperplasia are synonymous. Complex hyperplasia (previously known as adenomatous hyperplasia) can occur with or without cytological atypia. The atypia may be severe enough to create difficulty in distinguishing the hyperplastic state from a well-differentiated carcinoma.

To diagnose hyperplasia histologically, there should be an increase in the glands-to-stromal ratio. The glands may vary in size and shape or they may branch abnormally. Cytological atypia includes a loss of polarity of cells within the glands, an increase in the nuclear–cytoplasmic ratio, and nuclear irregularity with hyperchromatic changes, chromatin clumping and prominent nucleoli. This atypia is the only feature distinguishing benign endometrial lesions from those with invasive potential.

Simple hyperplasia often occurs in anovulatory teenagers and in the perimenopausal years. Atypical hyperplasia coexists with endometrial carcinoma in 5–10% of cases, and many will progress to carcinoma. This progression depends on the severity of atypia and it is thought that about 20% will develop carcinoma within 10 years.

Hyperplasia is usually discovered by endometrial biopsy as part of the investigation of abnormal uterine bleeding. There are no other symptoms or physical signs. It is common to treat hyperplasia with progestogens in young women but to consider hysterectomy, particularly if there are atypical changes, in those who have completed their family.

Endometrial carcinoma

Endometrial adenocarcinoma can have a variety of histological appearances depending upon whether it is purely glandular, or has areas of squamous differentiation (which may appear malignant or benign), or whether it demonstrates a papillary or clear cell pattern. The latter two forms are associated with a poorer prognosis.

Endometrial sarcoma

Endometrial sarcoma is very rare. It tends to be a locally aggressive tumour that metastasizes early and is generally characterized by a poor prognosis.

Prognostic factors

Endometrial cancer is falsely regarded as a less aggressive tumour than other gynaecological malignancies but this is simply because it more commonly presents at an earlier

Table 22.1					
FIGO staging of endometrial carcinoma					
Stage	**Definition**	**Stage at presentation**	**Pelvic nodes involved**	**5-year survival**	
I_A	Tumour limited to the endometrium				
I_B	Growth that has invaded <50% of myometrial thickness	73%	<20%	85%	
I_C	Growth that has invaded >50% of myometrial thickness				
II_A	Endocervical glandular involvement only	11%	20%	65%	
II_B	Cervical stroma involved				
III_A	Invades seroserosal surface of uterus, ± adnexa, ± positive washings				
III_B	Vaginal metastases	13%	35%	40%	
III_C	Metastases to pelvic or para-aortic nodes				
IV_A	Tumour invasion of bladder and/or bowel				
IV_B	Distant metastases including intra-abdominal and/or inguinal lymph nodes	3%	50%	10%	

Histopathology: degree of differentiation
Uterine adenocarcinoma should be grouped according to the degree of differentiation as follows:
G1 – 5% or less of a solid growth pattern
G2 – 6–50% of a solid growth pattern
G3 – more than 50% of a solid growth pattern

stage **(Table 22.1)**. Stage for stage, endometrial cancer has a prognosis similar to that of cancer of the cervix. There are many factors that affect the prognosis, the most obvious being the stage of disease. This is an indication of how far the cancer has spread, as well as how aggressive the tumour is. The histological type of endometrial cancer is also important. Papillary serous cancer which is more common in older women, spreads in a manner similar to cancer of the ovary and, is associated with a significantly poorer prognosis. Other factors which affect the prognosis are outlined in **Box 22.2**.

Treatment

Endometrial carcinoma is staged using the FIGO scheme (Table 22.1). This is a surgico-pathological system based on the histology results from the excised uterus, tubes, ovaries and lymph nodes and the results of peritoneal cytology. Before operation, however, in addition to the usual preoperative investigations, the patient should have a chest X-ray and liver function tests to look for evidence of metastases.

Other possible preoperative investigations to search for metastases include ultrasound scan and magnetic

Box 22.2

Prognostic factors in endometrial cancer

■ Histological type
■ Histological differentiation
■ Stage of disease
■ Myometrial invasion
■ Peritoneal cytology
■ Lymph node metastasis
■ Adnexal metastasis

resonance imaging (MRI). Ultrasound examination can determine the size of the tumour and predict the presence of myometrial invasion. It is also useful in determining the presence of advanced disease. MRI, which is becoming more commonly used, is able to assess the condition of the myometrium more specifically and also to determine the extent of myometrial invasion. More importantly, MRI may be used to determine whether the cervix has been invaded by the tumour **(Fig. 22.5)**. If there is no cervical involvement, a staging laparotomy may be carried out.

In addition to a hysterectomy and bilateral salpingo-oophorectomy, there is debate as to whether the pelvic lymph nodes should be removed, sampled or left alone.

radiotherapy to the vault of the vagina (brachytherapy) may prevent recurrence developing in this area. Radiotherapy to the whole pelvis (teletherapy) will also prevent local disease recurring in this area, but, surprisingly, does not improve overall survival. An argument for performing formal lymphadenectomy is that if the nodes are free of tumour, then radiotherapy can be avoided in cases that might otherwise have been irradiated.

Radiotherapy may be used for treatment of local disease if the patient is medically unfit for major surgery. However, this is becoming less common as most patients' co-morbidity can be optimized for surgery. For more advanced lesions, whole pelvic radiotherapy may be used.

If disease is widespread, chemotherapy may be considered. The drugs most helpful in this situation are cis-platinum and doxorubicin. Once again, their influence on survival is controversial, as response rates to measurable disease are only of the order of 20%.

Recurrence

Most relapses occur early (i.e. within 2 years of primary treatment). Recurrences are commonest in the vault of the vagina, but may also be in the lungs, bone, vagina, liver, and inguinal and supraclavicular nodes. It should be remembered that 80% of those with recurrent disease will die within 2 years, and care should be taken to maximize the quality of life over this time rather than subject the patient to treatments with high morbidity and a slim chance of success.

Those with a recurrence who have not received radiotherapy should be considered for this treatment. For the remainder, the choice is between hormonal therapy and chemotherapy. The main hormonal option is high-dose progestogens, which may give a response in around 30% of patients. Chemotherapy can produce tumour shrinkage in some cases but toxicity is considerable, not least because these patients are often frail and have severe coexistent medical disorders.

Summary

Endometrial cancer is often considered to be easily treatable, but, stage for stage, its survival approximates that of ovarian cancer. It is fortunate that most women present with postmenopausal bleeding in the early stages of the disease.

To ensure the best possible outcome, women who present with bleeding 6 months or more after their last menstrual period should be referred urgently for a gynaecological opinion. From there, referral to a cancer centre specializing in the treatment of gynaecological cancer is likely to be beneficial.

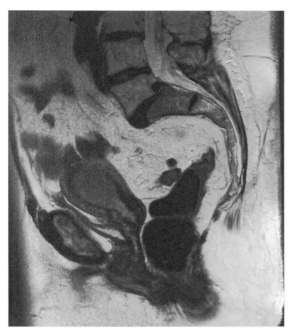

Fig. 22.5 A sagittal image through the uterus, showing the endometrial cavity distended by tumour. The tumour extends into the endocervical canal and is invasive posteriorly at the fundus. (Courtesy of Dr S Swift, Department of Radiology, St James's Hospital, Leeds.)

Any of these strategies is acceptable and none is mandatory. Nevertheless it would seem sensible to have at least some indication if there is a risk of retroperitoneal disease, although the risk of this can be predicted from other factors such as tumour grade and depth of myometrial invasion. As with any tumour, the more lymph nodes which are removed the more likely it is that metastases will be found. There are, however, potential complications to lymphadenectomy and the risks of surgery should be weighed against the benefits. If the tumour is of high grade, or there is deep myometrial invasion, extrapelvic spread is more likely and a surgical assessment of the para-aortic lymph nodes may be appropriate.

If, during the preoperative investigations or at the time of laparotomy, the disease is discovered to have spread beyond the uterus, treatment should be individualized. Treatment of disease in the fallopian tubes or ovaries is relatively easy to manage and for stage III disease has a relatively good prognosis. More widespread tumour, however, should be managed depending on the degree and location of spread and the condition of the patient.

The treatment of those with endometrial cancer after surgery is related to the stage of the disease (Table 22.1). Radiotherapy may be used as adjuvant (postoperative) treatment if the tumour invades the myometrium deeply, as there is a high risk of extrauterine disease. Local

Key points

- Endometrial cancer is the second most common gynaecological cancer in the UK, after cancer of the ovary, and is generally a postmenopausal disease.
- The aetiology is not fully known, but exposure to unopposed oestrogens is known to increase the risk of developing the disease.
- Endometrial cancer classically presents with postmenopausal bleeding or irregular premenopausal bleeding. Less commonly the presentation can be with vaginal discharge.
- Diagnosis is made by biopsy of the endometrium. The cavity can be directly visualized with a hysteroscope, and the tissue sampled by curettage or using an outpatient sampling device. Postmenopausally, endometrial carcinoma is very unlikely if the transvaginal endometrial thickness is less than 4 mm.
- Treatment is generally surgical (hysterectomy and removal of the ovaries), and in some cases lymphadenectomy may be advisable. In advanced or recurrent disease, radiotherapy is the treatment of choice.

23

Disorders of the vulva

Introduction

The vulva consists of the mons pubis, labia majora, labia minora, clitoris and the vestibule Fig 3.1. It is covered with keratinizing squamous epithelium, unlike the vaginal mucosa which is covered with non-keratinizing squamous epithelium. The labia majora are hair-bearing and contain sweat and sebaceous glands: from an embryological viewpoint, they are analogous to the scrotum. Bartholin's glands are situated in the posterior part of the labia, one on each side of the vestibule. The lymphatics of the vulva drain to the inguinal nodes and then to the external iliac nodes. The area is richly supplied with blood vessels.

Examination of the vulva

Before direct examination of the vulva, a general dermatological examination may be useful, particularly:

- the nail beds for signs of pitting (found in psoriasis)
- the extensor surfaces (elbows and knees) also for features of psoriasis
- the flexor surfaces for lichen planus and dermatitis
- the mouth for other features of lichen planus.

The vulva may than be inspected under a good light, as described on page 29. If necessary, closer inspection is possible using the colposcope.

Simple vulval conditions

Urethral caruncle

A urethral caruncle is a polypoidal outgrowth from the edge of the urethra which is most commonly seen after the menopause. The tissue is soft, red and smooth and appears as an eversion of the urethral mucosa. Most women are asymptomatic, but others experience dysuria, frequency, urgency and focal tenderness. If there are any suspicious features, an excision and biopsy may be required to exclude the very rare possibility of a urethral carcinoma.

Bartholin's cysts

The greater vestibular, or Bartholin's, glands lie in the subcutaneous tissue below the lower third of the labium majus and open via ducts to the vestibule between the hymenal orifice and the labia minora. They secrete mucus, particularly at the time of intercourse. If the duct becomes blocked, a tense retention cyst forms, and if there is superadded infection, a painful abscess develops. The abscess can be incised and drained, usually under general anaesthesia, with the incision on the inner aspect of the labium so that secretions bathe the introitus rather than the outside of the vulva. To prevent the cyst reforming, the fistula is kept open by suturing its edges to the surrounding skin, a procedure known as marsupialization **(Fig. 23.1)**. Bartholin's gland carcinoma is rare.

Small cysts

The commonest small vulval cysts are usually either inclusion cysts or sebaceous cysts. Inclusion cysts form because epithelium is trapped in the epidermis, usually following obstetric trauma or episiotomy. They are usually asymptomatic and need no treatment. Sebaceous cysts are usually multiple, mobile, non-tender, white or yellow, filled with a cottage cheese-like substance and more common in the anterior half of the vulva. Excision may be requested by the patient.

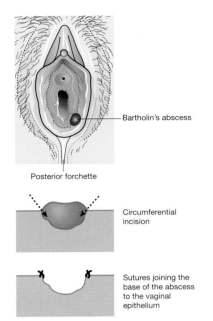

Bartholin's abscess

Posterior forchette

Circumferential incision

Sutures joining the base of the abscess to the vaginal epithelium

Fig. 23.1 Marsupialization of a Bartholin's abscess. The lower part of the abscess cavity granulates and heals during the subsequent weeks. (From Pitkin J, Peattie A, Magowan BA. *Obstetrics and Gynecology. An Illustrated Colour Text.* Churchill Livingstone, Edinburgh, 2003.)

Cysts in an episiotomy scar can be tender and need excision. Infected cysts need to be excised and drained, and recurrent infections should be treated by excision in their non-acute phase.

Moles

Vulval moles are usually asymptomatic but become more pigmented at puberty. Any other change in a vulval naevus is an indication for removal. There is a good case to be made for removing all vulval moles, as approximately 2% of malignant melanomas in women arise from the vulva.

Fibroma, lipoma, hidradenoma

Fibromas and lipomas are benign, mobile tumours of fibrous tissue and fat, respectively. Hidradenomas are rare tumours of sweat glands near the surface of the labia. All are benign, but the diagnosis is usually only made once they have been excised.

Haematoma

The commonest cause of a vulval haematoma is vaginal delivery. It may also occur following any vulval operation, or by 'falling astride' accidents, particularly in children. The possibility of sexual assault should be borne in mind in this situation. Vulval haematomas usually present with severe pain, and evacuation under general anaesthesia is often required.

Simple atrophy

Elderly women develop vaginal, vulval and clitoral atrophy as part of the normal ageing process of skin. In severe cases, the thin vulval skin, terminal urethra and fourchette cause dysuria and superficial dyspareunia, the labia minora may fuse and bury the clitoris. Introital stenoses can make coitus impossible. A simple effective moisturizer rubbed into the vulva is effective, although some advocate topical oestrogen replacement. There is a small amount of systemic absorption with topical oestrogen therapy, and, if this route is chosen, treatment should be for no more that 2 or 3 months without either a break or a short course of progesterone to prevent endometrial stimulation.

Ulcers

These may be:

- aphthous (yellow base)
- herpetic (exquisitely painful multiple ulceration, pp. 124,131)
- syphilitic (indurated and painless, p. 132)
- associated with Crohn's disease ('like knife cuts in skin')
- a feature of Behçet's syndrome (a chronic painful condition with aphthous genital and ocular ulceration)
- malignant (see below)
- associated with lichen planus (see below) or Stevens–Johnson syndrome
- tropical (lymphogranuloma venereum, chancroid, granuloma inguinale).

Treatment depends on the cause. The management of Behçet's syndrome is difficult, but the combined oral contraceptive or topical steroids may be tried.

Infection

Candida, vulval warts, herpes, lymphogranuloma venereum, scabies, granuloma inguinale, tinea, chancroid and syphilis are discussed in Chapter 13.

Hidradenitis suppurativa is a chronic unrelenting infection of the sweat glands. The glands become obstructed and chronic inflammation follows. Long-term antibiotics reduce further attacks, but the only cure is local excision.

Dermatoses

Vulval 'dystrophy' is an abnormality of vulval epithelium. Epithelial growth may be hypoplastic, hyperplastic, or abnormal in some other way.

Lichen sclerosus

This chronic and recurrent condition can present at any age, but is more common in the older patient and usually presents with pruritus. Less commonly, presentation is with dyspareunia or pain. It is an autoimmune condition and there is an association with other autoimmune disorders, including pernicious anaemia, thyroid disease, diabetes mellitus, systemic lupus erythematosus (SLE), primary biliary cirrhosis, and bullous pemphigoid. Histologically, the epidermis appears thin, with loss of rete ridges. The superficial dermis is hyalinized and a band of chronic inflammatory cells is seen beneath it.

Clinically, the skin appears white, thin and crinkly, but may be thickened and keratotic if there is coexistent squamous cell hyperplasia **(Fig. 23.2).** There may also be clitoral or labial adhesions. Diagnosis is by biopsy. Lichen sclerosus is non-neoplastic but may coexist with vulval intraepithelial neoplasia and there is an association with subsequent development of vulval squamous cell carcinoma in 2–5% of cases. Although long-term follow-up is considered appropriate by some clinicians, patients with a problem will usually present directly (often between appointments) if a problem occurs.

Treatment is required particularly if the condition is symptomatic, and initially is usually with a potent topical steroid cream (e.g. Dermovate b.d.), reducing gradually to a milder preparation (e.g. 1% hydrocortisone b.d., o.d. or less) as symptoms require. An emollient such as Oilatum or Diprobase is symptomatically beneficial. The patient should also cut her nails to try to break the itch–scratch–itch cycle. Vulvectomy has no role, the recurrence rate after surgery being around 50%.

Squamous cell hyperplasia

Squamous epithelial hyperplasia is characterized by thickened hyperkeratotic skin with white, itchy plaques. Pruritus is usually severe. Diagnosis is again by biopsy, and treatment is as for lichen sclerosus.

Other dermatoses

Allergic/irritant dermatosis

The vulval skin, especially the introitus, is not uncommonly affected by dermatitis. The dermatitis is either due to an irritant (non-immunological) or a true allergy (immunological aetiology). The chemicals causing hypersensitivity of the vulval skin include cosmetics, perfumes, contraceptive lubricants, sprays and douches. Detergents, dyes, softeners, bleaches, soaps and chlorine used to clean undergarments can also cause irritation. In severe cases hypersensitivity may develop to local anaesthetic creams and even steroid preparations.

Women with contact dermatitis have a red inflamed vulva with features of eczema, and patch testing may identify local irritants. Temporary relief may be obtained with vulval moisturizers (e.g. Emulsiderm in a daily bath), emollients (e.g. topical aqueous cream) and topical corticosteroids (e.g. a month's course of topical Dermovate). As before, lesions that do not respond should be biopsied to confirm the diagnosis.

Psoriasis

Psoriasis manifests as a dry red papular rash that is usually well circumscribed and extends to the thigh. The diagnosis is easier to make if bleeding occurs when the classic silvery scales are removed. Because the vulva is often moist, it is often difficult to distinguish psoriasis from candidal infection or dermatitis. Candida should be excluded. The lesions may be treated topically with coal tar preparations, ultraviolet light, steroid creams or other suitable formulations.

Intertrigo with candida

Intertrigo refers to a moist inflammatory dermatitis which can occur in any body fold because of apposition and chafing of skin surfaces. Skin folds are more likely to rub together in those who are overweight and in those who use occlusive clothing.

The skin is sore, macerated and often red, inflamed and cracked. Weight loss, local hygiene, and ventilation should be encouraged, for example the use of stockings and cotton underclothes rather than tights and nylon pants. Dusting powder (e.g. talcum powder), astringents (e.g. zinc) or barrier preparations may also be helpful.

Candida often complicates intertrigo and should be treated as on page 126. Providing there is no candidal infection, steroid creams may be used to relieve inflammation.

Lichen planus

Lichen planus is a chronic papular rash with a dark blue hue, involving the vulva and flexor surfaces. It can affect other flexor surfaces and oral mucous membranes, and the diagnosis is supported by the finding of other lesions. It is usually idiopathic, but can be drug related. Treatment is with potent topical steroids or ultraviolet light, and it tends to resolve within 2 years. Surgery should be avoided.

Pruritus

Pruritus describes an intense itching with a desire to scratch. It is commoner in those aged over 40 years, and symptoms are often most severe under times of stress or depression. There are numerous aetiologies **(Box. 23.1).**

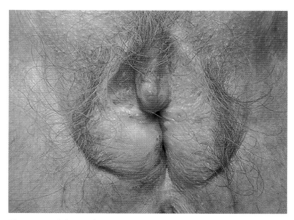

Fig. 23.2 Lichen sclerosus. The skin is white, with some reddened areas, and adhesions have significantly narrowed the introitus.

Causes of pruritus vulvae

- Infection (candida, pediculosis, thread worms)
- Eczema
- Dermatitis (consider patch testing)
- Irritation from a vaginal discharge
- Lichen sclerosus
- Lichen planus
- Vulval intraepithelial neoplasia (VIN)
- Vulval carcinoma
- Medical problems, e.g. diabetes mellitus, uraemia or liver failure
- Psychogenic

A biopsy may be necessary to establish the diagnosis, and patch testing may be of help. If no cause is found, it may be worth considering the possibility of previous sexual abuse or psychosexual problems.

It is important to break the scratch/itch cycle and strong short-term topical steroids will reduce the local inflammation caused by scratching. Application of a strong steroid cream twice daily for 3 weeks, followed by hydrocortisone cream 1% daily as maintenance, is useful, as is the use of soap substitutes (e.g. Oilatum). Irritants and bath-water additives should be avoided, soap substitutes used, the area dried gently (e.g. with a hairdryer), loose cotton clothing worn and nylon tights avoided. Antihistamines may also be of help. Co-existing depression may also warrant treatment.

Vulvodynia

This is chronic vulvar discomfort, especially that characterized by the complaint of burning, stinging, irritation or rawness. There may also be pruritus. No one factor can be identified as the specific cause. It may also occasionally be associated with previous sexual abuse. There may be a response to low-dose tricyclic antidepressants (e.g. amitriptyline).

Vulvar vestibulitis is a chronic clinical syndrome with erythema, severe pain on entry or to vestibular touch, and tenderness to pressure localized within the vestibule. If symptoms are of less than 3 months' duration, there is often response to topical corticosteroids. If the condition is chronic, treatment is empirical and symptomatic, with surgical resection being considered only as a last resort.

Vulval intraepithelial neoplasia (VIN)

Vulval intraepithelial neoplasia refers to the presence of neoplastic cells within the confines of the vulval epithelium. There are three types of VIN: squamous; melanoma in situ; and non-squamous.

Squamous VIN (Bowen's disease, bowenoid papulosis)

This is classified as grade I, II or III depending on the severity, and it is considered, much like with cervical intraepithelial neoplasia (CIN), that the human papilloma virus may be important in the aetiology. Many are asymptomatic, although pruritus is present in perhaps one- to two-thirds and pain is an occasional feature. Lesions may be papular and rough surfaced, resembling warts **(Fig. 23.3)**, or macular with indistinct borders. White lesions represent hyperkeratosis, and pigmentation is common. The lesions tend to be multifocal in women under 40 and unifocal in the postmenopausal age group.

Diagnosis is by biopsy, which may be taken at vulvoscopy, using 5% acetic acid as at colposcopy, under either local or general anaesthesia. The opportunity should be taken to look at the cervix at the same time, as there is an association with CIN. As the natural history is so uncertain, treatment is controversial. Regression has been observed (particularly with low-grade VIN) but progression of high-grade VIN to invasion may occur in approximately 5% of cases, and up to 15% of those with VIN III may have superficial invading vulval cancer.

Treatment of VIN may be indicated in those over the age of 45, those who are immunosuppressed and those with multifocal lower genital tract neoplasia. Such treatments include surgical excision, Nd-YAG laser therapy or imiquimod cream (Aldara).

Non-squamous VIN (Paget's disease)

In this uncommon condition, there is a poorly demarcated, often multifocal, eczematoid lesion, associated in 10% with adenocarcinoma either in the pelvis or at a distant

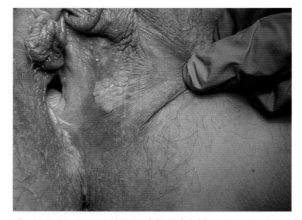

Fig. 23.3 Squamous VIN III of the left labia majora. In this case the lesion is rough surfaced, not unlike the appearance of wart virus infection, but lesions are also commonly macular with indistinct borders.

site. Treatment is by wide local excision. Recurrences are common.

Vulval carcinoma

Vulval cancer is relatively uncommon. Squamous cell carcinoma accounts for 90% of vulval cancers. Approximately 5% of vulval malignancies are malignant melanomas and the others include Bartholin's gland cancer, basal cell carcinomas and sarcomas. It is usually a disease of older women (60+ years) and, like cervical cancer, is commoner in cigarette smokers and women who are immunocompromised.

Clinical presentation

Most women will present with a history of long-standing vulval irritation or pruritus, and some will have had a previous history of lichen sclerosus. A lump or ulcer is common **(Fig. 23.4)**. As the disease advances, the tumour grows and focal necrosis may cause discharge and pain. The diagnosis is confirmed by histological examination of a biopsy.

Pathophysiology

Squamous cell carcinoma spreads to the inguinal nodes and from there to the external iliac nodes in the pelvis **(Table 23.1)**. Unless the lesion has only penetrated the basement membrane by <1 mm, node involvement is common and may include both the superficial and deep inguinal lymph node systems. Clitoral lesions have extensive lymphatic drainage and cells may embolize along the inferior vesical vessels and drain directly to the internal iliac nodes.

Surgical management

The treatment of vulval carcinoma is usually some form of surgical excision, either a wide local excision or vulvectomy. The decision about whether to undertake additional groin node exploration depends on whether there are any clinically suspicious groin nodes, the grade of tumour (more likely if poorly differentiated), and the depth of invasion on the initial specimen. It may be appropriate to carry out only a unilateral exploration if the lesion is well lateralized. Distant metastases are not a contraindication to radical vulval surgery, as death from a large fungating genital neoplasm or erosion of the femoral artery or vein by metastatic groin nodes is very unpleasant.

The groin explorations are carried out through separate incisions, and the wound will often be drained for around 7–10 days under suction, as lymph fluid accumulates and breakdown is common. If there is significant groin node involvement, it may be necessary to give adjuvant pelvic node radiotherapy as well.

The commonest complication of a radical vulvectomy is breakdown of the wound, which may take weeks to heal. In addition, these women are often elderly, immobile, and have had surgery on their pelvic vessels close to the femoral vein, leaving them at a high risk of venous thromboembolic disease. Long-term sequelae of surgery include vulval mutilation and lymphoedema. The 5-year survival is around 80% if groin nodes are negative and 40% if positive.

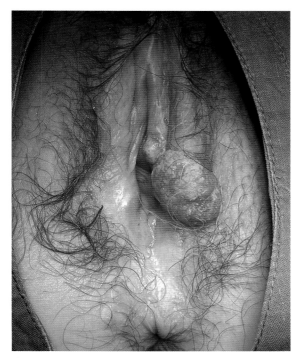

Fig. 23.4 A stage II left-sided squamous vulval carcinoma.

Table 23.1	
FIGO staging of vulval carcinoma	
Stage	**Definition**
I$_A$	Tumour less than 2.0 cm in dimension and less than 1 mm of stromal invasion. No lymph vascular space invasion (LVSI) and no nodal disease
I$_B$	Tumour less than 2.0 cm in dimension but with more than 1 mm of stromal invasion
II	Tumour of more than 2.0 cm dimension confined to vulva or perineum with negative nodes
III	Tumour of any size with spread to lower urethra, ± vagina, ± anus, ± unilateral groin lymph node metastases
IV$_A$	Tumour invades any of the following: upper urethra, bladder mucosa, rectal mucosa, pelvic bone ± bilateral groin nodes
IV$_B$	Any distant metastases including pelvic nodes

Recurrence

Recurrence of the excised tumour at the primary site is unusual providing a 10mm margin has been achieved. The epithelium is likely to be unstable, however, and new vulval tumours may arise. Treatment of recurrence is surgical, although interstitial radiotherapy may be appropriate. A check should be made at follow-up for signs of tumour spread to nodes.

Key *points*

- A swollen symptomatic Bartholin's gland or abscess should be marsupialized and not simply incised.
- Lichen sclerosus is associated with squamous carcinoma of the vulva in around 2–5% of women.
- Vulval intraepithelial neoplasia (VIN) is analogous to intraepithelial neoplasia in the cervix (CIN). Treatment of VIN is local excision of severely dysplastic lesions with careful follow-up.
- Vulval carcinoma is usually of squamous cell type and tends to afflict the more elderly population. The treatment is excision ± unilateral or bilateral inguinal lymphadenectomy. Pelvic radiotherapy may also be indicated if there is a significant chance of nodal spread.

24

Cervical neoplasia

Introduction

Cervical cancer is the most common cancer among women in many developing countries, and worldwide there are over 450,000 cases each year. The overall lifetime risk is about 5% in parts of Africa, India and Latin America, compared with 1% in Europe and North America. About 3000 cases of cervical cancer are diagnosed each year in the UK, and 1300 of these women will die from the disease.

Fortunately cervical cancer has a premalignant phase and many of the criteria for a suitable screening programme are fulfilled. The aim of this screening is to detect premalignant cervical disease by means of a 'smear test' and treat the premalignant disease before invasion occurs. Both the incidence and mortality have fallen considerably since the introduction of this screening programme.

Cervical intraepithelial and cervical cancer screening

Transformation zone

Cervical intraepithelial neoplasia (CIN) develops in the transformation zone of the cervix. Understanding the transformation zone is the key to understanding cervical cancer screening. The endocervix is lined by columnar epithelium and the ectocervix by squamous epithelium. Under the influence of oestrogen, part of the endocervix everts, thereby exposing the columnar epithelium to the chemical environment of the upper vagina **(Fig. 24.1)**. The change in pH, along with other factors, causes the delicate columnar epithelium cells to transform into squamous epithelium through the process of metaplasia. CIN develops in this transformation zone and it is this area which is sampled cytologically.

Cells shed from the surface may be sampled by a variety of devices, so that cells from both the endocervix and ectocervix can then be examined microscopically for cytological abnormalities. Cellular abnormalities are classified into different degrees of 'dyskaryosis'. Although dyskaryosis is a cytological diagnosis **(Fig. 24.2)**, the degree of dyskaryosis correlates to some degree with the degree of cervical intraepithelial neoplasia, which is a histological diagnosis **(Figs 24.3 and 24.4)**. As well as examining the desquamated cervical cells, cervical smear reports may also identify infection such as candidal, trichomonal or wart virus infection. Rarely they may identify cells from other parts of the genital tract, such as malignant endometrial or ovarian cells.

The precise rates of progression and spontaneous resolution of the disease are unknown. Roughly one-third of lesions will progress to the next stage (CIN I to II, CIN II to III, etc.), a third will remain unchanged, and a third will regress. The duration of progression to invasive carcinoma is variable, but the average is perhaps around 10 years.

Screening recommendations

In the UK there is an organized systematic computerized screening programme with national recommendations to screen from the ages of 20 to 65 years. Different regions, however, have different protocols, and England has recently recommended screening from the age of 25 years.

Colposcopy

Significant dyskaryosis on a cervical smear is an indication for further assessment with colposcopy. This is a procedure by which the cervix is examined in more detail using a type of binocular microscope referred to as a colposcope **(Fig. 24.5)**. Although moderate and severe dyskaryosis are absolute indications for colposcopy, controversy exists as to whether it is required for mild dyskaryosis. Some believe it is important, while others are concerned it may lead to overtreatment of lesions which will often regress spontaneously. The indications for colposcopy are listed in **Box 24.1**.

Pre-pubertal   **Pubertal**

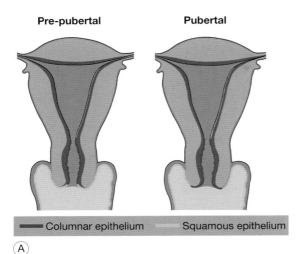

Columnar epithelium   Squamous epithelium

(A)

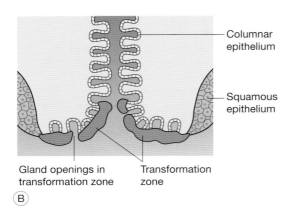

Columnar epithelium

Squamous epithelium

Gland openings in transformation zone   Transformation zone

(B)

Fig. 24.1 The transformation zone. (A) The cervix everts at puberty, exposing the columnar epithelium of the endocervical canal. **(B)** This epithelium, referred to as the transformation zone, gradually undergoes metaplasia to squamous epithelium.

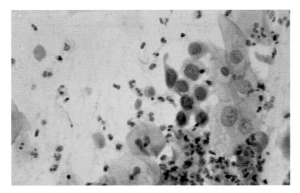

Fig. 24.2 Slide prepared from a cervical smear. There is moderate dysplasia with hyperchromasia, irregular nuclei and multinucleation. This slide also shows *Trichomonas vaginalis*, leucocytosis and a spermatozoon.

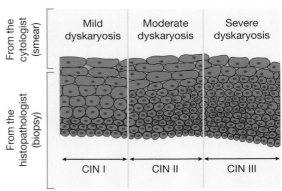

From the cytologist (smear)

| Mild dyskaryosis | Moderate dyskaryosis | Severe dyskaryosis |

From the histopathologist (biopsy)

| CIN I | CIN II | CIN III |

Fig. 24.3 The CIN grading system.

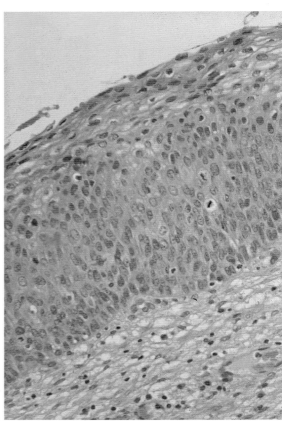

Fig. 24.4 CIN II in a biopsy specimen. There are abnormal cells arising from the basal layer, but not extending to the full thickness of the epithelium.

The patient is placed in the lithotomy position and a bivalve speculum is then inserted to allow visualization of the cervix. It is important to identify the squamocolumnar junction (SCJ). Abnormal epithelium, such as CIN, contains an increased amount of protein and lower levels of glycogen than normal epithelium. If acetic acid is applied

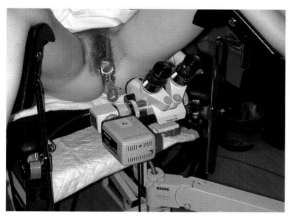

Fig. 24.5 **Colposcopy, using a high-powered microscope, allows detailed examination of the cervix.**

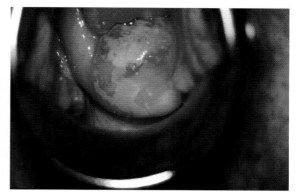

Fig. 24.6 **Acetic acid coagulates protein, and the abnormal cells, which have more protein, appear 'aceto-white'.**

Box 24.1

The indications for colposcopy

1. Abnormal cervical cytology

Smear result	Action
Severe dyskaryosis	Colposcopy
Moderate dyskaryosis	Colposcopy
Mild dyskaryosis	Repeat cytology/ colposcopy
Borderline	Repeat cytology
Glandular dyskaryosis	Colposcopy

2. Clinical suspicion of invasive disease
3. Mild or borderline on two occasions 6 months apart

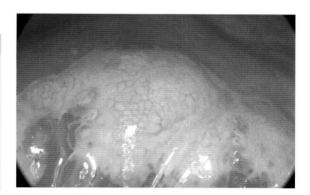

Fig. 24.7 **Patches of aceto-white may be separated by areas of blood vessels, creating a mosaic pattern.**

to the cervix, the protein coagulates and the abnormal cells appear 'aceto-white' **(Fig. 24.6)**. There may also be a mosaic pattern with patches of aceto-white separated by areas of red vessels **(Fig. 24.7)**. Some of the vascular patterns may appear punctated if the vessels are viewed end-on. The inter-vessel distance increases with more severe lesions, and bizarre branching with coarse punctation and atypical vessels suggests invasive disease. Lugol's iodine (Schiller's iodine) stains glycogen mahogany brown, and the abnormal cells, which have less glycogen and therefore take up less iodine, can also be viewed in this way.

Treatment of CIN

High-grade CIN (CIN II and III) requires treatment. With CIN I there is more controversy and generally a period of cytological surveillance will be employed as many of these lesions will spontaneously resolve. If high-grade CIN is suspected colposcopically, the options are to treat immediately (termed 'see-and-treat') using an excisional method (e.g. large loop excision) or to biopsy to confirm high-grade CIN and treat thereafter. This depends on the certainty of the colposcopic findings and the likelihood that the patient will attend for the follow-up.

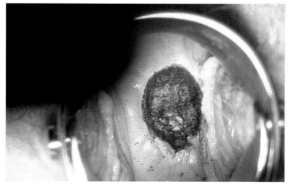
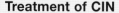

Fig. 24.8 **An area of CIN II has been excised using a loop** (Table 24.1). The cauterized area heals spontaneously.

The cervix is infiltrated directly with local anaesthetic, and a loop diathermy excision or some other form of excision is performed **(Fig. 24.8)**. The alternative of ablating the area has the disadvantage that the histological assessment is less complete (see **Table 24.1**). As smoking is an aetiological factor, its cessation should be discussed with the patient.

Table 24.1
Treatment modalities for CIN

Method	Summary of method	Pros	Cons
Loop excision of the transitional zone	Wire loop with high-frequency current	Easy outpatient procedure. Tissue is available for pathology	Small association with cervical incompetence and stenosis
Radical electrodiathermy	Cervical cautery using a monopolar high-frequency current	Easy outpatient procedure	No tissue available for pathology. Depth of tissue destruction not known
Cryotherapy	Freezing the cervix with a nitrogen probe	Easy outpatient procedure	No tissue available for pathology. Depth of tissue destruction not known
Laser vaporization	Destruction with CO_2 laser	Easy outpatient procedure. Known depth of tissue destruction	No tissue available for pathology
'Cold' coagulation	Heating to approx 100°C	Easy outpatient procedure	No tissue available for pathology. Depth of tissue destruction not known
Cone biopsy	Surgical excision, often under anaesthesia	Large specimen obtained. Tissue is available for pathology	Often needs general anaesthesia. Associated with cervical incompetence and stenosis

Follow-up

Any woman who has had CIN, whether treated or not, continues to be at risk of developing cervical cancer due to either incomplete treatment of her CIN or the development of new disease. Follow-up is therefore important and this is usually carried out cytologically by repeating smears. Colposcopy can also be used. Protocols vary, but, following successful treatment of CIN, it is reasonable to arrange a follow-up smear after 6 months, and then annually for 5–10 years, before returning to the national screening programme if the smears have been negative.

Success of the UK cervical screening programme

The aim of screening is to identify women at high risk of cervical cancer to enable intervention at a time that allows treatment to substantially reduce this risk. The screening programme, although successful, will not be able to prevent all cervical cancers. It is estimated that for the UK cervical screening programme, for women aged between 25 and 49 years, 3-yearly screening prevents 84 cervical cancers out of every 100 that would develop without screening.

Cervical cancer

Aetiological factors

Cervical cancer arises from areas of CIN, as noted above. At least 30% of patients with CIN III, if left untreated, will probably go on to develop invasive disease over a period of 5–20 years.

Sexual behaviour

Cervical cancer is usually a disease of sexually active women and has been linked mainly to human papillomavirus (HPV). Women with cervical cancer are likely to have had more sexual partners and to have started intercourse earlier, and are less likely to have used barrier methods of contraception, compared with other women. The sexual behaviour of their partners may also be important. The disease is more frequent in parous women.

Human papillomavirus

A strong association has been observed between HPV serotypes 16 and 18, pre-invasive disease, and invasive cervical cancer. It is believed that certain serotypes of HPV are important cofactors in the development of cervical cancer and may act by producing proteins (E6/7) which affect the action of the p53 gene product. The p53 gene is important in repairing DNA, and, if damaged, may predispose to malignant change. HPV is present in around a third of all women in their 20s in the UK.

The combined oral contraceptive pill

Studies have shown that prolonged use of the oral contraceptive pill increases the risk of cervical cancer up to fourfold, but only in women who carry HPV. It can be argued that this effect is attributable to differences in sexual behaviour rather than to the pill itself.

Smoking

Women who smoke are also at increased risk of developing cervical cancer. This may be due to alterations in immune function in the cervical epithelium or chemical carcinogenesis.

Future prevention

As certain subtypes of HPV are now known to be the main aetiological factors associated with the development of cervical cancer, there has been significant effort to develop a vaccine to these virus subtypes. Two separate vaccines have been developed with the aim of protecting an individual from the common oncogenic HPV subtypes. Cevarex and Gardasil have now passed through clinical trials and are available in many countries. It is thought that for these vaccines to be most effective, girls should be inoculated before they have become sexually active. Routine inoculation of girls at the age of 12–13 has commenced in the UK. The intended benefit is to reduce the incidence of cervical carcinoma by 70%. As not every cervical cancer will be prevented, however, it is important that cervical screening continues.

Presentation

Patients with cervical cancer may present with postcoital bleeding, intermenstrual bleeding, menorrhagia or an offensive vaginal discharge. In early cases there may be no symptoms, and the diagnosis is made only after abnormal cervical cytology is discovered. Other symptoms such as backache, referred leg pain, leg oedema, haematuria or alteration in bowel habit are usually associated with advanced-stage disease. General malaise, weight loss and anaemia are also late features.

Three categories of clinical appearance are described:

1. The most common is an exophytic lesion **(Fig. 24.9)**. It usually arises on the ectocervix, often producing a large friable polypoid mass which bleeds easily. It can also arise from within the endocervical canal so that the canal becomes distended and 'barrel shaped'.
2. An infiltrating tumour that shows little ulceration or exophytic growth but tends to produce a hard indurated cervix.
3. An ulcerative tumour which erodes a portion of the cervix and vaginal vault, producing a crater with local infection and seropurulent discharge.

Pathology

The majority of cervical cancers are squamous, and may be of keratinizing (the commonest), large cell, non-keratinizing and small cell subtypes. Around 10–25% are adenocarcinomas. There may also be coexistent squamous metaplasia or neoplasia (adenosquamous carcinoma).

Spread

Cervical cancer spreads by direct extension into adjacent structures and via the draining lymphatics. Blood-borne metastases are rare. Direct invasion beyond the cervix is usually into the upper vagina, parametrium and pelvic

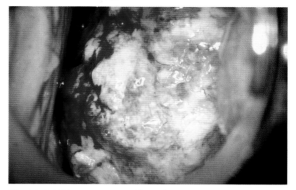

Fig. 24.9 This squamous cell carcinoma was staged II$_A$.

sidewall, and this tumour may lead to ureteric obstruction. There may also be invasion of the bladder and rectum.

There is no predictable pattern of lymphatic spread, with paracervical, parametrial and both internal and external iliac nodes potentially involved. There may also be spread to the common iliac, para-aortic and left supraclavicular area.

The risk of lymph node metastases correlates with both stage and tumour volume. Around 10% of patients with stage I disease have pelvic node involvement, rising to around 35% in those with stage III disease. The incidence of para-aortic node involvement is less, at around 5% of patients with stage I disease and 25% with stage III disease.

Staging, investigation and prognostic factors

Cervical cancer is staged (FIGO) by clinical examination **(Table 24.2)**, which is often carried out under anaesthetic, and the diagnosis confirmed histologically by biopsy. The examination should include a rectovaginal examination to assess parametrial involvement. The stage is not altered by subsequent radiological (e.g. MRI or CT) or surgico-pathological findings (although in early disease the histological dimensions of the tumour are important). Although this may seem inconsistent, it is to maintain consistency with other parts of the world where the disease is more common but where 'high tech' imaging is not always available. The use of ultrasound, MRI and CT scanning has replaced the use of cystoscopy and intravenous urography (IVU) in many centres. If nodes are radiologically suspicious, for example, it may be more appropriate to avoid surgery and treat with chemotherapy and radiotherapy.

Although in developed countries a greater proportion of cases present with stage I disease, in worldwide terms the majority (>75%) of women with cervical cancer present with advanced stage (stage III/IV) disease. The prognosis for patients with early-stage disease is relatively good **(Table 24.2)** but the prognosis for patients with advanced-stage disease is poor.

Table 24.2

FIGO staging of cervical cancer

Stage	Invasion	Prognosis 5-year survival	Treatment
I_{A1}	Depth of invasion ≤3 mm and width ≤7 mm (includes early stromal invasion of up to 1 mm)	84–90% if tumour <3 cm; 85% will have negative pelvic nodes and 95% of these patients will be 'cured'	Local excision; if margins of a cone clear (i.e. no residual tumour or CIN) then conization is adequate, with no need for pelvic lymphadenectomy
I_{A2}	Depth of invasion 3.1–5 mm and width ≤7 mm		Simple hysterectomy and pelvic lymphadenectomy
I_{B1}	Tumour confined to cervix and diameter less than 4 cm	66% if tumour > 3 cm	
I_{B2}	Tumour confined to cervix and diameter more than 4 cm		Radical hysterectomy or chemo–radiotherapy
II_A	Upper third of vagina	62%	
II_B	Upper two-thirds of vagina plus parametrial disease		Radical hysterectomy or chemo–radiotherapy
III_A	Lower third of vagina		
III_B	Pelvic side wall and/or hydronephrosis	40%	Chemo–radiotherapy
IV_A	Bladder, rectum	15%	Chemo–radiotherapy
IV_B	Beyond pelvis		

Management

Stage I_{A1}–I_{A2}

Stage I_{A1} can be cured by simple excision. If preservation of fertility is required, a cone biopsy with close cytological follow-up may be adequate treatment; where preservation of fertility is not important, simple hysterectomy is preferable. In all other cases of stage I disease more aggressive treatment with either radical radiotherapy or radical surgery is required. With stage I_{A2} there is around 5% chance of nodal involvement. In these patients, local excision, as above, would be combined with formal pelvic lymphadenectomy. If these nodes are positive, adjuvant radiotherapy would be required too.

Stage I_B–II_A

The choice between radical hysterectomy and radical radiotherapy is determined by the clinical condition of the patient. There is no difference in survival between the two methods but there are significant differences in morbidity.

Radical hysterectomy and pelvic lymphadenectomy involve total hysterectomy, excision of the parametria, upper third of the vagina and paracolpos, as well as dissection of the pelvic lymph nodes. The key surgical principle is to obtain a satisfactory surgical margin and to be able to histologically assess the draining lymphatics. Oophorectomy may be performed if appropriate, but the ovaries are rarely the site of metastatic spread and usually can be safely conserved. The operative mortality is less than 1%, although potential morbidity includes infection, thromboembolic disease, haemorrhage and vesicovaginal fistulae. There are also medium-term problems with reduced bladder sensation and voiding difficulties, together with long-term problems of high residual urinary volumes, recurrent urinary infections, stress incontinence and lymphocyst formation.

Radical radiotherapy usually consists of external beam therapy (teletherapy) to the pelvis and local vaginal therapy (brachytherapy). There is now evidence that combining this with cisplatin chemotherapy increases the survival rate and this has become the standard of care. Teletherapy is delivered in fractions over a number of weeks to treat the pelvic lymphatics, whereas with brachytherapy a vaginal delivery system is inserted and left in situ for 12–18 hours to irradiate central disease. The radiation dose which can be given is limited by the size of the lesion and the proximity of the bladder and bowel, both of which are particularly susceptible to radiation damage. The principal morbidity results from vaginal dryness, which can lead to sexual dysfunction, radiation cystitis, proctitis and vaginal stenosis. As this morbidity often gets worse with time, surgery is considered to be more suitable for those patients who are younger. In those found to have positive pelvic nodes postoperatively, it is usual to offer adjuvant chemotherapy and radiotherapy (chemo–radiotherapy).

Patients with stage I_{B1} will be offered either surgery or chemo–radiotherapy. In most modern cancer centres, patients will be extensively imaged. If there is a suggestion of extension outwith the cervix, then chemo–radiotherapy would be advised rather than surgery. There are two reasons for this: firstly, the morbidity associated with radical surgery plus chemo–radiotherapy is significantly greater that with the latter alone and secondly, if the cervix has been removed, it is not possible to give the high doses, via brachytherapy, that are required to achieve local control.

Similarly, for patients with stage I_{B2} and stage II_A, chemo–radiotherapy would now normally be advised. The reason for this is that even if radical surgery was to be successful, the likelihood of an unsatisfactory margin or positive nodes is sufficiently great to make adjuvant treatment likely.

For patients with small stage I_{B1} lesions that have been assessed in detail with MRI/CT imaging, and in whom future fertility is important, there is the possibility of radical local treatment. This is called radical trachelectomy and lymphadenectomy. The cervix is removed along with the paracervical tissues but the uterus is left in situ with a special suture left to maintain 'cervical competence'. The lymph nodes are also removed. This approach is still being evaluated – although it offers the patient the potential of future pregnancy, it is not without significant problems.

Stage II_B–IV

The treatment of advanced-stage disease usually involves radical radiotherapy in combination with cisplatin chemotherapy. Failure to cure inoperable cervical cancer may result from suboptimal treatment of the central disease or the existence of lymph node metastases. With large lesions, the sensitivity of adjacent structures to radiation may prevent use of curative radiation doses at the tumour periphery, and, furthermore, some tumours may be radio-resistant.

Recurrent disease

Those patients with recurrence have a 1-year survival of around 10–15%. Most recurrences are suitable for palliative care only. If the patient has not been previously treated with radiotherapy, this may be a treatment option, but the majority of patients will have already had radical radiotherapy. Patients with a central pelvic recurrence may be cured by pelvic exenteration (excision of vagina/uterus with the bladder or rectum or both). With careful selection, up to 60% of these cases may survive 5 years, but the operation is associated with major morbidity.

The remaining patients may benefit from chemotherapy to palliate symptomatic recurrence or radiotherapy to palliate recurrence involving bone or nerve roots. The most active chemotherapy agents are cisplatin and ifosfamide, and combinations based on these drugs cause initial tumour shrinkage in up to 70% of cases. The main benefit from chemotherapy is the relief of disease-related symptoms, such as pelvic pain, but chemotherapy itself can cause considerable toxicity and does not improve survival in these women.

Key *points*

- Cervical cancer is the most common cancer among women in many developing countries and worldwide there are over 450,000 cases each year.
- The risk of cervical cancer is related to sexual behaviour. Early age of first intercourse and a high number of sexual partners are risk factors. Smoking may also increase the risk.
- An important causative agent appears to be human papillomavirus serotypes 16 and 18.
- Screening is possible because of a relatively long precancerous phase and involves a programme of regular cervical smears. Cytological abnormalities on smears (dyskaryosis) correlate to some degree with histologically abnormal cervical intraepithelial neoplasia (CIN).
- When cervical smears demonstrate dyskaryosis, colposcopy allows identification of abnormal epithelium suggestive of CIN to be located, biopsied and treated.
- Although cervical cancers are mainly of squamous type, around 10–25% are adenocarcinomas.
- FIGO staging of cancer is from stage I to IV. Stage I can be treated by surgery or radiotherapy. More advanced cancer can be treated by radiotherapy ± chemotherapy.

Gestational trophoblastic disease

Introduction

Gestational trophoblastic disease (GTD) is a term used to describe a number of conditions characterized by an abnormal proliferation of trophoblastic tissue. There are premalignant and malignant forms: the premalignant form is subdivided into partial and complete hydatidiform moles, and the malignant form into invasive moles, choriocarcinoma, and placental site trophoblastic tumours **(Table 25.1)**. GTD has a number of important differences from other forms of malignancy in its aetiology, genetic make-up, pathophysiology and responsiveness to treatment. Fortunately, the malignant forms of the disease are extremely sensitive to chemotherapy, and treatment routinely results in cure, even in patients presenting with widespread disease.

Even molar pregnancy, which is the most common form of GTD, is a relatively rare condition, with an estimated worldwide incidence of around 1–3 cases for every 1000 live births. The incidence has previously been thought to vary across different geographical regions and racial groups, with estimates from the 1960s showing a near 10-fold higher incidence in Korea, the Philippines and China compared with Europe and the United States. Recent data, however, show a more uniform comparison.

The incidence of molar pregnancies is higher at the extremes of reproductive age, at approximately 1 in 30 in those aged under 15 and as high as 1 in 5 in those in their late 40s. As these extremes of the reproductive age group make up only a very small proportion of the women who become pregnant, over 90% of cases occur in women aged 18–40.

In view of the rarity of the condition, ongoing management is best provided by those in a few specialist centres.

Trophoblast cells in health and disease

In a healthy pregnancy the trophoblast cells make up a key component of the placental tissue. Their role is to promote invasion of the conceptus into the lining of the uterus, invade into the uterine blood vessels, promote angiogenesis and produce human chorionic gonadotrophin (hCG).

The malignant forms of GTD, both those arising from molar pregnancies and those arising from malignant transformation of cells in healthy placentae, share many of these characteristics. In addition to the abilities to invade into the lining of the uterus and stimulate new blood vessels, however, the malignant cells are also able to spread to other organs of the body and grow at a very fast rate without any limit on their division. Fortunately, despite these changes, the production of hCG is always retained, and this is extremely helpful in establishing a diagnosis and in monitoring the response to treatment.

Premalignant GTD (Table 25.1)

Premalignant GTD is divided into partial and complete molar pregnancies. The original derivation of the term hydatidiform mole, from the Greek *hydatis* meaning a watery vesicle and the Latin *mola* meaning a shapeless mass, is an accurate description of the appearance of a complete molar pregnancy evacuated after the first trimester. With the near-universal use of first-trimester ultrasound, however, this florid appearance is now rarely seen in well-resourced countries.

Partial hydatidiform mole

Molar pregnancies occur as the result of an error in either the production of the oocyte or at the time of fertilization. Normally, fertilization combines a 23,X set of haploid chromosomes from the ovum with either a 23,X or 23,Y haploid set from the sperm, the result being a diploid 46,XX or 46,XY zygote which has the correct balance of maternal and paternal genes. In contrast, a partial molar pregnancy has 69 chromosomes, 23 from the mother and the other 46 paternally derived, usually from the entry of two separate sperm into the ovum **(Fig. 25.1)**.

In a partial molar pregnancy there is usually an embryo, and it may be seen on an early ultrasound. The ultrasound may have been 'routine', or have been carried out because of vaginal bleeding, vaginal discharge, abdominal pain or excessive morning sickness. Although structurally abnormal, there may be no obvious ultrasound features of this in the early first trimester and the diagnosis may therefore not become apparent until histological tissue examination is carried out after a failed pregnancy. The features are of

Table 25.1			
Classification of gestational trophoblastic disease			
Classification	**Pathology**	**Usual karyotype**	**Clinical features**
Premalignant			
Partial hydatidiform mole	Focal hyperplasia of villi Benign	69,XXY: two paternal haploid sets and one maternal haploid set	Difficult to diagnose on ultrasound as a fetus can be present during the first 8–10 weeks. Most present as failed pregnancies. Less than 1% require additional treatment after evacuation
Complete hydatidiform mole	Generalized hyperplasia Benign	46,XX: two haploid sets, both paternal ('androgenically diploid')	Uterine cavity filled with vesicular mole tissue on ultrasound without an embryo. Approximately 10–15% become malignant and require additional therapy
Malignant			
Invasive mole	Features of invasion	Virtually all are androgenically diploid	Molar tissue invading the myometrium and may cause uterine rupture if not treated
Choriocarcinoma	Is histologically differentiated from a hydatidiform mole by the absence of villi	Contains maternal and paternal chromosomes (unlike choriocarcinoma of ovarian origin)	Most follow a live birth, stillbirth, miscarriage or ectopic pregnancy, but can arise from a hydatidiform mole. There is frequently metastatic spread. Highly curable with chemotherapy
Placental site trophoblastic tumour (PSTT)		Contains maternal and paternal chromosomes	Slow-growing malignancy invading the myometrium and potentially metastasizing to the lung. hCG levels are less elevated than in choriocarcinoma. Usually treated with surgery and chemotherapy

focal hyperplasia and swelling of the villi, though many areas do not have these obvious changes and distinguishing a partial mole from a hydropic miscarriage can be difficult. Fortunately, the risk of malignant change after a partial molar pregnancy is less than 1%, and very few patients end up requiring chemotherapy.

Complete hydatidiform mole

In contrast to partial molar pregnancies, complete molar pregnancies have the correct number of chromosomes, with the majority having a 46,XX karyotype. In complete molar pregnancies, however, all the nuclear genetic material is from the father and they are therefore termed androgenetic in origin.

There appears to be two mechanisms by which this genetic combination arises:

- The maternal 23,X haploid set of chromosomes in the ovum may be lost at the time of fertilization and the 23,X haploid paternal chromosomes from the fertilizing sperm may duplicate themselves, giving rise to the 46,XX cell.
- Alternatively, an 'empty' ovum may be fertilized by two separate spermatozoa (dispermy), which also leads to a paternally derived karyotype.

In a complete molar pregnancy there is never any fetal material, and the placental tissue has marked hyperplasia and gross vesicular swelling of the villi. The classical macroscopic 'bunch of small grapes' appearance of a complete molar pregnancy generally occurs only in the second trimester; thus, as most are usually diagnosed in the first trimester, this appearance is less often seen in well-resourced countries **(Fig. 25.2)**. In areas without routine ultrasound, presentation may be with a large-for-dates uterus (from the bulk of the tumour), or with hyperemesis, or, more rarely,

with thyrotoxicosis resulting from the supraphysiological levels of hCG.

Approximately 10–15% of complete molar pregnancies become malignant and will require chemotherapy after their surgical evacuation.

Malignant GTD (Table 25.1)

Invasive mole

Invasive molar pregnancy is rare but occurs when the molar tissue invades predominantly into the myometrium. The clinical presentation is with a uterine mass and an elevated hCG level. As a result of the myometrial invasion, the tumour can lead to uterine rupture and present with abdominal pain and bleeding. Histologically, invasive mole has a similar appearance to a complete molar pregnancy and usually responds well to chemotherapy.

Choriocarcinoma

Choriocarcinoma is a highly malignant tumour arising from malignant transformation of the trophoblast cells, and histologically is characterized by haemorrhage, necrosis and intravascular growth. It lacks the villous structure of the normal trophoblast or molar pregnancy. The disease is very rare, with approximately 1 case per 50,000 live births. Choriocarcinoma may become apparent shortly after a pregnancy or can present after an interval of up to 20 years after the causative pregnancy.

Presentation is usually with persistent vaginal bleeding and a markedly raised hCG (the serum hCG level, which is usually less than 100,000 IU/l at the time of delivery, should

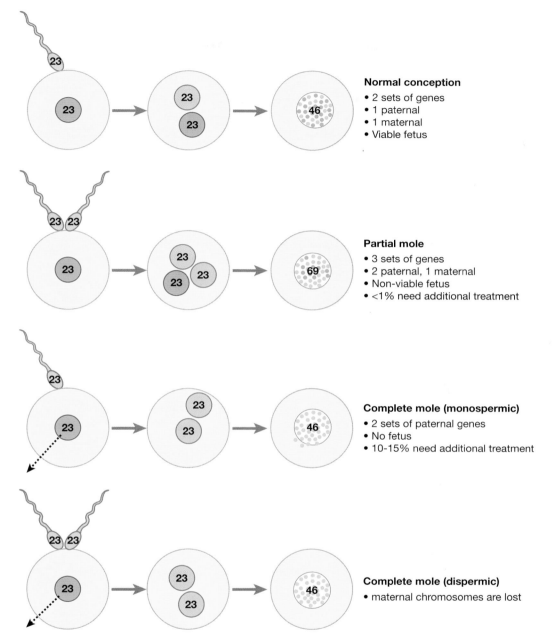

Fig. 25.1 Genetic make-up of normal pregnancy and partial and complete molar pregnancies.

fall to normal within 3 weeks postpartum). Diagnosis can also follow presentation of a metastasis in:

- the lung, causing haemoptysis or dyspnoea
- the brain, leading to neurological abnormalities
- the gastrointestinal tract, causing chronic blood loss or melaena
- the liver, leading to jaundice
- the kidney, causing haematuria.

The finding of an elevated hCG level in a woman with cancer is highly suggestive of choriocarcinoma.

In contrast to molar pregnancies, there do not appear to be any risk factors or higher-risk groups for the development of choriocarcinoma.

Placental site trophoblastic tumour (PSTT)

PSTT is the least frequent type of gestational tumour, with approximately 1 case for every 200,000 live births. In contrast to choriocarcinoma, PSTT is believed to arise from the intermediate trophoblastic cells, which have a lower capacity

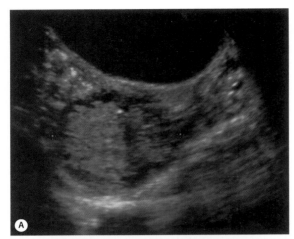

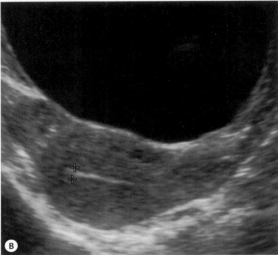

Fig. 25.2 Complete molar pregnancy. (A) Ultrasound appearance of recurrent complete molar pregnancy tissue in the uterus prior to chemotherapy treatment. **(B)** Follow-up scan performed 6 weeks after chemotherapy completion.

to invade and also make relatively less hCG than the syncytiotrophoblast cells that give rise to choriocarcinoma.

The presentation of PSTT is similar to that of choriocarcinoma, though interestingly it occurs only after the delivery of a female infant and is more likely to be associated with hCG-induced amenorrhoea. It usually presents rather later than choriocarcinoma, tends to grow more slowly and is less chemosensitive.

Management of molar pregnancies

Following an ultrasound scan suggestive of a molar pregnancy, the first step is to arrange a uterine evacuation. In a complete molar pregnancy, where there are no fetal parts, the evacuation should be performed by a suction procedure. The risks of bleeding and perforation during surgical evacuation are significant, however, and the procedure should be performed by a senior surgeon and with cross-matched blood available. Medical evacuation may be appropriate for a partial mole, particularly if larger fetal parts are present, but this should be followed with a surgical evacuation of any retained products of conception. It is recommended that oxytocin is avoided until after the uterine evacuation is completed, to minimize the risk of distant spread by uterine contractions.

Following the evacuation, the diagnosis is confirmed on histological examination and supported, if needed, by cytogenetic studies of the trophoblast cells. The registration and follow-up of molar pregnancy is discussed below.

Follow-up after a molar pregnancy

Following the evacuation of a complete molar pregnancy there is an approximately 10% chance of persistent disease and the development of malignancy, whilst after a partial molar pregnancy the risk is less than 1%. There is no effective prospective method of determining which patients will develop persistent disease and will therefore require further treatment, but hCG follow-up after the evacuation allows this group to be identified.

To ensure that this is meticulously carried out, in the UK, follow-up of molar pregnancies is organized through three central laboratories (in London, Sheffield and Dundee). Each case of molar pregnancy is registered with the nearest laboratory, which will then organize the hCG follow-up directly. This system has been a major factor in ensuring the extremely high cure rates now seen for the disease, and the clinical experience in these centres has led to most of the therapeutic developments in these rare tumours.

In the majority of patients with molar pregnancies, the hCG values fall to normal within 2 months and relapse after this is very rare. The current advice is that follow-up is needed for only 6 months from the time of the evacuation or for 6 months from the first normal hCG level in those where the rate of fall is slower. It is recommended that women postpone a further pregnancy during the follow-up period, as the hCG from this pregnancy could mask the hCG from relapsed disease, and this would delay diagnosis and treatment. There is also advice to avoid the contraceptive pill during this time and to use barrier methods of contraception.

There is an increased risk of a further molar pregnancy in a subsequent pregnancy, a risk estimated to be approximately 1:75. For women unfortunate to have two molar pregnancies, the risk of a third in a later pregnancy is in the order of 1:10. Follow-up is therefore recommended after all subsequent pregnancies.

Management of malignant GTD

Following evacuation of a molar pregnancy there are a number of indications for further treatment **(Box 25.1)**. The most frequent of these is a rise or a plateau in the hCG levels after the evacuation. The majority of patients receive treatment with chemotherapy, which has a high cure rate and is generally well tolerated. A few women who have completed their families and have no evidence of spread may opt instead for a hysterectomy, but they still require careful follow-up as occult extrauterine disease may exist and chemotherapy could still be required.

In contrast, all patients with choriocarcinoma occurring after a pregnancy require chemotherapy; surgery in this group is rarely useful. As the disease is so exquisitely sensitive to chemotherapy, the majority of patients with GTD occurring after a molar pregnancy can be treated with low-toxicity single-agent chemotherapy using methotrexate. This is well tolerated, has minimal side-effects, does not cause hair loss or significant sickness, and there is minimal risk of neutropenia. In contrast, some GTD patients, particularly those with choriocarcinoma after a normal pregnancy, require treatment with a more toxic combination chemotherapy regimen, usually EMA-CO.

To help determine which type of treatment is required, the FIGO scoring system can be used **(Table 25.2)**. This allows the calculation of a score based on eight variables. Patients scoring 6 points or fewer receive simply methotrexate chemotherapy, whilst those scoring 7 and above start with combination chemotherapy. Overall cure rates of 99% for those in the low-risk treatment group, and approximately 90% for those in the high-risk group – even for those patients presenting with advanced disease **(Fig. 25.3)** – can be expected. The majority of the patients who are difficult to cure present with choriocarcinoma and have had a long interval from their causative pregnancy.

After the completion of chemotherapy, most patients recover fairly rapidly and in nearly all cases fertility is retained. An interval of 12 months from the completion of chemotherapy to the next pregnancy is usually recommended, and the majority of women are able to have further children. There is thought to be little excess risk of fetal abnormalities in this post-chemotherapy group.

Box 25.1

Indications for chemotherapy treatment after a molar pregnancy

- Brain, liver, or gastrointestinal tract metastases, or lung metastases >2 cm on chest X-ray
- Histological evidence of choriocarcinoma
- Heavy vaginal bleeding or gastrointestinal/intraperitoneal bleeding
- Pulmonary, vulval or vaginal metastases unless the hCG level is falling
- Rising hCG in two consecutive serum samples
- hCG >20,000 IU/l more than 4 weeks after evacuation
- hCG plateau in three consecutive serum samples
- Raised hCG level 6 months after evacuation (even if falling)

Table 25.2

FIGO prognostic score system for gestational trophoblastic disease

	Score			
	0	1	2	4
Age	<40	≥40	–	–
Antecedent pregnancy	Mole	Miscarriage	Term	–
Interval	<4 months	4–6 months	7–13 months	≥14 months
Pretreatment hCG (IU/l)	<1000	1000–10,000	10,000–100,000	>100,000
Largest tumour size	<3 cm	3–5 cm	>5 cm	–
Site of metastases	Lung	Spleen, kidney	Gastrointestinal tract	Brain, liver
Number of metastases	0	1–4	5–8	>8
Previous chemotherapy	–	–	Single agent	Two or more drugs

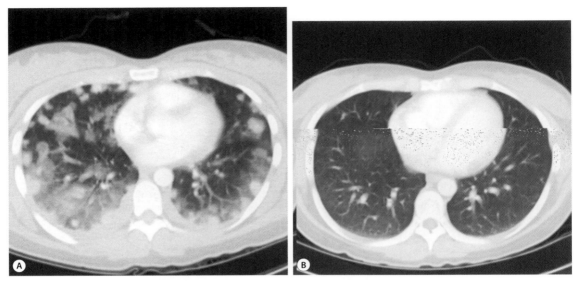

Fig. 25.3 Choriocarcinoma. (A) CT scan of the chest, demonstrating extensive pulmonary metastases and haemorrhage, in a patient with choriocarcinoma presenting 1 month after a normal delivery. **(B)** A CT scan performed 6 months later shows the complete resolution of the disease in response to chemotherapy.

Key *points*

- Gestational trophoblastic disorders represent an abnormal proliferation of trophoblastic tissue and may be benign (molar pregnancy) or malignant (invasive mole, a choriocarcinoma, or a placental site trophoblastic tumour).
- Trophoblastic tumours always produce hCG, and this acts as an excellent marker for follow-up.
- A hydatidiform mole may be complete or partial. A complete mole is diploid (but all the chromosomes are paternally derived) and there is no fetal tissue (only trophoblast). A partial mole is usually triploid (with 46 of the 69 chromosomes being paternally derived) and there may be a fetus.
- The diagnosis of a molar pregnancy is often suggested by ultrasound in which there is homogeneous solid tissue with a vesicular appearance. The diagnosis is confirmed by histopathological examination of tissue.

- The initial management of a molar pregnancy is to carry out an evacuation of the uterus, and follow-up is required to ensure that the hCG level is falling. Further treatment, usually chemotherapy, is required if the hCG rises progressively following the uterine evacuation, or if the pathology is reported as choriocarcinoma.
- Choriocarcinoma can occur after any type of conception, including a normal pregnancy, miscarriage or hydatidiform mole.
- All the malignant forms of gestational trophoblastic disease, including choriocarcinoma, are exquisitely sensitive to chemotherapy and the cure rate is high.
- Following a molar pregnancy there is a modest increase in risk of further molar pregnancy in any subsequent pregnancies.

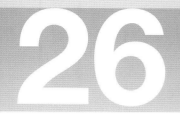

The physiology of pregnancy

Introduction

Pregnancy brings huge physiological changes and, teleologically, it is assumed that these changes are in the fetal interest (see **Box 26.1**). The changes are proactive; in other words, they are not proportional to the size of the fetus, such that by the end of the first trimester many systems are functioning at levels close to those at term. The systems are reviewed in order below.

Respiratory system

Oxygen consumption is increased by around 15–20%. The requirement for this is partly maternal – to satisfy the increase in cardiac output, renal function and other metabolic requirements, including respiratory function, breast and uterine development. Around 40% of the increased oxygen requirement is for the fetoplacental unit. To supply this increased oxygen requirement the mother hyperventilates, increasing minute ventilation by about 40% above the normal 7 l/min. This increase in ventilation is far greater than the increase in oxygen consumption, effectively providing a safety net.

The increase is predominantly achieved by increasing tidal volume rather than respiratory rate – in other words, the mother breathes more deeply. This is more efficient than increasing the respiratory rate, as there is less dead-space movement (i.e. that air which is outwith the alveoli and hence not involved in gas exchange). Maternal serum CO_2 falls, favouring CO_2 transfer from the fetus to the mother. These changes are thought to be mediated by progesterone, as a smaller but similar effect is noted in patients taking progestogen-containing contraceptives **(Fig. 26.1)**.

Dyspnoea is a common symptom in pregnancy. This dyspnoea is perceptual rather than a reflection of inadequate gas exchange, and is often worse at rest. In late pregnancy, the gravid uterus may restrict diaphragmatic movement, exacerbating any feelings of breathlessness. Nevertheless it is important to consider pathological causes of breathlessness, particularly pulmonary thromboembolic disease.

Cardiovascular system

In pregnancy there is an increase in cardiac output and a decrease in peripheral vascular resistance.

Cardiac output rises by about 40%, from around 3.5 l/min to 6 l/min, from increases in both stroke volume and cardiac rate. As with the respiratory system, these changes are disproportionately greater than required. The fall in peripheral vascular resistance mediated by vasodilatation is not quite compensated for by the increased cardiac output, so the overall effect is a slight fall in blood pressure in the second trimester, sometimes as much as 5 mmHg systolic and 10 mmHg diastolic. The blood pressure may rise slightly again in the third trimester and it may be difficult to separate this from the pathological state of pre-eclampsia. The hyperdynamic circulation of pregnancy can often reveal functional flow murmurs of little clinical significance, as well as changing the cardiac axis on ECG and X-ray.

This high blood flow maximizes PO_2 on the maternal side of the placenta and maximizes O_2 transfer to the fetal circulation. The plasma volume expansion and increased cardiac output may also help heat loss by increasing blood flow through the skin, thus compensating for the increased metabolic rate of pregnancy. Peripheral vasodilatation causes a feeling of warmth and a tolerance to cold, and

Box 26.1

Teleology

A 'teleological' explanation for an event is one where the explanation is sought directly from the effects. For example, if a change in PCO_2 favours the fetus, it is teleological to say that the reason for the change is fetal advantage. The change has arisen by natural selection, and is therefore assumed to be in the fetal interest.

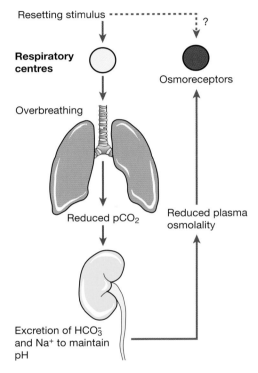

Fig. 26.1 The postulated events leading to the resetting of the respiratory centre in pregnancy.

Table 26.1

Blood changes in pregnancy

	Non-pregnant	Pregnant
Haemoglobin (g/dl)	12–14	10–12
Red cell count (×10¹²/l)	4.2	3.7
Haematocrit (venous)	40%	34%
MCV (fl)	75–99	80–103
MCH (pg)	27–31	No change
MCHC (g/dl)	32–36	No change
White cell count (×10⁹/l)	4–11	9–15
Platelets (×10⁹/l)	140–440	100–440
ESR (mm/h)	<10	30–100

ESR, erythrocyte sedimentation rate; MCH, mean corpuscular haemoglobin: MCHC, mean corpuscular haemoglobin concentration; MCV, mean corpuscular volume.

Blood, plasma, and extracellular fluid volume

On average the total red cell mass increases steadily throughout the pregnancy by 25%, from around 1300 ml to 1700 ml. The circulating plasma volume, however, increases by 40%, from around 2600 ml to 3700 ml. Because the plasma volume increases proportionately more than red cell mass, there is a dilutional drop in the haemoglobin concentration and in the haematocrit, such that a haemoglobin level of 10.5 g/l would be normal in a healthy pregnancy.

Plasma colloid osmotic pressure falls in pregnancy; as a result, fluid shifts into the extravascular compartment, causing oedema. Not only do almost all pregnant women have some dependent oedema, but so also do non-pregnant women in the postovulatory (high progesterone) phase of the cycle.

Blood constituents and anaemia

The typical changes in the full blood count in pregnancy are shown in **Table 26.1**. Iron requirements are increased **(Table 26.2)** to meet the requirements of the larger red cell mass, developing fetus, and the placenta, and the serum ferritin level therefore falls. The fetus gains iron from maternal serum by active transport across the placenta, mostly in weeks 36 to 40. It has been found that the haemoglobin drop mentioned above can be minimized by giving iron supplements, and some authors have concluded that there must therefore be a pathological iron deficiency. Despite this, trials of supplementation have not demonstrated a reduction in any important adverse pregnancy outcome, and observational data indicate that maternal and perinatal

may be a factor in the palmar erythema and spider naevi of pregnancy.

The cardiac output may rise by a further 2 l/min in established labour; this may in part be due to uterine contractions dispelling blood from the uterus, and thereby increasing venous return. Following delivery the uterus contracts, reducing cardiac output to 15–25% above normal, which over the next 6 weeks gradually returns to the pre-pregnancy state.

Late in pregnancy the mass of the uterus is liable to press on, and partially occlude, the inferior vena cava. This reduced venous return leads to a reduced cardiac output and may lead to hypotension, the so-called 'supine hypotensive syndrome'. Mothers are therefore often supported on a left lateral tilt during labour to relieve this pressure by displacing the gravid uterus. This is an important fact to remember in an emergency situation.

Table 26.2
The requirements of elemental iron during pregnancy

Fetus and placenta	500 mg
Red cell increment	500 mg
Postpartum blood loss and 6 months' lactation	360 mg
Total	**1360 mg**
Saving from amenorrhoea approximately	**360 mg**
Net increased demand approximately	**1 gram**

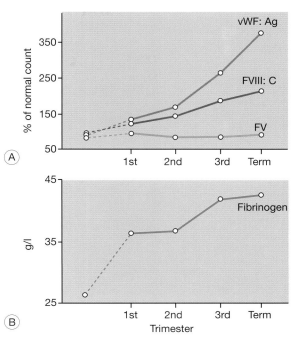

Fig. 26.2 The levels of the procoagulants (A) factor VIII, von Willebrand factor and (B) fibrinogen rise in pregnancy. FV, factor V.

mortality do not rise with low Hb concentrations until levels fall below 7 g/dl. Despite these reservations, it is likely that iron deficiency does occasionally occur, particularly if iron stores are low before pregnancy. The World Health Organization (WHO) has suggested iron supplementation at haemoglobin levels below 10.5 g/dl.

Folate metabolism

The daily folate requirement rises from 50 mg to 400 mg, and folate deficiency may occur. It is usually possible to meet this increased requirement through a normal diet, although intake in those with a poor diet is likely to be inadequate. Daily folic acid supplementation from before conception reduces the risk of neural tube defects. There are no known teratogenic effects from folate supplementation.

Haemostasis in pregnancy

Pregnancy is a hypercoagulable state, with an increase in procoagulants (particularly fibrinogen, but also platelets, factor VIII, von Willebrand factor) and a reduction in naturally occurring anticoagulants (e.g. antithrombin III). Fibrinolysis is also increased, so there is an increased net turnover of coagulation factors **(Figs 26.2 and 26.3)**. Fibrinolytic activity returns to normal within 1 hour of placental delivery, suggestive that inhibition of fibrinolysis is mediated by the placental unit.

The reason for this hypercoagulable state is presumably, teleologically, to minimize blood loss at delivery, but the disadvantage is the increased risk of thromboembolic disease. Until the advent of blood transfusion, haemorrhage was a much more important cause of maternal mortality than was thromboembolic disease, and it is therefore likely that hypercoagulability offered an evolutionary advantage.

Compared with the changes in coagulation and fibrinolysis, platelet changes are small. The platelet count falls only slightly but there is an increased aggregability, probably in relation to prostaglandin changes **(Fig. 26.4)**.

Renal system

Renal blood flow and glomerular filtration rate (GFR) increase by about 60% from early in the first trimester to around 4 weeks postpartum. This causes a fall in plasma creatinine from around 73 to 47 mmol/l and urea from 4.3 to around 3.1 mmol/l. It is important to be aware of this fact when assessing renal function, as values that would appear normal pre-pregnancy may in fact indicate impairment in the pregnancy state. The increased GFR is not matched by increased tubular reabsorption and there would therefore be a tendency to lose sodium were it not for a compensatory increase in aldosterone levels. Glycosuria is common because the filtered load of glucose is greater than the tubular reabsorption capacity. Although glycosuria is often normal in pregnancy, it may still be pathological – evidence of gestational diabetes.

Dilatation of the renal pelvis and ureters is caused by both progesterone and local obstruction by the gravid uterus. It occurs from early in the first trimester and results in urinary stasis, which increases the likelihood of urinary tract infection; this may be further exacerbated by the presence of glycosuria.

Endocrine system

Pregnancy influences endocrine functioning in two main ways: placental hormonal production, and by increased protein binding.

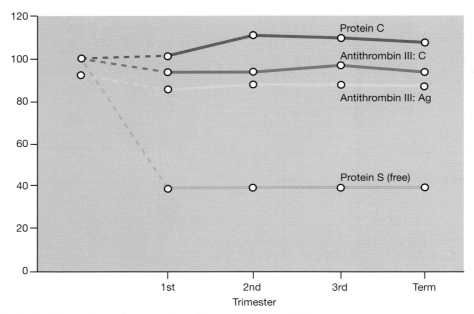

Fig. 26.3 The levels of the anticoagulants antithrombin III and protein S fall in pregnancy.

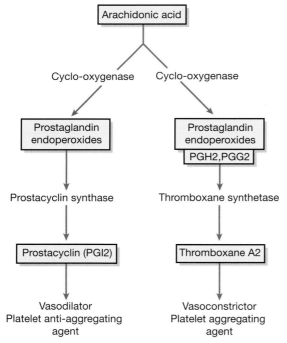

Fig. 26.4 Prostaglandin metabolism. In normal pregnancy there is increased biosynthesis of eicosanoids – particularly prostacyclin (PGI$_2$), a vasodilator with platelet inhibitory properties, and thromboxane A$_2$, a vasoconstrictor with a tendency to stimulate platelet aggregation. As both usually increase in proportion to each other, there is a net neutralization and homeostasis is maintained. This homeostasis is disrupted in pre-eclampsia because of a relative deficiency in prostacyclin owing to either a decrease in its synthesis and/or an increase in the production of thromboxane A$_2$. This imbalance leads to vasoconstriction, hypertension, and platelet stimulation.

Placental hormonal production

The placenta produces a number of hormones, including oestrogen, progesterone (which relaxes smooth muscle), human placental lactogen (which increases maternal glucose and lipids), and human chorionic gonadotrophin (which prevents disintegration of the corpus luteum in early pregnancy) **(Table 26.3)**. The placenta also produces corticotrophin-releasing hormone, which in turn stimulates maternal production of ACTH leading to increased aldosterone and cortisol, which in turn contribute to the maternal fluid changes described above.

Thyroid function

In pregnancy there is increased iodine uptake activity and the total serum levels of T$_3$ and T$_4$ are also raised. Only the unbound portion of thyroxine is metabolically active, however, and as oestrogens also induce synthesis of thyroid-binding globulin, the levels of free T$_3$ and T$_4$ remain within the normal range or may even fall slightly.

Pituitary function

Oestrogen stimulates the release of thyrotrophin-releasing hormone, which in turn increases prolactin production by the anterior pituitary. Prolactin stimulates breast growth antenatally, but lactation is inhibited by progesterone until after delivery of the placenta, when the prolactin acts with oxytocin from the posterior pituitary to stimulate milk production. Pituitary prolactin production is increased to such an extent in pregnancy (around 10 times the pre-pregnancy level) that the pituitary increases in size by around 135%.

Table 26.3	
Roles of selected placental hormones	
Hormone	**Role**
Human chorionic gonadotrophin (hCG)	Initially maintains the corpus luteum's secretion of progesterone and oestrogen; later it may have a role in regulating placental oestrogen secretion and in modulating the maternal immune response
Oestrogen	Over 90% is in the form of oestriol; it is involved in uterine growth, cervical changes, and breast development
Progesterone	Smooth muscle relaxation, acting on the uterus, gastrointestinal tract and ureters. Also has a role in regulating maternal physiological changes
Human placental lactogen (hPL)	Mobilizes maternal free fatty acids, improving glucose availability for the fetus

Gastrointestinal system

There is a general reduction in gut motility and a slowing of transit times. This may benefit the fetus by increasing the absorption of certain nutrients. Delayed gastric emptying and gastric relaxation are a feature of pregnancy, especially with highly osmotic foods (e.g. glucose), and are particularly marked in labour. This altered state becomes clinically important if the woman requires a general anaesthetic, because of the risk of aspiration pneumonia (Mendelson's syndrome – history box), and acid-reduction medications are therefore routinely prescribed prior to caesarean section.

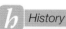 *History*

Mendelson's syndrome describes chemical pneumonia caused by aspiration during anaesthesia, especially during pregnancy. It is named after Curtis Lester Mendelson (b. 1913), an American obstetrician, who gave up his New York Professor's career aged 46 for life on the tiny West Indian Abaco islands.

Nausea and vomiting are common in early pregnancy. It is not clear whether they are caused by rising human chorionic gonadotrophin (hCG) or oestrogen or some other factor; management is discussed further on page 245. Most pregnant women report increased appetite and thirst, and many have cravings for, or aversions to, certain foods. Perhaps the most common aversions are to tea and coffee. Pica, a craving for non-food substances such as coal, chalk or soap, is rare but well known. The cause is unknown.

Gastric acid secretion is reduced in pregnancy, which is presumably the reason why peptic ulcer disease commonly improves. In contrast, reflux oesophagitis is likely to be more severe, and results from a combination of reduced tone in the lower oesophageal sphincter and increased intra-abdominal pressure.

Many women report constipation in pregnancy and this is usually attributed to the relaxing effect of progesterone on gut smooth muscle. There is, however, little good evidence that constipation really is more common in pregnancy. If it occurs it should be managed, as in the non-pregnant state, with increased dietary fibre and stool-bulking agents.

Rectal haemorrhoids probably result from a combination of increased straining and increased intra-abdominal pressure, and as part of the generalized vasodilatation mentioned above.

Liver and bile ducts

Normal pregnancy is a mildly 'cholestatic' state. Biochemical tests of liver function, however, lie within the normal range, with the exception of alkaline phosphatase levels, which are approximately doubled. Most of this increase comes from placental secretion of this enzyme rather than from the liver. Pathological cholestasis is discussed on page 259.

Oestrogen increases the serum cholesterol and this is translated into bile salt production, which supersaturates the bile. Since progesterone also reduces gall bladder emptying, pregnancy predisposes to gallstone formation.

Skin and appendages

The skin participates in the generalized increase of blood flow in pregnancy. Increased pigmentation is also seen in the nipples and in the midline of the abdomen (linea nigra), as a result of placental melanocyte-stimulating hormone production. Striae gravidarum, or stretch marks, occur in the presence of high oestrogen levels, in skin subject to stretching, such as that over the breasts and abdomen. Initially reddish/purple, they fade after delivery to a faint silvery colour. There is no effective prevention or treatment.

The cycle of hair growth is altered in pregnancy, with a greater proportion (95% vs 85%) of hairs in the actively growing phase. As a result there are many over-aged hairs at the end of pregnancy, which fall out and lead to the common symptom of hair coming out 'in handfuls' postnatally. This change is temporary.

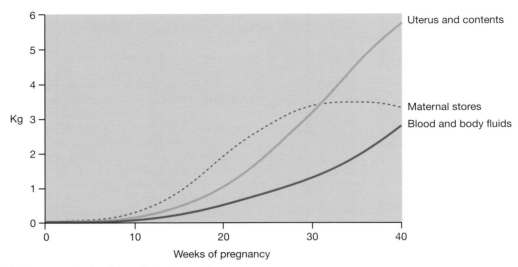

Fig. 26.5 Components of weight gained in normal pregnancy.

Metabolic changes

Extra energy is required not only for the developing fetus but also to fuel the increase in maternal physiological parameters. The resting metabolic rate is increased by around 20% and weight increases on average by around 12 kg **(Fig. 26.5)**. Initially there is an increased sensitivity to insulin, which leads to increased glycogen synthesis, increased fat deposition and an increase in amino acid transfer into cells. After mid-pregnancy there is a degree of insulin resistance. The serum glucose level at this stage may therefore rise, a change presumably in the fetal interest as fetal glucose levels will also rise. The insulin resistance also leads to increased levels of serum lipids which can be used by the mother as an alternative energy source to glucose. Although maternal amino acid levels fall, there is increased transport across the placenta.

Pregnancy is a diabetogenic state. Cortisol, progesterone, oestrogen and human placental lactogen are all insulin antagonists, and tend to increase the glucose level. If the pancreatic islet β-cells are unable to produce sufficient insulin to balance this increase, or if there is maternal insulin resistance, the maternal glucose level may rise pathologically **(Fig. 26.6)**. This is discussed further on page 254.

Calcium homeostasis

Fetal skeletal development requires 20–30 g of calcium, and this need is met by increasing maternal intestinal absorption. There is usually, therefore, no maternal bone demineralization. Calcium transfer across the placenta is an active process occurring against a concentration gradient and it is therefore not surprising that maternal free calcium levels are not significantly changed. Serum protein and albumin fall as part of the plasma dilution of pregnancy so that total calcium is reduced.

Placental transfer

The placenta provides a functional and immunological barrier and is an organ of:

- respiration
- nutrient transfer, also providing the mechanism for waste excretion
- hormonal synthesis.

The mechanisms of transfer across the placenta are outlined in **Table 26.4**. The nuclei and other intracellular organelles in the syncytiotrophoblast come to lie in groups to form areas of thick metabolically active tissue which are probably the sites of active diffusion. Between them are other areas with only a very fine layer separating maternal and fetal blood, the vasculosyncytial membrane, and these are where most passive gas transfer occurs.

Respiration

The following changes maintain the diffusion gradient:

1. The high O_2 affinity of fetal haemoglobin. The dissociation curve of fetal haemoglobin is shifted to the left so that at a given PO_2 the percentage saturation is higher than for adult haemoglobin **(Box 26.2)**. More importantly for the fetal interest, at a given level of oxygen transfer the PO_2 will be lower (see **Fig. 26.7**).
2. The high fetal Hb (normal 14–20 g/dl) also results in a lower PO_2 for a given saturation.
3. Finally, the passage of CO_2 from fetus to mother helps increase maternal oxygen dissociation and fetal association. This shift of the maternal oxygen dissociation curve to the right caused by CO_2 accumulation is called the Bohr effect **(Fig. 26.7)**.

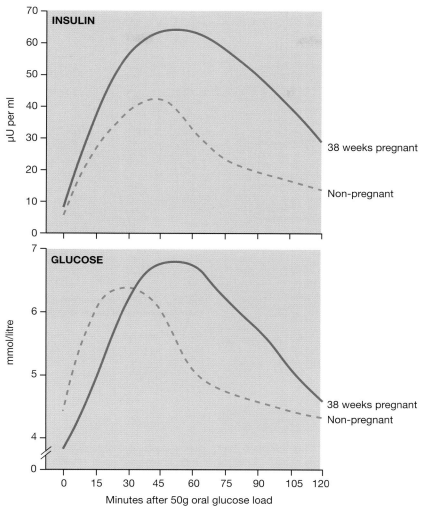

Fig. 26.6 The patterns of change of insulin and plasma glucose following a 50 g oral glucose load in the non-pregnant woman compared to late pregnancy.

Table 26.4	
Some examples of the mechanism of placental transfer	
Mechanism	**Substance**
Passive diffusion	CO_2, O_2, water
Facilitated diffusion	Glucose (by a carrier molecule)
Active transport by enzymatic action	Amino acids, Ca, Fe, vitamins B and C, free fatty acid
Organelle transport by pinocytosis	IgG

The CO_2 dissociation curves are similar in fetal and maternal blood. Although most CO_2 is carried as bicarbonate, bicarbonate is a charged molecule and cannot cross the placenta. Only dissolved CO_2 can cross the placenta, and this is again by diffusion. This transfer is facilitated by maternal hyperventilation, which lowers maternal PCO_2, and lower fetal concentrations of carbonic anhydrase, which slows the establishment of equilibrium between CO_2 and HCO_3^-. Furthermore, as maternal Hb gives up oxygen, its CO_2 affinity increases (the Haldane effect), and the opposite (reverse Haldane effect) decreases CO_2 affinity of fetal haemoglobin as it in turn takes up oxygen.

Nutrition

The developing fetus requires energy, largely provided by glucose, amino acids and fatty acids. These are mostly transported across the placental membrane by active processes as outlined in **Table 26.4**. In later pregnancy, excessive glucose is converted into glycogen and fat, such that by term, 15% of the body weight is fat. In preterm babies and those with in-utero growth restriction, these energy stores are lower.

Box 26.2

Maternofetal oxygen equilibrium

Consider the hypothetical situation of the fetomaternal circulation at oxygen equilibrium with a PO_2 of 4 kPa (30 mmHg), maternal Hb 11 g/dl and fetal Hb 17 g/dl. Maternal haemoglobin will be 60% saturated and fetal 80% saturated. Each gram of fully saturated haemoglobin carries 1.38 ml of oxygen. Maternal oxygen carriage (saturation × haemoglobin concentration × 1.38) is thus $0.6 \times 11 \times 1.38 = 9.1$ ml/dl, while fetal oxygen carriage is $0.8 \times 17 \times 1.38 = 18.8$ ml/dl. The oxygen molecules would therefore equilibrate in a ratio of 2:1 in favour of the fetal circulation. In practice, although equilibrium may be reached locally on either side of the vasculosyncytial membrane, it is not achieved overall. Firstly there is functional shunting in both circulations, and secondly the fetal PO_2 remains well below maternal levels because of local oxygen consumption by the placenta. This is to the fetal advantage since a high PO_2 would stimulate premature closure of the ductus arteriosus. During fetal life the ductus arteriosus connects the pulmonary artery to the aortic arch, allowing most of the blood from the right ventricle to bypass the fetal lungs.

The final result of all this is that even though the PO_2 is much lower in the fetus, the O_2 content of fetal blood is higher than in the mother's blood. Fetal umbilical venous blood (Hb 17 g/dl) at a PO_2 of 4 kPa (30 mmHg) will be 75% saturated and carry $0.75 \times 17 \times 1.38 = 17.5$ ml/dl of oxygen. Maternal uterine venous blood (Hb 11 g/dl), even at a higher PO_2 of 5.3 kPa (40 mmHg), will be only 70% saturated and carry $0.7 \times 11 \times 1.38 = 10.6$ ml/dl.

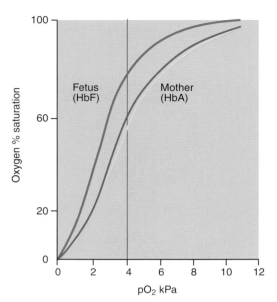

Fig. 26.7 Fetal haemoglobin has a higher affinity for O_2 than does maternal haemoglobin. The dissociation curve of fetal haemoglobin (blue) is shifted to the left so that at a given PO_2 the percentage saturation is higher than for adult haemoglobin. More importantly for the fetal interest, at a given level of oxygen transfer the PO_2 will be lower. As CO_2 passes from the fetus to the mother, so the maternal dissociation curve shifts to the right (red curve to yellow curve). This is the Bohr effect.

Immunology

Most human cells have a gene on chromosome 6 that codes for a particular protein called the human leucocyte antigen or 'HLA'. Each of us has a unique HLA gene and the protein synthesized from this gene coats the surface of all the cells in our body, allowing our immune cells to recognize 'self' cells. If leucocytes identify a 'non-self' code, they initiate a process of cell destruction. The fetus is genetically unique and will have a different HLA complement from that of either parent. If a skin graft is taken from a child and grafted onto its mother, the graft will be rejected. Yet while the fetus is 'grafted' onto the lining of the maternal uterus, it is not rejected. There must therefore be some protective mechanism, or mechanisms, to prevent immunological fetal rejection.

HLA has different subtypes. The classical genes, HLA-A, -B and -C, provide the highly individual molecules coding for 'self', and these molecules are absent on many of the placental cells. This would render these placental cells less susceptible to maternal leucocyte recognition and therefore less liable to destruction. Some immunological reaction, however, may be important to prevent placental over-invasion, and some placental cells do express the classical genes, particularly HLA-C. Further modulation of this uneasy fetomaternal immune relationship may be modified by another HLA molecule, HLA-G, specific only to placental tissue. Much more work is required before these mechanisms are understood more clearly, particularly as it is becoming apparent that immunological disparity may lie behind recurrent miscarriage, fetal growth restriction, and pre-eclampsia.

Summary

Women who are pregnant overbreathe, retain fluid and calories, and increase the perfusion of most organs. In the process, many blood parameters change, and there may be anaemia, glycosuria, constipation and cholestasis. Nevertheless, most of the changes are, directly or indirectly, in the fetal interest. Minor symptoms, and blood values outside the normal non-pregnant range, do not necessarily require treatment. Other than reassurance and correct interpretation.

Key points

- Pregnancy exerts profound physiological changes on a mother's body in virtually every organ system.
- The ventilation rate increases by 40%. The alveolar ventilation rate increases, and there is a fall in the physiological dead space. These changes in respiratory function provide additional oxygen for the developing fetoplacental unit, and for the mother's additional requirements.
- Cardiac output increases during pregnancy by approximately 40% through increases in both stroke volume and heart rate. Blood pressure falls in early pregnancy but by late pregnancy it returns to normal again or may even be slightly raised.
- The red cell mass increases by 25%, but a 40% increase in circulating plasma volume leads to a dilutional fall in haemoglobin concentration and the haematocrit. A policy of routine iron supplementation for healthy women with singleton pregnancies is not appropriate, but supplementation is useful in the presence of iron-deficiency anaemia.
- Progesterone concentrations rise in pregnancy and have effects in many parts of the body. They can cause constipation, delayed gastric emptying, reflux oesophagitis, urinary frequency and urinary stasis, and have the effect of exacerbating varicose veins. Some women may develop impaired glucose tolerance in pregnancy.

27 Strategies to improve global maternal and neonatal health

Estimates of global maternal and neonatal mortality

It is estimated that 536,000 women worldwide die each year from the complications of pregnancy and childbirth, with 99% of these occurring in developing countries – that is one every minute. Just over half of all maternal deaths occur in the sub-Saharan Africa region alone (270,000), followed next by South Asia (188,000). It has also been estimated that for every one woman who dies, around 20 women have serious ill-health and lifelong disability as a result of these same complications.

One of the eight Millennium Development Goals (MDGs) adopted in 2000 following the Millennium Summit is MDG 5, which sets a target of reducing maternal mortality by 75% between 1990 and 2015. Country estimates of maternal mortality are therefore needed to inform planning of health programmes. As many of these deaths occur in resource-poor countries, or in countries where there is no system of birth and death registration, the numbers are by necessity only approximate. Nonetheless, a methodology has been developed by the World Health Organization (WHO), the United Nations Children's Fund (UNICEF), the United Nations Population Fund (UNFPA), the World Bank, and the United Population Division (UNPD) to calculate country, regional and global estimates. These are expressed either as a maternal mortality ratio, or as maternal mortality rates, or sometimes as 'the lifetime risk of dying' (which also takes the fertility rate into account) **(Table 27.1)**.

At least 80% of all maternal deaths in Africa and Asia are probably from direct obstetric causes, and result from five complications that are well understood and can be readily treated: haemorrhage, sepsis, eclampsia, obstructed labour and complications of abortion **(Figs 27.1** and **27.2)**. We know how to prevent these deaths – there are relatively inexpensive and effective interventions.

Other conditions are sometimes documented as indirect causes of maternal death, for example severe anaemia (with or without additional haemorrhage) leading to cardiac failure, or sepsis post caesarean section in an HIV-positive patient.

In addition to this high number of maternal deaths, an estimated 4 million neonatal deaths also occur each year; this accounts for almost 40% of all deaths under 5 years **(Fig. 27.3)**. The health of the neonate is closely related to that of the mother, and the majority of deaths in the first month of life could also be prevented if interventions were in place to ensure good maternal health: birth injuries, birth asphyxia and most neonatal tetanus could be prevented with skilled professional conduct of the delivery. Similarly, many cases of sepsis in the neonate are directly linked to the health of the mother and/or the care she received during childbirth.

Obstetric causes of maternal mortality

The five main obstetric causes of direct maternal mortality are discussed here.

Haemorrhage

Haemorrhage is probably the cause of the majority of maternal deaths in resource-poor areas. This may be because of antepartum bleeding (e.g. abruption of the placenta), bleeding during delivery (e.g. with a ruptured uterus) or postpartum (e.g. from an atonic uterus or retained placenta).

The risk of dying from haemorrhage is higher if women are already anaemic in pregnancy (Hb <11.0 g/dl). Oxytocics are effective in preventing postpartum haemorrhage (active management of the third stage), as well as in treating uterine atony, but such oxytocics may not be routinely used

Table 27.1

Estimates of maternal mortality rate, annual number of maternal deaths, and lifetime risk of maternal death by United Nations MDG region for 2005 (2007 report)

Region	Maternal mortality rate (deaths per 100,000 live births)	Annual number of maternal deaths	Lifetime risk of maternal death
Africa	820	276,000	1:26
Oceania	430	1000	1:62
Asia	330	241,000	1:120
Latin America and Caribbean	130	15,000	1:290
Countries of the Commonwealth States	51	2000	1:1200
Developed regions	9	1000	1:7300
World total	400	536,000	1:92

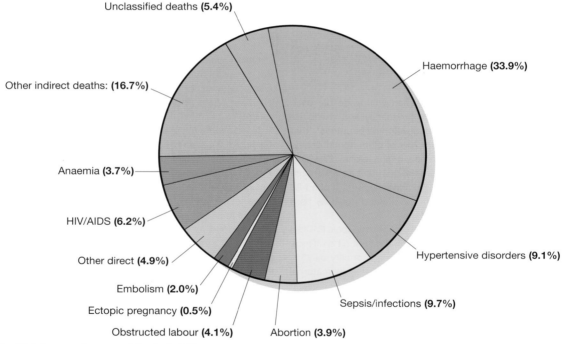

Fig. 27.1 Causes of maternal deaths in Africa.

and/or available. Vaginal and cervical tears can be surgically repaired if materials, instruments and skilled staff are available. The ability to give intravenous fluids, safe blood transfusion and anaesthesia is extremely important when pregnancy or delivery is complicated by haemorrhage. It is estimated that non-availability of blood for transfusion accounts for about a quarter of these haemorrhage deaths.

Obstructed labour

The most common cause of maternal death from obstructed labour is attributable to true cephalopelvic disproportion, though malpresentation is also important (**Figs 27.4** and **27.5**). Sometimes labour is not 'obstructed' per se but there is failure of adequate uterine contractions. In those with a longitudinal lie, timely intervention with appropriate oxytocic therapy can improve uterine contractions and allow a vaginal delivery. The correct use of a simple accurately documented partogram, with an 'action line' to prompt a response if labour does not progress normally, has been shown to be very helpful in making the diagnosis of obstruction (**Fig. 27.6**).

In many cases women are referred to a health facility late and only after prolonged labour (more than 12 hours). The presenting part may be deeply impacted in the pelvis and a vaginal examination may demonstrate gross fetal caput and

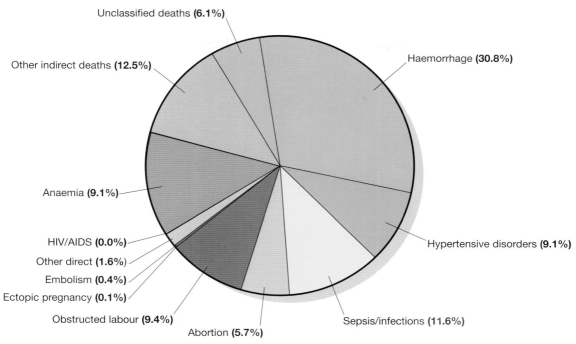

Fig. 27.2 Causes of maternal deaths in Asia.

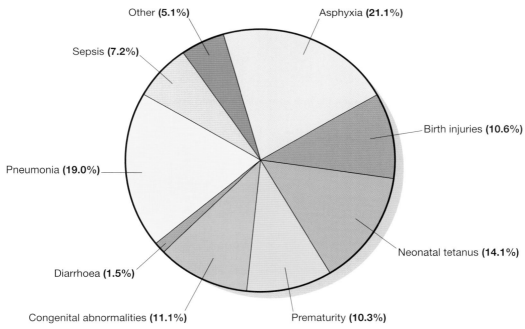

Fig. 27.3 Causes of neonatal mortality.

moulding; there are also associations with the mother being short, malnourished, pyrexial, dehydrated and exhausted. She may be in severe pain from a tonically contracted uterus, or there may be pain, bleeding and shock from a uterine rupture. With a ruptured uterus the fetal heartbeat is usually absent and the fetal parts can often be palpated easily abdominally.

Management depends on whether the baby is alive or dead: if alive, a caesarean section should be performed; if dead, a craniotomy or other destructive procedure may be

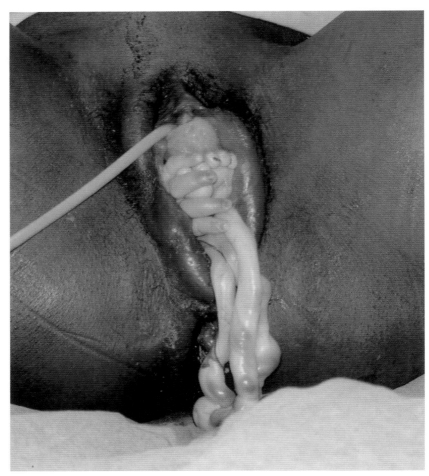

Fig. 27.4 Obstructed labour from a transverse lie, with an arm, leg and cord prolapse.

more appropriate. If uterine rupture is suspected, a laparotomy will be required; a repair may be possible, but it is often necessary to carry out a hysterectomy.

If the presenting part has been impacted in the pelvis for many hours, pressure necrosis of the genital tract, as it is compressed between the baby's head and the bony pelvis, may lead to obstetric fistulae. Vesicovaginal fistulae are the most common, but rectovaginal and ureterovaginal fistulae also occur. Such fistulae may also occur after difficult obstetric abdominal surgery. Women who suffer from fistulae often become outcasts from their society, and may live in poverty; very many are unable to access suitable care.

In order to try to prevent fistulae, or to encourage small fistulae to close spontaneously, it is important that all women who have survived prolonged or obstructed labour (with or without a caesarean section) should be treated initially by continuous bladder drainage and preferably with antibiotics to minimize the risk of urinary tract infection. Spontaneous closure can occur within 6–8 weeks of this conservative management, but many fistulae do not heal spontaneously and require specialized surgical management. Such

surgery requires considerable expertise and many specialists (obstetricians, gynaecologists and urologists) will need to seek additional training to be able to offer a good surgical repair. Equally important is the provision of good nursing care, physiotherapy and steps towards reintegration into their society.

Sepsis

Bacterial genital tract sepsis following prolonged membrane rupture or retained products of conception may lead to overwhelming septic shock, multisystem failure and death. Early antibiotic treatment is important, and forms part of the EOC package. If there are retained products of conception, e.g. after an incomplete miscarriage or an unsafe abortion, manual vacuum aspiration (MVA) of retained products of conception can be life-saving **(Fig. 27.7)**. This has, in many countries, replaced the traditional technique of dilatation and curettage (D&C), which requires general anaesthesia: using good technique, MVA can be performed in early pregnancy under local anaesthesia.

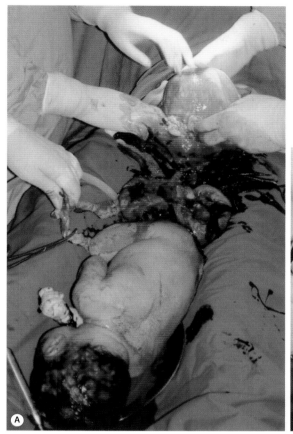
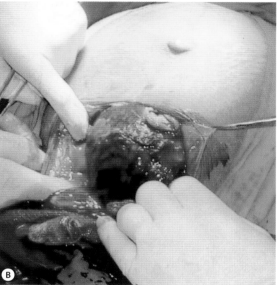

Fig. 27.5 Uterine rupture following obstructed labour with cephalopelvic disproportion.

Unrecognized rupture of the membranes during pregnancy risks ascending infection and this can lead to chorioamnionitis, premature delivery and major systemic sepsis. Prophylactic antibiotics, therefore, must always be given after prolonged membrane rupture or after caesarean section.

Untreated sexually transmitted infections (STIs) are common during pregnancy in resource-poor countries and may contribute to sepsis. Similarly, underlying impairment of the overall immune response, for example with HIV infection, carries an increased risk of opportunistic infections and also makes it more difficult to treat sepsis when it occurs.

Eclampsia

Eclampsia, especially if a fit is prolonged, can lead directly to maternal death. As the hypertensive disorders of pregnancy affect many systems, however, the exact cause of a death can often be difficult to ascertain. Cerebral haemorrhage is probably the most common, but renal or hepatic failure, respiratory failure, coagulopathy or HELLP syndrome may also contribute (page 296).

Recognition of pre-eclampsia by measurement of blood pressure and testing of urine for protein should be available for all women during pregnancy and after delivery. Once recognized, magnesium sulphate reduces the incidence of seizures in women with severe pre-eclampsia and is the preferred treatment drug for an eclamptic fit. The only real treatment for pre-eclampsia and eclampsia, however, is delivery; this obviously requires the means to induce labour, or to deliver by operative means. Adequate drug control of the blood pressure is important to prevent cerebral accidents, and good monitoring in a high-dependency area of the ward of such a sick woman is very useful in preventing and treating further complications.

Unsafe abortion

As abortion is illegal in many countries, such as in most of Africa, Latin America, the Middle East and many Asian countries, attempts at abortion are often carried out by unskilled practitioners outwith any recognized medical resource. Unsafe abortion may lead directly to maternal death through uterine perforation, sepsis and haemorrhage, and

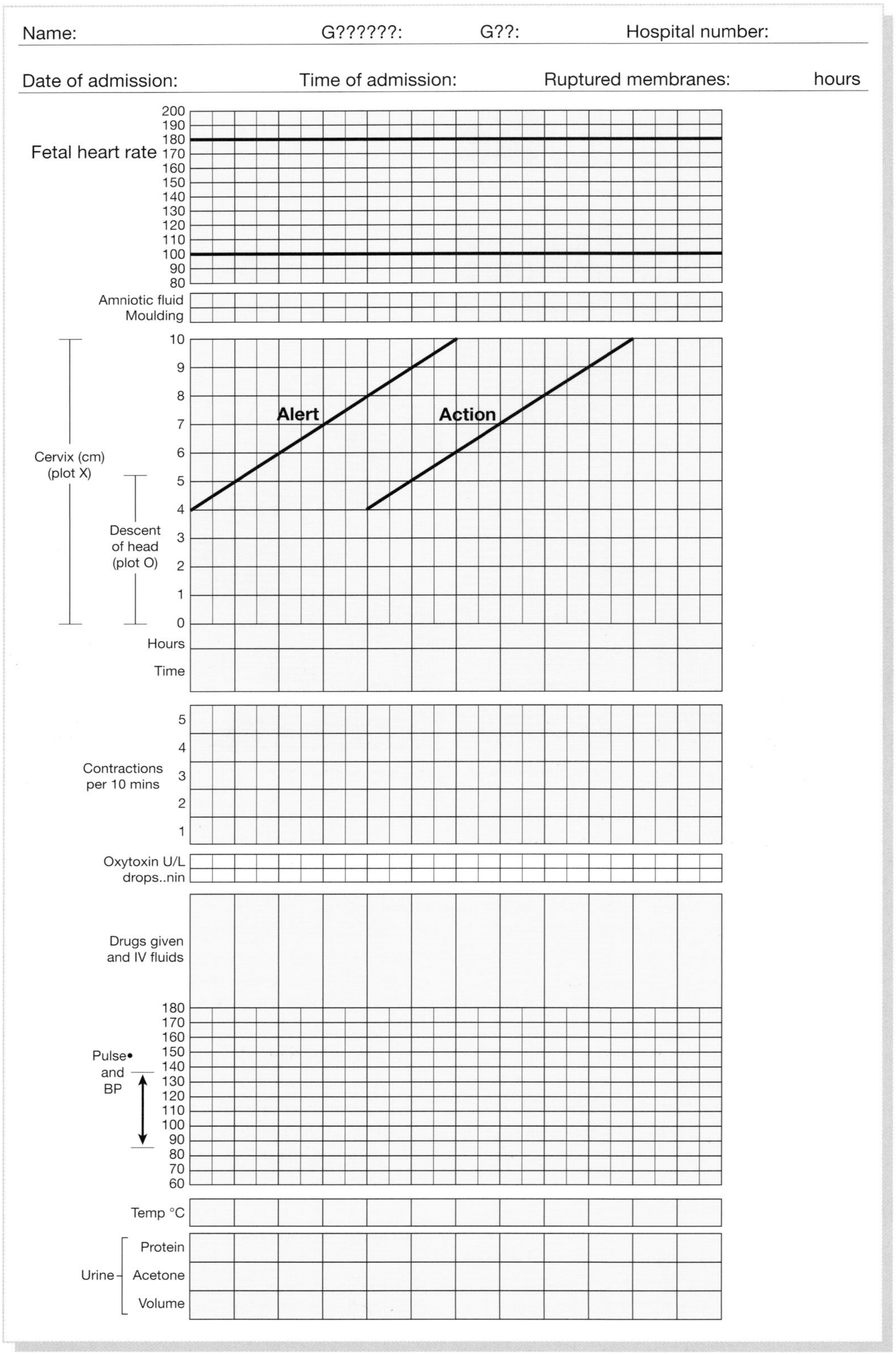

Fig. 27.6 WHO modified partogram. The 'alert' and 'action' lines can be used to prompt referral or intervention if delay in progress of labour is apparent.

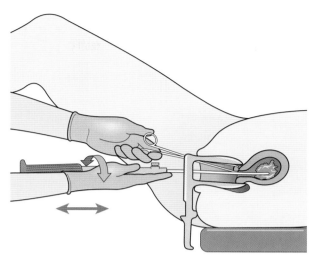

Fig. 27.7 Manual vacuum aspiration (MVA).

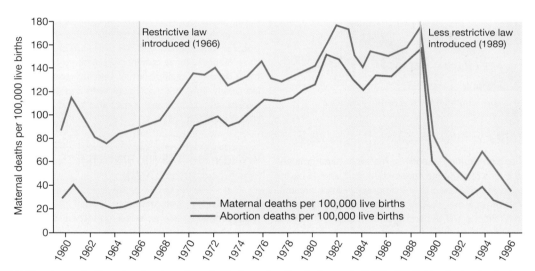

Fig. 27.8 The change in the rate of maternal mortality from abortion in Romania (1960–1996). Unsafe abortion is also strongly linked to the non-availability of contraception.

is clearly associated with the non-availability of abortion services **(Fig. 27.8)**.

Unsafe abortion is also strongly linked to the non-availability of contraception **(Fig. 27.9)**. Many women do not have access to a full range of contraceptives and in some instances they may not be able to use contraceptives without permission from their husbands and/or family in law.

Medical conditions contributing to maternal mortality and morbidity

In addition to the main obstetric cause of death, there are often underlying endemic medical conditions which exacerbate risks.

Anaemia

It has been estimated that over half the pregnant women in the world have a haemoglobin level indicative of anaemia. This is usually a chronic anaemia and the mother is frequently asymptomatic at rest, but she may decompensate easily in labour and, in the event of an obstetric haemorrhage, she is much more likely to die.

Relatively few studies have comprehensively assessed the aetiological factors responsible for anaemia in pregnancy, but it is likely that there are multiple factors, which will vary between geographical areas and by season. These factors include malaria, micronutrient deficiency (iron, vitamin A), parasitic infestation, recurrent bleeding in pregnancy, chronic infections and infection with HIV.

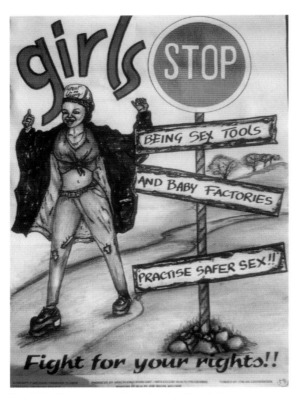

Fig. 27.9 Many women have few fertility choices.

Malaria

As well as contributing directly to maternal death, malaria is also a cause of maternal anaemia. Malaria should be the first diagnosis considered in any pregnant woman presenting with fever in a malaria-prone area. The symptoms and any complications will depend on the intensity of malaria transmission and the level of acquired immunity (higher immunity in areas of moderate or high transmission). Pregnant women with severe malaria are particularly prone to hypoglycaemia, pulmonary oedema, anaemia and coma.

A thick (blood) film will help detect the parasite, and a thin film will identify the species. Of the four types of human malaria, *Plasmodium vivax* and *P. falciparum* are the most common and *P. falciparum* is the most lethal. If facilities for testing are not available, empirical treatment should be commenced. Treatment depends on the sensitivity profile of the local species. In countries where malaria is common, all pregnant women are recommended routine prophylaxis during pregnancy.

HIV/AIDS

Worldwide, about 40 million people are living with HIV infection and about half of all affected adults are female. Those with AIDS have an increased susceptibility to infective conditions and are therefore at higher risk of maternal mortality.

Mother-to-child transmission has been by far the most important cause of infection in the estimated 5 million HIV-positive children. Pregnant women should be offered screening for HIV early in pregnancy because appropriate antenatal interventions are needed both to treat the mother and to reduce maternal-to-child transmission of HIV infection. This includes antiretroviral therapy (ARV), a caesarean section and avoidance of breastfeeding where indicated. Choice and type of ARV is dependent on viral load and CD4 count; it is also very important to recognize and treat opportunistic infections, including STIs, tuberculosis and *Pneumocystis carinii*.

In many countries, being HIV positive carries a very significant 'stigma' and many women (and men) do not undergo testing. Antiretroviral therapy is also far from widely available in many countries.

Tuberculosis (TB)

TB is the biggest killer of young people and adults in the world today: it kills more women than all causes of maternal mortality put together. It is also the leading cause of death in those affected by HIV/AIDS. One-third of the world population is infected with TB, although only 10% of these have disease, most commonly pulmonary disease. Treatment involves multiple drug therapy, usually rifampicin, isoniazid, ethambutol, pyrazinamide and streptomycin (all except streptomycin are considered safe in pregnancy and with breastfeeding).

Requirements for maternal and newborn health

There are two key strategies that, if implemented, will reduce maternal and neonatal mortality and morbidity:

- the provision of skilled birth attendance (SBA)
- the availability of essential (or emergency) obstetric care (EOC) and newborn care (NC).

Skilled birth attendance

A skilled birth attendant (SBA) is someone with the midwifery skills necessary to manage normal deliveries and diagnose, stabilize, and refer obstetric complications. Skilled birth attendance means the availability of a skilled birth attendant plus the enabling environment, i.e. the necessary drugs, equipment, transport system and supportive health-care system in which the skilled birth attendant works. For each country, the higher the percentage of women who have a skilled birth attendant at delivery, the lower the maternal mortality ratio in that country **(Fig. 27.10)**.

Two-thirds of women in the least developed countries deliver without the help of a skilled birth attendant. While many of 'traditional birth attendants' are very capable, they are limited in their ability to act appropriately in emergency

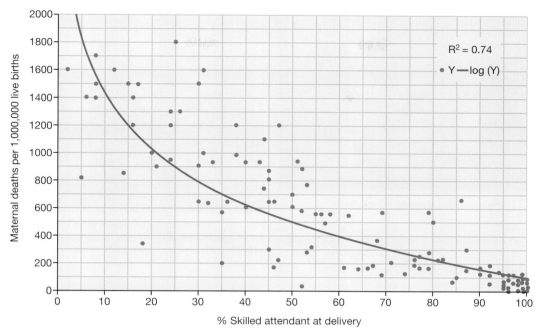

Fig. 27.10 The availability of a skilled birth attendant is strongly associated with a lower maternal death rate.

situations and may use therapies that are not likely to be helpful. A few illustrative examples are outlined below:

During the antenatal period, dangerous herbal medicines and potions may be administered, e.g. some have oxytocic properties.

- Some essential foods are withheld because of nutritional taboos.
- During labour, the abdomen may be massaged in a certain way to change the position of the fetus.
- In obstructed labour, the abdomen may be pressed hard or forcefully massaged to aid the delivery of the baby. This is harmful and can lead to uterine rupture. In some societies obstructed labour is even considered to be a punishment for marital infidelity.
- Postpartum haemorrhage is sometimes seen as cleansing the woman of 'bad blood' and may therefore not be considered dangerous.
- Maternal and fetal illness is at times attributed to evil spirits or bad omens, thereby delaying or preventing proper medical attention.

Essential (emergency) obstetric care

To reduce maternal mortality, it is important that all women have access to emergency (or essential) obstetric care (EOC) when an obstetric complication occurs. There is unified agreement on two levels of this care **(Box 27.1)**: basic emergency obstetric care (BEOC) and comprehensive emergency obstetric care (CEOC). The UN agencies recommend that at least four BEOC facilities and one CEOC facility should be

---

Box 27.1

Levels of emergency obstetric care

Basic emergency obstetric care (BEOC)

- Parenteral antibiotics to treat sepsis
- Parenteral oxytocics to treat haemorrhage
- Parenteral anticonvulsants to treat (pre-) eclampsia
- Manual removal of a retained placenta
- Removal of retained products of conception by manual vacuum aspiration (MVA)
- Assisted vaginal delivery (vacuum extraction, forceps)

Comprehensive emergency obstetric care (CEOC)

All six BEOC functions, plus:
- Obstetric surgery
- Blood transfusion

---

available for a population of 500,000. In many countries this minimum level of coverage is not available.

Magnesium sulphate is relatively inexpensive, but it may simply not be available or local clinicians may not be familiar with its use. Cheaper broad-spectrum oral antibiotics are generally available, but intravenous antibiotics and other more expensive preparations (which may be needed for drug-resistant strains) may not be available in remote locations; also, when doctors are not around, the nurse/midwife may not be licensed to give even a starting dose of parenteral antibiotics.

Manual vacuum aspiration can be easily carried out with a manually operated hand-pump, but this needs to be purchased, the device maintained, and sufficient numbers of healthcare providers need to be trained in its use.

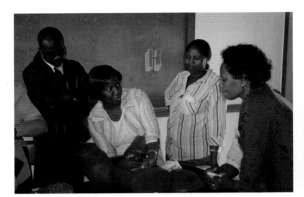

Fig. 27.11 Obstetric skills training in Swaziland.

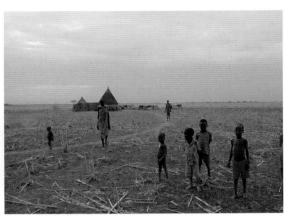

Fig. 27.12 The obstacles to providing an infrastructure for emergency obstetric care to this remote area of Sudan, especially after so many years of civil war, are huge.

Blood is almost always in short supply. Often it can be given only if a relative or a friend provides it, or replaces it, and relatives not uncommonly decline no matter how healthy the potential donor may be. It may be possible to purchase blood from a 'private' blood bank; however, since these frequently rely on paid donors, the chance of receiving unscreened blood –with its potential risk of transmission of HIV or hepatitis B – may be high.

In-depth assessments of availability and coverage of EOC have shown that in many cases structures are in place, and equipment and consumables are available, but that staff lack the competency and skills to provide EOC and essential newborn care. Healthcare professionals, as well as health-service managers, have a crucial role in implementing these interventions and ensuring they are accessible to all pregnant women and newborns. The combination of lack of knowledge and of skills is a key reason why many beneficial evidence-based practices are still not used in many resource-poor settings.

As there is often a migration of doctors from the poorer rural parts of many countries to the wealthier cities, and a migration of doctors from under-resourced countries to those countries with greater income potential, there is often sense in focusing training on those most likely to remain resident where the need is greatest **(Fig. 27.11)**. This will often involve training local medical officers and local midwives, or sometimes up-skilling training traditional birth attendants.

The poor performance of health services in under-resourced countries is also often compounded by broken equipment, poor logistical support, and shortages of drugs and equipment. Countries therefore need balanced investment, not only in human resources, but also in infrastructure, drugs, logistics and other supportive services that will enhance the capacity to deliver healthcare **(Figs 27.12 and 27.13)**.

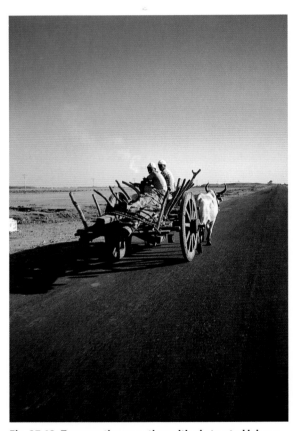

Fig. 27.13 Transporting a mother with obstructed labour to hospital. Bihar, North India.

Challenges of delivering healthcare

In 2007 the global conference 'Women Deliver' in London celebrated 20 years of the Safe Motherhood Initiative. But has progress been made and can the 5th Millennium Development Goal mentioned above (to reduce maternal mortality) actually be achieved? Medically speaking, the answer is yes: we know what is needed and we know what to do in case of complications of pregnancy and childbirth. In particular, we know that the availability of skilled birth attendance and emergency obstetric care, basic neonatal care, and family planning are seen as key: it has been estimated that this would cost about US$3 per person per year. It would, however, require a political will that is unlikely to arise suddenly, especially in those countries which afford women a lesser social status than men.

In 1750, contrasting the rich splendor of the French aristocracy and the desperate poverty of the wider population, the French philosopher Jean-Jacques Rousseau wrote:

'It is obviously contrary to the law of nature ... for a handful of people to gorge themselves on superfluities while the starving multitude lacks necessities.'

The world we live in now is far richer than 18th century France, but, if anything, there is more poverty and more inequality than in the world of Rousseau. Although we live in a world of plenty, a huge number of people on the planet live in conditions of deep poverty and food insecurity. As fortunate members of a wealthy society in a world that contains such need, can we justify the comforts we enjoy? If poverty and radical inequality are unjust, as Rousseau argues they are, then are *we* unjust in supporting a system that affords us such benefits?

The fact that more than a billion people on our planet live in extreme poverty is not simply an unfortunate feature of our world, *it is our problem*. It can be very tempting, as doctors, to focus exclusively on the medical aspects of disease and ignore the much more glaring roots of morbidity and mortality such as this huge wealth inequality.

As a profession we have at least as great a duty to address these issues as we have to find medical cures for medical diseases. Solutions include generous well-directed aid, action against corruption, the encouragement of proper governance, education, and support for both a free press and an independent judiciary. We, as clinicians, must support these goals.

Key points

- Worldwide, approximately 536,000 women die each year from pregnancy- or childbirth-related complications. 99% of these deaths occur in the developing world and most are avoidable.
- The five main causes of direct maternal mortality are haemorrhage, obstructed labour, sepsis, eclampsia and complications of abortion. Indirect causes include severe anaemia, malaria, HIV/AIDS and tuberculosis.
- There are two key strategies that, if implemented, will reduce maternal and neonatal mortality and morbidity—the provision of skilled birth attendance (SBA) and the availability of essential (emergency) obstetric care (EOC).
- Improving maternal health is one of the eight Millennium Development Goals (MDG) adopted by the international community at the UN Millennium Summit in 2000. MDG 5 aims at reducing the maternal mortality ratio (MMR) by three-quarters between 1990 and 2015.
- Between 1990 and 2005, the MMR declined by only 5%. In order to achieve MDG 5, the progress needs to be accelerated.

28

Antenatal care

Introduction

Most pregnancies are uneventful and uncomplicated and would progress normally without medical intervention. There are three main purposes to antenatal care: health promotion, preparation for labour and parenthood, and surveillance of risk. The purpose of the latter is to provide appropriate surveillance for all pregnancies in the hope of identifying the small number that do develop complications, with the aim of optimizing the outcomes for both the mother and her baby.

This should be achieved with as little interference as possible and tailored to a woman's individual risk factors. Care, however, is often based on a traditional arrangement of antenatal visits. The schedule varies, with the initial, or 'booking', visit ideally between 8 and 10 weeks, with subsequent visits often 4-weekly until 30 weeks, 2-weekly until 32 weeks, and then weekly thereafter. While there is ongoing debate about rearranging this care according to evidence-based practice which indicates a less frequent attendance, the incentive for change from parents and care providers is often weak.

In western societies, antenatal care is provided by a variable combination of midwives, obstetricians and family doctors depending on local preferences and resources.

Care may be shared, and may include some hospital visits and some more local visits to other practitioners, allowing the hospital to focus on those who need more intensive input. Some women will receive their antenatal care solely at home.

In the resource–poor countries, many mothers have little or no antenatal care. Access to healthcare is limited by poverty, lack of facilities, lack of education, and cultural resistance.

The booking visit

The purpose of the antenatal booking visit is to detect any risk factors that may indicate the necessity of extra surveillance above that provided to low-risk women. It is also an opportunity to identify any social difficulties and to discuss the parents' own wishes for the pregnancy and delivery.

Past obstetric history

A detailed account of the previous pregnancies and labours should be documented including gestation at delivery and whether the labour was induced or of spontaneous onset. The duration of labour, mode of delivery, birth weight, sex, neonatal outcome and any postnatal complications should also be noted.

Women who have experienced obstetric difficulties in a previous pregnancy are often keen to talk these through and consider the likelihood of recurrence. This is frequently a listening exercise so that anxieties can be expressed, especially in cases of previous fetal or neonatal loss. An explanation followed by discussion of possible recurrence risks and a plan for the next pregnancy is useful.

Medical and surgical history

This should include details of previous operations, particularly gynaecological procedures such as a previous cone biopsy that may predispose to cervical incompetence, and include a history of whether blood transfusions have been received. Questions should be asked about relevant medical disorders such as hypertension, diabetes, heart disease, renal disease, epilepsy, asthma or abnormal thyroid dysfunction.

Family history

The family history should enquire of potential inherited conditions such as thalassaemia, cystic fibrosis, sickle cell anaemia, and also chromosomal disorders and previous congenital structural abnormalities.

History of present pregnancy

The date of the first day of the last menstrual period and details of the menstrual cycle prior to conception should be noted. Correlation with early pregnancy ultrasound dating is important.

Social and drug history

It is essential to note all drugs and medications taken by the mother during the pregnancy as some preparations may be teratogenic. Alcohol, smoking and drug misuse should also be noted and discussed, with referral to appropriate support and/or cessation services. Evidence of socioeconomic deprivation is relevant since women may require additional support during pregnancy. Identification of matters relating to child protection necessitates referral to the social work department.

Examination

A general examination is performed to include measurement of pulse rate, blood pressure, baseline weight and height. Weight and height are measured to assess body mass index (BMI). A BMI >30 indicates the potential for complications. Abdominal examination provides an approximate indication of the uterine size, and may identify abnormal masses and other abnormalities. There is no indication to carry out a routine vaginal examination, although it remains sensible to perform cervical cytology if overdue.

Ultrasound scan

This key investigation establishes fetal viability, gestational age, and excludes or identifies multiple pregnancy. It may also be an opportunity to measure the nuchal translucency (see p. 266) and to diagnose some gross fetal anomalies, e.g. anencephaly.

Urine analysis

The urine is analysed for the presence of protein and glucose.

Booking blood samples

- Full blood count to exclude maternal anaemia and thrombocytopenia (p. 260).
- Blood group to determine the ABO and rhesus status of the mother and to detect the presence of any red cell antibodies (p. 313).
- Rubella status to identify those mothers who are not immune to rubella and are therefore at risk of a primary rubella infection during pregnancy. Such women are offered rubella vaccination after delivery (p. 274).
- Haemoglobin electrophoresis may be offered to all women, or restricted to those of certain ethnic origin, particularly those of Asian, Afro-Caribbean or Mediterranean origin, and will identify those mothers who may be carriers of sickle cell anaemia or thalassaemia.
- Hepatitis B status allows for counselling of the woman and her family together with neonatal vaccination if the result is positive.
- Serological testing for syphilis. Those with positive tests should receive referral to a genitourinary medicine specialist and treatment with penicillin.
- HIV (see p. 234).

Screening discussion

It is essential to use the booking visit to discuss screening options for chromosomal and structural abnormalities. This is often an emotive area and parents should be made aware of the implications of any tests they decide to take or decline.

Antenatal planning

Mothers at the extremes of reproductive age are at increased risk of obstetric complications, particularly hypertensive disorders, and they also carry an increased risk of perinatal mortality.

The incidence of proteinuric pre-eclampsia in a second pregnancy is 10–15 times greater if there was pre-eclampsia in the first pregnancy compared to those with a normal first pregnancy, although pre-eclampsia tends to be less severe in subsequent pregnancies. It has been suggested that low-dose aspirin taken from early pregnancy (<17 weeks and probably from the first trimester) may reduce the incidence of fetal growth restriction or perinatal mortality in those with previous severe disease.

Those who have had a previous instrumental delivery usually have a straightforward delivery next time around, but may occasionally request an elective caesarean section. This is controversial, and careful consideration of the advantages and disadvantages is required. In general, those with a previous caesarean section for a non-recurrent indication, e.g. breech, fetal distress or relative cephalopelvic disproportion secondary to fetal malposition should be offered vaginal birth after caesarean (VBAC), although repeat elective caesarean section may be recommended in certain circumstances. With spontaneous onset of labour, women can be quoted an approximate 70% likelihood of achieving a vaginal birth when undertaking VBAC, with the principal risk of uterine rupture occurring in approximately 1 in 300 attempts at VBAC.

In situations where there has been previous fetal growth restriction or an intrauterine death, subsequent management depends on the cause and the estimated likelihood of recurrence. More intensive antenatal monitoring is usually offered and the outcome is usually good, particularly when the loss was 'unexplained'.

Smoking is associated with low-birth-weight babies, probably related to fetal hypoxaemia and ischaemia from both carbon monoxide and nicotine. Although there is no evidence to support an association with fetal abnormality, long-term follow-up has demonstrated intellectual and emotional impairment. Smoking is also associated with an increased risk of placental abruption, preterm labour, intrauterine fetal demise and sudden infant death syndrome. Alcohol and drug misuse carry significant fetal risks and these should be avoided in pregnancy.

Women whose work environment exposes them to radiation, hazardous gases or specific chemicals should be appropriately counselled. There is no evidence that video display units (VDUs) are harmful, or indeed that work itself is harmful to the mother or fetus. The mother should be advised that she can continue working providing she is not unduly tired. Moderate exercise is likely to be of benefit and should be encouraged, but should probably be avoided if there are significant complications such as hypertension, cardiorespiratory compromise, antepartum haemorrhage or threatened preterm labour.

Antenatal surveillance

Subsequent visits are then used to identify obstetric complications.

Gestational hypertension and pre-eclampsia

The blood pressure and a urinalysis should be checked at every visit, and there should be a low threshold for acting on any abnormalities (see Ch. 34).

Fetal growth restriction (FGR) and small for gestational age (SGA) (see also Ch. 33)

'Small for gestational age' describes the baby whose birth weight is below the centile for a specified gestation, most commonly the 10th centile. The term 'fetal growth restriction' describes 'a fetus which fails to reach its genetic growth potential'. In practice it may be difficult to differentiate the two antenatally, but fetal growth restriction carries a significant risk of antenatal and intrapartum asphyxia, intrauterine death, neonatal hypoglycaemia, long-term neurological impairment and perinatal death. It is therefore important to identify these babies at an early stage to enable more intensive monitoring or delivery.

Screening for small babies is by clinical palpation and objective measurement of symphysis fundal height with a tape measure; this is recognized to identify 40–50% of the babies that are SGA. Ultrasound will identify 25–90% of small babies, depending on the criteria used, but there is currently no evidence to support the routine use of third-trimester ultrasound size measurements in low-risk pregnancies.

Impaired glucose tolerance and diabetes

Some centres offer a glucose tolerance test to women who fulfil certain criteria such as family history of diabetes, previous large-for-gestational-age baby or persistent glycosuria, whilst other centres screen all women by checking random blood sugar measurements. Yet other centres offer a glucose tolerance test to all women. The choice in part depends on the prevalence of the condition in the relevant population, and the significance of the diagnosis is discussed further on page 253.

Haemolytic disease

Maternal IgG antibodies to fetal red cell antigens cross the placenta and may lead to fetal haemolysis, anaemia and hydrops fetalis. Initial sensitization usually occurs at the time of previous delivery, but may also occur with vaginal bleeding at any stage, amniocentesis, external cephalic version or at some unrecognized event (silent fetomaternal transfusion). The most significant antibody is to the rhesus antigen, which rhesus-negative mothers may develop against rhesus-positive fetal cells. All women should be screened for anti-red cell antibodies at booking and again in the third trimester. Those with antibodies require further investigation (p. 313). Rhesus-negative women without sensitization (the vast majority) are routinely recommended to receive two doses of anti-D at 28 and 34 weeks to minimize the risk of sensitization from unrecognized fetomaternal transfusions.

Breech presentation

The incidence of breech presentation is 40% at 20 weeks, 25% at 32 weeks, and 3% at term, with the chance of spontaneous version after 38 weeks being less than 4%. It is associated with multiple pregnancy, bicornuate uterus, fibroids, placenta praevia, polyhydramnios and oligohydramnios. Planned caesarean section at term is associated with less perinatal mortality and less serious neonatal morbidity than is planned vaginal birth, making it important for breech presentation to be identified prior to the onset of labour. This allows the option of external cephalic version, and a more planned delivery.

Breech presentation can be suspected following clinical palpation and confirmed by ultrasound scan. For further management, see page 355.

Anaemia

As there is a physiological fall in haemoglobin (Hb) as pregnancy advances, there is often uncertainty about the value of treating mild anaemia (e.g. Hb 9–10 g/dl). Iron supplements may lead to gastrointestinal side-effects and have no proven benefits in the absence of demonstrable iron deficiency. Most maternity units will recommend oral FeSO4 if the Hb is <10 g/dl or if the mean corpuscular volume (MCV) is low (<80 fl), but it may be worth checking serum folate, vitamin B12 and ferritin before deciding on therapy. Oral iron is well absorbed and the only indication for parenteral iron is when there are concerns regarding compliance or there are prohibitive side-effects with the oral route. Parenteral iron should never be given in thalassaemia.

Polyhydramnios

In the second and third trimesters, liquor is produced by fetal kidneys and is swallowed by the fetus. Excess liquor, polyhydramnios, is suspected by clinical examination – the uterus feels tight fetal parts are difficult to palpate and the symphysis fundal height is above the 90th centile for gestational age. Polyhydramnios is diagnosed with ultrasound and may be described by:

- a single pool >8 cm in depth, and/or
- an amniotic fluid index >90th centile. This is a measurement of the maximum depth of liquor in the four quadrants of the uterus **(Fig. 28.1)**.

Polyhydramnios occurs in 0.5–2% of all pregnancies and is associated with maternal diabetes (~20%) and congenital fetal anomaly (~5%) **(Table 28.1)**.

Even in the absence of an identifiable cause (>60%), polyhydramnios is associated with an increased rate of:

- placental abruption
- malpresentation
- cord prolapse
- carrying a large-for-gestational-age infant
- requiring a caesarean section
- perinatal death.

It is important to arrange a growth and detailed ultrasound scan, glucose tolerance test, and fetal well-being assessment. Antibody titres should be checked to exclude

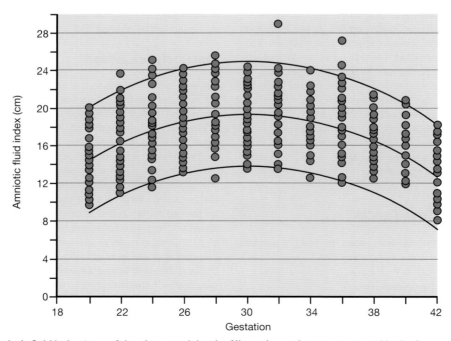

Fig. 28.1 Amniotic fluid index (sum of the ultrasound depth of liquor in centimetres measured in the four quadrants of the uterus) according to gestation.

Table 28.1	
Polyhydramnios	
Cause of polyhydramnios	**Pathology**
Increased production from high urine output	Macrosomia, diabetes, recipient of twin–twin transfusion, hydrops fetalis
Gastrointestinal obstruction	Oesophageal atresia, duodenal atresia, bowel obstruction or Hirschsprung's disease
Poor swallowing because of neuromuscular problems or mechanical obstruction	Anencephaly, myotonic dystrophy, maternal myasthenia, facial tumour, macroglossia or micrognathia

alloimmune haemolytic disease (p. 313). Only rarely does it become necessary to aspirate liquor for maternal comfort. If it is aspirated, it quickly reaccumulates. Increased antenatal fetal surveillance is important, as is an increased awareness of the risks of intrapartum complications. A paediatrician should examine the baby for congenital anomalies, particularly oesophageal atresia or tracheo-oesophageal fistula.

Prolonged pregnancy (>42 weeks)

This is defined as pregnancy beyond 42 weeks' gestation. It occurs in 10% of pregnancies and is associated with an increase in perinatal mortality due to 'unexplained' intrauterine death, intrapartum hypoxia and meconium aspiration syndrome.

Monitoring of post-dates pregnancy

Routinely monitoring pregnancies over 40 weeks with ultrasound or cardiotocography (CTG) confers no demonstrable benefit.

Sweeping the membranes

This involves performing a vaginal examination and inserting a finger through the internal os to separate the membranes from the uterine wall, thus releasing endogenous prostaglandins. It may be uncomfortable for the mother. If a sweep is carried out once after 40 weeks' gestation, it increases the incidence of spontaneous labour before 42 weeks, especially in those with a low Bishop score.

Induction of labour

Induction of labour after 41 weeks reduces the incidence of fetal distress and meconium staining compared with pregnancies managed conservatively with monitoring; there is

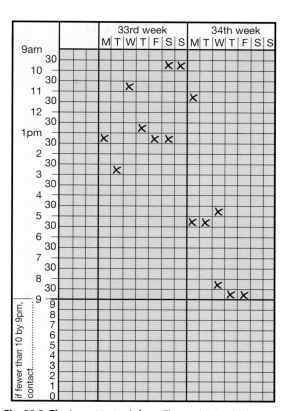

Fig. 28.2 The 'count to ten' chart. The mother is asked to start recording fetal movements at 9.00 a.m. and to contact the hospital for further tests if she has not recorded a total of 10 movements by 5.00 p.m.

also a reduction in the caesarean section rate. It is estimated that 500 inductions of post-dated pregnancies are required to prevent one perinatal death.

Antenatal assessment of fetal well-being

Many hospitals have 'Day Unit' facilities for mothers who require additional assessment after their routine antenatal screening has identified a potential problem, most commonly pre-eclampsia or fetal growth restriction. Fetal monitoring may be by fetal movement charts, cardiotocography, biophysical profile scoring and Doppler flow velocity studies.

Fetal movement counting

This is used as a screening test for further investigations (**Fig. 28.2**). The woman is asked to choose a starting time (usually 9 a.m.) and record how long it takes to feel 10 separate movements. If there have been <10 movements by 5 p.m., she is asked to contact the hospital for further tests. There is great variation in what may be considered as normal and 'a change in the usual movements' may be more important than absolute numbers. The value of routine movement counting is uncertain and a number of studies have failed to demonstrate any benefit.

Fetal cardiotocography (CTG)

The interpretation of CTGs is discussed on page 332. The CTG gives an indication of fetal well-being at a particular moment but has little longer-term predictive value. The routine use of antenatal CTG in low-risk pregnancies is not associated with an improved perinatal outcome.

Fetal biophysical profile (BPP)

In the standard biophysical score, five parameters are assessed, each scored out of 2, and the total out of 10 is used to give an indication of fetal well-being **(Table 28.2)**. Of all the parameters, liquor volume is probably the most predictive of fetal well-being. A major disadvantage of the BPP is that it is potentially time-consuming, requiring up to 30 minutes of scanning time. As most babies with an abnormal BPP score also have abnormal umbilical artery Doppler flow, it is more appropriate to use Doppler studies. Furthermore, Doppler abnormalities usually precede abnormalities in the BPP.

Doppler flow velocity studies

Doppler ultrasound examination of the umbilical arteries is used as an assessment of downstream placental vascular resistance. It semi-quantitatively assesses blood flow, and reduced blood flow in fetal diastole correlates with fetal compromise. In severe compromise, diastolic flow may stop altogether or may even reverse. There is probably no useful screening role for routine Doppler studies in low-risk pregnancies.

Doppler examination of the umbilical arteries is useful in pregnancies considered at risk of hypoxia due to impaired placental function. In particular, a normal waveform would suggest that a small-for-gestational-age fetus was constitutionally small rather than growth restricted due to impaired placental function. Abnormal waveforms (absent or reduced end diastolic flow) are associated with an increased risk of structural and chromosomal abnormalities, and detailed sonography is indicated to avoid inappropriate iatrogenic morbidity.

Common antenatal problems

Backache

This occurs as ligaments relax, and a support brace, a firm mattress, and flat shoes may be of help. Symptoms of nerve involvement warrant careful clinical examination with referral to physiotherapy in the first instance.

Pelvic girdle pain (PGP)

This is pregnancy-associated pain, instability and dysfunction of the symphysis pubis joint caused by asymmetrical movement of the pelvic bones. It is a common complaint, affecting 14–22% of pregnant women. Referral to obstetric physiotherapists should be considered and advice provided on positioning and appropriate pain relief. Discussions on mode of delivery should take place, and whilst planned caesarean section may be considered for extreme cases, vaginal birth is advocated for most women.

Carpal tunnel syndrome

The median nerve passes under the flexor retinaculum and receives sensation from the radial half of the hand. Oedema of the carpal tunnel frequently results in compression, leading to paraesthesia of the thumb, index finger and lateral aspect of the middle finger. Holding the wrist hyperflexed for 2 minutes reproduces the symptoms. Treatment is by resting with the arm elevated, the use of splints, application of ice, therapeutic ultrasound, a local hydrocortisone injection, or, in severe cases, surgical division of the retinaculum.

Constipation

Constipation is a common complaint in pregnancy and can be exacerbated by iron therapy. Usually, dietary advice with recommendation of adequate intake of fibre and fresh fruit and vegetables is all that is required. Laxatives may be used, although bowel stimulants should be avoided due to the potential for stimulation of the uterine smooth muscle.

Haemorrhoids

The weight of the gravid uterus reduces venous return and this predisposes to haemorrhoids. Treatment is by avoiding constipation, and local application of proprietary creams. Rarely, thrombosed and/or prolapsed haemorrhoids require surgical treatment.

Table 28.2	
Parameters of the biophysical profile	
CTG	More than two accelerations of 15 bpm lasting longer than 15 seconds in 20 minutes
Fetal breathing	Lasting more than 30 seconds in 30 minutes
Fetal movements	More than three limb or trunk movements in 30 minutes
Fetal tone	One return to flexion (of neck) after extension, or one hand opening and closing
Liquor	More than 3 cm depth in two planes

Heartburn

Relaxation of smooth muscle by high circulating levels of pregnancy hormones (particularly progesterone) causes relaxation at the gastro-oesophageal junction and reduces lower oesophageal sphincter pressure. This can result in the passage of acidic gastric juice into the lower oesophagus. It is helpful to avoid large meals, spicy meals, fatty foods, alcohol and cigarette smoking. Sleeping in a more upright posture can also help. Aluminium- and magnesium-based antacids appear to be safe during pregnancy and there has been no reported teratogenicity with the H_2 antagonist ranitidine.

Itching

This may be localized to the perineum or may be generalized. Localized itching may be due to infection (particularly candidiasis, but less commonly pediculosis pubis or *Trichomonas vaginalis*). Generalized itching may occur with eczema, urticaria or scabies. If there is a systemic rash, consider one of the four pregnancy-associated dermatoses (see **Table 28.3**). Itching may also be due to intrahepatic cholestasis of pregnancy, particularly if on the palms of the hands (see p. 259).

Leg cramps

This affects a third of women in pregnancy and will be severe in 5%. Elevating the end of the bed 20 cm or so may help. Salt supplements are of unproven benefit and quinine should not be used. Calcium supplements may be of benefit to a minority of women.

Nausea and vomiting

This commonly starts at approximately 6 weeks' gestational age and, while it usually settles at 12–16 weeks, it occasionally continues throughout the pregnancy. It is sometimes referred to as 'morning sickness' but often persists throughout the day. The sickness often takes the form of retching, rather than true vomiting, and seldom affects the mother's health. The cause of vomiting is unknown, but the onset and resolution of symptoms may mirror the rise and fall of human chorionic gonadotrophin (hCG) in maternal serum. Furthermore, conditions associated with high levels of hCG, for example multiple pregnancies or molar pregnancies, may be associated with more severe symptoms.

Those admitted to hospital due to excessive vomiting are said to have 'hyperemesis gravidarum'. Inability to keep down fluids or solids leads to weight loss, dehydration and electrolyte disturbances, and may very rarely lead to vitamin B deficiency (and polyneuropathy). Liver failure, renal failure, and fetal or maternal death are rare. On admission the urine should be tested for ketones and blood sent for urea, electrolytes and haematocrit (urea and haematocrit may be elevated in dehydration). Liver function tests may also be deranged in severe hyperemesis, with reduced albumin and increased transaminase levels. It is appropriate to perform an ultrasound scan if the woman has not previously undergone a scan.

Treatment with intravenous fluids is usually sufficient in itself to reduce nausea and should be the only initial management. Antiemetics may be used but only if the vomiting is not settling. No antiemetics are licensed for use in pregnancy, but the risk of teratogenesis is probably very low with metoclopramide, cyclizine or prochlorperazine.

Table 28.3					
Dermatoses of pregnancy					
	Incidence	**Features**	**Usual timing of onset**	**Fetal problems**	**Treatment**
Polymorphic eruption of pregnancy	1:240	Abdominal urticaria and vesicles (with no bullae), rarely occurring in the periumbilical area, sometimes extending to the proximal limbs	32 weeks' gestation to term	None	Antihistamines and topical steroids
Prurigo of pregnancy	1:300	Excoriated pustules on extensor surfaces	25–30 weeks' gestation	None	Antihistamines and topical steroids
Pruritic folliculitis		Acneiform rash	16–40 weeks' gestation	None	Topical steroids
Pemphigoid gestationis	1:10,000	Pruritic erythematous papules, plaques and wheals spreading from the periumbilical area to the breasts, thighs and palms. Diagnosed by the presence of immunofluorescence on biopsy	9 weeks' gestation to 7 weeks postpartum	Fetal growth restriction and increased incidence of fetal abnormality	Antihistamines, topical steroids, systemic steroids and rarely plasmapheresis

Only rarely is vitamin B supplementation, enteral feeding or parenteral feeding required.

Vaginal discharge

Physiological vaginal discharge may be heavier during pregnancy, but pathological causes should be excluded. Candidiasis (thrush) is common and is typically a thick white or cream discharge with a cottage-cheese-like appearance. It may cause vulval itching. When a heavy vaginal discharge is noted, appropriate swabs should be taken to confirm the presence of infection and to suggest appropriate treatment.

Varicose veins

Varicose veins and ankle oedema are common, as the weight of the gravid uterus impairs venous return. They seldom improve until after delivery. Symptomatic relief in pregnancy may be gained from rest, elevation of the legs at rest, and the use of support stockings or tights.

Patient education (parentcraft)

This important function is most often undertaken by nominated midwives but may also have input from delivery suite staff, obstetricians and anaesthetists. Many women request guidance and information about normal and abnormal antenatal events and what to expect during the antenatal period, in labour and after delivery. The knowledge gained and the opportunity to discuss her pregnancy with an interested midwife can make a significant difference to the mother's perception of the pregnancy.

Parentcraft provides education for primigravidae, who have had no previous experience of pregnancy and labour, and advice is given about diet, dental care, stopping smoking and reducing alcohol intake. Multigravidae may request 'refresher' classes. Labour, normal and abnormal, can be explained. Visits to the delivery ward are offered, allowing women to become familiar with the delivery rooms, and provide the first contact with the staff of the delivery suite. Information about analgesia is provided so that women may make an informed decision as to their preference, although they should be encouraged to keep an open mind.

Parentcraft classes targeting a particular group are becoming popular, e.g. multiple pregnancy or teenage classes, where women can meet others in similar circumstances to themselves. In this way, particular difficulties experienced by a group can be discussed and addressed.

Drug misuse

The prevalence of drug misuse is increasing and particularly in women of childbearing age. Serious problem misuse and poly-drug misuse are associated with socioeconomic deprivation and an increase in obstetric complications including miscarriage, antepartum haemorrhage, fetal growth restriction, intrauterine death and preterm labour. Care must usually be directed firmly towards social factors before any impact on obstetric problems can be achieved. Pregnancy may provide a window of opportunity to provide real help, breaking a cycle of poor parenting that might otherwise in turn lead to further problems in the next generation.

The history should cover:

- type of drug **(Table 28.4)**
  - street drugs, e.g. heroin, amphetamines
  - pharmacological preparations (usually illicit and/or prescribed), e.g. benzodiazepines, buprenorphine and analgesics, particularly DF118 and other codeine compounds
  - prescribed preparations, usually methadone
- pattern of use, dose, route, frequency, and method of financing supply
- social support, the other children, partner, family, friends, social work involvement, clothing, food, shelter and transport
- impending legal problems
- risks of infection including HIV, hepatitis B/C counselling with or without testing
- domestic abuse – this is a common occurrence within all groups of pregnant women, and all women should be asked about this at the initial or booking visit.

There may be poor self-esteem following a lack of trusting relationships, lack of positive body image, and concerns about the woman's abilities to be a parent.

Management

Social factors

Illegal drugs are expensive and addicts often become involved in theft or prostitution (with its risks of violence and sexually transmitted diseases). In addition, lifestyle may be erratic and pregnancy outcome is compounded by various additional nutritional and social factors. Attendance for antenatal care may often compete with more immediate problems (e.g. seeing the social worker or lawyer, or getting money/drugs etc.) but if such care can be delivered locally with truly flexible access and be combined with confidentiality, non-judgemental consistency, access to social workers and legal aid, then fuller and more holistic care can be achieved.

Users of opiates/opioids

For opiate/opioid users it is worth considering transfer to methadone (which is metabolized more slowly, and therefore has more stable levels, and less risk of fetal distress and preterm labour associated with sudden withdrawals or fluctuations in serum opiate levels). Those stabilized on methadone alone probably have a lower neonatal mortality than those still taking heroin. There may also be improved prenatal attendance.

Table 28.4	
Fetal effects of drugs	
Drug	**Effect on fetus**
Alcohol	There is no clear dose relationship. Fetal alcohol syndrome is rare (fetal growth restriction, microcephaly, craniofacial abnormalities and mental retardation). Consumption of even small amounts of alcohol has been associated with a reduction in birth weight and intellectual impairment
Amphetamines	There is no good evidence of fetal abnormality. Fetal thrombocytopenia is very rare
Benzodiazepines	Neonatal withdrawal occurs at levels associated with abuse, even after quite brief use. 'Floppy infant syndrome' may occur if high doses have been given to a non-abusing mother in the 15 hours prior to delivery
Ecstasy	No increased risk has been demonstrated
Cannabis (hash, marijuana)	There have been no demonstrable teratogenic effects, but there is almost certainly fetal growth restriction
Opiates/opioids (e.g. heroin, methadone, DF118, buprenorphine)	Methadone and heroin are also associated with fetal growth restriction, and heroin is also associated with amenorrhoea (±anovulation) and preterm labour. Buprenorphine and DF118 probably have similar associations to heroin, but with DF118 there is increased severity of withdrawal
Cocaine and 'crack'	There is an increased risk of abruption, premature rupture of membranes, and possibly fetal growth restriction and sudden infant death syndrome
Nicotine	There is an association with fetal growth restriction, preterm labour, perinatal death and delayed development. Tobacco use, if heavy, may lead to neonatal withdrawal symptoms
LSD	No increased risk has been demonstrated

Detoxification

There are theoretical fetal risks from very rapid opiate/opioid detoxification but in practice the true fetal risks from even 'cold turkey' detoxification are relatively small. Despite this, patients undergoing rapid detoxification should be managed on an obstetric unit, or at least under the close supervision of an obstetrician with an interest and experience in substance misuse. It has been suggested that the risks of detoxification (whether rapid or gradual) may be higher in the first and third trimesters, but practical experience does not bear this out. The goal should be to reduce drug use to a level compatible with stability (e.g. with methadone), not necessarily aiming for abstinence. It may be more acceptable for a mother taking a moderate dose of methadone to top up with very small amounts of a similar non-injected substance (e.g. smoking heroin) than increasing methadone doses to very high levels in a futile attempt to achieve total abstinence from illicit drugs. If, however, women attempt unrealistic reductions in methadone and top up with other drugs, the dose of methadone should be increased. Topping up with benzodiazepines is particularly inadvisable.

Neonatal complications

There is an increased incidence of low birth weight due to fetal growth restriction, preterm delivery and sudden infant death syndrome. Neonatal withdrawal problems are particularly associated with opiates/opioids and benzodiazepines, and are worse if they have been used together. Severity is dose related and timing depends on the rate of drug metabolism, e.g. heroin and morphine are metabolized rapidly and signs usually develop within 1 day, whereas methadone is metabolized more slowly and signs usually occur at between 3 and 5 days. Classically, babies are hungry but feed ineffectually. There is CNS hyperexcitability (increased reflexes and tremor), gastrointestinal dysfunction (finger sucking, regurgitation, diarrhoea) and respiratory distress. Treatment options include replacement for those who have been taking opiates/opioids, but it is not appropriate for benzodiazepine withdrawals. The severity of withdrawal symptoms is reduced by breastfeeding.

Key points
• Pregnancy is a physiological event, not an illness, and medical interference should be limited to those women who are most likely to benefit. Nonetheless, complications can arise in 'low-risk' women. • Antenatal care is a multifaceted screening programme aimed at identifying problems at an early stage to minimize the risks to mothers and their babies.

29

Postnatal care

The puerperium is defined as being from delivery of the placenta to the end of the sixth postnatal week. This arbitrary definition, however, has no true physiological basis as some pregnancy changes revert to the pre-pregnancy state within a few minutes whereas others never revert.

The uterus contracts within a few minutes of delivery from a cavity capable of containing 4 or 5 litres to a space barely able to contain an adult's fingers. It involutes over the next 4 weeks, its weight reducing from 1000 g to just 50–100 g, with the lochial discharge changing from red to brownish pink and finally cream/white. Maternal weight reduces, plasma volume, red cell mass and haemostasis revert to normal, and the other systemic, endocrine and metabolic adaptations return to the pre-pregnancy state. Lactation, instigated by the falling progesterone levels and maintained by oxytocin, can inhibit the return of menstruation and fertility until weaning.

Routine postnatal assessment is useful to help provide the mother with support as she cares for her baby, and to identify any puerperal complications at an early stage.

Normal puerperium

For those giving birth in hospital, the postnatal stay should be tailored to each individual mother. The length of this stay depends largely on maternal wishes and on her clinical condition, and may be anything from an immediate discharge to several days or longer. Difficulties with establishing breastfeeding or bonding, the development of medical problems, poor social circumstances or lack of home support may all warrant additional inpatient support.

If the woman is rhesus negative, a Kleihauer test should be sent and the baby's blood group determined to establish whether anti-D prophylaxis is required. The mother should also be offered rubella vaccination if she is known not to be immune.

Early postnatal checks

In the UK, the midwife sees the woman regularly after birth, based on individual needs, and checks on:

- general emotional and physical well-being
- infant feeding and care – breastfeeding should be encouraged if possible
- urinary and bowel function (see below)
- lochia – this may continue for up to 4–8 weeks
- contraceptive plans.

In the early postnatal days, all women should be given the opportunity to discuss their birth with the appropriate healthcare professional.

On examination, the following should be checked as a matter of routine:

- Pulse, blood pressure and temperature, looking for signs of haemorrhage, anaemia or sepsis.
- Abdominal examination to ensure that the uterus is involuting and non-tender. On the first day after birth the uterine fundus should be palpable at the umbilicus and it gradually reduces in size until, by the 10th–14th day it is no longer palpable above the symphysis pubis.
- The perineum, looking particularly for evidence of wound breakdown in those who have had perineal trauma and/or sutures. Cool gel packs may be applied intermittently, although ice packs are not advocated. Simple analgesia can be prescribed and local anaesthetic gels or sprays may sometimes be of help.

The midwife will see a woman for a minimum of 10 days and up to 28 days. In some regions the duration of postnatal visits has been extended to 6 weeks, to incorporate the 6-week examination.

Late postnatal check

This usually takes place around 6 weeks after birth and should be a chance to review the birth, address any doubts or questions, and place these in context for future births.

It is important to assess the baby and how well the mother is coping, looking particularly for tiredness or depression.

The maternal haemoglobin may be checked and cervical cytology performed as appropriate. Contraception is discussed and enquiries made about whether intercourse has resumed and whether there were any specific problems.

Postnatal problems

Anaemia

The incidence of postnatal anaemia is 25–30%. It is reasonably simple to treat non-symptomatic anaemia with oral iron, reserving transfusion for those with significant symptoms.

Bowel problems

Constipation may be due to a number of factors, including fear of defecation following perineal trauma, reduced mobility, oral medication such as iron or codeine, or narcotic analgesia in labour. Constipation is reported by up to 20% of women in the puerperium. Haemorrhoids also affect around 20% of women and these often persist for some time after birth. They are more common in primiparous women and after instrumental delivery.

Breast problems

Two-thirds of women will have some problem, including nipple pain, engorgement, mastitis, *Candida albicans* (thrush), cracks, abscesses and bleeding. For women who are not breastfeeding, suppression of lactation is the main problem with engorgement being the main symptom. For breastfeeding women, problems can largely be prevented by proper advice regarding positioning of the baby's mouth and supportive counselling. Mastitis, if it occurs, is usually the result of a blocked duct, although it can occur secondary to infection (e.g. with *Staphylococcus aureus*).

Episiotomy breakdown

This is not uncommon, but long-term problems are rare. If the wound is clean, resuturing should be considered. If there is any suggestion of infection, however, it is probably better to allow healing by secondary intention and antibiotics should be considered.

Incontinence

In the first year after birth, 3–5% of women experience urinary tract infection and about 5% report urinary frequency for the first time. Low-grade urinary tract infection is possible especially after catheterization.

At least 20% of women suffer from stress incontinence if assessed 3 months after birth. This is mostly from neurapraxia and commonly resolves spontaneously. A few women will still be incontinent a year later.

Inability to control flatus or faeces occurs in around 5% of women after birth, but as it is often embarrassing, women frequently do not report it. According to ultrasound studies, 35% of primiparae have demonstrable damage to the anal sphincter although many do not have symptoms **(Fig. 29.1)**. Both direct perineal trauma and nerve damage following spontaneous or instrumental delivery contribute to the problem. Investigation and treatment of symptoms is warranted.

Psychiatric problems in the puerperium

These range from 'the blues', which can be so common as to be normal, to the much more serious puerperal psychosis, which is rare and can have fatal consequences.

'The postnatal blues'

This occurs in over 50% of women, usually beginning on days 2–4, peaking at days 4–6 and lasting for 2–7 days. It is a mood disturbance rather than a mood illness, which may have a hormonal basis, and it is unrelated to obstetric or cultural factors. There is emotional lability, tearfulness, sadness, sleep disturbance, poor concentration, restlessness and headaches. The mother may feel vulnerable and/or rejected, and may show undue concern for the baby. Treatment is with reassurance and support. Antenatal preparation may be of help.

Postnatal depression

The incidence of postnatal depression is between 10% and 25% in the first postnatal year, with the peak onset around weeks 3–4. In two-thirds, the illness is self-limiting; in one-third it may be sustained or severe. There are the usual features of depression, but particularly increased irritability, tiredness, decreased libido, guilt at not loving or caring enough for the baby, inability to cope with the baby, or undue anxieties over the baby's health and feeding. There is no biochemical explanation for postnatal depression but there are likely to be a number of social and psychological factors. It may also be associated with a past history of depression. Encouraging women to talk about their feelings to a non-judgemental person has been demonstrated to increase their likelihood of early recovery. Treatment depends on severity, circumstances and patient preferences, but includes brief psychotherapy, supportive psychotherapy, counselling and antidepressants. The outcome is generally good.

Puerperal psychosis

This has an incidence of 1:500–1:800 deliveries, beginning around days 3–7 and peaking at 2 weeks. There may be serious risks to both the mother and child. One study has suggested that 5% of affected women commit suicide and 4% kill their baby. There are variable psychotic symptoms, sometimes superimposed upon postnatal blues. The clinical picture is a shifting one, often ushered in by one or two

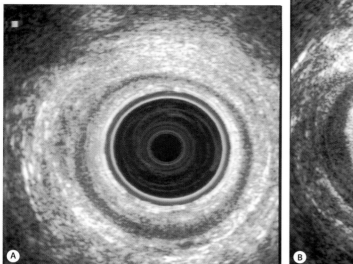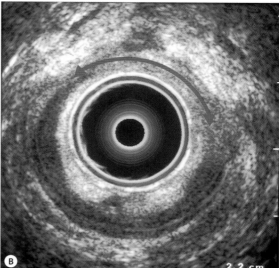

Fig. 29.1 Anal sphincter damage on endoanal ultrasound. (A) Normal anal sphincter scan. **(B)** Anterior anal sphincter defect between the 10 o'clock and 3 o'clock position.

nights' insomnia. Mood abnormality is common and the mother may be suspicious, sometimes denying the pregnancy and baby. There may be delusions, hallucinations, confusion and cognitive impairment. The condition is associated with a past history of psychosis (especially manic depression), with being unmarried, having a caesarean section, developing an infection or suffering a perinatal death. Mother and baby should be admitted to hospital, ideally to a specialized mother and baby unit. The prognosis is good for the incident episode, particularly if the family is supportive, but 20% of those who become pregnant again will develop a further puerperal psychosis. 50% will have another psychotic episode at some time in their life.

Puerperal pyrexia

This is defined as a temperature of >38°C on any occasion in the first 14 days after birth or miscarriage (a slight fever is not uncommon in the first 24 hours). Pyrexia is usually due to urinary or genital infections (including endometritis) but may also be related to infection in the chest or breast. Deep venous thrombosis and pulmonary thromboembolism should be considered. After a full clinical examination (including breasts, legs, perineum, chest, and abdominal palpation of the uterus) a midstream specimen of urine, and endocervical and wounds swabs, as appropriate, are sent for microbiological analysis. A suggestion of a chest infection necessitates physiotherapy and sputum should also be sent for culture. Blood cultures are taken if the woman is systemically unwell.

In general, if the mother is well and the temperature only mildly elevated, conservative treatment may be warranted. If she is unwell and the source of infection is not clear, treatment should be started with a broad-spectrum antibiotic. Antibiotic therapy may also be required for breast infections; breastfeeding or hand expression should continue if possible. A breast abscess may require surgical incision and drainage.

Secondary postpartum haemorrhage

See page 282.

Superficial thrombophlebitis

This affects about 1% of women. There is a painful, erythematous and tender (usually varicose) vein. Treatment is with support stockings and anti-inflammatory drugs.

Key *points*

- The puerperium is a time of major physiological change, and a time of major emotional and personal upheaval.
- Postnatal checks are useful to assess both the mother and baby. The major maternal complications are sepsis, haemorrhage, thromboembolic disease and depression.

30

Medical disorders in pregnancy

Medical disorders are relatively common in pregnancy and often have no implications for the mother or her baby. However, the alteration in maternal physiology which occurs during pregnancy may affect the medical condition, or the medical condition itself may affect the pregnancy and the baby. Treatment options for the mother may be limited by concerns for fetal welfare and there is therefore the potential for difficult clinical decision-making.

The following conditions will be considered, but see also hypertension (p. 291), and infection in pregnancy (p. 273):

- diabetes mellitus
- venous thromboembolic disease
- cardiac disease
- connective tissue disease
- epilepsy
- hepatic disorders
- renal disorders
- respiratory disorders
- thrombocytopenia
- thyroid disorders.

Diabetes mellitus

Diabetes mellitus may be diagnosed before pregnancy or may be discovered for the first time during pregnancy. Discovery during pregnancy is rare for type 1 (insulin-dependent) diabetes but not uncommon for type 2 (non-insulin-dependent) diabetes. In addition to these, a transient self-limiting state of hyperglycaemia may occur in pregnancy as a result of maternal endocrine changes.

Glucose homeostasis is maintained by the balance between insulin, which reduces glucose levels by increasing cellular uptake, and other hormones such as glucagon and cortisol, which increase glucose production. In pregnancy the placenta produces additional cortisol as well as other insulin antagonists such as human placental lactogen, progesterone and human chorionic gonadotrophin, all of which tend to increase the maternal glucose level. If the pancreatic β islet cells are unable to produce sufficient insulin to balance this increase, or if there is maternal insulin resistance, the mother may develop a state of hyperglycaemia referred to as 'gestational diabetes'. A lesser rise in glucose levels that does not reach the criteria required for a diagnosis of gestational diabetes is termed 'impaired glucose tolerance of pregnancy'.

Women with pre-existing diabetes mellitus may have high glucose levels in the first trimester at the time of organogenesis, and there is a consequent increase in the rate of congenital abnormalities. The abnormalities are principally cardiac defects, neural tube defects and renal anomalies and are more likely to occur if the diabetic control has been poor. Although the mechanism of this teratogenesis is unclear, there is evidence that improved pre-pregnancy and early pregnancy blood glucose control reduces the risk of congenital abnormality.

Fetal glucose levels closely reflect those of the mother, with glucose crossing the placenta through facilitated diffusion. Maternal insulin does not cross the placenta and the fetus produces its own insulin from around 10 weeks' gestation. This insulin is recognized to have a significant role in promoting fetal growth. As maternal levels of glucose are higher in mothers with diabetes, fetal levels are also increased and, in turn, there is increased fetal insulin production. This fetal hyperinsulinaemia often results in macrosomia (large babies) and organomegaly as well as increased erythropoiesis and neonatal polycythaemia.

In addition to the risk of congenital abnormality there is also a risk of unexplained intrauterine fetal death, possibly because fetal hyperinsulinaemia leads to chronic hypoxia and lactic acidaemia. A macrosomic fetus may be more at risk of these complications because of its increased oxygen demands.

Although fetal growth restriction can occur in pregnancies of diabetic women, only 15% weigh less than the 50th centile. Labour and delivery may therefore be complicated by dystocia and in particular shoulder dystocia. Neonates may have hypoglycaemia, hypocalcaemia, hypomagnesaemia and polycythaemia. There is also an increased incidence of hyaline membrane disease.

Effects of pregnancy on diabetes

Insulin requirements may be static or decrease during the first trimester. They typically increase during the second and third trimesters and may reduce slightly towards 40 weeks. Pregnancy may exacerbate diabetic retinopathy, and the fundi should be assessed for signs of proliferative retinopathy, with laser treatment advised as necessary.

Effects of diabetes on pregnancy

The incidence of pre-eclampsia is increased. There is also an increased incidence of maternal infection, particularly of the urinary tract. Polyhydramnios, which probably results from fetal polyuria, may result in unstable lie, malpresentation and preterm labour.

Screening for impaired glucose tolerance and gestational diabetes

This is a controversial subject. National (UK) guidelines recommend offering a 75 g glucose tolerance test (GTT) at 24–28 weeks to women with risk factors, including a family history of diabetes, a raised BMI (>30), a previous macrosomic baby (>4.5 kg), or those with previous gestational diabetes (GDM). For those with previous GDM, early self-monitoring or a GTT should be offered at 16–18 weeks and, if normal, repeated at 28 weeks.

The normal fasting plasma glucose is <5.5 mmol/l. For an oral GTT, patients should fast overnight. Venous blood is taken for fasting blood glucose and a 75 g glucose drink is given. Further venous blood samples are taken after 1 hour and 2 hours. The World Health Organization (WHO) non-pregnant diagnostic criteria are:

- diabetes: fasting glucose ≥7.0 mmol/l and/or 2-hour level ≥11.1 mmol/l
- impaired glucose tolerance: fasting glucose <7.0 mmol/l and the 2-hour level 7.8–11.1 mmol/l.

When these criteria are applied to a European population in the third trimester of pregnancy, 10% will have impaired glucose tolerance.

Management of impaired glucose tolerance and gestational diabetes

The management is also controversial. There is some evidence that treatment is beneficial with a 2-hour value of 7.8–11.1 as well as when the criteria for diabetes are reached. Treatment with dietary advice and adjustment should be the first step, and to consider insulin if the target levels below are not achieved. Insulin treatment should aim to keep the preprandial glucose less than 6 mmol/l. There is also growing evidence for the use of the oral hypoglycaemic agent metformin.

Up to 70% of women with impaired glucose tolerance in pregnancy go on to develop diabetes mellitus in the subsequent 25 years. Recurrence of GDM in subsequent pregnancies is up to 75% (especially if treatment with insulin was required).

Antenatal management of established diabetes

At pre-pregnancy counselling, advice should be given about good diabetic control, diet, smoking and high-dose (5 mg) folate supplements. If possible, pregnancy management should be in a combined obstetric/diabetic clinic with frequent visits planned as required. Blood glucose should be measured several times a day at home, aiming for tight control (e.g. with preprandial levels 3.5–5.9 mmol/l and 1-hour postprandial levels of <7.8 mmol/l). Glycosylated haemoglobin (HbA1c) should be checked monthly when planning a pregnancy and in early pregnancy, aiming for levels towards 6.1%.

Insulin is commonly given as a short-acting analogue three times a day (with meals), with an intermediate- or long-acting insulin once or twice a day as background. Ketoacidosis should be avoided as it is associated with an increased risk of perinatal mortality.

Maternal renal function and optic fundi should be examined in early pregnancy, and a detailed anomaly scan offered at 18–22 weeks. The maternal abdomen should be examined for polyhydramnios, macrosomia or fetal growth restriction (measurement of symphysis–fundal height), and serial ultrasound fetal biometry is frequently requested.

Routine third-trimester assessments of fetal well-being (cardiotography [CTG] or biophysical profile) are not of demonstrable benefit and should be restricted to pregnancies with complications other than maternal diabetes alone. With regard to delivery, each case should be considered individually. There is no need for intervention before 38 weeks if there is no evidence of complications, and there is no indication for elective caesarean section on the basis of diabetes alone. If preterm labour occurs, steroids may be given as for the non-diabetic patient, but will lead to marked deterioration in diabetic control unless insulin doses are increased appropriately.

Delivery

Concern regarding fetal macrosomia and the potential for shoulder dystocia in particular may necessitate a planned caesarean section. The inherent inaccuracy of ultrasound estimations of fetal weight (±15%) limits the clinician's ability to provide advice on the most appropriate mode of delivery. All diabetic women delivering vaginally should be attended by a midwife or obstetrician familiar with and preferably skilled in the manoeuvres required to overcome shoulder dystocia.

There are numerous different regimens of intravenous dextrose and insulin, but the aim of all is to maintain tight intrapartum control whether during labour or for caesarean section. In the immediate postpartum period insulin requirements rapidly return to pre-pregnancy levels and the previous subcutaneous regimen can be re-established. For women with GDM, insulin should be discontinued following delivery.

Venous thromboembolic disease

Antenatal

In pregnancy the balance of the clotting system is altered towards clot formation. There are increased levels of fibrinogen, prothrombin and other clotting factors, together with reduced levels of endogenous anticoagulants. This tendency to clot formation is only in part offset by an increase in fibrinolysis. In addition to the clotting system changes, the gravid uterus causes a degree of mechanical obstruction to the venous system and leads to peripheral venous stasis in the lower limbs.

Venous thromboembolic disease appears to be very rare in Africa and the Far East but is the commonest direct cause of maternal mortality in the UK. The reason for such wide racial difference may be that the factor V Leiden mutation and prothrombin gene variants are rare in African and Asian populations. In the UK, over 50% of maternal deaths from thromboembolism occur antenatally, mostly in the first trimester.

Over 80% of deep venous thromboses (DVTs) in pregnancy are left-sided, in contrast to only 55% in non-pregnant woman. The underlying explanation is not established, but difference may reflect compression of the left common iliac vein by the right common iliac artery and the ovarian artery, which cross the vein on the left side only. Furthermore, over 70% of DVTs in pregnancy are iliofemoral compared to the non-pregnant rate of around 9%, and are therefore more likely than lower calf vein thromboses to give rise to pulmonary embolism.

Thromboembolism may be asymptomatic but usually presents with the traditional symptoms and signs such as calf tenderness, cough and chest pain. It may also present with lower abdominal or groin pain. It is essential to make a definitive diagnosis if at all possible, not just for management of the current pregnancy but because there are major implications for subsequent pregnancies as well.

Haematological testing for D-dimers is not helpful in pregnancy. Radiological investigations are required if there is clinical suspicion. Duplex Doppler ultrasound is particularly useful for identifying femoral vein thromboses although iliac veins are less easily seen **(Fig. 30.1)**. It is safe and should be the first-line investigation. X-ray venography is more specific, but has the disadvantage of radiation exposure. Venography or MRI is appropriate if Doppler studies give equivocal results. Pregnancy is not a contraindication to carrying out a chest X-ray and/or a ventilation–perfusion $(\dot{V}/\dot{Q})$ scan – any radiation risks are outweighed by the benefits of accurate diagnosis **(Fig. 30.2)**. A normal scan virtually excludes the diagnosis of pulmonary embolism. A computerized tomography pulmonary arteriogram (CTPA) may also be appropriate, especially if a large pulmonary embolism is suspected.

Treatment of DVT or pulmonary embolism in pregnancy is with intravenous (i.v.) or subcutaneous (s.c.) heparin, continued into labour. Low-molecular-weight heparin (LMWH) is appropriate in most instances, although i.v. unfractionated heparin is still appropriate for those with a major pulmonary embolus. LMWH carries a lower risk of thrombocytopenia and of osteoporosis. After delivery the woman may choose to continue with s.c. heparin or commence warfarin, continuing anticoagulation for 6–12 weeks as decided by timing of onset and clinical severity of the thrombosis. Once anticoagulants are stopped, women should be screened for thrombophilias **(Box 30.1)**.

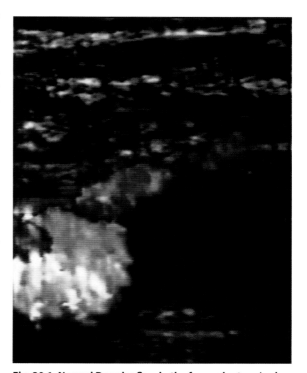

Fig. 30.1 Normal Doppler flow in the femoral artery (red, left) with no flow through the occluded femoral vein (black, right).

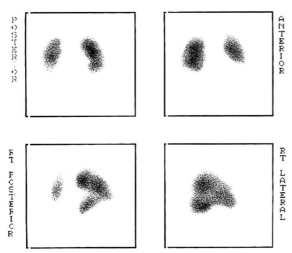

Fig. 30.2 Positive Q̇ scan. Note the lack of perfusion in the right lower lobe. The ventilation scan was normal. (From Pitkin J, Peattie A, Magowan BA. Obstetrics and Gysnecology. An Illustrated Colour Text. Churchill Livingstone, Edinburgh, 2003.)

The optimal management of those with a previous history of thromboembolism is more uncertain. Women who have experienced a single episode of thromboembolism should be screened for thrombophilia. If the screen is negative, and the event occurred outside pregnancy and was not severe, antenatal thromboprophylaxis may not be required. Postnatal thromboprophylaxis with LMWH should be recommended for 6 weeks. If the screen is positive, or there are other risk factors or a positive family history, antenatal and postnatal prophylaxis with LMWH should be offered.

Postnatal risk assessment

The risks of thromboembolism should be reassessed in all women after delivery (see **Box 30.2**), and those at risk (previous thrombosis, thrombophilia, emergency caesarean section, or any two of the other risk factors) offered thromboprophylaxis with LMWH (e.g. enoxaparin 40 mg once daily).

Cardiac disease

Heart disease of variable types complicates less than 1% of all pregnancies but accounts for around 16% of maternal deaths in the UK. Rheumatic heart disease remains a significant problem in the developing world and it is also encountered with increasing frequency in western countries as a result of migration. There are increasing numbers of fertile women who have had surgery as children for congenital heart disease. Maternal mortality is highest in conditions where pulmonary blood flow cannot be increased to compensate for the increased demand during pregnancy – particularly Eisenmenger's syndrome, where maternal mortality rates reach 40–50%.

Unfortunately, many symptoms and signs similar to those of heart disease occur commonly in normal pregnancy, making a clinical diagnosis difficult. Breathlessness and syncopal episodes are present in 90% of normal pregnancies, atrial ectopic beats are common, and up to 96% of normal women may have an audible ejection systolic murmur. Further investigation should be considered if the murmur is loud (>2/6), if a precordial thrill is present, or if there are any other suspicious features, especially in immigrant women.

If problems are discovered, a cardiologist should be involved during the antenatal period. If there is no haemodynamic compromise (e.g. congenital mitral valve prolapse), the prognosis is good and there is often no requirement for cardiac follow-up. If there are potential haemodynamic problems, very close follow-up by a multidisciplinary team is mandatory and a careful plan should be made for delivery. Serious consideration of pregnancy termination is advisable in women with Eisenmenger's syndrome, primary pulmonary hypertension, or pulmonary veno-occlusive disease. With atrial fibrillation, anticoagulation is required to prevent atrial clot forming and subsequent embolic problems. If the maternal PO_2 is decreased, the fetus is at

Cardiac disease and delivery

- Labour should be conducted in a high-dependency or intensive care unit, possibly with central venous catheter monitoring, aiming for a vaginal delivery. Hypotension, hypoxia and fluid overload should be avoided.
- Epidural analgesia may be used in some circumstances.
- Antibiotics should be given if required for endocarditis prophylaxis.
- The second stage should be kept short. For the third stage, Syntocinon should be given slowly – rather than Syntometrine, which leads to hypertension.
- Particular care is required in the immediate postpartum period as the increased circulating volume following uterine retraction may lead to fluid overload and congestive failure.

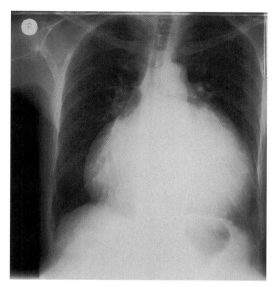

Fig. 30.3 Postpartum cardiomyopathy after twin delivery in a mother aged 42 years.

risk from hypoxia and fetal growth restriction, and should be monitored closely.

Severe cardiac disease can cause problems at delivery, particularly in those with prosthetic valves, aortic stenosis, severe mitral stenosis, left ventricular dysfunction, or pulmonary hypertension **(Box 30.3)**.

Myocardial infarction is rare in pregnancy but is the commonest cardiac cause of maternal mortality. Peripartum cardiomyopathy is also rare (<1:5000), but carries a 5% mortality and is associated with hypertension in pregnancy, multiple pregnancy, high multiparity and increased maternal age. It presents with sudden onset of heart failure and on chest radiology or echocardiography there is a grossly dilated heart **(Fig. 30.3)**.

Connective tissue disease

These diseases are not uncommon and, as they often affect women during their childbearing years, they are not infrequently found in association with pregnancy. See also the antiphospholipid syndrome page 101.

Systemic lupus erythematosus (SLE)

Pregnancy does not affect the long-term prognosis of SLE. There is probably an increased chance of an exacerbation of the disease (flare-up) occurring in pregnancy, and during the postnatal period. Women should be discouraged from becoming pregnant when their disease is active to minimize problems. Active SLE nephritis during pregnancy is associated with significant maternal and perinatal mortality and morbidity, and in particular with a risk of pre-eclampsia.

SLE is associated with increased fetal loss rates from spontaneous miscarriages and preterm delivery. This is particularly so in those with antiphospholipid antibodies. There is an increased incidence of pre-eclampsia and this may be difficult to differentiate from a disease flare, as both are associated with hypertension and proteinuria. There is no increase in the rate of fetal abnormalities, although there is a risk of fetal congenital heart block associated with the presence of anti-Ro and anti-La antibodies **(Fig. 30.4)**. Neonatal lupus may rarely occur and is characterized by haemolytic anaemia, leucopenia, thrombocytopenia, discoid skin lesions, pericarditis and congenital heart block.

If lupus anticoagulant or anticardiolipin antibodies are present, low-dose aspirin should be given, and in women with a previous history of thromboembolic disease or adverse pregnancy outcome, low-molecular-weight heparin is indicated. Careful monitoring of renal function is appropriate. Flare-ups should be managed where possible with oral prednisolone and there should be regular ultrasound fetal biometry owing to the increased risk of fetal growth restriction.

Epilepsy

A seizure in pregnancy should be assumed to be eclampsia until proven otherwise. Around a third of pregnant women with epilepsy have an increase in seizure frequency independent of the effects of medication. For women with epilepsy on treatment, the fall in anticonvulsant levels due to dilution, reduced absorption, reduced compliance and increased drug metabolism is partially compensated for by reduced protein binding (and therefore an increase in the level of free drug). There is an increased incidence of fetal anomalies in association with antiepileptic drugs (AEDs) (6% vs 3% in the general population) **(Fig. 30.5)**. Single-drug regimens are less teratogenic than multidrug therapy **(Table 30.1)** and sodium valproate carries the highest risk of teratogenesis.

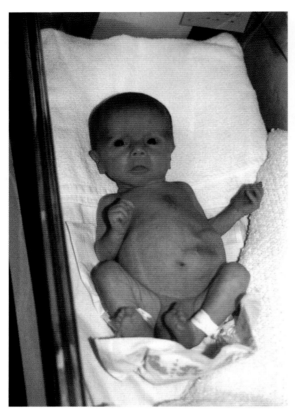

Fig 30.4 Pacemaker in a baby with congenital heart block in association with anti-Ro antibodies.

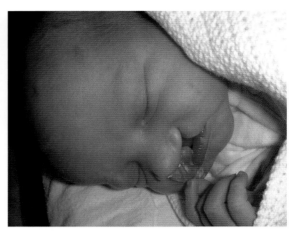

Fig. 30.5 Anticonvulsants are associated with neural tube, cardiac and craniofacial defects (with permission).

Hepatic disorders

There are a large number of potential causes of liver dysfunction in pregnancy **(Tables 30.2** and **30.3)**. A history of a prodromal illness, overseas travel or high-risk group for blood-borne illness may suggest viral hepatitis. Itch is suggestive of cholestasis. Abdominal pain is associated with gallstones, HELLP syndrome (p. 297) or acute fatty liver. Clinical signs are often unhelpful in diagnosis. Urea and electrolytes (U&Es), urate, liver function tests (LFTs), blood glucose, platelets and coagulation screen should be performed and blood sent for hepatitis serology. Abdominal ultrasound of the liver and gall bladder may show obstruction or fat infiltration. It is normal for the alkaline phosphatase level to increase in pregnancy (1.5–2 times normal).

Renal disorders

In pregnancy there is a physiological increase in the size of both kidneys as well as dilatation of the ureter and renal pelvis. This dilatation is greater on the right than on the left because of the dextrorotation of the uterus. There is also an increase in creatinine clearance owing to the increased glomerular filtration rate (maximal in the second trimester). In pregnancy the normal serum urea is <4.5 mmol/l and creatinine <75 μmol/l.

Infection

Urinary tract infections (UTIs) occur in 3–7% of pregnancies and, if untreated, may lead to septicaemia and preterm labour. Asymptomatic bacteriuria should be treated since there is a 30–40% risk of developing a symptomatic UTI. Pyelonephritis should be treated aggressively.

Obstruction

Acute hydronephrosis is characterized by loin pain, ureteric colic, sterile urine and a renal ultrasound scan showing dilatation of the renal tract greater than normal for pregnancy **(Fig. 30.6)**. If the symptoms are not settling and the ultrasound scan does not demonstrate the cause of the obstruction, a limited intravenous urogram should be considered. Treatment is with ureteric stenting or nephrostomy. There may be no obvious cause of obstruction and complete resolution may occur following delivery. Renal tract calculi are associated with an increased incidence of UTIs but otherwise do not usually affect pregnancy (unless obstruction is severe).

Chronic renal impairment

With chronic renal disease in pregnancy, the fetal prognosis is best if maternal renal function and blood pressure (BP) are optimized. If the plasma creatinine is <125 μmol/l, the maternal and perinatal outcome is usually good. If pregnancy occurs with a creatinine >250 μmol/l, there is a high risk of renal deterioration. Between these levels women should be advised that pregnancy may cause their renal function to deteriorate and that there are also risks to the

Table 30.1	
Management of epilepsy in pregnancy	
Pre-pregnancy counselling	Monotherapy ideal. Folate supplementation should be continued until at least 12 weeks
Anticonvulsant dosage	Anticonvulsant doses adjusted on clinical grounds. There are fetal risks from the anticonvulsant medication as well as from not taking the drugs (from increased fit frequency) Checking plasma levels is usually not necessary, but can occasionally be useful to check compliance and exclude toxicity ('free' drug levels rather than 'total' drug levels are ideal)
Detailed ultrasound scan at 18–22 weeks	Neural tube, cardiac and craniofacial abnormalities, as well as diaphragmatic herniae, are more common
Vitamin K for women on enzyme-inducing anticonvulsants	Oral vitamin K should be given daily from 36 weeks (some anticonvulsants are vitamin K antagonists and increase the risk of haemorrhagic disease of the new-born). The baby should be given intramuscular vitamin K stat at birth and the paediatrician alerted to the possibilities of anticonvulsant drug withdrawal
Seizures	Most seizures in pregnancy will be self-limiting; if prolonged, however, rectal or intravenous diazepam or intravenous lorazepam IV with or without ventilation may be required
Postnatal	The mother may breast-feed safely (drugs pass into the milk but neonatal levels are low). Advice should be given about safe and suitable settings for feeding, bathing etc. Carbamazepine, phenytoin, primidone and phenobarbitone induce liver enzymes, reducing the effectiveness of the standard-dose combined oral contraceptives, and a higher-dose oestrogen preparation or alternative form of contraception is therefore required

Table 30.2	
Liver disorders specific to pregnancy	
Hyperemesis gravidarum	This may occasionally be associated with abnormal LFTs
Obstetric cholestasis	Usually presents after 30 weeks' gestation possibly due to a genetic predisposition to the cholestatic effect of oestrogens. Pruritus affects the limbs and trunk, and it is often severe. There may be a positive family history in up to 50% of cases Serum total bile acid concentration is increased early in the disease and is the optimum marker for the condition. Transaminases may be increased (less than three-fold). Bilirubin is usually <100 μmol/l, and there may be pale stools and dark urine There are no serious long-term maternal risks but there is a risk of preterm labour, fetal distress and intrauterine fetal death. Delivery at 37–38 weeks is appropriate in an effort to prevent fetal death. Maternal vitamin K is recommended and antihistamine treatment often prescribed for symptomatic relief
HELLP syndrome	See page 297
Acute fatty liver of pregnancy	This is very rare, carries a high maternal and fetal mortality, and may progress rapidly to hepatic failure. It usually presents with vomiting in the third trimester associated with malaise and abdominal pain followed by jaundice, thirst and alteration in consciousness level. LFTs are elevated, urate is very high and there is often profound hypoglycaemia. There may be hypertension and proteinuria. Coagulopathy, hypoglycaemia and fluid imbalance should be corrected and the fetus delivered. Following delivery there is a risk of postpartum haemorrhage and liver dysfunction may be prolonged. Hepatic encephalopathy may develop and liver transplant is occasionally necessary. If the patient recovers, there is no long-term liver impairment

fetus (mainly fetal growth restriction and preterm delivery). Some renal diseases carry a poorer prognosis than others and specialist advice is required.

Women with chronic renal disease should receive pre-pregnancy counselling. The woman should be seen frequently antenatally, particularly in the third trimester. Hypertension should be treated aggressively, U&Es, plasma protein, urinalysis and midstream urine (MSU) samples checked at each visit, and a 24-hour urine collection or protein–creatinine ratio sent each month to quantify proteinuria. Close fetal monitoring is important in the third trimester. It is difficult to distinguish pre-eclampsia from increasing renal compromise, as both may present with hypertension and proteinuria.

Table 30.3	
Liver disorders coincidental to pregnancy	
Viral hepatitis	This is the commonest cause of abnormal LFTs in pregnancy. Serology should be performed for hepatitis A, B and C as well as for cytomegalovirus (CMV), Epstein Barr virus (EBV) and toxoplasmosis (see p. 274)
Gallstones	Asymptomatic gallstones do not require treatment. Cholecystitis should be managed conservatively if possible
Cirrhosis	In severe cirrhosis there is usually amenorrhoea. If pregnancy occurs, and the disease is well compensated, there is usually no long-term effect on hepatic function. The main risk is bleeding from oesophageal varices
Chronic active hepatitis	This is usually associated with amenorrhoea. Pregnancy does not usually have any long-term effect on liver function. Obstetric complications are common and fetal loss rate is high. Immunosuppressant therapy with prednisolone and azathioprine should be continued in those with autoimmune disease
Primary biliary cirrhosis	This is variable in severity. The prognosis for mother and fetus is good in mild disease. It may present during pregnancy for the first time in a similar way to obstetric cholestasis

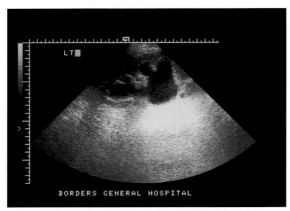

Fig. 30.6 Ultrasound of left kidney with ureteric obstruction and calyceal clubbing. There was a calculus in the lower third of the ureter.

Pregnancy should be discouraged in women on dialysis as the fetal prognosis is poor. Pregnancy in women who have had a renal transplant is increasingly common and usually successful with good allograft function.

Respiratory disorders

Breathlessness due to the physiological increase in ventilation is a common symptom in pregnancy. Although there is an increased tidal volume from early pregnancy, the exact cause of the feeling of breathlessness is unclear. Investigation should be considered only if there is excess breathlessness, or if there are clinical signs. It should be remembered that breathlessness can also be a feature of pulmonary thromboembolic disease and heart failure.

Asthma is a common condition. In most women the disease is unchanged in pregnancy. Treatment is similar to that outside of pregnancy and women already established on treatment should continue. Inhaled beta-sympathomimetics and inhaled steroids are considered safe. Oral steroids should be given if clinically indicated.

Thrombocytopenia

Maternal thrombocytopenia in pregnancy

In the second half of normal pregnancies there is a mild thrombocytopenia (platelet count $100-150 \times 10^9/l$) in 8% of women which is not associated with any additional risk to the mother or fetus. The platelet count may be reduced in pre-eclampsia.

Autoimmune thrombocytopenic purpura (AITP) is the commonest cause of thrombocytopenia in early pregnancy (but can also arise in later pregnancy) and may be acute or chronic. Antiplatelet antibodies may be detected. These may cross the placenta and, rarely, cause fetal thrombocytopenia, although this seldom is associated with long-term morbidity (cf. alloimmune thrombocytopenia below). No treatment is required in the absence of bleeding, providing the platelet count remains above $50 \times 10^9/l$. If the platelet count falls below this level, steroids and/or immunoglobulin can be given. Specialist haematological advice is appropriate before considering specific treatment.

Fetal (alloimmune) thrombocytopenia

This is a rare disorder in which there are maternal antibodies to fetal platelets. This has some similarities with rhesus disease in which there are maternal antibodies to the fetal red cells. The maternal platelet count is normal but there may be profound fetal thrombocytopenia and antenatal or intrapartum fetal intracranial haemorrhage. The diagnosis should be suspected when a previous child has experienced neonatal thrombocytopenia and maternal antiplatelet antibodies have been identified (often to the HPA-1a antigen).

Antenatal therapy is either with fetal platelet transfusion and/or maternal immunoglobulin and elective caesarean section.

Thyroid disorders

1% of pregnant women in the western world are affected by thyroid disease, with hypothyroidism being commoner than hyperthyroidism. The fetal thyroid gland secretes thyroid hormones from the 12th week and is independent of maternal control.

Hypothyroidism

This may present with fatigue, hair loss, dry skin, abnormal weight gain, poor appetite, cold intolerance, bradycardia and delayed tendon reflexes. If untreated there is an increase in the rate of spontaneous miscarriages and stillbirths compared to the euthyroid population, as well as a risk of fetal neurological impairment. There is minimal fetal risk if the mother is treated and is euthyroid. Thyroid function should be regularly monitored, aiming to keep TSH and free T4 within the normal range for pregnancy. If the woman is already on treatment and euthyroid at booking, the dose probably need not be increased. Fetal hypothyroidism may occur when the mother carries antithyroid antibodies or is receiving antithyroid medication.

Hyperthyroidism

Thyrotoxicosis presents with weight loss, exophthalmos, tachycardia and restlessness. It is usually due to Graves' disease but may occur secondary to a toxic thyroid adenoma or multinodular goitre. Untreated thyrotoxicosis is associated with a high fetal mortality and a risk of maternal thyroid crisis at delivery. Well-controlled hyperthyroidism is not associated with an increase in fetal anomalies but there is a tendency for babies to be small for gestational age. Graves' disease usually improves during pregnancy.

Carbimazole and propylthiouracil cross the placenta and can potentially cause fetal thyroid suppression, but in low doses this is rarely significant. Radioactive iodine is contraindicated in pregnancy and surgery is indicated only for those with a very large goitre or poor compliance with oral therapy.

Postpartum thyroiditis

This occurs following 5–10% of all pregnancies, with initial hyperthyroidism followed by hypothyroidism and then recovery. Because the hypothyroidism occurs at around 1–3 months, the condition may be confused with postnatal depression. Symptoms of hyperthyroidism may be treated with propranolol (antithyroid drugs accelerate the appearance of hypothyroidism). Hypothyroidism should be treated with thyroxine as above, withdrawing around 6 months after delivery. A small proportion of affected women may require long-term treatment or may develop hypothyroidism later in life.

Key points

- Diabetes carries increased risks of congenital abnormality, macrosomia and intrauterine death for the fetus. Good peri-conceptual and maternal glycaemic control is the cornerstone of management.
- Pregnancy-related venous thromboembolic disease is the commonest direct cause of maternal mortality in many western countries. Relevant symptoms should be appropriately investigated. Thromboembolic prophylaxis is important in both obstetrics and gynaecological practice.
- Anticonvulsants, particularly sodium valproate and polytherapy, increase the risk of fetal abnormality.
- Abnormal liver function tests may be related to the pregnancy, but are commonly due to incidental viral infections.
- Asymptomatic UTIs should be treated.
- Well-controlled thyroid disease poses little serious risk to the mother or fetus.

31

Prenatal diagnosis

Introduction

The finding of some 'abnormality' in pregnancy transforms what was previously an exciting and joyous event into a worrying and distressing time. Tact, understanding and reassurance (if appropriate) are paramount. The very greatest of care should be taken in explaining any findings to parents. The advice given to parents is of such importance that it will frequently be necessary to involve senior members of the obstetric team as well as members of other specialties, particularly paediatricians, and clinical geneticists and radiologists.

The aims of prenatal diagnosis are fourfold:

- the identification at an early gestation of abnormalities incompatible with survival, or likely to result in severe handicap, in order to prepare parents and offer the option of termination of pregnancy (TOP)
- the identification of conditions which may influence the timing, site or mode of delivery
- the identification of fetuses who would benefit from early paediatric intervention
- the identification of fetuses who may benefit from in-utero treatment (rare).

It should not be assumed that all parents are going to request TOP even in the presence of lethal abnormality. Many couples have opted to continue pregnancies in the face of severe defects which have resulted in either intrauterine or early neonatal death, and have expressed the view that they found it easier to cope with their grief having held their child. Others say that they were glad of the opportunity to terminate the pregnancy at an early stage and that they could not have coped with going on. More controversial still are the problems of chronic diseases with long-term handicap and long-term suffering for both the child and the parents. The parents themselves must decide what action they wish to take – it is they who will have to live with the decisions they make. It is our role to advise, guide and respect their final wishes, irrespective of our own personal views.

Non-directive counselling

When parents are found to have an abnormal baby they often know little or nothing about the abnormality, about termination or about recurrence risks. They need information, and it is the role of obstetricians and genetic counsellors to inform accurately and in language that is clear to understand. Often parents ask the doctor what he or she would do, but it remains important to encourage the couple towards their own decision.

Non-directive counselling has to be truly non-directive. The sentence 'the risk of handicap is 5%' sounds worse than 'the baby has a 95% chance of being normal'. Expressions like 'high risk' or 'severe handicap' imply a value judgment and should be avoided if possible. 'Common' may be interpreted as anything from 1% to 99%, depending on the context and the listener.

It is sometimes helpful to give information in writing, as well as verbally. Parents may need time to take in information, and it is often important that they take time to consider any decisions carefully. It can be extremely useful to arrange a review a day or two after the initial appointment.

The spectrum of congenital abnormality

Although most congenital abnormalities are individually rare, together they cause an enormous burden of suffering. Approximately 2% of newborn babies have a serious abnormality detectable at, or soon after, birth. The main ones are listed in **Box 31.1**.

Assessing the risk

In general, the risks for most couples are very small, although the risk of Down syndrome (history box) increases with increasing maternal age. In some instances, however, there may be a family history of an inherited condition – for example, Duchenne muscular dystrophy, cystic fibrosis, sickle cell disease or myotonic dystrophy. Consanguinity increases the risk of genetic problems, particularly in relation to autosomal recessive conditions. Structural abnormalities are also usually slightly more likely to occur in those with a family history; for example, a woman who has had

a child with spina bifida has an approximately 2% risk of a recurrence compared to the background risk of ≈0.2%.

History

John Langdon Down (1828–1896) was a liberal Victorian physician who defended the higher education of women, opposed slavery, and supported the unity of mankind. In a paper entitled 'Observations on the Ethnic Classification of Idiots' he put forward the theory that it was possible to classify different types of conditions by ethnic characteristics. He listed several types, including Down syndrome, which he classified as the 'Mongolian type of Idiot'.

In addition, it is important to consider medical conditions. Those with diabetes have an increased risk of cardiac and neural tube defects, and those with epilepsy are also at increased risk of structural problems, particularly if taking potentially teratogenic anticonvulsants. The majority of structural and chromosomal problems, however, occur in those who have no predisposing history or recognized risk factors, and screening tests are offered to those at apparently low risk.

Screening for fetal abnormalities

The decision to screen for abnormality rests with each individual couple. Some wish no screening tests at all, others may be keen to consider all of the options below. A number of screening strategies are available **(Table 31.1)**.

Ultrasound scanning

Structural anomalies are seen on ultrasound scan and most clinicians advocate that all mothers should be offered a detailed ultrasound at around 18–21 weeks' gestation. This has the advantage that those with major or lethal anomalies (e.g. spina bifida or renal agenesis) can be offered termination, and it also allows planned deliveries of those conditions which may require early neonatal intervention (e.g. gastroschisis or transposition of the great arteries).

Scanning has the limitation, however, that many defects are not identified. It is likely, for example, that less than 50% of cardiac defects are recognized and the false reassurance provided by a scan may become a source of parental resentment. Furthermore, a 'soft marker' may be uncovered, the significance of which is often unclear. These soft markers are ultrasound appearances which in themselves are not an abnormality, but which may point to other problems, particularly chromosomal abnormalities. They are found in approximately 5% of all pregnancies at a second-trimester scan and cause of a lot of parental anxiety. Such markers include choroid plexus cysts **(Fig. 31.1)**, mild renal pelvic dilatation, echogenic cardiac foci **(Fig. 31.2)**,

---

Box 31.1

Selected congenital abnormalities

Genetic disorders

- Down syndrome (trisomy 21)
- Edwards syndrome (trisomy 18)
- Patau syndrome (trisomy 13)
- Triploidy
- Sex chromosome abnormalities
- XO (Turner syndrome)
- XXY (Klinefelter syndrome)
- XYY
- XXX
- Apparently balanced rearrangements (translocations or inversions)
- Unbalanced chromosomal structural abnormalities
- Gene disorders (e.g. fragile X syndrome, Huntington's chorea, Tay–Sachs disease)

Structural disorders

- Congenital heart disease
- Neural tube defects (e.g. anencephaly, encephalocele, spina bifida)
- Abdominal wall defects (e.g. exomphalos, gastroschisis)
- Genitourinary abnormalities (e.g. renal dysplasia, polycystic kidney disease, pyelectasis, posterior urethral valves, Potter syndrome)
- Lung disorders (e.g. pulmonary hypoplasia, diaphragmatic herniae, cystic fibrosis)

Congenital infection

- Toxoplasmosis
- Rubella
- Cytomegalovirus
- Herpes simplex virus
- Chickenpox
- Erythrovirus
- Hepatitis
- *Listeria monocytogenes*
- Syphilis
- Beta-haemolytic streptococci – group B

Table 31.1

Overview of potential screening programmes for chromosomal and structural abnormalities

Programme	Advantages	Disadvantages
NT and serum at 11–14 weeks	Good detection of Down syndrome at early gestation (11–14 weeks)	Use of CVS may increase miscarriage rate Minimal detection of structural abnormalities
NT and serum at 11–14 weeks and FDS at 18 weeks	Good detection of Down syndrome at early gestation (11–14 weeks) Good detection of structural abnormalities	Use of CVS may increase miscarriage rate
FDS at 18 weeks	Good detection of structural abnormalities	Minimal detection of Down syndrome
Serum screening alone at 16 weeks	Good detection of Down syndrome Amniocentesis may be safer than CVS Reasonable detection of open lesions, particularly neural tube defects	Minimal detection of other structural abnormalities
Serum screening at 16 weeks with FDS at 18 weeks	Good detection of Down syndrome Amniocentesis may be safer than CVS Good detection of structural abnormalities	Down syndrome not identified until relatively late (17–18 weeks)

CVS, chorionic villus sampling; FDS, fetal detailed scan; NT, nuchal translucency.

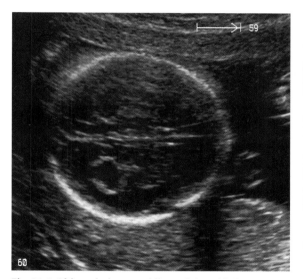

Fig. 31.1 Although there are bilateral choroid plexus cysts, the baby was karyotypically normal.

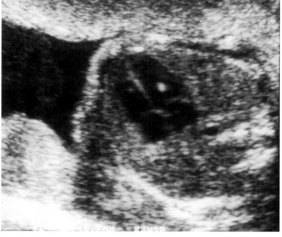

Fig. 31.2 Echogenic focus in the left ventricle of a four-chamber cardiac view.

and mild cerebral ventricular dilatation. If the soft marker is isolated, the risk of chromosomal problems is low, but if more than one is found, or if there are any other structural defects, the risk of a chromosomal problem is very much higher.

Unlike structural abnormalities, chromosomal abnormalities can be much more difficult to identify on ultrasound scan. Around two-thirds of fetuses with Down syndrome (trisomy 21) will have a normal appearance at 18 weeks, and the remaining third may demonstrate only minor defects which are not pathognomonic of the condition. Most fetuses with the less common trisomies, e.g. Edwards syndrome (trisomy 18 – history box) or Patau syndrome (trisomy

13 – history box), do show some abnormality, although the abnormality is again often neither specific nor diagnostic. As Edwards and Patau syndromes are usually lethal in the perinatal period, there are fewer lifelong implications than for Down syndrome. Much of the screening work has therefore been directed at Down's, in particular measuring specific markers in the maternal blood (serological screening), or measuring the thickness of nuchal fluid behind the fetal neck (nuchal translucency assessment).

Serological screening

This is used almost exclusively to detect two abnormalities: spina bifida and Down syndrome. Alpha-fetoprotein (αFP) is an alpha-globulin of similar molecular weight to albumin

John Hilton Edwards (1928–2007) was an English physician and medical geneticist who is credited with the first description, in 1960, of Edwards syndrome.

History

Klaus Patau (1908–1975), a German-born American human geneticist, named the syndrome caused by an extra chromosome 13 as Bartholin–Patau syndrome after Thomas Bartholin (1616–1680), discoverer of the lymphatic system, and who first observed clinical features of trisomy 13.

which is synthesized by the fetal liver. If there is a break in the fetal skin (for example with spina bifida), αFP escapes into the maternal circulation and the maternal serum level becomes elevated.

Normal serum αFP levels rise with advancing gestation and most laboratories report results as multiples of the median (MoM) for unaffected pregnancies at the gestation of sampling. A level of 1.0 is normal, and for screening purposes levels raised to more than 2.0–2.5 MoM indicate the need for detailed scanning to look for neural tube defects, twins, gastroschisis or intrauterine death. As there is a large overlap between normal and affected pregnancies, a raised level of maternal serum αFP is therefore only a screening test and not a diagnostic test. The scan provides the diagnosis.

It has also been observed that the level of maternal serum αFP is lower than expected when the fetus has Down syndrome. The reason for this remains unclear but the result can be combined with maternal age to give an estimated risk of the fetus being affected. This risk can be further modified by measuring human chorionic gonadotrophin (hCG; raised in Down's) and unconjugated oestriol (low in Down's) – the so-called 'triple test'. Again, there is considerable overlap between the levels in unaffected and affected pregnancies, so any test which uses these markers can only give an estimation of risk, not a definite diagnosis. Unfortunately, as we have seen, there is no simple ultrasound test for Down syndrome and the parents have to weigh up the risks of the more invasive tests of amniocentesis and chorionic villus sampling (CVS).

Nuchal translucency

Screening for Down syndrome is also possible by measuring the fetal nuchal translucency (NT) on first-trimester ultrasound scanning **(Fig. 31.3)**. The risk of Down syndrome increases with larger NT measurements. NT measurement is combined with first trimester biochemistry in order to provide an estimate of risk of Down syndrome. CVS may then be used to establish an earlier diagnosis than with amniocentesis

(see below), thereby allowing an early surgical termination of pregnancy rather than a late medical termination. There is, however, evidence to suggest that parental psychological morbidity is independent of whether a diagnosis is made in the first or second trimester, and indeed medical termination may carry less psychological morbidity than surgical (even if medical complications are higher).

Increased nuchal translucency is also a marker for structural defects, particularly cardiac, renal, abdominal wall as well as diaphragmatic herniae.

Diagnosis of chromosomal abnormalities

Diagnostic tests are offered if screening tests suggest that the mother is above a certain risk level of carrying a baby with a chromosomal abnormality. A risk threshold of 1 in 250 or higher is commonly used.

Amniocentesis

Diagnostic amniocentesis may be performed after 15 weeks' gestation. A 22-gauge needle is inserted into the amniotic cavity under ultrasound control and 10–15 ml of amniotic fluid are drawn off **(Fig. 31.4)**. Rhesus-negative women are given anti-D immunoglobulin to prevent immunization. The risk of miscarriage is around 1%.

Karyotype results are usually available within 3 weeks, but rapid FISH (fluorescence in-situ hybridization) or quantitative PCR (polymerase chain reaction) techniques may be used to exclude the commoner aneuploidies; the result is available within 72 hours.

Chorionic villus sampling

CVS or placental biopsy may be performed any time after 10 weeks' gestation. Either a flexible cannula is passed through the cervix, or a needle is passed transabdominally – both under ultrasound control **(Fig. 31.5)**. Results are usually available within 72 hours, the full karyotype within 3 weeks. CVS may carry the same complication rate as an amniocentesis, but for most practitioners CVS probably carries a higher risk of miscarriage (2%).

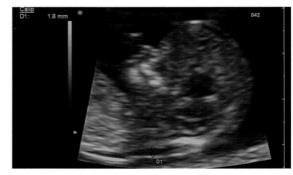

Fig. 31.3 This is the view required to measure the nuchal translucency (between the on screen calipers).

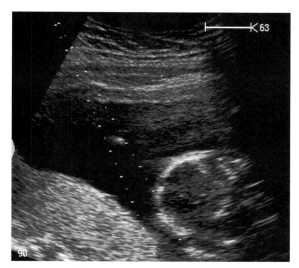

Fig. 31.4 Amniocentesis is carried out under direct ultrasound guidance. The tip of the needle can be seen between the dotted guidelines 2 cm above the fetal head.

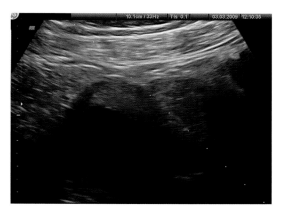

Fig. 31.5 Chrionic Villus Sampling is performed under direct, real time ultrasound imaging. Here, the needle follows the on screen needle guide dots. (Courtesy of Dr M Ledingham, Glasgow.)

Structural and chromosomal abnormalities

Down syndrome (trisomy 21)

The overall incidence is 1:650 live births, but the incidence increases with increasing maternal age:

20 years 1:2000
30 years 1:900
35 years 1:350
36 years 1:240
38 years 1:180
40 years 1:100
44 years 1:40

Most Down syndrome children, however, are born to younger mothers, as there are overall many more younger mothers than older ones. Although walking, language and self-care skills are usually attained, independence is rare. There is mental retardation (with a mean IQ around 50) and an association with congenital heart disease. Gastrointestinal atresia is common, and there is early dementia with similarities to Alzheimer's disease. 20% die before the age of 1 year and 45% by the age of 60 years.

95% of cases are due to non-dysjunction, with translocation 14:21 accounting for 2%, other translocations accounting for 2% and mosaicism 1%. Half of the translocations occur de novo. The recurrence risk for non-dysjunction is ≈1:100 if the mother is less than 35 years old and approximately four times the baseline risk if she is more than 35 years old. If there is a 14:21 translocation in the mother, the recurrence risk is 1:10, and if in the father, 1:50.

Edwards syndrome (trisomy 18)

The incidence is around 1:2500 live births and most are due to non-dysjunction. The baby has intrauterine growth restriction (IUGR), a small elongated head (strawberry-shaped on ultrasound), severe mental retardation, rocker bottom feet, and an increased incidence of gastrointestinal and renal anomalies. Virtually all have congenital heart disease, often a ventriculoseptal defect. 50% die before the age of 2 months and 90% before the end of the first year.

Patau syndrome (trisomy 13)

This is rare, at around 1:5000 live births. There is IUGR, severe mental retardation, and an increased incidence of cleft palate, gastrointestinal atresias and holoprosencephaly. Again, most have congenital heart disease. The majority of children die before the age of 3 months, and survival is rare after the age of 1 year.

Triploidy

These children rarely survive to birth and there is no survival beyond the neonatal period.

Turner syndrome (XO)

This occurs in around 1:3000 live births: 60% are pure XO; just over 15% are mosaics (usually XO/XX); and the rest are deletions, rings or isochromosomes of Xq or Xp. The incidence is increased with increasing paternal age and decreased with increasing maternal age. Antenatally there may be a cystic hygroma ± generalized oedema and cardiac defects **(Fig. 31.6)**. The child may have short stature, cubitus valgus, coarctation of the aorta, a bicuspid aortic valve, streak gonads and only occasionally a lowered IQ. A small proportion may have fertility (particularly mosaics and deletions), although the incidence of premature ovarian failure is high.

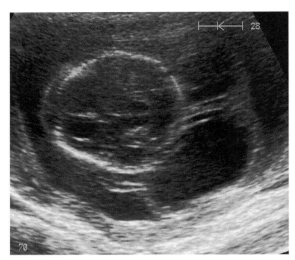

Fig. 31.6 Cystic hygroma. There is a massive loculated cystic swelling behind the fetal neck.

XXX

The incidence of 1:1000 live births is doubled or tripled when the maternal age is more than 40 years. The phenotype and fertility are normal and the abnormality frequently goes unnoticed. There is, however, an increased risk of sex chromosome abnormalities (≈4%) and premature menopause in the offspring. XXX+ (i.e. more than three X chromosomes) is rare. Dysmorphism and mental retardation in this group are common, as is menstrual dysfunction. The individual may be fertile.

Klinefelter syndrome (XXY)

This is uncommon, at around 1:700–2000 live births (history box). The individual is phenotypically a tall male, with occasionally a reduced IQ, sparse facial hair and gynaecomastia. It is the commonest single cause of male hypogonadism and is usually diagnosed in the investigation of male infertility. There is an association with hypothyroidism, diabetes and asthma. Azoospermia is usual.

 History

The second most common extra chromosome condition is named after Harry Klinefelter (b. 1912), an endocrinologist from Massachusetts, who first described it in 1942.

XYY

Again, this is uncommon, at around 1:700 live births, and there is no association with maternal age. The IQ and fertility are usually normal and the suggestion of increased impulsive behaviour may be biased by the population sampled. Individuals are usually tall. The risk of sex chromosome abnormalities in offspring is ≈4%.

Apparently balanced rearrangements (translocations or inversions)

If apparently balanced rearrangements are found at amniocentesis, it is essential to check the karyotype of both parents. If one parent has the translocation and is phenotypically normal, it is likely that the fetus will be phenotypically normal as well. There is a chance that other offspring (or offspring of the fetus) will have an unbalanced translocation, and counselling ± karyotyping should be offered. In general, the smaller the section of chromosome involved, the greater the likelihood of a fetus surviving to term with an unbalanced translocation. Offspring may, of course, also have normal karyotypes without the translocation. If the translocation has occurred de novo, the overall risk of phenotypic abnormality is in the order of 10%, but as some chromosomal rearrangements are normal population variants, genetic advice should always be sought.

Unbalanced chromosomal structural abnormalities

Many chromosomal structural abnormalities are well characterized, but it is often difficult to be specific. Parental karyotyping is required and genetic advice should be sought. Mental impairment is common, and physical abnormality is possible.

Cystic hygroma (see Fig. 31.6)

Cystic hygromas are fluid-filled swellings at the back of the fetal neck which probably develop because of a defect in the formation of lymphatic vessels. It is likely that the lymphatic and venous systems fail to connect and lymph fluid accumulates in the jugular lymph sacs. Larger hygromas are frequently divided by septae and may be associated with skin oedema, ascites, pleural and pericardial effusions, and cardiac and renal abnormalities. There is also an association with aneuploidy (particularly Turner's, Down's, Edwards') and it is appropriate to offer karyotyping. If generalized fetal hydrops is present, the prognosis is bleak. Isolated hygromas may be surgically corrected postnatally and have a good prognosis. Only rarely are they so large as to result in problems with labour.

Congenital heart disease

This is the commonest congenital malformation in children and affects about 5–8:1000 live births. Of defects diagnosed antenatally, about 15% are associated with aneuploidy, most commonly trisomies 18 and 21.

The four-chamber view of the heart can be used as a screening test **(Fig. 31.2)** and will identify 25–40% of all major abnormalities, particularly ventriculoseptal defect, ventricular hypoplasia **(Fig. 31.7),** valvular incompetence and arrhythmias. Moving above the four-chamber view allows the aorta and pulmonary artery to be visualized **(Fig. 31.8)**. This increases the sensitivity to identify over 60% of cardiac defects by screening for Fallot's tetralogy (history box) and transposition of the great arteries. At 18 weeks, most of these major connections can be seen, but high-risk pregnancies (e.g. those with diabetes, or women taking anticonvulsants, or who have a personal or family history of congenital heart disease) should be re-scanned at 22–26 weeks for more minor defects.

History

Etienne-Louis Arthur Fallot (1850–1911) was a professor of forensic medicine and hygiene in Marseille. He had a reputation as an astute clinician and for accurate careful physical examination.

Neural tube defects

The neural tube is formed from the closing of the neural folds, with both anterior and posterior neuropores closed by 6 weeks' gestation **(Fig. 31.9)**. Failure of closure of the anterior neuropore results in anencephaly or an encephalocele, and failure of posterior closure results in spina bifida. The European incidence of neural tube defects is around 1:1000 pregnancies.

Anencephaly   The skull vault and cerebral cortex are absent. The infant is either stillborn or, if live born, will usually die shortly after birth.

Encephalocele   There is a bony defect in the cranial vault through which a dura mater sac (± brain tissue) protrudes **(Fig. 31.10)**. This may be occipital or frontal. Small isolated encephaloceles carry a good prognosis, whereas those with microcephaly secondary to brain herniation carry a very poor prognosis.

Spina bifida (Figs 31.11 and 31.12)   This may take the form of a meningocele or a myelomeningocele. In a meningocele the meninges of the neural tissue bulge through a posterior spinal wall defect, whereas in a myelomeningocele the central canal of the cord is also exposed. Those with spinal meningoceles usually have normal lower limb neurology and 20% have hydrocephalus. Those with myelomeningoceles usually have abnormal lower limb neurology and many have

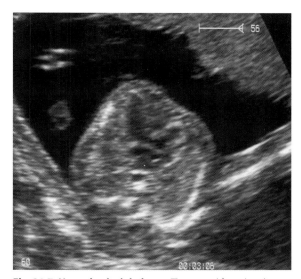

Fig. 31.7 Hypoplastic right heart. The normal four chamber view is not obtained. the baby died in the early neonatal period.

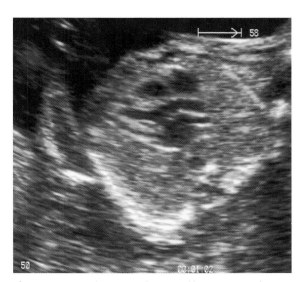

Fig. 31.8 Aorta. The aorta in this normal heart is seen to be arising exclusively from the left ventricle, excluding the diagnosis of Fallot's tetralogy.

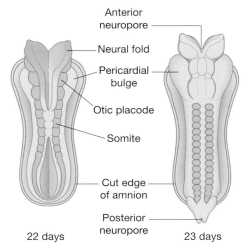

Anterior neuropore

Neural fold

Pericardial bulge

Otic placode

Somite

Cut edge of amnion

Posterior neuropore

22 days

23 days

Fig. 31.9 Dorsal view of embryo on days 22 and 23, demonstrating neural tube closure.

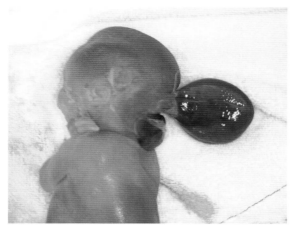

Fig. 31.10 Encephalocele. There is a defect in the posterior aspect of the skull, allowing brain tissue to herniate into the sac.

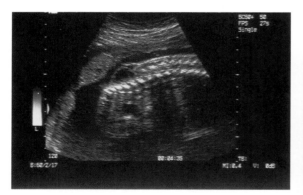

Fig. 31.11 Spina bifida. There is a large lumbosacral defect, with the sac of the myelomeningocele clearly visible.

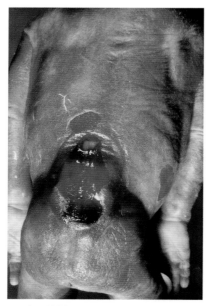

Fig. 31.12 Spina bifida.

hydrocephalus. In addition to immobility and mental retardation, there may be problems with urinary tract infection, bladder dysfunction, bowel dysfunction, and social and sexual isolation.

Daily folic acid taken from before conception reduces the recurrence risk of neural tube defects in those who have had a previously affected child. A pre-conceptual prophylactic dose for all women who are planning a pregnancy probably also offers some protection.

Abdominal wall defects

Exomphalos (Fig. 31.13)

This occurs following failure of the gut to return to the abdominal cavity at 8 weeks' gestation and results in a defect through which the peritoneal sac protrudes. The sac may contain both intestines and liver. There are chromosomal abnormalities in 30% (especially trisomy 18) and 10–50%

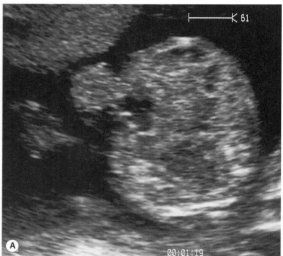

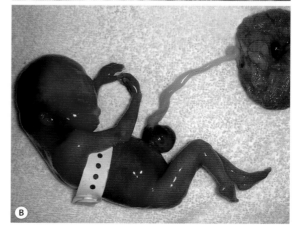

Fig. 31.13 Small exomphalos in a fetus terminated for multiple abnormalities.

have other lesions, particularly cardiac and renal. There is also an association with ectopia vesicae and ectopia cardia (midline bladder and cardiac herniae). If the exomphalos is isolated (i.e. no other structural abnormalities), the chromosomes are normal and there is no bowel atresia or infarction, the prognosis is good (>80% long-term survival). The sac rarely ruptures at vaginal delivery.

Gastroschisis (Fig. 31.14)

There is an abdominal wall defect usually to the right and below the insertion of the umbilical cord. Small bowel (without a peritoneal covering) protrudes and floats free in the peritoneal fluid. Gut atresias and cardiac lesions occur in 20% but the association with chromosomal abnormality is very small (probably <1%). The prognosis is good if the bowel is viable, although 10% end in stillbirth despite apparently normal growth. Gut dilatation may be associated with bowel obstruction or ischaemia but is not directly linked to prognosis. These babies are usually small for dates and require very close surveillance. The recurrence risk is less than 1%.

Genitourinary abnormalities

Multicystic dysplastic kidneys

The kidneys have large discrete non-communicating cysts with a central, more solid core and are thought to follow early developmental failure **(Fig 31.15)**. The inheritance is sporadic. If the cysts affect only one kidney, the other is normal, and there is adequate liquor, the prognosis is good. If the cysts are bilateral and the liquor is reduced, the prognosis is poor.

Polycystic kidney disease

Adult polycystic kidney disease has an autosomal dominant inheritance and is relatively benign, often not producing symptoms until the fifth decade of life. Many individuals have ultrasonically normal kidneys at birth.

Infantile polycystic kidney disease has an autosomal recessive inheritance. There is a wide range of expression, with the size of cysts ranging from microscopic to several millimetres across. Both kidneys are affected, and there may also be cysts present in the liver and pancreas. Ultrasound features of oligohydramnios, empty bladder, and large symmetrical bright kidneys **(Fig. 31.16)** may not develop until later in pregnancy. If there is survival beyond the neonatal period, there may be later problems with raised blood pressure and progressive renal failure. Long-term survival is rare.

Pyelectasis (Fig. 31.17)

Renal pelvic dilatation may be unilateral (79–90%) or bilateral. It is probably caused by a neuromuscular defect at the junction of the ureter and the renal pelvis, and presents with increasing pelvic dilatation in the presence of a normal ureter. As there is an association with postnatal urinary tract infections and reflux nephropathy, it is reasonable to start all affected neonates on prophylactic antibiotics and arrange postnatal radiological follow-up. Even in those with mild dilatation (≥5mm and <10mm) there is vesicoureteric reflux in 10–20%, although only a small proportion require surgery.

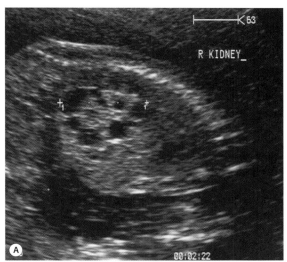

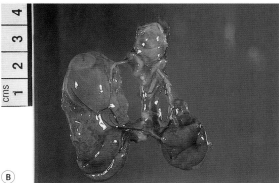

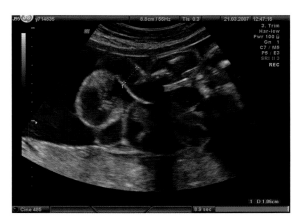

Fig. 31.14 Gastroschisis, with multiple loops of bowel free in the amniotic fluid.

Fig. 31.15 Dysplastic renal scan. Note the enlarged kidney containing fluid-filled cysts: **(A)** ultrasound; **(B)** postmortem specimen.

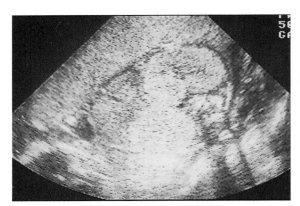

Fig. 31.16 Infantile renal cystic scan. Note anhydramnios and bright renal echoes from the microscopically small cysts.

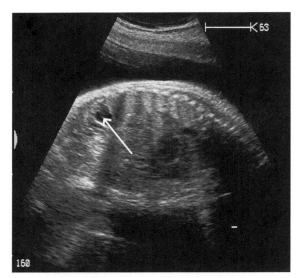

Fig. 31.17 Pyelectasis. The renal pelvis is markedly dilated, although the renal cortex looks well preserved.

Posterior urethral valves

In this condition, folds of mucosa at the bladder neck prevent urine leaving the bladder. The fetus is usually male, there is often oligohydramnios, and on ultrasound there are varying degrees of renal dysplasia. There is a chromosomal abnormality in 7% of isolated defects, and in one-third of those with other abnormalities. It may be possible to insert a 'pigtail' shunt between the bladder and amniotic cavity to relieve the obstruction, but the long-term prognosis is still poor as the renal damage may not be reversible.

Potter syndrome

Bilateral renal agenesis (Potter syndrome – history box) is associated with extreme oligohydramnios which leads to the Potter's sequence of pulmonary hypoplasia (see below) and limb deformity (due to fetal compression). The condition

is lethal. The recurrence risk is approximately 3% although autosomal dominant forms with variable penetrance have been described.

 History

Edith Louise Potter (1901–1993), from Iowa, described this syndrome. Importantly, she had the insight to realize that teratogenic syndromes involving apparently unrelated organs might result from the timing of a specific teratogenic influence.

Lung disorders

Pulmonary hypoplasia

Liquor is important for alveolar maturation, particularly in the second trimester. Without liquor there will be pulmonary hypoplasia. Severe oligohydramnios occurs if there is very preterm pre-labour membrane rupture or Potter syndrome (see above). Pulmonary hypoplasia also occurs with diaphragmatic herniae as there is no room for lung expansion.

Diaphragmatic hernia

Stomach, colon and even spleen can enter the chest through a defect in the diaphragm, usually on the left. The heart is pushed to the right and the lungs become hypoplastic. The incidence of aneuploidy is 15–30% and there is an association with neural tube defects, congenital heart disease, and renal and skeletal abnormalities. The overall survival for left-sided diaphragmatic herniae (which accounts for about 80% of cases) diagnosed antenatally in North America and Europe is around 70–80%; the prognosis for right-sided herniae is less good. Current research is looking at the best ways to predict those that have a higher mortality and morbidity, and to consider fetal therapy in this group. Polyhydramnios, mediastinal shift and left ventricular compression are poor antenatal prognostic factors. Postnatal surgery aims to reduce the hernia and close the diaphragmatic defect.

Single gene disorders

There is a very large number of single gene disorders, and many of these are amenable to prenatal diagnosis. A few of these are described below to illustrate some of the diagnostic issues.

Cystic fibrosis

The UK gene frequency for cystic fibrosis is 1:20 (i.e. heterozygote frequency) and the estimated overall couple risk for a live birth is around 1:2500 (there is probably an increased miscarriage rate in homozygotes). Clinically there is respiratory, gastrointestinal, liver and pancreatic dysfunction and azoospermia is usual in males. The prognosis is very variable – although death around the age of 20–30 still occurs, the prognosis is improving and many affected individuals now live considerably longer. The health of an affected sibling is not a prognostic guide to the health of other siblings. Four mutant alleles account for 85% of the gene defects in the UK (the commonest being DF508), and antenatal screening for these is possible using saliva specimens, with CVS offered if both parents are gene carriers.

Fragile X syndrome

This is the commonest cause of moderate mental retardation after Down syndrome and the commonest form of inherited mental handicap. It is X-linked. Males are usually more severely affected than females. Speech delay is common and there is an associated behavioural phenotype with gaze aversion. The condition is caused by the expansion of a CGG triplet repeat on the X chromosome. Normal individuals have an average of 29 repeats, but for an unexplained reason this may increase to a pre-mutation of 50–200 repeats. Those with a pre-mutation are phenotypically normal, but the pre-mutation is unstable during female meiosis and can expand to a full mutation of more than 200 repeats. There is an approximately 10% chance of this occurring (in the absence of a full mutation in that generation already). This causes the fragile X phenotype in 99% of males and around 30–50% of females. Parental screening is possible and CVS may be used to identify the degree of amplification of the CGG repeats in potential offspring.

Huntington's chorea

The onset of this autosomal dominant condition is usually after the age of 30, although it may present as early as 10–15 years of age (history box). There is dementia, mood change (usually depression) and choreoathetosis, progressing to death in approximately 15 years. It is caused by a CAG trinucleotide expansion on chromosome 4p and this allows accurate carrier and prenatal testing. There are major ethical issues around testing both mothers and their offspring.

History

George Huntington (1778–1858), from Long Island, first observed this syndrome as a child while riding with his father (also a physician) on his rounds. 'Driving with my father through a wooded road leading from East Hampton to Amagansett, we suddenly came upon two women bowing, twisting, and grimacing. I stared in wonderment, almost in fear. What could it mean? From this point on my interest in the disease has never wholly ceased.'

Tay–Sachs disease

The gene frequency is 1:30 in Ashkenazi Jews, but is rare in other groups (history box). There is a build-up of gangliosides within the CNS, leading to mental retardation, paralysis and blindness. By the age of 4 years, the child is usually dead or in a vegetative state. Carriers may be screened by measuring the level of hexosaminidase A in leucocytes.

History

Warren Tay (1843–1927), an ophthalmologist from Yorkshire, and Bernard Sachs (1854–1944), a neurologist and psychiatrist of Jewish descent from Bavaria, described this syndrome. It was originally named as 'Amaurotic Familial Idiocy'.

Prenatal congenital infection

Infections in pregnancy are especially important because of potential risks to the fetus. A number of agents are known to be teratogenic, particularly in the first and early second trimesters. Others carry the risk of miscarriage, premature labour, severe neonatal sepsis or long-term carrier states.

Risk factors

Farm workers are at risk of chlamydial infection (which causes abortion in sheep) and listerial infection, both of which can cause abortion in humans. Care is required particularly at lambing time. Toxoplasma may also be acquired from cows, sheep and domestic cats. Certain foods have also been implicated in congenital infection **(Table 31.2)**.

Specific infections (see also Table 31.3)

Infections in general raise the maternal levels of immunoglobulins of both the IgG and IgM variety. Maternal IgG crosses the placenta, while IgM, a much larger molecule, does not. The fetus does not make IgM until beyond 20 weeks' gestation and its presence in fetal or early neonatal blood implies infection. Infection does not necessarily mean that the infection has caused a problem, and absence of fetal or neonatal IgM at sampling does not completely exclude intrauterine infection.

Table 31.2	
Foods that carry potential infection risks in pregnancy	
Soft cheeses	Unpasteurized milk and its products may contain listeria. Those made from pasteurized milk are safe
Raw eggs	Must be avoided as there is a risk of salmonella (including puddings)
Meat or pâté	Undercooked meat may transmit toxoplasma or rarely listeria
Fruit	This should always be washed before eating as it may be contaminated with salmonella, toxoplasma or one of several intestinal parasites

Chickenpox at term (see Table 31.3 **for chickenpox in early pregnancy**)

Severe and even fatal cases of chickenpox can occur in neonates whose mothers develop chickenpox just before delivery, as the baby is born before maternal IgG production has increased sufficiently to allow passive transplacental protection. If maternal infection occurs 1–4 weeks before delivery, up to 50% of babies are infected and approximately a quarter of these develop clinical varicella. Severe infection is most likely to occur if the infant is born within 7 days of onset of the mother's rash, when cord blood IgG is low.

Table 31.3

Infections in pregnancy

Agent	Epidemiology	Maternal features	Fetal, neonatal and infant features	Risk	Treatment/ Prevention
Rubella	Person to person. UK immunity now 97% and congenital infection is rare	Asymptomatic or mild maculopapular rash	Miscarriage IUGR, ↓ platelets, hepatosplenomegaly, jaundice, deafness, congenital heart disease, mental retardation, cataracts, microphthalmia, microcephaly, cerebral palsy	Risk of affected fetus: <4 weeks 50% 5–8 weeks 25% 9–12 weeks 10% >13 weeks 1%	Consider TOP if <12 weeks. Postnatal maternal vaccination if she is not immune
Toxoplasmosis (protozoan – *Toxoplasma gondii*)	From cats, uncooked meats and unwashed fruits	May have fever, rash and lymphadenopathy, but most are asymptomatic	Hydrocephalus, chorioretinitis, intracranial calcification, ↓ platelets	<12 weeks: transmission is 10–25%, of which 75% will be severely affected 12–28 weeks: transmission is 54%, of which 25% will be severely affected >28 weeks: transmission is 65%–90%, of which <10% will be severely affected	Consider TOP only if primary infection <20 weeks
CMV (herpesvirus)	Person to person	Nearly always asymptomatic	Hepatosplenomegaly, ↓ platelets, IUGR, microcephaly, sensorineural deafness, chorioretinitis, hydrops fetalis, exomphalos, cerebral palsy	40% fetuses infected. Risk is unaffected by gestation. Of these, 90% are normal at birth, although 20% develop late sequelae. Of the 10% who are symptomatic, 33% die and the rest have long-term problems	Primary infection carries a 10–25% risk of severe abnormality.
Erythrovirus	Respiratory transmission.	Erythema infectiosum (slapped cheek disease). May be asymptomatic	Aplastic anaemia, hydrops fetalis (Fig. 31.18) and myocarditis ± fetal loss (if <20 weeks). Transmission <20 weeks ≈10%, of which ≈10% are lost. If >20 weeks, transmission ≈60%, but no adverse effects have been demonstrated	If <20 weeks and fetus survives the infection (≈90%), it is likely to result in a healthy live birth	Intrauterine transfusion may be possible to correct hydrops fetalis
Chickenpox (varicella zoster virus)	Person to person	Papules and pustules	Limb hypoplasia, skin scarring, IUGR, eye abnormalities, neurological abnormalities and hydrops fetalis	25% transmission. Probably <1–2% have problems if <20 weeks. No structural problems if >20 weeks. See also 'Chickenpox at term' p. 274	Give ZIG (zoster immunoglobulin) to the mother if <10 days from contact or <4 days from onset of rash, (although the benefits are not proven).

If delivery occurs within 5 days of maternal infection, or if the mother develops chickenpox within 2 days of giving birth, the neonate should be given passive varicella zoster immunoglobulin and the infant should be monitored for around 2 weeks. If neonatal infection occurs, it should be treated with aciclovir.

Hepatitis

Hepatitis A has not been associated with significant complications in pregnancy. All mothers should be screened antenatally for hepatitis B virus. The initial serological response to infection is with HBsAg, followed by HBeAg, a marker of high infectivity. Vertical transmission to the fetus is most likely to occur with acute infection (especially third trimester) or in the presence of HBeAg, and may lead to neonatal infection or long-term carriage. The baby should be given passive hepatitis B immunoglobulin at birth as well as an active hepatitis B immunization.

With hepatitis C, vertical transmission is related to viral load but is unlikely in the absence of detectable RNA. There is no evidence that treatment during pregnancy reduces the chance of transmission, and ribavirin is probably teratogenic. Hepatitis E infection in pregnancy, whilst uncommon, carries a 30% maternal mortality rate and possible risk of fetal loss.

Herpes simplex virus

An acute attack of primary genital herpes shortly before delivery may lead to a localized or systemic neonatal infection, including encephalitis. The risk of infection is greatest with a primary infection, but can occur with recurrence, although this risk decreases with time from the first attack. Screening is of no proven value, but caesarean section may be indicated in the presence of a primary infection.

Rubella

Rubella infection is outlined in **Table 31.3** but its importance lies in the potential for prevention through vaccination. Immunity from natural infection is lifelong. Seroconversion and lifelong immunity occur in about 95% of vaccinated individuals and, as the benefits of herd immunity have been clearly demonstrated, many countries now immunize all pre-school children. Rubella antibodies are commonly checked at the first antenatal visit and postnatal vaccination is offered to those with low titres.

In common with other prenatal infections, it can be difficult to predict which fetuses are going to be infected, and which of these infected fetuses will be affected. Furthermore, the very process of sampling fetal blood in utero for such tests may encourage transplacental transmission.

Erythrovirus (previously called Parvovirus B$_{19}$)

Erythrovirus infection in the first half of pregnancy can cause aplastic anaemia in the fetus, leading to high output cardiac failure and fetal demise **(Fig. 31.18)**. The use of fetal middle cerebral artery Doppler studies in this situation has been

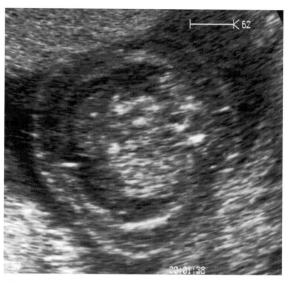

Fig. 31.18 Hydrops fetalis caused by infection with erythrovirus. There is ascites and marked skin oedema in this ultrasound image of a cross section of the fetal abdomen.

extremely valuable since the Doppler velocity correlates well with the degree of anaemia and allows an accurate determination of those who require in-utero transfusion. Transfusion is usually very successful and the outlook for babies receiving transfusion is excellent.

Listeria monocytogenes

This is a rare bacterial infection transmitted by food, usually soft ripe cheeses, pâté, cooked–chilled meals and ready-to-eat foods that have not been thoroughly cooked. Following an initial gastroenteritis, which may be fleeting, bacteraemia results in bacilli crossing the placenta and causing amnionitis, preterm labour (which may result in stillbirth) or spontaneous miscarriage. There may be meconium, neonatal jaundice, conjunctivitis or meningoencephalitis. Diagnosis is made by blood culture or by culture of liquor or placenta. Treatment is with high-dose amoxicillin or erythromycin.

Beta-haemolytic streptococci – group B

Between 5% and 20% of women carry this organism in the vagina. It is associated with preterm rupture of the membranes. About 50% of babies become colonized at delivery but only about 1% of these develop infection. The neonatal mortality from infection may be as high as 80%, with 50% of those surviving meningitis having subsequent neurological impairment. Antenatal screening is not recommended in the UK (initial screen positives may become negative and vice versa) but those with known colonization should receive intrapartum penicillin. There is no evidence to support antenatal treatment of asymptomatic carriers, as carriage is rapidly re-established following treatment.

Syphilis

Congenital syphilis is rare, and those identified antenatally with positive serology should be treated with penicillin.

Termination for abnormality

Prenatal diagnoses are often made relatively late in pregnancy and termination is by inducing labour, rather than by surgical means. This needs to be handled sensitively. Parents may initially be reluctant to see the baby, but should be offered the opportunity. Many mothers are later comforted that they underwent a delivery and saw and named the baby. Photographs of the baby can also be taken for the parents.

Postmortem examination should be encouraged, and if parents decline, they may accept a limited postmortem investigation with X-rays, clinical photographs and specimens for karyotype studies instead. Follow-up to discuss the results and their implications for subsequent pregnancy is important.

Key points

- Approximately 2% of newborn babies have a serious abnormality detectable at, or soon after, birth. Many of these can be diagnosed antenatally.
- There are a number of different strategies for prenatal screening programmes. Adequate verbal and written information is essential PRIOR to undermarking screening.
- Parents are often confronted with difficult decisions: Explanations may require to be repeated and often involve experts from several disciplines.

32

Obstetric haemorrhage

Introduction

Obstetric haemorrhage is one of the leading causes of maternal mortality worldwide, and even in the more affluent societies with ready access to resuscitation, oxytocics, blood transfusion and surgery, deaths still occur. Haemorrhage may be of rapid onset. It is important to recognize its severity promptly, institute effective therapy and keep ahead of the loss.

A vaginal examination should never be performed in the presence of vaginal bleeding without first excluding placenta praevia – 'No PV until no PP'.

Definitions

Vaginal bleeding associated with intrauterine pregnancy is divided into the following categories:

- threatened miscarriage – up to 24 weeks' gestation
- antepartum haemorrhage – from 24 weeks' gestation until the onset of labour
- intrapartum haemorrhage – from the onset of labour until the end of the second stage
- postpartum haemorrhage – from the third stage of labour until the end of the puerperium.

Antepartum haemorrhage

Causes

Antepartum haemorrhage is further classified according to the source of the bleeding.

Local

There may be local bleeding from the vulva, vagina or cervix. Bleeding from the cervix is not uncommon in pregnancy and may be provoked by sexual intercourse. A cervical ectropion is often found, and only very rarely is there a carcinoma. Later in pregnancy a 'show' of mucus along with a small amount of blood may simply herald the onset of labour as the cervix becomes effaced or 'takes up'.

Placental

Placenta praevia

This is defined as a placenta encroaching on the lower segment, with the lower segment arbitrarily defined on ultrasound scanning as extending 5 cm from the internal os. Placenta praevia is commoner in older mothers and those with a previous caesarean section. It is classified either as major or minor, or graded I–IV **(Table 32.1, Fig. 32.1)**.

It is not possible to avoid haemorrhage in labour with a major placenta praevia, but it may be possible to deliver successfully with a minor degree of praevia. In the assessment of suitability for such a delivery, engagement of the presenting part is probably more important than the actual distance of the placenta from the internal os on ultrasound scan **(Fig. 32.2)**. Those who do not have an at least partially engaged head should be delivered by caesarean section. These sections should be personally supervised or performed by a senior obstetrician, and a large blood loss should be anticipated.

A low-lying placenta may be identified in an asymptomatic woman at the time of an ultrasound scan early in pregnancy. As the uterus grows from the lower segment upwards, the placenta appears to move upwards with advancing gestation. 2% of those with a low-lying placenta before 24 weeks, 5% of those at 24–29 weeks and 23% of those at 30+ weeks will still have a placenta praevia at term. This is not a reflection of placental migration, but simply a feature of uterine growth. When a low-lying placenta is detected on ultrasound scanning early in pregnancy, it is reasonable to repeat the scan early in the third trimester and then review the management if the placenta is still low.

The risk of placenta praevia is of a sudden, unpredictable, major haemorrhage and some clinicians advocate hospital admission from 30–32 weeks onwards so that facilities for resuscitation and delivery are immediately available. This can be socially difficult for the woman, particularly if she has existing children at home, and immobility in hospital may predispose to thromboembolic disease. There is therefore a trend towards outpatient management, particularly for those who have had no bleeding, or just light bleeding, and who live close to the hospital. Those who have had heavy bleeds, or who live further away, are often advised

Table 32.1		
Classification of placenta praevia		
Minor	I	Encroaches on lower segment
	II	Reaches internal os (marginal)
Major	III	Covers part of os (partial)
	IV	Completely covers the os (complete)

to stay in hospital. Elective delivery is usually planned for 38–39 weeks, but may be earlier if there is a major haemorrhage.

If the placenta invades the myometrium it is termed 'placenta accreta', and this markedly increases the chance of severe haemorrhage.

Placental abruption

Placental abruption is defined as retroplacental haemorrhage and usually involves some degree of placental separation. Its management depends on the amount of bleeding, the maturity of the baby, and the fetal condition. It is essential to remember, however, that with placental abruption the amount of 'revealed' bleeding from the vagina may not reflect the degree of internal retroplacental bleeding and, indeed, a woman may have considerable internal bleeding without any external loss at all – a 'concealed abruption' **(Fig. 32.3)**. Maternal cigarette smoking is the principal risk factor for abruption.

Light bleeding from the edge of a normally situated placenta does not normally compromise the fetus and can be treated by a short spell of rest with subsequent close supervision of fetal growth and placental function until normal labour.

Major revealed haemorrhage is obvious, and urgent delivery is usually required. A major concealed abruption is inferred from the degree of pain, uterine tenderness and evidence of shock; again, urgent delivery may be required. The decision between vaginal delivery and caesarean section can be difficult, but depends on the severity of bleeding and the fetal condition.

If there is no fetal heartbeat, vaginal delivery is indicated, as the mother should not be subjected to an unnecessary caesarean section if the baby is dead. However, it is very likely that there will have been a major degree of blood loss. Hypovolaemic shock may develop and may progress to multisystem failure if not corrected. In addition, release of thromboplastins from the damaged placenta may lead to disseminated intravascular coagulation with depletion of platelets, fibrinogen and other clotting factors. Waiting for vaginal delivery therefore carries risks, and caesarean section may occasionally be indicated to minimize these systemic risks. The decision is further complicated by the risks of carrying out an operation in the presence of disseminated intravascular coagulation.

Unknown cause

A specific explanation for the bleeding is often not found, even after the pregnancy is over, and it is then presumed to have come from a normally situated placenta. Bleeding

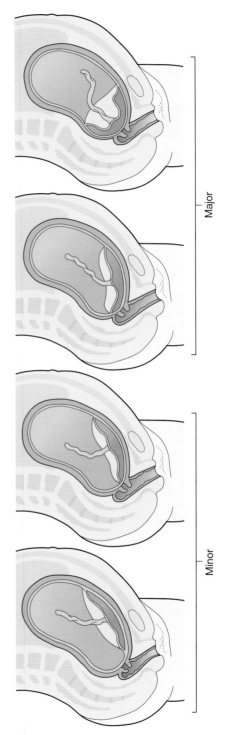

Fig. 32.1 Classification into 'major' and 'minor' placenta praevia depends on the distance of the placenta from the internal os. It is also important to note whether the placenta is anterior or posterior, as caesarean section is more difficult through an anterior placenta.

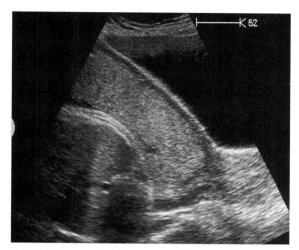

Fig. 32.2 An anterior placenta praevia extending to just beyond the internal os.

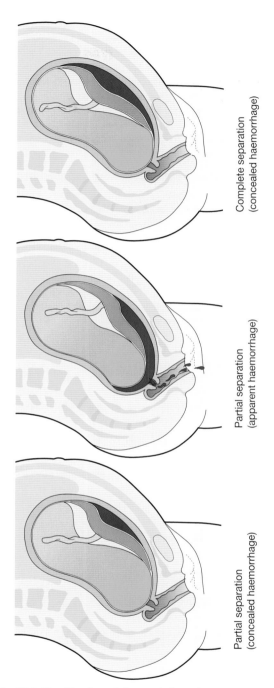

Fig. 32.3 Classification of placental abruption.

with no explanation is the commonest clinical scenario and, in the absence of maternal or fetal compromise, is managed expectantly.

Clinical presentation

Bleeding can be light, moderate or severe, and can occur with or without pain. Admission to hospital is advised, as even light bleeding may be a sign of premature labour, or a warning of further haemorrhage to come.

An attempt should be made to determine the cause of the bleeding. In practice, history and initial examination are carried out simultaneously. It is relevant to ask when the bleeding started, how much blood has been lost, and when the baby was last felt to move. Observation will tell if the mother is in pain, which suggests abruption or labour, and there may be visible blood on the bed or legs or floor. If she is pale, with low blood pressure and rapid pulse, there is probably hypovolaemic shock. With an abruption the uterus is hard and tender ('Couvelaire' uterus – history box) and there may be no discernible fetal heartbeat. When the bleeding has been from a placenta praevia, the uterus is usually soft, the presenting part will be free, and the fetal heartbeat is usually present. Subsequent management depends on the estimated severity of haemorrhage.

 History

Alexandre Couvelaire (1873–1948) was the first to describe extensive haemorrhage into the myometrium; he recognized that it was impairing the myometrium's ability to contract, such that in the case he reported, a caesarean hysterectomy was required. He also was an early proponent of caesarean section for placenta praevia.

Light bleeding, with a soft uterus and normal cardiotocography

An ultrasound scan should be arranged to check the placental site and, providing the placenta is not low-lying, a speculum examination should be performed to look for cervical effacement or dilatation, an ectropion or a carcinoma. If all is normal, it is common practice to admit the woman until the bleeding settles. Many clinicians, however, will not admit the patient if the bleeding is light and seen to be coming from an ectropion. Women who are rhesus negative should be given prophylactic anti-D.

If there is a placenta praevia and the patient is at more than 37–38 weeks' gestation, it is reasonable to arrange for delivery. If less than this gestation, a conservative approach is usually appropriate.

Light bleeding, but with a hard tender uterus

The diagnosis is probably a concealed abruption, and management is undertaken as above. The route of delivery will depend on a number of factors, including evidence of fetal distress and the presence of any coagulopathy. Resuscitation will be required.

Heavy bleeding

Whether the diagnosis is placenta praevia or an abruption, delivery is likely to be required irrespective of gestation. Resuscitation will again be required.

Intrapartum haemorrhage

Abnormal bleeding during labour must be distinguished from a 'show' that may occur during cervical dilatation. In a previously low-risk pregnancy, intrapartum bleeding would be an indication for continuous electronic fetal monitoring. Placental abruption can occur during labour, but the possibility of uterine rupture (especially if history of previous delivery by caesarean section) also needs to be considered.

Causes

Uterine rupture

Uterine rupture is relatively rare, and is discussed on page 373.

Vasa praevia

This is very rare, and occurs when cord vessels run in the fetal membranes and cross the internal os. These vessels may rupture in early labour and this leads to rapid fetal exsanguination. It may be that the cord is inserted into the membranes rather than directly into the placenta **(Fig. 32.4)**, or that the vessels are running from the placenta to a separate succenturiate placental lobe. The condition presents as severe fetal distress or fetal death following a relatively small intrapartum haemorrhage. A Kleihauer test on a sample of the blood may distinguish fetal from maternal red cells, but in practice the baby is usually delivered immediately because of the fetal distress and the diagnosis is made retrospectively by examination of the placenta and membranes.

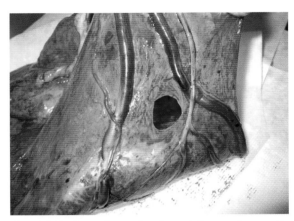

Fig. 32.4 Cord vessels running through the membranes. If these vessels overlie the internal os, they are termed 'vasa praevia'.

Postpartum haemorrhage

It is impossible to predict with certainty which patients will have a postpartum haemorrhage, and it is important to appreciate that a major haemorrhage can very rapidly lead to maternal death.

Definitions

There is always some bleeding during the third stage of a normal delivery, usually around 200–300 ml.

- A primary postpartum haemorrhage is defined as a blood loss of 500 ml or more within 24 hours of the delivery of the baby.
- A secondary postpartum haemorrhage is any significant loss between 24 hours and 6 weeks after the birth.

Primary postpartum haemorrhage

This occurs in around 5% of all deliveries. It is more common in grand multiparity (five deliveries or more), multiple pregnancy, women with fibroids, polyhydramnios. placenta praevia, and in those who have had a long labour. It may also follow an antepartum haemorrhage and is more likely in women with a past history of postpartum haemorrhage.

Prevention

It is important to treat anaemia in the antenatal period (haematinic supplements), particularly if the woman has risk factors for postpartum haemorrhage. It is usual to give a uterotonic such as Syntocinon 5 IU or Syntometrine (Syntocinon + ergometrine) with delivery of the baby. Active management of the third stage of labour is associated with a lower incidence of postpartum haemorrhage.

Causes

- *Atony* – including retained placenta (90%). Normally, contraction of the uterus in the third stage of labour causes compression of intramyometrial blood vessels,

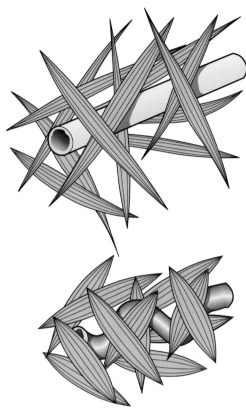

Fig. 32.5 Postpartum haemostasis is achieved largely because the contracting myometrial fibres constrict the vessels within the uterine wall.

and bleeding usually settles promptly **(Fig. 32.5)**. If there is uterine atony, this compression does not occur. Atony is more likely if part or all of the placenta is retained, as its physical presence prevents contraction occurring and partial placental separation permits bleeding.

- *Trauma* (7%). Bleeding may come from an episiotomy, a vaginal or cervical laceration **(Fig. 32.6)**, or a rupture in the uterine wall. Lacerations of the genital tract are more common after an instrumental delivery than after a spontaneous one.
- *Coagulation problems* – usually disseminated intravascular coagulation (DIC) (3%). DIC may be present due to a number of different causes.
- *Multiple causes* may be present.

Clinical presentation

The bleeding is usually obvious, but, occasionally, an atonic uterus can fill up without obvious external loss and the first real sign can be cardiovascular collapse. A less dramatic, prolonged trickling of blood may go unnoticed, the significance of which may not be appreciated. With blood-soaked pads and bedding, it is easy to underestimate the real loss. The most critical factors are the signs of shock, pallor, rising pulse and falling blood pressure.

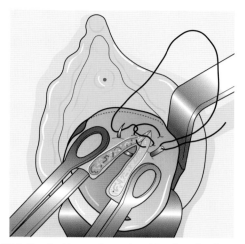

Fig. 32.6 Cervical lacerations often bleed profusely. They are best repaired under general anaesthesia.

The key questions are:

1. Has the placenta been delivered and is it complete?
2. Is the uterus firmly contracted?
3. If so, is the bleeding due to trauma?

Management

A controlled reassuring presence is important.

Assessment

- Make a rough but realistic estimate of the loss.
- Check the pulse and blood pressure.
- Palpate the abdomen to assess the size and tone of the uterus.

Treatment

- If the uterus is atonic, a contraction can be 'rubbed up' by abdominal massage. Bimanual compression may also be tried **(Fig. 32.7)**.
- Intravenous access should be established with *two* wide-bore cannulae and blood taken for haemoglobin, haematocrit, platelets, clotting and a red cell crossmatch (the number of units depends on volume lost).
- Syntocinon 10 IU stat i.v. should be given to further contract the uterus, followed by a Syntocinon infusion.
- Crystalloid and/or colloid should be rapidly infused to maintain the circulating volume. A catheter should be inserted to aid contraction or compression of the uterus and to measure urine output.
- If the placenta has not been delivered, a gentle attempt at controlled cord traction should be tried. If still retained, a regional block or general anaesthetic will be required for a manual removal. If the placenta is pathologically adherent (placenta accreta) in the presence of haemorrhage, a hysterectomy may be required.
- Further oxytocics may be given, e.g. Syntocinon i.v., ergometrine i.m., carboprost i.m. or intramyometrially, or misoprostol rectally.

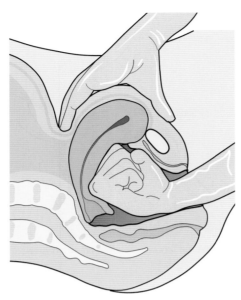

Fig. 32.7 Bimanual compression may be very helpful to aid uterine contraction in postpartum haemorrhage.

- If there is ongoing loss, a general anaesthetic will allow assessment for vaginal or cervical lacerations.

If the haemorrhage continues:

- A CVP line should be considered and a blood transfusion commenced. Group-specific un-crossmatched blood or even O negative blood may be used in extreme emergency.
- The coagulation defects of DIC should be corrected with fresh frozen plasma or cryoprecipitate, depending on specialist advice. Rarely, recombinant factor VIIa can be used.
- Techniques to stop haemorrhage are aimed at either maintaining compression of the uterus or applying pressure on the placental bed. A brace suture, e.g. B Lynch suture, involves sutures placed through the lower part of the uterus from front to back that are then looped over the fundus and tied. This maintains compression. Balloons in the uterus, e.g. Rusch balloon, apply pressure to the placental bed. This can also be achieved with intrauterine surgical packs. Hysterectomy (or subtotal hysterectomy) may be indicated, especially if there is a non-lower-segment uterine rupture or placenta accreta. Internal iliac artery ligation is only likely to be suitable for atony, is of less use with placenta accreta, and is of no use for uterine lacerations.
- Radiologically directed arterial embolization is also an option for uncontrolled haemorrhage, provided the woman is stable for transfer to the radiology theatre suite (**Fig. 32.8**).

Secondary postpartum haemorrhage

This is defined as bleeding between 24 hours and 6 weeks postnatally. It is usually due to infection or retained products of conception or both, rarely to a vulval haematoma and

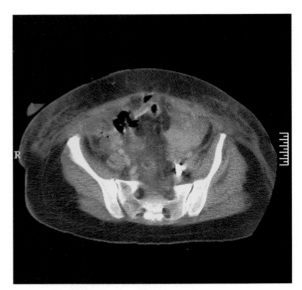

Fig. 32.8 Radiologically guided internal iliac artery embolization can be life-saving in severe postpartum haemorrhage. The embolizing 'coils' are visible as a bright area anterior to the left side of the sacrum, just behind a large intra-abdominal haematoma.

exceptionally to trophoblastic disease. Checks should be made of pulse, blood pressure and temperature, the uterus palpated for tenderness, and an endocervical swab sent for culture.

In practice, the decision is usually between conservative management with antibiotics, or arranging for an evacuation of retained products with antibiotic cover under anaesthesia. In the first week the evacuation can often be carried out digitally without the need to instrument the uterus and risk perforation. Clinical judgment is important, often giving broad-spectrum antibiotics in the first instance if the bleeding is not severe, and arranging an evacuation if it does not settle. Ultrasound scans can be unhelpful as many normal women have asymptomatic retained products after entirely normal deliveries and the temptation may be to carry out an unnecessary and potentially hazardous uterine evacuation. However, in the presence of persistent bleeding, ultrasound can be used to observe the spontaneous resolution of intrauterine haematomas and identify retained products.

> **Key** *points*
>
> - Obstetric haemorrhage is one of the leading causes of maternal mortality worldwide.
> - It can be rapidly fatal, and it is extremely important to establish adequate i.v. access, resuscitate, and identify the cause of the bleeding.
> - A mother who has experienced an obstetric haemorrhage is often apprehensive about a subsequent pregnancy, particularly if the bleeding has been severe. The chance of recurrence is relatively small.

33

Small babies

Introduction

Babies are born with a wide range of birth weights. While those born prematurely are more likely to be of low birth weight, the focus of this chapter is on fetuses and neonates who appear to be, or are, small for their gestational age (SGA). These babies may simply be small, in other words they are normal babies who just happen to be at the smaller end of a normal range (constitutionally small), or are small for a pathological reason. These latter fetuses are referred to as being affected by intrauterine growth restriction (IUGR).

The key issues are how to screen a low-risk population in order to identify these small fetuses and, once identified, how best to identify those that are risk of developing problems in utero or in labour.

Accuracy of dating

It is not possible to reliably diagnose SGA or IUGR without accurate knowledge of gestation. Menstrual dating has significant inherent inaccuracies. The dates may be inaccurately recalled, the cycle may be irregular, and bleeding in early pregnancy may be mistaken for menses. Gestation is most accurately determined by an ultrasound scan undertaken before 20 weeks' gestation, as it is a reasonable approximation to assume that all fetuses are of similar size up until this point. The natural variation in size after this stage makes accurate dating very difficult. The most reliable measurements are based on the crown–rump length between the 8th and 14th weeks, and the biparietal diameter (across the head) between the 16th and 20th weeks.

The estimated date of delivery is taken as 40 weeks after the date of the start of the last menstrual period (LMP) providing the cycle length is 28 days. A correction may be made for those with regular longer or shorter cycles; for example, if the cycle is 35 days long, then 7 days should be added to the date of the LMP. Abdominal palpation is an inaccurate way of establishing gestational age, as is the date that fetal movements were first noted. The rest of this chapter will assume that gestational age is known.

Small for gestational age (SGA)

Small for gestational age describes the baby or fetus whose birth weight or estimated fetal weight is below a specified centile for its gestation at birth. The chosen centile may be the 10th, 5th or 3rd, depending on different policies, and this choice reflects a trade-off between sensitivity and specificity. If the 10th centile is chosen, it will correctly identify most babies liable to be at risk on account of their small size but will also include many other babies who are not at risk. If the 3rd centile is chosen, then specificity will be good, in other words a greater proportion of identified babies will be at risk, but more 'at-risk' babies might be missed. The most commonly used threshold is the 10th centile.

Intrauterine growth restriction (IUGR)

The term intrauterine growth restriction indicates 'a fetus which fails to reach its genetic growth potential'. IUGR presents as a fetus whose growth on serial ultrasound scanning falls below a certain threshold. This threshold is poorly defined and is often implied as the crossing of centiles on a chart of fetal biometry (see later).

Babies with IUGR appear thin as measured by the ponderal index (the ratio of body weight to length) and their skinfold thickness, a measure of subcutaneous fat, is reduced. There is clearly an overlap in the categorization of small and/or growth-restricted fetuses; a proportion of SGA fetuses will be growth restricted but the majority will be constitutionally small, i.e. genetically determined to be small. Some growth-restricted fetuses will not be SGA, i.e. their growth is failing but they do not have a size below the 10th centile.

Factors affecting fetal growth

Fetal factors

- Genetic – depends on ethnic background and personal characteristics. Maternal genes are more relevant than paternal genes
- Chromosomal – decreased growth in association with fetal or placental aneuploidy
- Fetal anomaly

Maternal factors

- Nutrition
- Drugs/smoking
- Maternal disease, e.g. SLE, renal disease, pre-eclampsia.

Placental factors

- Adequate invasion
- Adequate vascular function

Aetiology

Fetal growth is determined by the baby's intrinsic genetic potential, which is then modified by various fetal, maternal and placental factors **(Box 33.1)**.

Fetal factors affecting fetal growth

The genetic make-up of the fetus is the main determinant of the intrinsic drive and is related to a number of factors, including ethnicity. Asian mothers, for example, have smaller babies than their European counterparts.

This intrinsic genetic drive is more related to the maternal genome than the genome of the father, and involves 'genomic imprinting'. It is well recognized that while large women often have correspondingly large babies, the correlation between large men and the size of their baby is poor.

Many developmentally abnormal fetuses are small, presumably as a result of a decreased intrinsic drive. This is particularly seen with chromosomal abnormalities, for instance trisomies 18, 13, 21 and triploidy. Small babies are also found in association with structural abnormalities of all the major organ systems as well as with fetal infection. These infections include toxoplasmosis, cytomegalovirus and rubella, but worldwide the main association is with malaria.

Maternal factors affecting fetal growth

Small variations in diet do not have a measurable effect on fetal growth, but extreme starvation does cause significant growth impairment. This was observed in the Dutch winter famine of 1944 and during the Siege of Leningrad from 1941 to 1944. There is no evidence, however, that food supplementation above a normal diet can improve growth in utero.

Oxygen supply is important. Babies born at high altitude are small, presumably as a result of the decreased oxygen content found in the rarefied atmosphere. This is also true of babies born to mothers with chronic hypoxia secondary to congenital heart disease. The fetus is able to partly compensate through placental hypertrophy, but this compensation is incomplete.

Drugs such as tobacco, heroin, cocaine and alcohol may decrease fetal growth. It has been estimated that smoking, for example, will decrease neonatal weight by an average of approximately 150 g. Maternal chronic disease also has an adverse effect on fetal growth, particularly if there is renal impairment.

Placental factors affecting fetal growth

Adequate placental function depends on adequate trophoblastic invasion. In the first trimester trophoblast cells invade the maternal spiral arteries in the decidua. In the second trimester a secondary wave of trophoblast extends this invasion along the spiral arteries and into the myometrium. This results in the conversion of thick-walled muscular vessels with a relatively high vascular resistance to flaccid thin-walled vessels with a low resistance to flow. In certain conditions, such as pre-eclampsia, it would appear that there has been failure of this secondary trophoblastic invasion, the consequences being subsequent placental ischaemia, atheromatous changes and secondary placental insufficiency. Why this failure should occur is unclear, but may be related to the immunological interface between the fetal and maternal cells. In pre-eclampsia there may be additional impaired placental flow from vasoconstriction. Local placental blood flow is under the control of prostacyclin and thromboxane A_2, with thromboxane causing vasoconstriction, and prostacyclin vasodilatation. There is a relative deficiency of prostacyclin in pre-eclampsia and an increase in the production of thromboxane A_2, the net result being placental vessel vasoconstriction. Release of thromboxane, which is produced and stored within platelets, can be suppressed by low-dose aspirin therapy and this offers the possibility of some useful intervention.

The overall effect of uteroplacental insufficiency, whatever the cause, is a decrease in the nutrient supply to the fetus. It is not surprising therefore that these fetuses are often found to be hypoxic, hypoglycaemic, and sometimes acidotic. To compensate for this hypoxia the fetus increases erythropoiesis in order to increase its oxygen-carrying capacity, and redistributes blood away from the peripheral circulation, gut and liver towards the brain, heart and adrenal glands.

The result is a baby with normal growth in length and brain development, but who is thin and has little or no subcutaneous fat. Glycogen stores are minimal. As these babies have relatively large heads compared to their bodies, their growth has in the past been described as 'asymmetrical', although the terms 'symmetrical' and 'asymmetrical' are no longer used to describe patterns of fetal growth or neonatal nutritional status.

Screening and diagnosis

A history may give some pointers towards the possibility of a small baby, particularly if there has been a previous small baby, an antepartum haemorrhage, or decreased fetal movements. The diagnosis should also be considered in any mother with signs of pre-eclampsia or history of a relevant pre-existing medical disorder. Usually, however, small babies are identified following routine clinical or ultrasound examination.

Clinical examination

Estimation of fetal weight from clinical examination is notoriously difficult. The fundus reaches the umbilicus by around 20–24 weeks and the xiphisternum by approximately 36 weeks. Some clinicians try to gain an impression of the fetal weight from bimanual abdominal palpation, while others prefer using a tape measure. After 20 weeks' gestation the height of the uterus, measured from the uterine fundus to the symphysis pubis in centimetres, is approximately equal to the gestation in weeks. Symphysis–fundal height (SFH) charts facilitate the interpretation of these measurements. An SFH less than the 10th centile is generally considered to be an indication for ultrasound fetal biometry.

Ultrasound examination

Ultrasound can be used to support the diagnosis of SGA or IUGR. Diagnosis of SGA or IUGR can be made with certainty postnatally, but this is of little value to the obstetrician and midwife in planning antenatal care/surveillance. Measurements can be made of the fetal head (circumference or biparietal diameter), the abdominal circumference and the femur length, and various equations have been used to estimate fetal weight. For practical purposes it is reasonable to consider the abdominal circumference alone, as measurements below the 10th centile have an approximately 80% sensitivity in the prediction of SGA neonates in high-risk pregnancies. There is no evidence that routine ultrasound screening is of value in low-risk women.

SGA or IUGR?

This is a key question and one which it is not always possible to answer. Those fetuses less than the 10th centile include those who are simply constitutionally small (perhaps around 70%) and those who have IUGR (perhaps 30%). The increased risks of stillbirth, birth hypoxia, neonatal complications and impaired neurodevelopment are likely to be in the IUGR group only, and it would be of great value to be able to reliably differentiate between the two groups. The diagnosis of SGA is straightforward, but the diagnosis of IUGR less so. Current clinical practice is to plot two or more fetal measurements on a chart of estimated fetal weight (or abdominal circumference) against gestational age. Examples of such plots in four fetuses are presented in **Figure 33.1**.

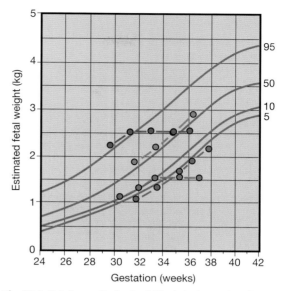

Fig. 33.1 Fetal growth charts. ● The baby is growing along the 50th centile. ● The baby is small for dates but does not have fetal growth restriction. ● The baby is latterly small for dates and has fetal growth restriction. ● The baby has fetal growth restriction but is not small for dates.

Charts of fetal size are not specifically designed for interpretation of serial measurements and the use of specifically constructed charts of fetal growth rates or velocity can improve diagnosis. An alternative strategy is to employ charts of fetal size which have been customized or individualized to a specific pregnancy. By calculating a 'term optimal fetal weight' based upon a number of easily obtained maternal and pregnancy physiological variables which have an influence upon fetal size – e.g. maternal weight, parity, ethnic origin – a customized 'growth' curve with centiles can be produced. This chart will be different for each pregnancy. A fetus with an estimated weight below the 10th centile of a customized chart is more likely to be genuinely growth restricted than a fetus which is small based on a population chart. The use of customized charts to improve the identification of growth restriction is recommended.

A detailed scan is warranted to look for any evidence of structural or chromosomal abnormality which makes IUGR more likely than SGA. A normal structural scan, however, does not prove the absence of IUGR, and it is then necessary to check other parameters of fetal well-being. These parameters are considered below. In practice, most fetuses less than the 10th centile require close observation and whether they have IUGR or are SGA only becomes apparent in retrospect.

Management

The main principle is to monitor the fetus and deliver at the appropriate time **(Box 33.2)**. No antenatal therapy is of proven benefit. The options for fetal monitoring include fetal

Clinical management of IUGR
- Screening by palpation
- Ultrasound confirmation that the baby is small
- Exclude fetal structural (± chromosomal) abnormality
- Consider whether the fetus is SGA or whether it has IUGR. Use Doppler studies.
- Monitor with Doppler studies and cardiotocography as appropriate
- Consider steroids if preterm
- Deliver if fetal demise is imminent; threshold strongly influenced by gestation

movement charts, fetal cardiotocography, biophysical scoring and Doppler blood flow studies. Of these, Doppler flow studies are the most valuable.

Fetal movement monitoring

A poorly nourished fetus will attempt to conserve energy by becoming less active and it may be useful to ask the mother about the frequency of perceived fetal movements. Most women experience a decrease in fetal movements as they approach term, but any sudden change in the pattern of movements may be of significance. The true value of routine fetal movement counting is uncertain since a number of studies have failed to demonstrate any material benefit.

Fetal cardiotocography

The interpretation of cardiotocographs (CTGs) is discussed on page 332. The CTG gives an indication of fetal well-being at a particular moment but has less longer-term value. The routine use of antenatal cardiotocography is not associated with an improved perinatal outcome and antenatal CTG monitoring should be restricted to specific indications.

Biophysical profile (BPP)

This is discussed in detail on page 244 but the predictive value in IUGR is low. The test takes a long time to carry out, sometimes up to an hour. As most fetuses with an abnormal BPP also have abnormal umbilical artery Doppler flow, it is more appropriate to rely on Doppler studies. A BPP may be helpful in certain circumstances such as when the Doppler waveform is already abnormal, but BPPs are seldom indicated in modern-day practice.

Doppler ultrasound

Doppler ultrasound of the umbilical artery is used as an assessment of placental vascular resistance further 'downstream'. A normal waveform indicates that an SGA fetus is constitutionally small rather than growth restricted because of impaired placental function. Reduction or loss of end-diastolic flow identifies a fetus at high risk of hypoxia, and absent end-diastolic flow has been shown to be a useful discriminator between those IUGR babies at high risk of

perinatal death and those at a lower risk **(Fig. 33.2)**. Other studies have shown that use of umbilical artery studies to monitor high-risk fetuses reduces perinatal morbidity and mortality.

Doppler studies of the fetal cerebral circulation can also provide additional useful information **(Fig. 33.3)**. As the growth-restricted fetus redistributes its blood flow away from the less vital organs towards the brain in response to hypoxia, it is reasonable to expect an increased cerebral flow. This is indeed observed to happen, with Doppler studies showing a decreased resistance of the middle cerebral artery. As the hypoxia becomes more severe, this resistance increases again, possibly secondary to cerebral oedema. Doppler examination of the fetal venous circulation is a relatively new development but can provide useful information when considering the timing of delivery. Doppler signals from the ductus venosus (a vein within the fetal liver) can be used to indirectly interpret the function of the right side of the fetal heart. Abnormal ductus venosus waveforms herald fetal demise.

In general, the sequence of changes observed with progressive fetal hypoxia is impaired growth, abnormal umbilical artery waveform, increased cerebral blood flow, abnormal ductus venosus flow followed by an abnormal fetal heart rate pattern and fetal demise. The rate of deterioration in fetal condition is unpredictable and this sequence of changes is not always present, but it does permit the development of a strategy for the outpatient management of the SGA/IUGR fetus.

Overall strategy

Figure 33.4 illustrates the probable sequence of events in fetal decompensation. As umbilical artery Doppler abnormalities are the first to appear, it is logical to use Doppler as the main screening tool. Thereafter, the optimal surveillance strategy in fetuses with absent or reduced end-diastolic flow is not established, but frequent monitoring with cardiotocography, biophysical profile and further Doppler studies is appropriate. The timing of the delivery will be decided by weighing up the risks of leaving the baby in utero against the risks of prematurity, but delivery is likely to be appropriate when the CTG becomes abnormal (decelerations or reduced variability), the biophysical profile becomes abnormal (e.g. <4) or there is reversal of end-diastolic flow. If IUGR is suspected before 34–36 weeks, it is appropriate to consider giving steroids to the mother to enhance fetal lung maturation (p. 302).

The actual mode of delivery depends on the individual circumstances, but it must be remembered that the placental reserve of some of these fetuses may be extremely low and careful monitoring in labour is required. Early recourse to caesarean section is appropriate if the monitoring shows signs of fetal compromise. Pre-labour caesarean section may be appropriate if there are significant pre-labour concerns about fetal well-being. A possible strategy for the outpatient management of women with SGA pregnancy is presented in **Figure 33.5**.

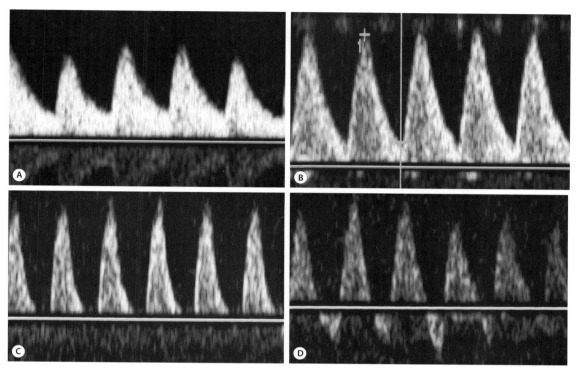

Fig. 33.2 Doppler ultrasound of the umbilical cord demonstrating (A) normal, (B) reduced, (C) absent and (D) reversed end-diastolic flow. Absent and reversed end-diastolic flow are associated with fetal compromise of placental origin.

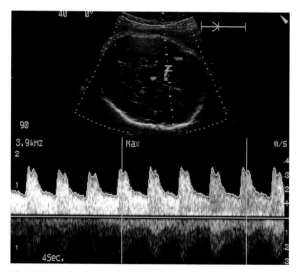

Fig. 33.3 In fetal growth restriction there is an increased flow in the middle cerebral artery.

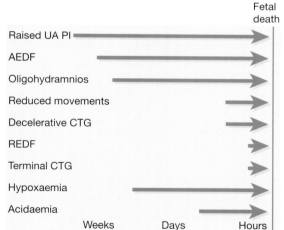

Fig. 33.4 The 'decompensation cascade' of fetal growth restriction. Absent end-diastolic flow (AEDF) is a relatively early sign of hypoxaemia, with reduced fetal movements, cardiotocographic abnormalities and reversed end-diastolic flow (REDF) late features. UA PI, umbilical artery pulsatility index.

Long-term implications of IUGR

Babies with IUGR are at increased risk of perinatal mortality and have a significant risk of stillbirth **(Box 33.3)**. Antenatal hypoxia may lead to long-term neurological handicap, as may more acute intrapartum hypoxia. Even if there is no overt evidence of handicap, studies of long-term development suggest that growth-restricted fetuses may be more clumsy and that their IQ may be 5–10 points lower than a normally grown sibling.

There is also evidence to suggest that IUGR predisposes babies to problems much later in life, particularly non-insulin-dependent diabetes and coronary heart disease. It may be that the fetus alters its metabolism to cope with poor nutrition in utero and is subsequently less able to cope

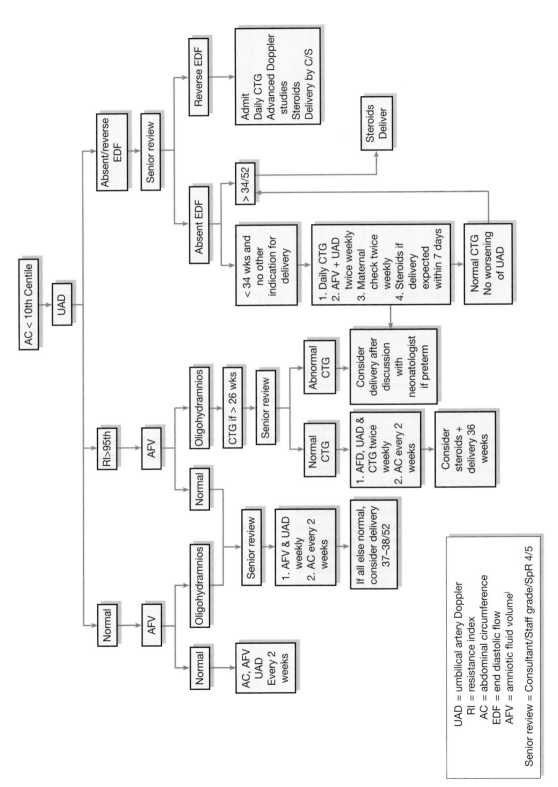

Fig 33.5 Flow chart for the management of an SGA fetus.

UAD = umbilical artery Doppler
RI = resistance index
AC = abdominal circumference
EDF = end diastolic flow
AFV = amniotic fluid volume

Senior review = Consultant/Staff grade/SpR 4/5

Box 33.3

Clinical significance of IUGR

Increased risk of:
- fetal anomaly
- perinatal asphyxia
- operative delivery
- perinatal death
- neonatal hypoglycaemia and hypocalcaemia
- necrotizing enterocolitis
- long-term handicap
- non-insulin-dependent diabetes and coronary heart disease in later life

with normal carbohydrate levels in later postnatal life. It is also possible that there are vascular compensatory changes with IUGR which predispose to later arterial disease.

Key points

- An accurate estimation of gestation is a prerequisite to the accurate diagnosis of fetal growth abnormality.
- Small for gestational age (SGA) refers to those fetuses whose weight is <10th centile for their gestational age. Most SGA fetuses are healthy.
- Intrauterine growth restriction (IUGR) refers to any fetus failing to achieve its growth potential. Not all SGA fetuses are growth restricted and not all growth-restricted fetuses are SGA. IUGR carries an increased risk of intrapartum asphyxia, neonatal hypoglycaemia and possible long-term neurological impairment. There is also an increased risk of perinatal mortality.
- Most screening tests attempt to diagnose SGA fetuses rather than growth-restricted fetuses. Diagnosis of IUGR requires at least two ultrasound scans. The use of customized or individualized charts of fetal size more reliably differentiates between the SGA fetus and the IUGR fetus.
- Successful management involves appropriate monitoring, with expedited delivery as necessary.

34 Pregnancy-induced hypertension, pre-eclampsia and eclampsia

Introduction

The term 'pregnancy-induced hypertension' (PIH) suggests a disorder of blood pressure that arises because of the presence of pregnancy. Such a simple view detracts from the fundamental pathological process that underlies this condition: PIH, pre-eclampsia and its variants are part of a multisystem disorder that can affect every organ system in the body and collectively are the second highest cause of direct maternal deaths in the UK.

Although pre-eclampsia is associated with abnormal trophoblast invasion in the first half of pregnancy, it is not until later in the pregnancy that the clinical syndrome of pre-eclampsia is seen. The mechanisms by which the abnormal placentation and subsequent impaired placental perfusion cause the widespread vascular endothelial dysfunction that characterizes pre-eclampsia are not fully understood.

Pre-eclampsia is defined as hypertension with proteinuria. It is, however, a very heterogeneous condition such that the timing of onset and the clinical course are unpredictable. In some, hypertension and proteinuria are the only manifestation, while others may present with severe renal or liver impairment, and in yet others the most prominent feature might be intrauterine fetal growth restriction secondary to placental disease.

Eclampsia is a generalized seizure that occurs during pregnancy in association with the features of pre-eclampsia. In a proportion of women with eclampsia, however, the features of pre-eclampsia are not evident at the time of the first seizure. The only cure for these conditions is delivery.

Definitions

Hypertension in pregnancy is common and affects up to 15% of pregnant women. Hypertension in pregnancy is classified into three groups, depending on the timing of onset and the associated clinical features:

- pre-existing (essential) hypertension (identified <20 weeks' gestation)
- pregnancy-induced hypertension (hypertension only, no proteinuria)
- pre-eclampsia (hypertension and proteinuria ± multisystem involvement).

Hypertension

In normal pregnancy the maternal blood pressure falls slightly during the first trimester, predominantly as a consequence of reduced systemic vascular resistance. Maternal blood pressure continues to fall during the second trimester and reaches a nadir at approximately 22–24 weeks' gestation. Thereafter, maternal blood pressure steadily increases during the third trimester to reach pre-pregnancy levels. Maternal blood pressure falls immediately after delivery of the baby, but then rises and peaks on the 4th postnatal day.

Maternal blood pressure should be measured in the sitting position with an appropriate-sized cuff that is placed on the upper arm at the level of the heart **(Fig. 34.1)**. Phase V Korotkoff sounds (i.e. 'disappearance' rather than 'muffling') should be used when measuring the diastolic blood pressure.

- Hypertension in pregnancy is defined as a blood pressure of ≥140/90 mmHg on two occasions more than 4 hours apart.
- A diastolic blood pressure of ≥110 mmHg on any one occasion or a systolic blood pressure of ≥160 mmHg on any one occasion is also significant hypertension.
- A systolic blood pressure of 30 mmHg above the booking systolic blood pressure or a diastolic blood pressure of 15–25 mmHg above the booking diastolic blood pressure are alternative and widely used criteria for the diagnosis of hypertension in pregnancy.

Hypertension in pregnancy may be pre-existing or related to pregnancy (PIH or pre-eclampsia). An increased maternal blood pressure in early pregnancy (before 20 weeks' gestation) is usually due to pre-existing hypertension, most commonly essential hypertension. In a young woman with pre-existing hypertension, consideration should be given to identify the rare secondary causes of hypertension such as renal disease, cardiac disease, phaeochromocytoma and endocrine disorders such as Cushing's syndrome. The diagnosis of essential hypertension may be made retrospectively if the maternal blood pressure has not returned to normal within 3 months of delivery of the baby.

PIH and pre-eclampsia rarely occur before 20 weeks' gestation unless associated with trophoblastic disease or fetal triploidy. The hypertension associated with pre-eclampsia usually resolves within 6 weeks of delivery.

Proteinuria

Proteinuria is defined as a urinary protein concentration of more than 300 mg/l, or a urinary protein excretion of more than 300 mg in 24 hours. These approximate to '1+' or more on urine dipstick testing.

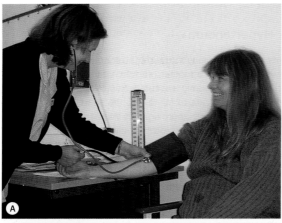

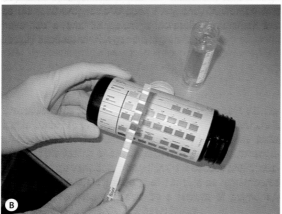

Fig. 34.1 Early detection of pre-eclampsia is important. (A) Measurement of blood pressure (reproduced with permission). **(B)** Testing for urinary protein.

Essential hypertension

Essential hypertension is more common in older women and the prognosis for pregnancy is generally good; the main risk is from superimposed pre-eclampsia. Women with essential hypertension are also at increased risk of placental abruption and intrauterine fetal growth restriction. Some women taking antihypertensive drugs may be able to discontinue their medication during pregnancy, particularly during the first and second trimesters. Drugs that are commonly used for the treatment of essential hypertension during pregnancy include methyldopa, labetalol and nifedipine. Diuretics and angiotensin-converting enzyme (ACE) inhibitors are contraindicated in pregnancy but may be used for the management of hypertension during the puerperium.

Pregnancy-induced hypertension (PIH), pre-eclampsia and eclampsia

Pathophysiology

Recognized risk factors for PIH and pre-eclampsia are shown in **Box 34.1**.

The precise aetiology and pathophysiology of PIH and pre-eclampsia remain unclear. It is established, however, that women who develop pre-eclampsia have a genetic or phenotypic susceptibility and that there are two distinct phases to the condition's development: first there is inadequate trophoblast invasion during early pregnancy, and secondly, in later pregnancy, there is reduced placental perfusion and uteroplacental ischaemia, which in turn gives rise to the clinical syndrome.

Box 34.1

Predisposing factors for developing PIH/pre-eclampsia

- First pregnancy
- Family history – mother/sister
- Extremes of maternal age
- Obesity
- Medical factors:
  - Pre-existing hypertension
  - Renal disease
  - Acquired thrombophilia – antiphospholipid antibodies
  - Inherited thrombophilia
  - Connective tissue disease (e.g. systemic lupus erythematosus)
  - Diabetes mellitus
- Obstetric factors:
  - Multiple pregnancy
  - Previous pre-eclampsia
  - Hydatidiform mole
  - Triploidy
  - Hydrops fetalis (immune and non-immune)
  - Inter-pregnancy interval of >10 years

The precise mechanism by which this abnormal placentation causes the multisystem disorder that characterizes pre-eclampsia is not known. It has been suggested that there is a trigger which promotes widespread vascular endothelial dysfunction in response to the reduced placental perfusion. This endothelial dysfunction subsequently causes metabolic changes, an exaggerated maternal inflammatory response and reduced organ perfusion.

Maternal susceptibility

The evidence for genotypic susceptibility to developing pre-eclampsia is strong. Large epidemiological studies demonstrate a three- to fivefold increased risk of pre-eclampsia in the first-degree relatives of affected women. While it is possible that a single maternal gene in some families may be important, no single gene has been identified. It may be that multiple genes (maternal, paternal and fetal) interact, and that environmental factors may affect their expression.

Certain phenotypes are also more susceptible. Women with insulin resistance and central obesity are at increased risk of developing pre-eclampsia, possibly on account of an exaggerated metabolic response. Those with connective tissue disease, such as systemic lupus erythematosus, are also at increased risk, possibly because of an exaggerated immune response. In addition, those with an inherited thrombophilia are more likely to develop pre-eclampsia. These associations suggest that the pathophysiology of pre-eclampsia involves a significant interaction between metabolic, immunological and coagulation processes, possibly mediated through vascular endothelial dysfunction and damage.

Phase 1 – abnormal placentation

In normal pregnancy, placentation occurs between 6 and 18 weeks' gestation. During normal placental development, major structural alterations of the spiral arteries occur, allowing an increase in blood supply to the placenta. Trophoblast invasion of the maternal spiral arteries causes the diameter of these arteries to increase approximately fivefold, converting a high-resistance, low-flow system to one with a low resistance and high flow. In women who develop pre-eclampsia, adequate trophoblast invasion does not seem to occur, or the trophoblast invasion is limited to the decidual portions of the vessels. The result is inadequate placental perfusion. This type of abnormal placentation is also associated with intrauterine fetal growth restriction that occurs independently of pre-eclampsia.

During early pregnancy, trophoblast invasion is regulated at the maternal decidual barrier by the action of factors expressed within the decidua and on the trophoblast cells. These regulatory factors include cell adhesion molecules (CAMs) and the extracellular matrix (ECM), proteinases and their inhibitors, growth factors and cytokines. Abnormalities in any one of these factors may lead to inadequate trophoblast invasion and subsequent pre-eclampsia.

It has been suggested that the primary factor in the aetiology of pre-eclampsia is immunological in origin. Abnormal placentation may be the result of maternal immune rejection of paternal antigens expressed by the fetus. HLA-G is a class 1B major histocompatibility antigen that is expressed by extra-villous trophoblast and may protect cells from natural killer cell lysis. Women who develop pre-eclampsia appear to have extra-villous trophoblast that does not express HLA-G. The predominance of pre-eclampsia in first pregnancies and the protective effect of parity further support an immunological mechanism for the condition.

Phase 2 – endothelial dysfunction

The second phase of pre-eclampsia is characterized by widespread endothelial damage and dysfunction. Women with pre-eclampsia have increased circulating levels of markers of endothelial dysfunction. Endothelial damage promotes platelet adhesion and thrombosis, and disturbs the normal physiological modulation of vascular tone, further amplifying the response.

The underlying pathophysiology of this second phase of pre-eclampsia is characterized by an exaggerated maternal systemic inflammatory response, with associated activation of leucocytes, platelets and the coagulation system. Pre-eclampsia is also associated with other markers of inflammation. Features of oxidative stress and dyslipidaemia are also evident and the overall effect is reduced organ perfusion.

Normal pregnancy is a state of systemic inflammation. In normal pregnancy there is a leucocytosis and an increase in leucocyte activation. Women with pre-eclampsia appear to have an excessive inflammatory response to pregnancy. Animal models have demonstrated that the administration of endotoxin during pregnancy can cause hypertension and proteinuria.

It has been suggested that the exaggerated maternal inflammatory response that is seen in pre-eclampsia may lead to endothelial dysfunction and damage. Other systemic metabolic changes that are associated with pre-eclampsia include hypertriglyceridaemia and a significant increase in free fatty acids. This atherogenic lipid profile may also be a contributor to endothelial dysfunction in women with pre-eclampsia.

Many of the features of the second phase of pre-eclampsia are the result of reduced organ perfusion caused by vasoconstriction, activation of the coagulation system and reduction of plasma volume. The resulting organ damage caused by hypoperfusion gives rise to the clinical features of pre-eclampsia, eclampsia and HELLP syndrome (see later) **(Table 34.1)**.

Normal pregnancy is associated with an increase in angiotensin II levels. Angiotensin II is a potent vasoconstrictor. However, during normal pregnancy, despite increased angiotensin II levels, peripheral vascular resistance falls. This appears to be because normal pregnant women are resistant to the effects of angiotensin II, a phenomenon that seems to be lost in women who develop PIH and pre-eclampsia. This suggests that abnormalities in the renin–angiotensin–aldosterone system may play a role in the pathogenesis of

Table 34.1

Potential secondary effects of the metabolic, inflammatory endothelial alterations in pre-eclampsia

CVS	Increased peripheral resistance leading to hypertension
	Increased vascular permeability and reduced maternal plasma volume
Lungs	Laryngeal and pulmonary oedema
Renal	Glomerular damage leading to proteinuria, hypoproteinaemia and reduced oncotic pressure which further exacerbates the hypovolaemia. May develop acute renal failure ± cortical necrosis
Clotting	Hypercoagulability, with increased fibrin formation and increased fibrinolysis, i.e. disseminated intravascular coagulation
Liver	HELLP syndrome
	Hepatic rupture
CNS	Thrombosis and fibrinoid necrosis of the cerebral arterioles
	Eclampsia (convulsions), cerebral haemorrhage and cerebral oedema
Fetus	Impaired uteroplacental circulation, potentially leading to FGR, hypoxaemia and intrauterine death

CVS, cardiovascular system; CNS, central nervous system; FGR, fetal growth restriction.

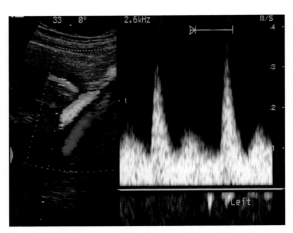

Fig. 34.2 Uterine artery Doppler notching at 24 weeks is predictive of pre-eclampsia and intrauterine growth restriction in high-risk mothers.

the condition. Women with pre-eclampsia are also more responsive to other vasoconstrictors such as vasopressin and noradrenaline and appear to be less responsive to vasodilators such as nitric oxide and prostacyclin (PGI2).

In pre-eclampsia, organ perfusion is further compromised by activation of the coagulation cascade. Altered platelet function is seen in most women with pre-eclampsia. In normal pregnancy there is increased biosynthesis of eicosanoids, particularly prostacyclin and thromboxane A_2. Prostacyclin is a vasodilator with platelet-inhibitory properties and thromboxane A_2 is a vasoconstrictor with a tendency to promote platelet aggregation. Prostacyclin and thromboxane A_2 usually increase in proportion to one another and consequently there is a net neutralization, and homeostasis is maintained. In women with pre-eclampsia, this homeostasis is disrupted due to a relative deficiency of prostacyclin. This occurs either because of a reduction in prostacyclin synthesis or because of an increased production of thromboxane A_2. This imbalance leads to platelet stimulation and also vasoconstriction and hypertension.

In pre-eclampsia, plasma volume is reduced as a consequence of increased capillary permeability. This further reduces organ perfusion.

Linking phase 1 and phase 2

It has been suggested that the reduced placental perfusion that is a feature of the first phase of pre-eclampsia is associated with oxidative stress. Women who develop pre-eclampsia have reduced levels of the antioxidant ascorbic acid, as well as increased levels of markers of oxidative stress. Furthermore, women who develop pre-eclampsia have increased cytotrophoblast levels of xanthine oxidase, a superoxide-generating enzyme. The oxidative stress that is associated with placental hypoperfusion may lead to leucocyte activation and/or cytokine production and subsequently the production of free radicals. Oxidative stress may also cause placental apoptosis and result in the shedding of placental debris into the maternal circulation. This debris, along with the free radicals produced by oxidative stress, may then lead to vascular endothelial damage that characterizes the maternal syndrome of the second phase of pre-eclampsia.

Screening and detection

Pre-eclampsia is an unpredictable condition and extremely variable in its manner of presentation. The aim of antenatal screening is to detect pre-eclampsia early enough to prevent disease progression, and hence both maternal and fetal complications, by timely delivery of the baby.

An important component of routine antenatal care for all pregnant women is directed towards screening for hypertension and proteinuria. Risk factors for pre-eclampsia can be identified at the booking visit. A number of additional screening tests for predicting pre-eclampsia have been proposed, but most are of limited clinical use. Abnormalities of the maternal uterine artery Doppler waveform between 18 and 24 weeks' gestation may identify a group of women at increased risk of developing severe pre-eclampsia that requires preterm delivery (<34 weeks' gestation) **(Fig. 34.2)**. Abnormalities of the maternal uterine artery Doppler waveform appear to be more significant if they are bilateral and if they persist into the third trimester of pregnancy.

In PIH and pre-eclampsia there are many non-specific symptoms and signs that are important indicators of

Box 34.2

Symptoms and signs of impending eclampsia

1. Unusual headaches, typically frontal
2. Visual disturbances (blurring of vision, diplopia, scotomas or flashes of light)
3. Restlessness or agitation
4. Epigastric pain, nausea and vomiting
5. Sudden severe hypertension and proteinuria
6. Fluid retention with reduced urine output
7. Hyperreflexia or ankle clonus
8. Retinal oedema, haemorrhages or papilloedema

Table 34.2

Investigations in PIH and pre-eclampsia

Investigation	Finding in pre-eclampsia
FBC	Reduced platelets, reduced haemoglobin, haemolysis on blood film
Renal function	Reduced urine output
	Increased urate, increased urea, increased creatinine
Coagulation system	Prolonged coagulation indices
Hepatic system	Elevated alanine transaminase (ALT) and aspartate transaminase (AST)

FBC, full blood count.

widespread multisystem involvement and these symptoms may herald the onset of severe pre-eclampsia **(Box 34.2)**.

Clinical management of hypertension in pregnancy without proteinuria

If the maternal blood pressure is found to be elevated, measurement should be repeated after 10–20 minutes. If it settles, no further action is needed; if still elevated, further assessment is required, ideally at an antenatal day care unit. The woman should be asked about the symptoms of pre-eclampsia (headaches, visual disturbance, epigastric pain, oedema), and the fetal size and well-being should be assessed clinically. Ultrasound can be used to assess fetal size, amniotic fluid volume and fetal umbilical artery Doppler waveform. Serum urate (which rises with pre-eclampsia), urea and electrolytes (U&Es), liver enzymes and platelets (which fall with pre-eclampsia) should also be checked **(Table 34.2)**.

In the absence of severe hypertension (160/110 or above), significant proteinuria or symptoms of pre-eclampsia, and if the biochemistry and haematology results are normal, then the woman can usually be managed as an outpatient. She should be seen at least twice weekly, for blood pressure and urinalysis checks. Serum biochemistry and haematology should also be repeated at least once a week. The woman should be advised to return to hospital if she feels unwell, or if there is any headache, visual disturbance or epigastric pain.

Treatment of the mother with antihypertensive drugs controls the hypertension but does not alter the course of pre-eclampsia. Treatment of hypertension may allow prolongation of the pregnancy and thereby may indirectly improve fetal outcome. Antihypertensive treatment is appropriate with consistent recordings of 150/100 or greater.

The only true 'cure' for pre-eclampsia is delivery of the fetus and placenta, but the timing of this will significantly influence the outcome for both the mother and the baby.

Clinical management of pre-eclampsia

In a woman with pre-eclampsia, it is important to consider the overall picture rather than make decisions on the basis of a single parameter. Progression of the disease is not consistent and further management should be tailored to the individual woman.

Indications for admission to hospital include:

- blood pressure >170/110 mmHg or >140/90 with 2+ proteinuria
- significant symptoms (headaches, visual disturbance, epigastric pain, oedema)
- abnormal biochemistry or haematology results
- significant proteinuria
- the need for antihypertensive treatment
- signs of fetal compromise.

The aim should be to prolong the pregnancy in order to reduce the risk to the baby, but this must be balanced against the risks to the mother. The decision to deliver and the method of delivery are dependent on many factors. There are usually fetal advantages to conservative management before 34 weeks if the blood pressure, laboratory values and fetal condition are stable.

The principles of management of pre-eclampsia are:

- To control the maternal blood pressure. Reduce the diastolic blood pressure to <100 mmHg using labetalol, nifedipine, hydralazine or methyldopa **(Table 34.3)**.
- To assess maternal fluid balance. Pre-eclampsia is associated with an increased vascular permeability and a reduced intravascular compartment. In women with pre-eclampsia, administering too little fluid risks maternal renal failure and giving too much fluid may cause pulmonary oedema. Fluid input and urine output should therefore be monitored. In severe pre-eclampsia the maternal oxygen saturation (SaO_2) should also be monitored, along with serum U&Es, urate, LFTs, haemoglobin, haematocrit, platelets and coagulation. If there is marked oliguria, central venous pressure monitoring may be helpful to differentiate intravascular volume depletion from renal impairment.
- To prevent seizures (eclampsia). The use of magnesium sulphate in severe pre-eclampsia halves the risk of subsequent eclampsia, and may reduce the risk of maternal death. Magnesium sulphate, given to those who have had an eclamptic seizure, also prevents further seizures.

■ To consider delivery. The timing of this depends on the maternal condition, the fetal condition and the gestational age. If preterm delivery is being considered, corticosteroids should be administered to the mother to reduce the risks associated with prematurity **(Fig. 34.3)**.

Management of eclampsia

Eclampsia occurs when there is a tonic-clonic convulsion in association with the features of pre-eclampsia (the word 'eclampsia' means 'lightning'). In the UK, the incidence of eclampsia is 4.9/10,000 maternities, with 38% of eclamptic seizures occurring antepartum, 18% intrapartum and 44% postpartum. Over a third of eclamptic seizures occur before proteinuria and hypertension have been documented. In the UK, the maternal mortality associated with eclampsia is 1.8%, with a neonatal death rate of 34/1000. In less-developed countries, incidences of up to 80/10,000 maternities have been reported, with maternal death occurring in approximately 10% of cases.

The treatment of eclampsia is outlined in **Box 34.3**.

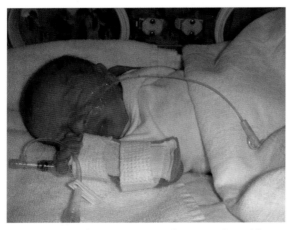

Fig. 34.3 This baby, born at 36 weeks to a mother with severe pre-eclampsia, weighed 1.6 kg. (Usual weight at 36 weeks: 2.2–3.3 kg.)

Prevention

Various preventive strategies have been employed in women considered to be at risk of developing pre-eclampsia. The estimated value of these interventions is shown in **Box 34.4**.

Box 34.3

Treatment of eclampsia

■ The patient should be turned onto her left side to avoid aortocaval compression. The airway should be secured and high-flow oxygen should be administered.
■ Magnesium sulphate ($MgSO_4$) should be administered intravenously to terminate the seizure and then by intravenous infusion to reduce the chance of further convulsions. The infusion should be continued for at least 24 hours following delivery or after the last seizure. $MgSO_4$ can depress neuromuscular transmission and the patient should be monitored for signs of toxicity. The respiratory rate and patellar reflexes should be monitored (reduced patellar reflexes usually precede respiratory depression). If there is significant respiratory depression, calcium gluconate can be used to reverse the effects of $MgSO_4$ and consideration given to ventilation.
■ Urgent delivery is necessary if the seizure has occurred antenatally or intrapartum.
■ Paralysis and ventilation should be considered if the seizures are prolonged or recurrent.

Box 34.4

Prevention of pre-eclampsia

Possibly of value

■ Low-dose aspirin
■ Calcium supplementation

Not of value

■ Diet with high protein content
■ Restriction of salt in diet
■ Restriction of weight gain
■ Vitamins C and E

Table 34.3

Drug treatment of hypertension in pregnancy

Drug	Action	Side-effects	Comments
Methyldopa (oral)	Central acting	Initial drowsiness	Safe; oral drug of choice. Slow onset of action. Not suitable if history of depression
Labetalol (oral/i.v.)	Alpha- and beta-antagonist	Postural hypotension, tiredness	Widely used in antenatal setting (oral) and hypertensive crisis (i.v.)
Hydralazine (oral/i.v.)	Direct-acting vasodilator	Precipitate hypotension	Widely used in hypertensive crisis (i.v.)
Nifedipine (orally/s.l.)	Calcium-channel antagonist	Flushing, headaches	Caution – interacts with $MgSO_4$. Watch for precipitous fall in blood pressure

Aspirin inhibits prostaglandin synthesis via cyclo-oxygenase and the dose of aspirin required to inhibit thromboxane synthesis is less than that required for prostacyclin inhibition. Low-dose aspirin should reduce the vascular and prothrombotic effects of thromboxane A_2 in women at risk of developing pre-eclampsia. Taking 75 mg aspirin daily from the first trimester of pregnancy leads to a 15% reduction in the incidence of pre-eclampsia. It should be offered to those women at high risk of developing pre-eclampsia and should be commenced on or before 12 weeks' gestation.

Calcium supplementation (>1 g/day) may also reduce the risk of hypertension by up to 30% and may reduce the risk of pre-eclampsia by up to 50%. Although calcium supplementation may reduce the rate of maternal mortality by up to 20%, it has no significant effect on preterm birth or stillbirth.

The use of antioxidants such as vitamin C and E is not useful for the prevention of pre-eclampsia. Likewise, restriction of salt intake and limiting weight gain during pregnancy are not useful in this regard.

HELLP syndrome

HELLP is the acronym for haemolysis, elevated liver enzymes (particularly transaminases) and low platelets. It is a variant of pre-eclampsia, and affects up to 12% of those with pre-eclampsia/eclampsia. HELLP syndrome is more common in multiparous women experiencing pre-eclampsia. Women with HELLP syndrome may present with epigastric pain, nausea and vomiting, and right upper quadrant tenderness may be evident on examination.

Aspartate transaminase (AST) rises first, followed by a rise in lactate dehydrogenase (LDH). A blood film may show burr cells and polychromasia consistent with haemolysis, although frank anaemia is uncommon. Platelet transfusion is only rarely required. HELLP syndrome is also associated with acute renal failure and disseminated intravascular coagulation (DIC), and there is also an increased incidence of placental abruption.

The management of HELLP syndrome is to stabilize the mother, correct any coagulation disorder, assess fetal well-being and assess the need for delivery. It is generally considered that delivery is appropriate for moderate or severe cases, but management may be more conservative (with close monitoring) if the condition is mild. Vigilance is required for at least 48 hours postpartum as deterioration in the maternal condition may occur. The risk of recurrence of HELLP syndrome in subsequent pregnancies is approximately 20%.

Key *points*

- Pre-eclampsia is a multisystem disorder, and is a major cause of maternal and perinatal morbidity and mortality.
- There are two phases; phase 1 is associated with abnormal placentation and phase 2 is characterized by an exaggerated maternal inflammatory response, endothelial dysfunction and reduced organ perfusion.
- The cure for pre-eclampsia is delivery of the fetus. Antihypertensive therapy does not fundamentally alter the progress of the condition.
- HELLP syndrome is a variant of pre-eclampsia; HELLP is an acronym for haemolysis, elevated liver enzymes and low platelets.

35

Prematurity

Introduction

Prematurity is defined as delivery between 24 and 37 weeks' gestation and occurs in 6–10% of births. Although preterm labour is more common in association with multiple pregnancy, antepartum haemorrhage, fetal growth restriction, cervical incompetence, amnionitis, congenital uterine anomaly, polyhydramnios and systemic infection, there is most often no apparent predisposing cause (idiopathic). Almost one-third of preterm births in the UK are iatrogenic following deliberate medical intervention when the risk of continuing the pregnancy for either the mother or the fetus outweighs the risks of prematurity.

To be born prematurely is a potentially serious hazard. Morbidity and mortality rates are inversely proportional to the maturity of organ systems, especially the lungs, brain and gastrointestinal tract, and it is exceptional to survive if delivered before 24 weeks' gestation. In the most recent perinatal mortality report from the Confidential Enquiry into Maternal and Child Health (CEMACH 2005), 48% of neonatal deaths were attributed to prematurity. Of those infants who survive, 10% will suffer some form of long-term handicap and a greater number may suffer from lesser developmental or behavioural problems; these proportions are higher with lower gestational ages.

Research into the mechanisms involved in preterm delivery and methods of preventing it has been relatively unsuccessful; as a result, prematurity is currently one of the most challenging problems facing both obstetricians and paediatricians.

Definitions

Preterm – a gestation of less than 37 completed weeks.

Very preterm – a gestation of less than 32 completed weeks.

Preterm labour – regular uterine contractions accompanied by effacement and dilatation of the cervix after 20 weeks and before 37 completed weeks.

Preterm pre-labour rupture of the membranes (PPROM) – rupture of the fetal membranes before 37 completed weeks and before the onset of labour.

Low birth weight (LBW) – birth weight of less than 2501 g. It is important to note that low-birth-weight infants may be preterm or growth restricted or both (p. 283).

Very low birth weight (VLBW) – birth weight of less than 1501 g.

Extremely low birth weight (ELBW) – birth weight of less than 1000 g.

Perinatal mortality rates – see Chapter 46.

Aetiology and predisposing factors

The incidence of preterm birth is 6–10% **(Table 35.1)** and approximately 1.5% will deliver before 32 weeks. Although only 0.5% deliver before 28 weeks, this latter group accounts for two-thirds of the neonatal deaths.

The aetiological factors that trigger spontaneous preterm labour are largely unknown, but may be mediated through cytokines and prostaglandins. In some instances, it is related to increased uterine size or to other hormonal factors. Infection has been implicated in preterm delivery and it may be that bacterial toxins initiate an inflammatory process in the chorioamniotic membranes, which in turn release prostaglandins. Bacteria may damage membranes by direct protease action, or by stimulating production of immune mediators like 5-hydroxytryptamine which stimulate smooth muscle cells. None of these postulated mechanisms satisfactorily explains every case of preterm labour and the aetiology is therefore considered to be multifactorial.

Table 35.1

Aetiology of preterm delivery

Spontaneous labour, cause unknown	35%
Elective delivery (iatrogenic), e.g. maternal hypertension, fetal growth problems, antepartum haemorrhage	25%
Preterm premature ruptured membranes	25%
Multiple pregnancy	15%

Box 35.1

Conditions during pregnancy associated with preterm delivery

Fetal and placental

- Congenital uterine anomaly
- Bleeding in the first or second trimester
- Antepartum haemorrhage
- Placenta praevia
- Intrauterine infection
- Pre-labour rupture of the membranes
- Fetal growth restriction
- Congenital fetal anomaly
- Multiple pregnancy
- Polyhydramnios

Maternal

- Severe maternal disease
- Pre-eclampsia
- Urinary tract infection, including asymptomatic bacteriuria
- Other infections and fevers, including malaria
- Bacterial vaginosis
- Psychological stress and domestic violence

Identifying women at increased risk of preterm birth

A number of techniques or strategies have been proposed to identify a group of pregnancies at increased risk of preterm birth. They include clinical risk scoring, bacteriological assessment of the vagina, cervical assessment and the measurement of fetal fibronectin (Ffn).

The 'risk scoring' is based on the recognized risk factors available from the maternal obstetric, gynaecological and medical histories together with smoking status, body weight and socioeconomic status. The strongest of these is history of previous preterm birth but this is not applicable to first-time mothers. Other recognized associations are presented in **Box 35.1**. Unfortunately, the performance of these scoring systems has been poor, with sensitivities quoted as less than 40%, but the system at least serves to highlight the potentially avoidable factors such as urinary tract infections, vaginal infections, smoking, drugs and lifestyle.

Screening for and treating vaginal infection has been considered as a mechanism to identify and treat those at high risk of preterm labour. Conflicting results have been demonstrated. Bacterial vaginosis, which is present in 10–20% of pregnant women, is associated with a doubling of the risk of preterm delivery if identified in the third trimester, but a fivefold increased risk if identified in the first or early second trimester. Unfortunately, clinical trials have not demonstrated that treating bacterial vaginosis reduces the risk of preterm labour. It is reasonable to treat bacterial vaginosis identified in early pregnancy, in those considered to have other risk factors for preterm labour.

Digital assessment of the cervix has also been proposed, with a high Bishop's scores (p. 342) judged to indicate an increased risk. This strategy performs poorly partly due to the difficulty in reliably assessing the length of the cervix. More recently, interest has focused on transvaginal measurement of the cervix. A normal cervical length is between 34 and 40 mm and there should be no funnelling at the internal os **(Fig. 35.1)**. A cervical length <15 mm at 23 weeks occurs in <2% of pregnancies but accounts for 90% of those who will deliver before 28 weeks. The risk of spontaneous preterm labour at less than 34 weeks' gestation with a cervical length less than 15 mm is 34%, rising to 78% if cervical length is less than 5 mm.

Fetal fibronectin is an adhesion molecule involved in maintaining the integrity of the choriodecidual extracellular matrix. It is usually not detectable in cervicovaginal secretions after 20 weeks until term or membrane rupture, but if it is found to be present it implies disruption of the extracellular matrix or an inflammatory process. The presence of fetal fibronectin measured at 23 weeks predicts 60% of spontaneous preterm births at <28 weeks in unselected pregnancies but the positive predictive ability is low, making it unsuitable for risk categorization in asymptomatic pregnancies.

Prevention of the onset of preterm labour

Antibiotics

Evidence suggests that screening for and treating asymptomatic bacteriuria can reduce the risk of preterm labour. Evidence with regards to screening for and treating vaginal organisms is more controversial. Meta-analyses have suggested that although organisms such as those causing bacterial vaginosis can be treated effectively with antibiotics, as yet evidence does not demonstrate an effect on reducing preterm delivery rates. Some studies have suggested that, in low-risk women, if such organisms are detected early in pregnancy, e.g. first trimester, then benefit can be gained by treating with clindamycin either vaginally or orally. It has been proposed that the demonstrated lack of effect of antibiotics in treating and preventing preterm labour is because of introduction of treatment after intrauterine bacterial colonization and the

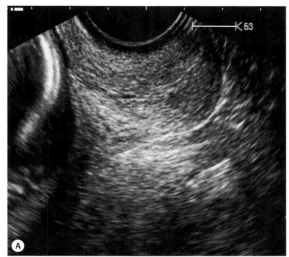

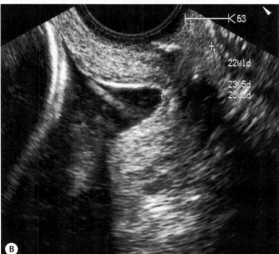

Fig. 35.1 Cervical length as measured by transvaginal scan. (A) Normal. **(B)** There is shortening of the cervix and funnelling at the internal os. Note the transvaginal cervical suture in situ.

subsequent inflammatory cascade have already become established.

Progesterone

Progesterone supplementation may reduce the risk of preterm birth. Potential mechanisms are reduced gap-junction formation, oxytocin antagonism (leading to relaxation of smooth muscle), maintenance of cervical integrity, and anti-inflammatory effects. Progesterone is administered intramuscularly or vaginally and is usually commenced around 20 weeks. Selecting the group of women who will benefit from progesterone supplementation is the subject of active research but women with previous preterm birth and/or a short cervix appear to benefit.

Cervical cerclage

There is some evidence that elective cervical cerclage (Shirodkar suture, McDonald suture – history box) performed in early second trimester is of benefit in those with a history of cervical incompetence (history of preterm birth and absence of painful uterine contractions). A Mersilene suture (or similar) is inserted transvaginally around the cervix under anaesthesia and removed electively after 38 weeks' gestation or as an emergency if labour establishes before that time (see **Fig. 35.1**). Transabdominal cervico-isthmic cerclage is a specialist procedure principally reserved for failed transcervical cerclage.

> ### History
>
> *Vithal Shirodkar (1899–1971) was an obstetrician and gynaecologist from Goa who proposed a purse-string suture of fascia lata around an incompetent cervical os to prevent second-trimester loss.*
> *Ian McDonald (1922–1990), from Australia, simplified the Shirodkar operation with the use of a silk purse-string suture around the cervix.*

'Rescue' cerclage refers to the emergency use of a suture in early preterm labour before or at the limit of viability where cervical incompetence is suspected. Careful selection criteria are employed since cerclage in the presence of clinical or subclinical infection can result in significant maternal morbidity.

Prophylactic tocolytics and bed rest are not effective interventions in the prevention of preterm labour and delivery.

Diagnosis and management of preterm labour

The definition of preterm labour is similar to the diagnosis of labour at term: regular painful contractions associated with progressive cervical dilatation. Diagnosis may be difficult in the early stages because in most cases, regular painful contractions may not progress to established labour. Labour may also be insidious, or heralded by a 'show', bleeding or abruption. Objective assessment may be helpful: a negative Ffn test means that approximately 1% of women will deliver within a week, permitting a high threshold for any interventions. Similarly, a cervical length of >20mm means that the contractions are likely to represent 'false' rather than 'true' preterm labour.

Maternal well-being is assessed by seeking evidence of infection or haemorrhage. The white cell count may be raised in infection, as may the C-reactive protein. Vaginal swabs and urine should be sent for culture.

The fetus can be assessed with cardiotocography, and then ideally with ultrasound to evaluate liquor volume, presentation, placental site and any evidence of fetal abnormality. If preterm delivery is likely, the paediatrician should be alerted and arrangements made for in-utero transfer if local facilities for resuscitation are insufficient.

Corticosteroids should be administered to the mother if delivery before 36 weeks is considered likely; they cross the placenta and increase the production and release of pulmonary surfactant by a complex receptor-mediated gene transcription mechanism. Betamethasone or dexamethasone 24 mg i.m. is given in divided doses over 24 hours and their use reduces the incidence of respiratory distress syndrome (hyaline membrane disease) by 50%. The incidence of necrotizing enterocolitis and periventricular haemorrhage is also reduced. No adverse neurological or cognitive effects following steroid treatment have been demonstrated. There is no identifiable increase in the incidence of maternal or fetal infection, but steroids are contraindicated if there is active maternal septicaemia. It is advisable to limit steroid administration to one 'course' during the pregnancy as there are some concerns regarding the effect repeated doses may have on the developing fetus, and there is no demonstrable benefit to repeated courses. Steroids should be used with caution in women with insulin-dependent diabetes, as they may precipitate ketoacidosis.

In preterm labour, intrapartum antibiotic prophylaxis (penicillin or clindamycin) is recommended to reduce the transmission of group B streptococcus. Prophylaxis in the mother may reduce the risk of early-onset neonatal group B streptococcal infection. If there is a clinical indication for antibiotics in the mother, such as a pyrexia, a broad-spectrum antibiotic should be used.

Inhibition of preterm labour

In view of the high morbidity and mortality associated with prematurity, an attempt may be made to stop preterm labour, particularly at gestations less than 33 weeks. The use of drugs to suppress uterine activity, 'tocolytics', will generate a delay of between 24 and 48 hours, which may be sufficient to allow steroid administration or in-utero transfer. On the other hand, if there has been an abruption or there is intrauterine infection, the risk of fetal compromise may be increased. Contraindications to tocolytic therapy are listed in **Box 35.2**.

A wide variety of drugs have been used for tocolysis, including calcium-channel blockers, cyclo-oxygenase inhibitors, an oxytocin antagonist and beta-sympathomimetics.

Calcium-channel blockers

There has been considerable research with nifedipine, a type 2 calcium-channel blocker, which inhibits inward calcium flow across cell membranes. Compared with beta-mimetics, nifedipine reduced the number of women delivering within 7 days of presentation and also reduced perinatal morbidity. The side-effects of dizziness, flushing and headache are all related to peripheral dilatation, but serious adverse effects are rare. There seem to be no obvious adverse fetal effects provided there is no precipitous fall in maternal blood pressure resulting in uterine underperfusion.

Box 35.2

Contraindications to tocolysis

Relative contraindications
- Significant vaginal bleeding
- Pre-eclampsia
- Fetal growth restriction

Absolute contraindications
- Fetal death
- Lethal congenital anomaly
- Chorioamnionitis
- Significant fetal distress
- Maternal condition requiring immediate delivery

Cyclo-oxygenase inhibitors

Most experience in this group of drugs is with indometacin. It inhibits cyclo-oxygenase, the enzyme which converts fatty acids into prostaglandin endoperoxidases, and it thereby reduces prostaglandin production. Trials have shown that indometacin reduces the frequency of delivery within 48 hours of presentation.

Indometacin may lead to maternal gastrointestinal irritation, thrombocytopenia, allergic reactions, headaches and dizziness but, in contrast to the beta-sympathomimetics, the main risks are to the fetus. The patency of the ductus arteriosus is prostaglandin-dependent and ductal constriction has been demonstrated in human fetuses from as early as 27 weeks' gestation in response to these drugs. There is also evidence that indometacin reduces fetal urine output, probably as a result of changes in proximal tubular reabsorption and the effect on fetal ADH. This results in reduced liquor volumes. Despite these two potential problems, significant adverse neonatal effects have not been convincingly demonstrated, but caution is nonetheless advised, particularly in cases with pre-existing oligohydramnios.

Oxytocin antagonist

Atosiban is a synthetic competitive inhibitor of oxytocin which binds to myometrial oxytocin receptors and leads to an inhibition of intracellular calcium release. It has been shown to be as effective as ritodrine, but has minimal maternal or fetal side-effects. Nausea and vomiting have occasionally been reported. Studies examining the effects of atosiban, however, failed to demonstrate its superiority over beta-mimetics or placebo in terms of tocolytic efficacy or infant outcomes, although the side-effect profile is favourable.

Beta-sympathomimetics

Ritodrine and salbutamol, which are chemically related to adrenaline (epinephrine) and noradrenaline (norepinephrine), cause stimulation of beta2-adrenergic receptors on myometrial cell membranes. This leads to a reduction in intracellular calcium concentrations and inhibition of the actin–myosin interaction necessary for smooth muscle contraction.

An intravenous infusion of ritodrine has been shown to reduce the proportion of deliveries within the first 48 hours. Beta-sympathomimetics stimulate the sympathetic nervous system and side-effects are common, including maternal (and fetal) tachycardia, visual disturbances, skin flushing, nausea, vomiting, hyperkalaemia and hyperglycaemia. Pulmonary oedema, hypotension and arrhythmias may occur, and maternal deaths have been reported. At a minimum there must be a calibrated infusion pump and good facilities for maternal monitoring. In general, most units in the UK would not use these drugs as a first-line therapy for tocolysis, preferring calcium-channel blockers or atosiban.

Delivery

If labour continues or tocolysis is unsuccessful, then close monitoring is important as a preterm fetus is more susceptible to intrapartum hypoxia and acidosis than is a fetus at term. Complications such as abnormal lie, cord prolapse, abruption and intrauterine infection are also more common.

The mode of delivery needs to be considered. While caesarean section may be indicated for an apparently compromised fetus, there is no evidence to support liberal use of caesarean section; indeed, preterm delivery by caesarean section may lead to significant fetal trauma. The vaginal route is preferred for those with cephalic presentation and there is no evidence to support the routine advocacy of epidurals, forceps or episiotomy. There is uncertainty about the most appropriate route of delivery in those presenting by the breech. In current clinical practice most preterm breeches before 26 weeks are delivered vaginally and many of those above this gestation are delivered by caesarean section.

Preterm pre-labour rupture of the membranes (PPROM)

This occurs in 2–3% of all pregnancies but in 20–50% of all spontaneous preterm deliveries and is more likely with polyhydramnios, twins, and vaginal infection. If the mother does not establish in labour, the problem is one of balancing the risks of chorioamnionitis with attendant maternal and fetal morbidity against the risks of prematurity.

The neonatal outcome is more guarded the earlier the membrane rupture occurs, on account of secondary pulmonary hypoplasia and severe skeletal deformities resulting from the absence of amniotic fluid (see **Box 35.3**). The amniotic fluid normally allows fetal movement and it circulates into the fetal lungs. Pulmonary hypoplasia occurs in 50% of cases with spontaneous membrane rupture before 20 weeks and in 3% after 24 weeks; reliable antenatal prediction of pulmonary hypoplasia remains elusive.

Chorioamnionitis is potentially extremely serious for both mother and baby as both may develop rapid and overwhelming fatal septicaemia. Infection supervenes after the membranes have ruptured in between 0.5% and 25% of

---

Box 35.3

Risks to the infant of preterm rupture of the membranes

- Cord prolapse
- Premature delivery
- Ascending intrauterine infection
- Pulmonary hypoplasia and skeletal postural deformities associated with oligohydramnios

---

cases, depending on criteria employed for diagnosis, and is more likely if vaginal examinations have been performed. Vaginal examinations are therefore contraindicated unless there is strong evidence of labour. It may be considered appropriate to carry out a sterile speculum examination to confirm the diagnosis, exclude cord prolapse and take a high vaginal swab (HVS), but an HVS is not a predictor of subsequent infection and the procedure may actually introduce infection.

The diagnosis of chorioamnionitis is suggested by maternal pyrexia, abdominal pain, uterine tenderness and a raised white cell count. It is also more likely if there has been a proven vaginal or urinary infection. It is therefore important to check the maternal temperature and white cell count, and send urine for microscopy. It should be noted that the white cell count rises after maternal steroid administration (see below), and C-reactive protein measurements are therefore preferred as a better predictor of infection.

Management of PPROM

Most mothers will establish in labour, with around 75% of those at 28 weeks' gestation delivering within 7 days. There is no evidence that tocolysis is beneficial. For those who do not establish in labour, regular fetal monitoring is essential. It is considered acceptable practice to manage these women on an outpatient basis following an initial inpatient stay and the woman is advised to take her own temperature at home four times a day. Delivery around 34–35 weeks strikes the appropriate balance between maturity and risk of chorioamnionitis but it is important to individualize management. As there is such a high risk of delivery, corticosteroids should be given if PPROM occurs at less than 36 weeks (see above). Prophylactic oral erythromycin has been shown to be associated with improved neonatal outcome when compared to placebo and is routinely recommended for 1 week post PPROM.

Key *points*

- Preterm labour occurs in 6-10% of pregnancies.
- Predicting preterm labour is difficult, but there are encouraging results from transvaginal ultrasound cervical assessment.
- Tocolytics are of limited efficacy.
- Antenatal steroids are effective in reducing respiratory distress syndrome and other complications of prematurity in the neonate.

36 Multiple pregnancy

Introduction

The natural incidence of twinning has a large geographical variation, ranging from 54/1000 in Nigeria, 12/1000 in the UK to 4/1000 in Japan. This difference is almost entirely due to variations in the rate of non-identical twins, while the incidence of identical twins remains remarkably constant at around 3/1000. In developed countries, the actual incidence of twin pregnancies is significantly greater than the natural incidence, due to in vitro fertilization and ovulation induction techniques. Around 25% of twin pregnancies, 50–60% of triplet pregnancies, and 75% of quadruplet pregnancies are a result of assisted reproduction techniques.

Overall, the perinatal mortality in twin pregnancies is four to five times higher than for singleton pregnancies, largely because of preterm delivery, fetal growth restriction, twin–twin transfusion syndrome (TTTS), and a slightly increased incidence of congenital malformations. Perinatal mortality rates rise exponentially with fetal number in higher-order pregnancies. The outcome of any multiple pregnancy is also significantly affected by its chorionicity (whether each fetus has its own or shares a placenta) **(Fig. 36.1)**.

The nature of twinning and chorionicity

'Zygosity' refers to whether the twins have come from the same ovum or from different ova – in other words whether they are identical or non-identical. 'Chorionicity' refers to the number of placentae **(Fig. 36.2)**.

Dizygotic twinning (non-identical)

Dizygotic twins account for approximately 70% of twins. This process occurs when two ova are fertilized and implant separately into the decidua. Each developing embryo will form its own outer chorion (chorionic membrane and placenta) and its own inner amniotic membrane. Dizygotic twin pregnancies are described as dichorionic and diamniotic.

Monozygotic twinning (identical)

Monozygotic twins (30% of twins) are derived from the splitting of a single embryo, and the exact configuration of placentation depends on the age of the embryo when the split occurs **(Fig. 36.2)**. A split that occurs at or before the eight-cell stage (3 days post-fertilization) will occur before the outer chorion has differentiated and will therefore give rise to two separate embryos that will each proceed to form their own chorion. These twin pregnancies, like dizygotic twins, will therefore be diamniotic and dichorionic. Embryo-splitting at the blastocyst stage (4–8 days post-fertilization)

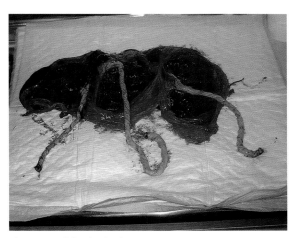

Fig. 36.1 Trichorionic placenta.

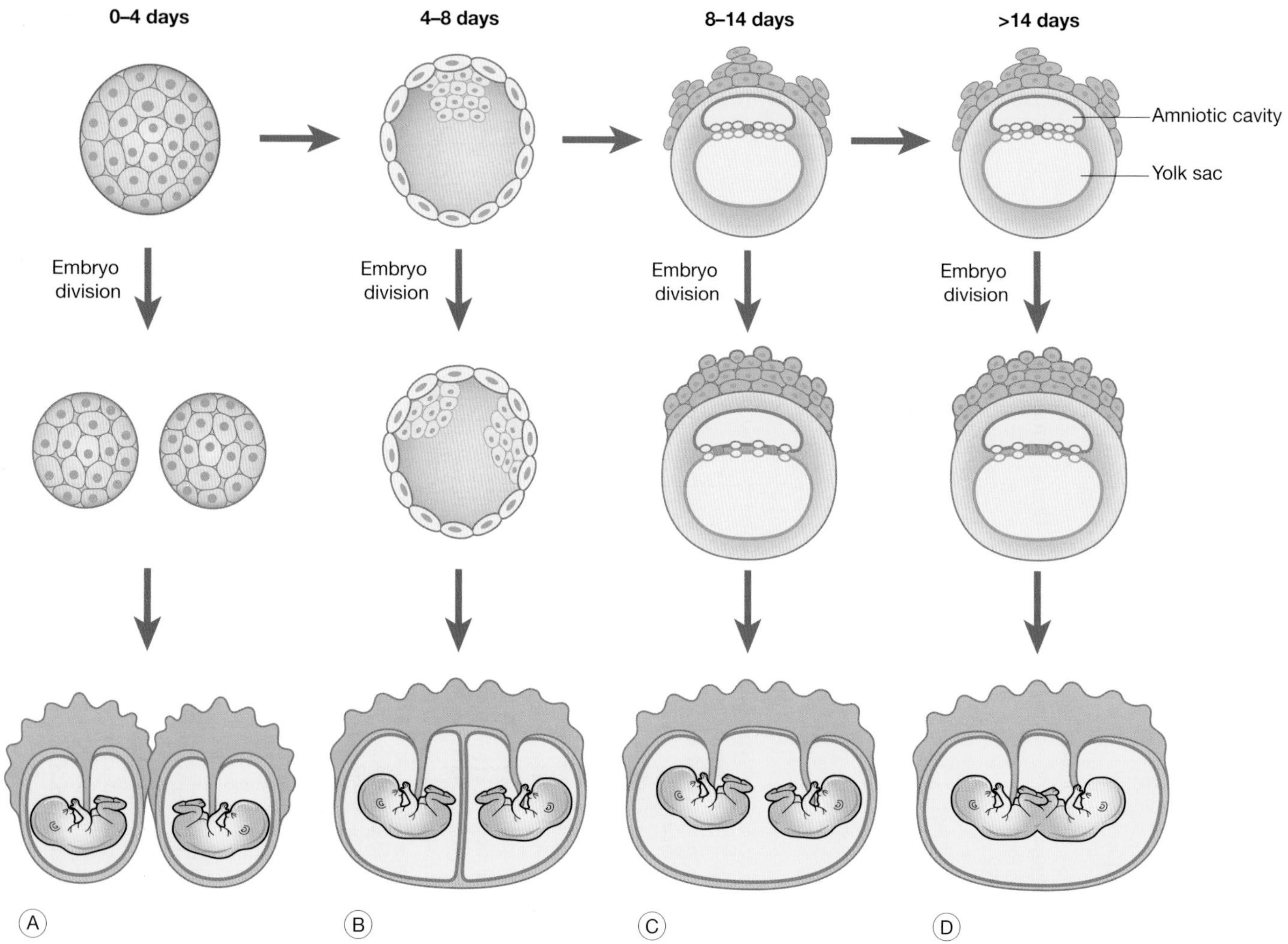

Fig. 36.2 Diagram of chorionicity. Monozygotic pregnancies may form any of the following combinations depending on the gestation of embryo division: **(A)** dichorionic diamniotic; **(B)** monochorionic diamniotic; **(C)** monochorionic monoamniotic; **(D)** conjoined twins.

Amniotic cavity

Yolk sac

0–4 days

4–8 days

8–14 days

>14 days

Embryo division

Embryo division

Embryo division

Embryo division

will occur after the chorion has started to differentiate and therefore the fetuses will share an outer chorion (placenta and outer chorionic membrane). This is the more common form of monozygotic twinning. Division of the embryo at between 8 and 14 days will result in the inner amniotic cavity and membrane being shared (monochorionic monoamniotic twins). Splitting beyond 14 days following fertilization is extremely rare, giving rise to conjoined twins **(Fig. 36.3; Table 36.1)**.

In monochorionic twins the shared placental mass inevitably contains a number of vascular anastomoses between the two fetal–placental circulations. The number and nature of these vascular connections places monochorionic twins at risk of specific complications and an increased perinatal loss and morbidity rate.

Chorionicity determination is therefore essential to allow risk stratification **(Table 36.2)**, and has key implications for prenatal diagnosis and antenatal monitoring. It is most easily determined in the first or early second trimester by ultrasound:

■ Widely separated first-trimester sacs or separate placentae are dichorionic.

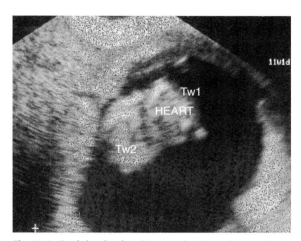

Fig. 36.3 Conjoined twins. Diagnosed at 12 weeks' gestation. This is a cross-sectional view through the thoraces of both of the twins. In view of the shared cardiac structures, termination was offered.

■ Those with a 'lambda' or 'twin-peak' sign at the membrane insertion are dichorionic **(Fig. 36.4A)**.
■ Those with a 'T' sign at the membrane insertion are monochorionic **(Fig. 36.4B)**.
■ Different-sex fetuses are always dichorionic (and dizygous).

Maternal complications

The incidence of all maternal complications is increased in multiple pregnancy.

Hyperemesis

The increased placental mass, and therefore increased maternal circulating human chorionic gonadotrophin (hCG) concentration, is associated with an increased and earlier incidence of hyperemesis.

Anaemia

There is a slight increase in the incidence of anaemia associated with multiple pregnancy, which is not completely explained by a haemodilutional effect of the increased plasma volume. The extra iron and folate requirement may justify routine supplementation.

Antepartum haemorrhage

Placenta praevia is more common with multiple gestation as a result of the larger placental surface. The management of this condition in multiple pregnancy is similar to that of a singleton pregnancy. Placental abruption also appears to be commoner in twin pregnancies.

Pre-eclampsia

The incidence of pre-eclampsia in twin pregnancy is three to four times greater than that in singleton pregnancies. It tends to develop earlier and may be more severe.

The mother is also at increased risk of gestational diabetes, general discomfort, varicose veins and dependent

Table 36.1			
Chorionicity in monozygous twins			
Timing of embryonic separation after fertilization	**Number of chorions**	**Number of amniotic sacs**	**Percentage of monozygous twins**
<4 days	Dichorionic	Diamniotic	30%
4–8 days	Monochorionic	Diamniotic	66%
8–14 days	Monochorionic	Monoamniotic	3%
>14 days	Monochorionic (conjoined)	Monoamniotic	<1%

Table 36.2

Fetal loss by chorionicity

	Dichorionic	Monochorionic
Fetal loss before 24 weeks	1.8%	12.2%
Fetal loss after 24 weeks	1.6%	2.8%
Delivery before 32 weeks	5.5%	9.2%

The high early fetal mortality in monochorionic pregnancy before 24 weeks is probably due largely to severe early-onset twin to twin transfusion sequence (see below).

oedema, delivery trauma, caesarean section, postpartum haemorrhage and breastfeeding challenges.

Fetal complications

Structural defects

The incidence of structural fetal abnormality is no different per fetus in a dichorionic pregnancy compared to a singleton pregnancy, but it is two- to threefold greater with monochorionicity. The mother therefore will have a two- to sixfold increased risk of carrying a fetus with a structural abnormality. In monochorionic twins it is thought that it is the process of embryo division which is inherently teratogenic. Characteristic abnormalities include cardiac defects, neural tube and other CNS defects, and gastrointestinal atresia. It is appropriate to offer all those with multiple pregnancies a detailed mid-trimester ultrasound scan. The abnormalities are usually confined to one twin (i.e. non-concordant); for example, if there is a neural tube defect in one twin, the other twin is normal in 85–90% of cases. Selective termination with intracardiac KCl is possible in dichorionic pregnancies only, and is most safely carried out before 16–20 weeks. The procedure, however, carries a 5% risk of miscarriage of both twins. In monochorionic twins, specialized cord occlusion techniques may be considered, but carry an increased risk of loss to the other twin due to the increased invasiveness of this procedure.

Chromosomal abnormalities

These are usually discordant in dizygotic twins and almost always concordant in monozygotic twins. The maternal age-related risk for carrying a fetus with Down syndrome is therefore approximately doubled in dichorionic twin pregnancies. Maternal serum screening for trisomy 21 performs poorly in twin pregnancy. Nuchal translucency measurement (without biochemistry) is a more useful screening test. If invasive diagnostic testing is indicated, amniocentesis of each amniotic sac is required in dichorionic pregnancies, and care must be taken to document which sample has come from which sac.

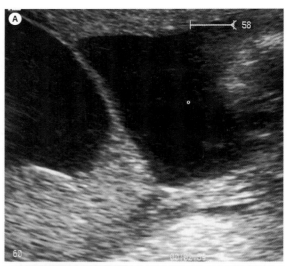

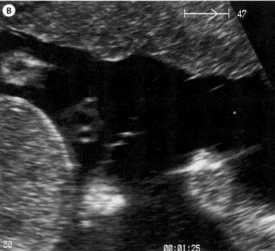

Fig. 36.4 Dichorionic twins – lambda sign (A), Monochorionic twins – no lambda sign (B). The two amniotic membranes form a 'T-sign' as they join the placenta.

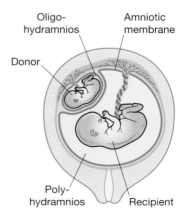

Fig. 36.5 Monochorionic twins demonstrating twin twin transfusion syndrome (Oligohydramnios—polyhydramnios Sequence).

Chorionic villous sampling is not usually appropriate for twin pregnancies as it is difficult to be sure that both placentae have been sampled, particularly if they are lying close together.

Premature birth

Twins typically deliver by 37–38 weeks' gestation and triplets by 32–34 weeks' gestation. Twins account for 25% of all premature births despite accounting for only 2% of births per year. Preterm delivery is higher in monochorionic compared to dichorionic twins **(Table 36.2)**. Increased uterine distension, early myometrial contractility and TTTS may be causative factors in premature labour in multiple pregnancy. At present there is no known effective treatment to prevent premature labour. Women should be advised to present early with any symptoms of suspected preterm labour so that corticosteroids can be administered to accelerate fetal lung maturation.

Intrauterine growth restriction

Twins typically reflect singleton size charts until 28–30 weeks' gestation and then growth slows. Approximately 30% of twins are small for gestational age by singleton standards and a significant difference in the growth of one twin compared to the other is seen in 12% of pregnancies. Placental dysfunction underlies intrauterine growth restriction in twin pregnancies as in singleton pregnancies. Abdominal palpation is not reliable to monitor fetal growth in multiple pregnancy. Serial ultrasound should be performed to measure fetal abdominal circumferences. If diagnosed, intrauterine growth restriction requires increased surveillance of fetal well-being with umbilical artery Doppler and cardiotocography (CTG) monitoring, so that delivery can be optimally timed. Monochorionic twins are at increased risk of intrauterine growth restriction, and require a lower threshold for delivery owing to the adverse consequences of a single intrauterine death in these twins.

Twins with one fetal death

First-trimester intrauterine death in a twin has not been shown to have adverse consequences for the survivor. This probably also holds true for the early second trimester, but loss in the late second or third trimester commonly precipitates labour such that 90% will have delivered both twins within 3 weeks of the loss. Prognosis for a surviving dichorionic fetus is then influenced primarily by its gestation. When a monochorionic twin dies in utero, however, there are additional risks of death (approximately 20%) or cerebral damage (approximately 25%) in the co-twin as a result of the shared fetal–placental circulations. As these are probably related to acute hypotension in the co-twin at the time of the other's death, early delivery of the surviving twin is unlikely to improve its outcome and may compound morbidity if performed at a premature gestation.

Antenatal problems specific to monochorionic twin pregnancies

Twin–twin transfusion syndrome (TTTS)

This complicates 10–15% of monochorionic multiple pregnancies and accounts for around 15% of perinatal mortality in twins. In this condition there is a net blood flow from one twin to the other through arterial to venous anastomoses in the shared placenta. The circulation of the recipient becomes hyperdynamic, with the risk of high-output cardiac failure and polyhydramnios. Conversely, the donor develops oliguria and oligohydramnios and often suffers growth restriction **(Figs. 36.5, 36.6)**. The ultrasound finding of the oligohydramnios/polyhydramnios sequence is the key to establishing an antenatal diagnosis.

Without treatment TTTS is associated with a greater than 80% pregnancy loss rate. Two interventions have proven useful: serial amniodrainage and laser ablation of the causative placental vascular anastomoses. Evidence has emerged that laser ablation is the most effective intervention (70% survival vs 50% survival with amnioreduction). Laser therapy is also associated with a lower rate of significant neurological morbidity in surviving twins compared to amnioreduction (5% vs 15%).

Monoamniotic twins

Twins who occupy a single amniotic sac, are at risk of cord entanglement in utero. Frequent CTG monitoring is required once they reach viability. Delivery is indicated if cord compression is subsequently diagnosed. Delivery is otherwise electively planned for 32 weeks' gestation. Delivery should be performed by caesarean section, as the risk of a cord accident is particularly high during labour.

Twin reversed arterial perfusion sequence

If the heart of one monochorionic twin stops, it may continue to be partially perfused by the surviving twin if large fetal arterial-to-arterial anastomoses exist in the shared placenta. The dead twin undergoes atrophy of its upper body and heart due to the especially poor oxygenation of these tissues, and becomes what has been described as an 'acardiac monster'. The condition is very rare and there is a high incidence of mortality in the donor twin due to intrauterine cardiac failure and prematurity. Cord ligation has been used with success in isolated cases.

Management of pregnancy

Initial visit

As many as 10% of twin pregnancies diagnosed in the first trimester will proceed only as singleton pregnancies and

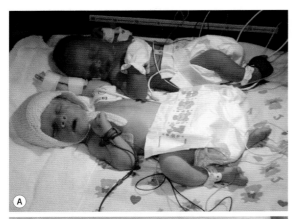

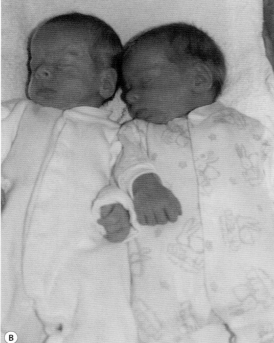

Fig. 36.6 Twin–twin transfusion sequence. These monochorionic twins were born at 37 weeks' gestation. Although their weights were almost identical, there was significant oligohydramnios around the recipient. **(A)** Pre-transfusion. **(B)** Post-transfusion. (With permission.)

parents should be made aware of this. It is important to ensure that chorionicity has been established at the first scan, as it becomes increasingly difficult to do so with advancing gestation. It may also be worth considering starting iron and folate supplementation at this stage.

The parents are often quite excited, and often shocked, so initial counselling should be brief and focus mostly on the positive aspects. The parents should however be asked to consider whether they want antenatal screening and should particularly consider the potential problems of finding one normal and one abnormal twin. Finally it

should be explained that more frequent antenatal visits will be required and that ultrasound will be used to monitor growth.

Subsequent visits

These are ideally performed at a dedicated twins clinic and timed to coincide with the ultrasound assessments, the schedule of which will depend on chorionicity.
Monochorionic twins:

- Every 2 weeks from 16 to 24 weeks to survey for TTTS.
- Detailed structural survey at 18 weeks' gestation.
- Detailed fetal cardiac scan at 20–22 weeks' gestation.
- Every 2 weeks from 24 weeks for fetal growth assessment.

Dichorionic twins:

- Detailed structural survey at 18 weeks' gestation.
- Every 2–4 weeks from 24 weeks for fetal growth assessment.

The mother should be monitored for complications such as pre-eclampsia and anaemia. Discussions about the risks and management of premature delivery and fetal growth problems are useful at 22–24 weeks' gestation. In uncomplicated pregnancies, discussion around mode of delivery and management of twin labour is useful at 32 weeks' gestation, when fetal presentations are unlikely to change. Tailored parentcraft advice or classes is worthwhile.

Management of twin delivery

Presentations at term are typically:

- cephalic/cephalic (40%)
- cephalic/breech (40%)
- breech/cephalic (10%)
- other, e.g. transverse (10%).

It is common practice to induce labour at 38–40 weeks in those who are suitable for vaginal delivery, and to carry out a caesarean section at 38 weeks in those who are not. In general with twins, providing the presentation of the first twin is cephalic, the balance of current evidence would suggest that vaginal birth is appropriate. Significant growth discordance may be a reason to consider caesarean section. If the labour is preterm (<34 weeks), many clinicians would also consider delivery by caesarean section.

The first stage of labour is managed as for singleton pregnancies and care should be taken to ensure that both twins are being monitored with CTG, rather than one twin twice. This is best achieved by monitoring twin I with a fetal scalp electrode and twin II abdominally.

An experienced obstetrician, an anaesthetist, two paediatricians and two midwives should be present for delivery, and, if not already required, a Syntocinon infusion should be ready in case uterine activity decreases after delivery of the first twin. After delivery of the first twin, it is often helpful to have someone 'stabilize' the lie of second twin to longitudinal by abdominal palpation while a vaginal examination is performed to assess the station of the presenting part. A portable, ultrasound machine is helpful to confirm the lie and presentation of the second twin. The membranes of twin II should not be broken until the presenting part has descended into the pelvis. If twin II lies transversely after the delivery of twin I, external cephalic or breech version is appropriate. If the lie is still transverse (particularly likely if the back is towards the fundus), the choice is between breech extraction (gentle continuous traction on one or both feet through intact membranes) and caesarean section. The CTG of twin II should be carefully monitored throughout and delivery expedited if suspected fetal distress is observed.

A maternal epidural is useful in the management of twin labour owing to the increased risks of obstetric intervention, particularly assisted delivery of twin II.

Triplets and higher multiples

In these cases, the perinatal mortality is high, mostly because of the high risk of premature labour, and it may be appropriate to discuss reducing the number of fetuses to twins at 12–14 weeks' gestation. With quadruplets or higher-order pregnancies, there is likely to be a greater chance of at least one or two survivors if fetal reduction is carried out, despite the miscarriage risk associated with the procedure itself. For triplets, the situation is less clear. The emotional and ethical problems associated with these decisions are considerable.

Triplets and higher-order multiple pregnancies require intensive antenatal care. These pregnancies are best delivered by caesarean section due to the inability to effectively monitor all fetuses in labour and the higher risk of fetal malpresentation.

Key *points*

- It is essential to establish chorionicity early to help advise about prenatal diagnosis and stratify subsequent care. Prenatal screening should only be undertaken after careful discussion of its implications.
- Monochorionic pregnancies are at further increased risk of preterm delivery and intrauterine growth restriction. They also have specific additional risks such as twin–twin transfusion syndrome and loss of co-twin complications.

37

Fetal haemolytic disease

Introduction

Haemolytic disease is likely to occur when maternal antibodies develop against fetal red blood cells. Red cells not infrequently cross from the fetus to the mother either antenatally or at some intrapartum event and, if they are antigenically different from the mother's red cells, there may be a maternal immune response with antibody production. IgG antibodies may cross in the opposite direction, back to the fetus, leading to haemolysis, anaemia, high-output cardiac failure and fetal death. There are numerous known red cell antigens but the rhesus D antigen accounts for approximately 85% of haemolytic disease.

Maternal rhesus isoimmunization exemplifies the achievements of systematic scientific and clinical research. In just 40 years it has been possible to unravel the pathophysiology, devise useful treatments and introduce an effective means to prevent a condition which had previously caused extensive fetal morbidity and mortality. Among populations with access to an anti-D prophylaxis programme, the fully developed clinical condition of haemolytic disease of the newborn is rare.

The blood group system

Blood groups are determined by antigens on the erythrocyte cell wall. In the ABO system the letter O is used to refer to those who lack both the A and B antigens. If the mother is group O and the fetus has paternally inherited the A or B antigen, the mother may, if exposed, develop antibodies to these fetal cells. In practice these antibodies rarely cause significant haemolytic disease and no antenatal investigations are warranted.

The next most important system is the rhesus system, which comprises at least 40 antigens, the most important of which are C, D and E. C and E have immunologically distinct isoforms which are designated 'c' and 'e', but it seems unlikely that a 'd' isoform exists. If there is a 'd' antigen, it

seems to have little if any immunogenic potential and the notation 'd' is used to indicate the absence of 'D'. A parent contributes one or other antigen (e.g. C or c) to the offspring from each of these three alphabetically designated pairs. An individual can therefore be homozygous or heterozygous for any of the six (e.g. Cde/cDE, cde/cdE). Those who carry the D antigen, which is inherited as an autosomal dominant, are referred to as rhesus D positive whether in the homozygous or heterozygous form.

Any of the rhesus antigens are capable of stimulating antibody formation but the D antigen is by far the most immunogenic, followed by c and E. If a rhesus-negative mother has a rhesus-positive baby and is at some stage sensitized to the baby's red cells, there is a chance of anti-D antibodies developing against the fetal cells. These antibodies may cross back to the fetus and lead to fetal haemolytic anaemia.

There are other significant antigens in addition to the ABO and rhesus systems. Many of these (e.g. Ce, Fya, Jka, Cw) are poorly developed on the red cell surface and usually stimulate only low levels of antibody production, often of the IgM category (which does not cross the placenta). Some, however, will cause significant haemolytic disease. One notable exception is the anti-Kell antibody, which seems to cause fetal bone marrow aplasia rather than haemolytic disease and is therefore much more complex to manage.

Incidence

This varies widely. Before the availability of anti-D prophylaxis, rhesus haemolytic disease was common in populations where there was a high prevalence of Rh (D)-negative individuals and where high parity caused an accumulation of isoimmunized women. In the UK, 17% of the population is Rh (D) negative and, assuming random mating without intervention, around two-thirds of Rh (D)-negative mothers would be expected to carry a rhesus-positive fetus.

Approximately 10% of pregnant women are therefore at risk of developing anti-D antibodies.

Since the effective use of prophylactic anti-D, the perinatal mortality from haemolytic disease has fallen from around 46/100,000 to 1.9/100,000. Newly sensitized cases are detected at a rate of approximately 1/1000 maternities.

Aetiology and predisposing factors

Transfer of fetal erythrocytes to the maternal circulation during pregnancy (fetomaternal haemorrhage) may occur without any obvious predisposing event and about 75% of women may be found to have fetal red cells circulating at some stage during the pregnancy or delivery. Fetomaternal haemorrhage is more likely, however, with disruption of the placental bed and this may occur with:

- miscarriage and ectopic pregnancy
- invasive intrauterine procedures, e.g. amniocentesis, CVS
- external cephalic version
- abdominal trauma
- antepartum haemorrhage
- labour and delivery, particularly with delivery of the placenta.

An immune response may, but does not inevitably, follow fetomaternal haemorrhage. The response depends in part on the volume of blood, its antigenic potential, and on the maternal responsiveness. ABO incompatibility between mother and fetus may paradoxically offer some protection, as the transfused cells are likely to be haemolysed by circulating maternal antibodies, reducing the risk of immunization. This observation illustrates the mechanism for the use of prophylactic anti-D immunoglobulin in that exogenous anti-D is used to bind and lyse any rhesus-positive fetal red cells that reach the maternal circulation.

Pathophysiology of haemolytic disease

Initial exposure leads to a small antigen-specific antibody response, largely of IgM (which does not cross the placenta). On subsequent exposure, for example in a second pregnancy, the already primed B cells produce a much larger response, this time with IgG, which does cross the placenta. In the fetal circulation it forms an antibody–antigen complex on the red cell membrane which provokes phagocytosis of the cell by the reticuloendothelial system and results in a reduction in fetal red cell numbers. This will lead to anaemia unless there is sufficient compensatory haemopoiesis from the marrow, spleen and liver.

Increasing anaemia causes progressive fetal hypoxia and acidosis leading to hepatic and cardiac dysfunction. Generalized oedema of skin develops, as well as ascites, a pericardial effusion and pleural effusions. This syndrome is known as immune hydrops fetalis and it may be fatal.

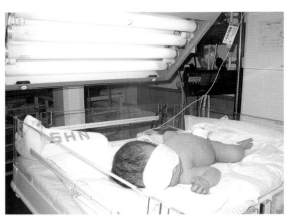

Fig. 37.1 Baby delivered at 37 weeks because of high anti-D levels. The bilirubin level rose steeply in the first 24 hours but, with phototherapy, exchange transfusion was avoided.

With haemolysis there is also an increased production of bilirubin, most of which passes across the placenta to the mother and is cleared by the maternal system. The fetus therefore does not become jaundiced antenatally, but after delivery its own liver is unable to metabolize bilirubin sufficiently quickly and the neonatal bilirubin level rises **(Fig. 37.1)**. If untreated, the bilirubin can rise to levels which endanger the nervous system. Bilirubin deposition in the basal ganglia leads to a condition called 'kernicterus'.

Although most fetal bilirubin is readily cleared, some also passes into the fetal urine and then into the amniotic fluid. The level of amniotic bilirubin is therefore an indicator of the severity of the haemolysis.

Prevention of haemolytic disease

Anti-D prophylaxis

The most effective preventive measure is the use of intramuscular anti-D to provide passive immunization of non-sensitized women around the time of exposure. A rhesus-negative mother who has a potentially sensitizing event (see **Box 37.1**) before 20 weeks' gestation should be given 250 IU of anti-D as soon as possible after the event, and certainly within 72 hours if possible. At more than 20 weeks the dose is 500 IU. At delivery a sample of fetal cord blood should be rhesus grouped and, if positive, a film made of the mother's blood for Kleihauer testing. The Kleihauer test estimates the volume of fetomaternal transfer and allows an appropriate dose of anti-D to be calculated.

As immunization can occur as a result of silent fetomaternal haemorrhage, prophylaxis is likely to be more effective if anti-D is given to all non-sensitized rhesus-negative mothers routinely in the third trimester (either 500 IU at 28 and 34 weeks, or a single larger dose early in the third trimester). This is standard practice in most areas.

Box 37.1

Indications for anti-D immunoprophylaxis

First trimester
- Ectopic pregnancy
- Surgical or medical termination of pregnancy
- Miscarriage with heavy loss or requiring surgical evacuation of products
- Chorionic villous sampling

Second trimester
- Amniocentesis
- Threatened miscarriage or antepartum haemorrhage
- Abdominal trauma

Third trimester
- Routine prophylaxis
- Antepartum haemorrhage
- External cephalic version
- Delivery
- Abdominal trauma

Table 37.1

Possible screening programme for antibodies in haemolytic disease of the newborn

All pregnant women (whether D +ve or D –ve)	ABO + Rh D group and antibody screen Rh D group and antibody screen	At 10–16 weeks At 28–36 weeks
Patients identified with alloantibodies Anti-D, c or Kell related	Antibody screen ± titre	At least monthly to 28 weeks, then 2-weekly to term
Other antibodies	Antibody screen ± titre	At 28–36 weeks, thereafter depending on the titre

Surprisingly, there is some evidence of benefit from anti-D prophylaxis even for women already mildly sensitized, in that subsequent children appear less severely affected by haemolytic disease than would otherwise have been expected.

Clinical presentation of haemolytic disease

Clinical symptoms and signs of fetal haemolytic anaemia occur late, are easily missed, and are of little help in management. In advanced disease, fetal movements may become feeble or even absent and there may be fetal growth restriction. Polyhydramnios, which is associated with fetal hydrops, may also be detected. In reality, however, detection is based on routine antenatal screening.

Routine maternal screening

All pregnant women at their first visit have serum sent for ABO and Rh (D) grouping with screening for irregular antibodies. The maternal serum level of any antibody discovered (usually anti-D) is used as an initial screening test for further action. There are regional variations, but an example of when to check for antibody levels is shown in **Table 37.1**.

Fetal assessment

If screening demonstrates the presence of an isoimmune antibody, further assessment is required to determine its significance. This depends in part on the clinical details and on the likely antigen status of the fetus. Additional investigation with middle cerebral artery Doppler may be warranted, and this may indicate the need for treatment by intrauterine transfusion. An important principle is that invasive procedures carry potential fetal risks and also increase the chance of fetomaternal haemorrhage which may exacerbate the isoimmune condition itself.

Clinical significance of the antibody

Red cell antigens vary in their likelihood of stimulating an immune response, with the D antigen being the most immunogenic. Most of the other antigens are less likely to lead to significant clinical problems and are not discussed further in this section. The D antibody titre in maternal serum can be measured and the level is recognized to correlate well with disease severity. Severe disease is rare if the maternal antibody level is <4 IU/ml, and additional specific intervention is probably not required. The risk of significant problems is only moderate between 4 and 15 IU/ml but above 15 IU/ml there is a risk of severe anaemia in 50% of fetuses. These higher levels call for further investigation, described below, and the management of these relatively uncommon cases should be centralized within specialized units. A sudden rise in levels, rather than a particular absolute level, is also likely to be significant.

The next stage is to assess the likely rhesus status of the baby by establishing the genotype of the putative father and remembering that the D antigen is inherited as an autosomal dominant. If the father is found to be d/d it is likely that anti-D antibodies in a rhesus-negative woman have developed from exposure to some other source of incompatible red cells, for example a previous blood transfusion or the fetus of a previous partner. Assuming confident paternity, the fetus will be unaffected and further specific action is unnecessary. If the father is homozygous for the D antigen, it follows that the fetus will also be rhesus D positive and will be at risk of haemolytic disease. Where the father is believed to be D/d, half of his offspring will be rhesus positive. In this situation it is important to establish the fetal blood group to determine whether or not the pregnancy is at risk. This can be done non-invasively by examining cell-free fetal DNA present in a maternal blood sample. Accuracies of 100% are reported for Rh D genotyping. DNA amplification of amniotic fluid should only be performed for fetal genotyping if the patient is already undergoing amniocentesis for other indications.

Non-invasive testing

Historically, serial amniocentesis and measurement of amniotic fluid bilirubin levels was the method of assessing at-risk pregnancies. However, this has been superseded by non-invasive testing utilizing fetal middle cerebral artery Doppler studies **(Fig. 37.2)**. A hyperkinetic circulation correlates very well with the degree of fetal anaemia, and can be used to predict the requirement for further therapy. In severe cases, there may be fetal hydrops with signs of ascites, a pericardial effusion, pleural effusions, and oedema of the skin.

Cardiotocography is also used and may reveal an unreactive pattern or even decelerations, but again only in advanced disease. A sinusoidal fetal heart pattern is thought to be fairly specific for severe anaemia. Between assessments, maternal counting of fetal movements may be of some use as they are usually reduced in severe fetal anaemia.

If ultrasound assessment is normal and the antibody level relatively low, a conservative approach with delivery at term is appropriate. If there are abnormal parameters, or a high antibody level, invasive testing by fetal blood sampling may be indicated.

Fetal blood sampling

This is carried out by inserting a needle into the baby's cord, at its point of placental insertion, and enables an immediate haemoglobin estimation to be made. It also provides a mechanism by which blood can be transfused in utero during the same procedure. Group O rhesus-negative blood is crossmatched to the mother's own serum prior to the procedure and, if the haemoglobin (or, in some centres, the

haematocrit) is low, a calculated volume may be transfused during the same sampling procedure. Intrauterine transfusion (IUT) carries the risk of cord haematomas, fetal bradycardia, intrauterine death, and further sensitization of the mother to fetal red cell antigens. It may need to be repeated on a number of occasions, depending on severity.

If an intravascular transfusion is too technically difficult, it is possible to inject the red cells directly into the peritoneal cavity, from which they are subsequently absorbed by the fetal lymphatic system.

Additional measures

In severe early cases, when hydropic change occurs before fetal transfusion is technically possible, repeated maternal plasma exchange may reduce the levels of maternal antibody. The technique requires special equipment to separate red cells from plasma and is both time-consuming and expensive. Maternal immunosuppression has also been tried in very severe cases.

Delivery

All babies with haemolytic disease should be delivered in a specialist unit with full neonatal intensive care facilities. If premature delivery is anticipated, maternal corticosteroid therapy is warranted. Babies in whom mild anaemia is suspected, or who have been successfully treated with IUT, can be delivered vaginally unless there are other obstetric indications for caesarean section. For cases managed with IUT, labour is induced at around 35 weeks' gestation. If a hydropic fetus requires delivery, this should be by caesarean section. Experienced paediatric attendance at delivery is essential and cord blood must be collected for assessment of haemoglobin, platelets, blood grouping, bilirubin and direct Coombs' testing. The neonate may require intensive support with measures to control anaemia, hyperbilirubinaemia and any associated cardiorespiratory problems.

Prognosis

For mildly affected fetuses in whom intrauterine therapy is unnecessary, the outlook, in experienced units, is excellent. Survival rates for non-hydropic fetuses undergoing IUT are ≥90%, compared with approximately 75% if hydrops is present.

Long-term sequelae

Early reports suggested serious neurological impairments, including cerebral palsy, abnormal development and hearing problems, especially in those children who were transfused in utero. Recent experience is very much more reassuring and suggests there are few, if any, additional risks beyond the well-recognized hazards of prematurity.

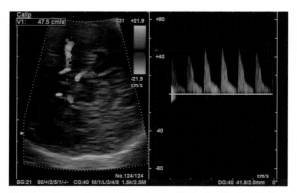

Fig 37.2 Measuring the blood velocity in the fetal middle cerebral artery correlates very well with the level of fetal anemia. This non-invasive assessment can be used to determine the need for intrauterine transfusion.

Key *points*

- Isoimmunization occurs when maternal antibodies develop against fetal red blood cells. These antibodies cross to the fetus and may lead to haemolysis, anaemia, high-output cardiac failure and fetal death. There are numerous known red cell antigens but the rhesus D antigen accounts for more than 85% of haemolytic disease.
- Entry of fetal cells to the maternal circulation is particularly likely with disruption of the placental bed, for example with antepartum haemorrhage. Passive immunization with anti-D IgG prevents sensitization in most cases.
- Appropriately regular serological screening of all pregnant women for irregular antibodies is essential to ensure timely detection of isoimmune fetal haemolytic disease.
- Treatment of severe disease is highly specialized and requires referral to appropriately experienced units. Assessment involves the use of Doppler ultrasound, and when fetal anaemia is suspected, fetal therapy with IUT is possible.

38

Labour

Introduction

Labour in humans is surprisingly hazardous. Evolution ought to have favoured those mothers who deliver without problems, and yet, for those without access to good medical care, the lifetime risk of dying from labour and postnatal complications may be 10% or more. Why has tens of thousands of years of natural selection not selected out those who labour poorly, favouring those who labour safely and go on to reproduce again?

Apes are able to give birth with little problem. Their pelvises are relatively large, the fetal head is relatively small and the fetus is born facing anteriorly. When the Australopithecines adopted an upright posture around 4 million years ago, the pelvic shape became narrower in the anteroposterior plane to allow more efficient weight transfer from the trunk to the femurs. As the fetal head was still relatively small, the Australopithecines were also able to deliver without much problem, although the head was this time in the transverse position.

With further evolution 1.5 million years ago to *Homo erectus* and then *Homo sapiens* the volume of the brain increased from around 500 ml to 1000–2000 ml. This increased the chance of the head being bigger than the pelvis (cephalopelvic disproportion) and to deliver successfully it became necessary for the head to rotate during delivery. The head entered the pelvic brim in the transverse position, as the inlet is widest in the transverse plane, but rotated at the pelvic floor to the anteroposterior plane, which is the widest diameter of the pelvic outlet.

This process requires efficient uterine activity and is aided by 'moulding' of the fetal head. Moulding is possible because the individual skull bones are unfused and can therefore move or even override each other to form the most efficient shape for delivery. The pelvic ligaments, particularly the cartilaginous joint of the symphysis pubis, relax antenatally under the influence of a hormone called relaxin, to maximize the pelvic diameters. Successful delivery also requires the fetus to enter the pelvis in the appropriate position. When these criteria are not met, problems may occur and these are discussed further in Chapter 42. The difficulty with human delivery, then, is related to the balance between our need to run (and therefore have a narrow pelvis) and our need to think (and therefore have a big head).

Primigravid compared to multigravid labour

There is a considerable difference between the labour of a primigravida (a mother having her first labour) and that of a parous woman who has had a previous vaginal delivery (Table 38.1). A first labour is one of the most profound emotional experiences any individual will experience. A successful well-managed vaginal delivery first time around usually leads to subsequent deliveries being relatively uneventful. Conversely, a poorly managed first labour can add to subsequent obstetric problems, and have emotional ramifications far beyond any obstetrical complications that may have occurred.

The uterus during pregnancy

The uterus is a thick-walled hollow organ, normally located entirely, in the non-pregnant state, within the lesser pelvis. The smooth muscle fibres interdigitate to form a single functional muscle which increases markedly during pregnancy mainly by hypertrophy (an increase in size of cells) and to a lesser extent by hyperplasia (an increase in the number of smooth muscle cells).

From early pregnancy onwards the uterus contracts intermittently, and the frequency and amplitude of these contractions increase as labour approaches. These 'Braxton Hicks' contractions are irregular, low frequency and high amplitude in character and are only occasionally painful. They normally begin at a 'pacemaker point' close to the junction of the uterus and the fallopian tube and spread from this point downwards. Intensity is maximal at the

Table 38.1

The difference between a normal primigravid and multigravid labour

Primigravida	Multigravida
Unique psychological experience	
Inefficient uterine action is common, therefore labour is often longer	Uterine action is efficient and genital tract stretches more easily, therefore labour is usually shorter
The functional capacity of the pelvis is not known – cephalopelvic disproportion is a possibility	Cephalopelvic disproportion is rare. If it does occur, it is usually secondary to some serious problem
Serious injury to the child is relatively more common. The incidence of instrumental delivery is higher	Serious injury to the child is rare. Furthermore, the risk of birth injury is less when the baby is born by propulsion rather than traction
Uterus is virtually immune to rupture	There is a small risk of uterine rupture, particularly if there is a pre-existing caesarean section scar

Box 38.1

Pro-pregnancy factors and pro-labour factors

Pro-pregnancy factors

- Progesterone
- Nitric oxide
- Catecholamines
- Relaxin

Pro-labour factors

- Oestrogens
- Oxytocin
- Prostaglandins
- Prostaglandin dehydrogenase
- Inflammatory mediators

fundus (where the muscle is thickest), intermediate at the mid-zone and least at the lower segment.

The initiation of labour

The mechanisms controlling the onset of labour are different for different mammals. In some mammals, it is the changing levels of oestrogen and progesterone which regulate the timing of onset. In other animals, for example sheep, there is some evidence that the fetal adrenal secretion of corticosteroids is the responsible trigger. In humans, however, there is no evidence of any sudden hormonal changes prior to the onset of labour and the precise trigger mechanism remains unclear. Any proposed mechanism must therefore be considered to be a hypothesis.

It seems that there is a balance between pro-pregnancy factors and pro-labour factors **(Box 38.1)**, the pro-pregnancy factors promoting pregnancy continuation and the pro-labour factors stimulating the onset of labour. Labour may be triggered when the pro-pregnancy factors become overwhelmed by increasing levels of the pro-labour factors, although why this should occur at one particular point remains uncertain. There is some limited evidence that the human fetus may play a role in regulating this balance, but the mother also has a role.

Pro-pregnancy factors

Progesterone is derived from the corpus luteum for the first 8 weeks or so of pregnancy and thereafter from the placenta. It has the direct effect of decreasing uterine oxytocin

receptor sensitivity and therefore promotes uterine smooth muscle relaxation. That it plays a significant pro-pregnancy role is illustrated by the fact that the progesterone antagonist mifepristone increases myometrial contractility, and has been successfully used to induce labour. Nitric oxide, a highly reactive free radical, is also a pro-pregnancy factor. Some studies have observed a fall in uterine nitric oxide synthetase activity as pregnancy advances, but these findings are not confirmed in other studies. Catecholamines act directly on the myometrial cell membrane to alter contractility and beta-sympathomimetics are used as tocolytics to suppress preterm labour. The specific roles for catecholamines in physiological terms and the role of the hormone relaxin are unclear.

Pro-labour factors

Oxytocin, a nonapeptide from the posterior pituitary, is a potent stimulator of uterine contractility. Circulating levels, however, do not change as term approaches. Oestrogen levels do increase, and oestrogens increase oxytocin receptor expression within the uterus. This gradual rise may be mediated in part by fetal adrenocorticotrophic hormone (ACTH). Prostaglandin levels also increase prior to the onset of labour. These are synthesized from arachidonic acid by cyclo-oxygenase (COX), and COX-2 enzyme expression in the fetal membranes has been observed to double by the time labour begins. Prostaglandins promote cervical ripening and stimulate uterine contractility both directly and by upregulation of oxytocin receptors, and there is some evidence that the increased levels may be mediated by maternal corticotrophin-releasing hormone (CRH) secretion.

Hypothesis

A proposed hypothesis for the onset of labour is that the uterus is under strong initial progesterone suppression but the rising oestrogen and CRH concentrations activate cell surface receptors and COX-2 activity. The increased myometrial activity is further promoted by an inflammatory

Summary of the mechanism of the labour

- Head at pelvic brim in left or right occipitolateral position
- Neck flexes so that the presenting diameter is suboccipitobregmatic
- Head descends and engages
- Head reaches the pelvic floor and occiput rotates to occipitoanterior
- Head delivers by extension
- Descent continues and shoulders rotate into the anteroposterior diameter of the pelvis
- Head restitutes (comes into line with the shoulders)
- Anterior shoulder delivered by lateral flexion from downward pressure on the baby's head; posterior shoulder delivered by lateral flexion upwards

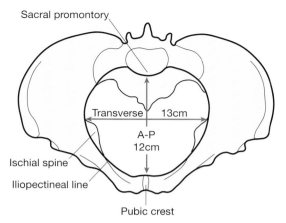

Fig. 38.2 The maternal pelvic inlet. The widest diameter is from one side laterally to the other.

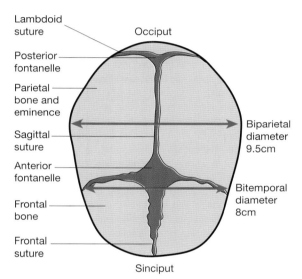

Fig. 38.1 The fetal skull. The widest diameter is anteroposterior.

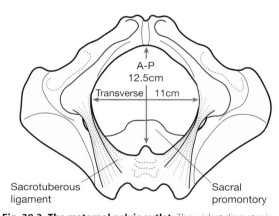

Fig. 38.3 The maternal pelvic outlet. The widest diameter is anteroposterior.

reaction in both the myometrium and the cervix, a process which also promotes cervical ripening. The actual timing of onset may therefore be determined by the oestrogen or CRH concentration reaching a sufficient level to overcome the pro-pregnancy suppression, but to what extent this is under maternal or fetal influence is unclear.

The mechanism of normal labour

(See also pelvic anatomy, Ch. 1.)

The mechanism of labour involves effacement and then dilatation of the cervix, followed by expulsion of the fetus by uterine contraction. The lower part of the uterus is anchored to the pelvis by the transverse cervical (or cardinal) ligaments as well as the uterosacral ligaments, allowing the shortening uterine muscle to drive the fetus downwards **(Box 38.2)**.

The cervix is composed of a network of collagen fibres embedded in proteoglycans and it needs to soften and efface before delivery can occur. Prostaglandins increase cervical ripening by inhibiting collagen synthesis and stimulating collagenase activity to break down the collagen. This collagenase activity comes in part from fibroblast cells but also from an influx of inflammatory cells, supporting the theory that labour is in part like an inflammatory process. Within the cervix the result is an overall reduction in the firm collagen fibres, leaving it softer and ready to dilate.

The fetus then needs to traverse the pelvis. The widest two points of the fetus are the head in the anteroposterior plane **(Fig. 38.1)** and the shoulders, laterally from one shoulder tip to the other (bis-acromial diameter). The head rotates from a lateral position at the pelvic brim to the anteroposterior position at the outlet **(Fig 38.2, 38.3** and **Fig 38.4)**. This rotation has the advantage that by the time the head is delivering through the outlet, the shoulders will be entering the inlet in the transverse position, maximizing the chance of successful delivery.

The position of the head as it traverses the canal is described according to the position of the occiput in relation

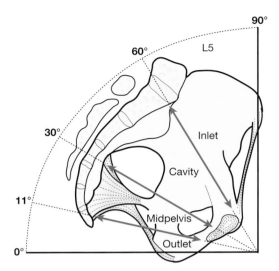

Fig. 38.4 Lateral view of the pelvis.

to the mother's pelvis The head usually enters the pelvic brim in either the right or the left occipitotransverse position **(Fig. 38.5A)**. The contracting uterus above causes the head to flex, so that the minimum head diameter is presented for delivery.

As the head descends it reaches the V-shaped pelvic floor at the level of the ischial spines **(Fig. 38.5B,C,D)** The V-shaped pelvic floor encourages the fundamentally important head rotation. **Figure 38.6** illustrates the tendency for the longest part of the head to fit into the lowest part of the V-shaped gutter, achievable only by a 90° rotation to either the occipitoanterior or occipitoposterior position. In most cases the head rotates anteriorly. The consequences of posterior rotation are discussed on page 359. The head, now occipitoanterior, descends beyond the ischial spines and extends, distending the vulva until it is eventually delivered **(Fig. 38.5E,F)**.

Meanwhile, at the pelvic inlet, the shoulders are now presenting in the transverse position. They too descend to the pelvic floor and rotate to the anteroposterior position in the V of the pelvic floor **(Fig. 38.5G)**. By this time the head has been completely delivered and it is free to rotate back to the transverse position along with the shoulders. The anterior shoulder can then be delivered by downward traction of the head, so that the lateral traction on the fetal trunk allows the shoulder to be freed from under the pubic arch **(Fig. 38.5G)**. The posterior shoulder is delivered with upward lateral traction and the rest of the baby usually follows without difficulty **(Fig. 38.5H)**.

The third stage of labour is from delivery of the baby until delivery of the placenta. The uterus contracts, shearing the placenta from the uterine wall, and this separation is often indicated by a small rush of dark blood and a 'lengthening' of cord. The placenta can then be delivered by gentle cord traction **(Fig. 38.5I)** but caution is required to avoid uterine inversion.

Diagnosis of labour

The diagnosis of 'labour' is important but often surprisingly difficult. The diagnosis is easy in retrospect, but of course a prospective diagnosis is required. The presence of palpable contractions does not necessarily mean that a woman is in labour, as Braxton Hicks contractions are common antenatally. For labour diagnosis there needs to be uterine contraction together with effacement and dilatation of the cervix.

Effacement has occurred when the entire length of the cervical canal has been taken up into the lower segment of the uterus, a process which begins at the internal os and proceeds downwards to the external os. This is analogous to pulling a polo-necked sweater over your head. It is of note that 'dilatation' refers only to the dilatation of the external os. Again, there is an important difference between primigravid and multigravid labours, as dilatation will not begin in a primigravida until effacement has occurred, whereas both may occur simultaneously in a parous woman **(Fig. 38.7)**.

If there are regular contractions and a fully effaced cervix, the woman can be said to be in labour. If, however, there are contractions with an only partially effaced cervix, further objective evidence must be sought in the form of either a 'show' or spontaneous membrane rupture. A 'show', or blood-stained mucous discharge, has occurred in approximately two-thirds of women by the time of presentation and supports the diagnosis in those with regular contractions. Spontaneous membrane rupture in the presence of regular contractions also confirms the diagnosis.

Pre-labour rupture of the membranes

In 6–12% of labours the membranes will rupture prior to the onset of uterine contractions or cervical dilatation. The mother will usually describe the feeling of 'water' leaking vaginally and, if a speculum examination is carried out, a pool of liquor is typically seen in the posterior vaginal fornix. A digital vaginal examination is not routinely indicated as this increases the risk of introducing infection. If managed conservatively, 70% of mothers will establish in labour spontaneously by 24 hours and 90% by 48 hours. This conservative management, however, carries a small risk of ascending infection, which may lead to chorioamnionitis. Rarely, chorioamnionitis may progress to a rapid overwhelming fetal and maternal sepsis.

Nonetheless, in view of the high chance of spontaneous labour over the first 48 hours a conservative approach may be appropriate. This is provided that the mother is apyrexial, the baby is in cephalic presentation, the liquor is clear and the fetal monitoring is normal. On the other hand, there is also evidence that induction of labour on admission may reduce the incidence of neonatal infection, with no increase in the rate of cae- sarean delivery. Women with pre-labour rupture of mem- branes should be counselled about their options and they and their partners should be involved in the deci- sion-making process. In those managed conservatively, women should be made aware of signs and symptoms of

infection and encouraged to record their temperature. If there is a clinical suspicion of chorioamnionitis with py- rexia or passage of meconium (see below), delivery must be expedited, usually by caesarean section unless labour is well established. Pain and discharge are late features of intrauterine infection.

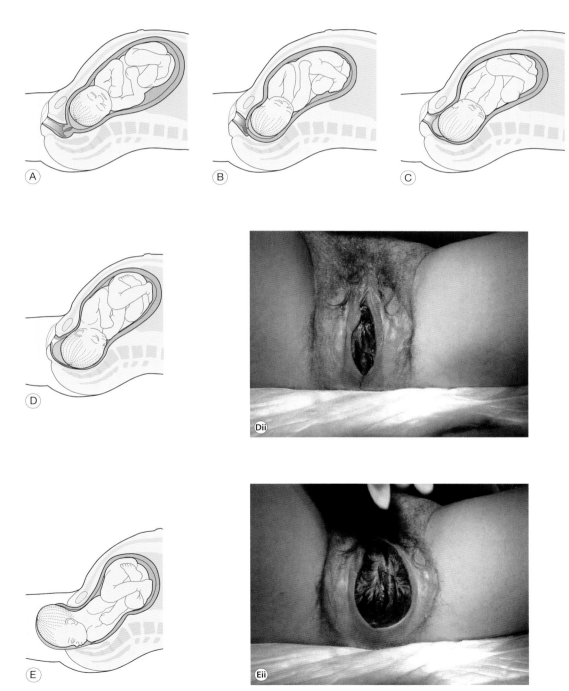

Fig. 38.5 Normal labour; A–I. See text.

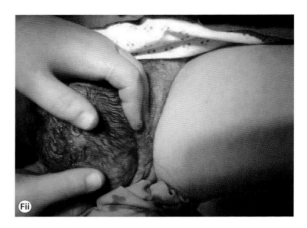

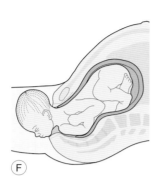

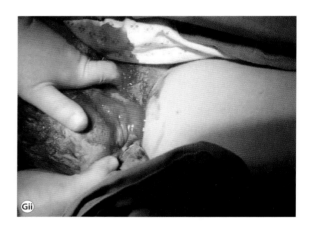

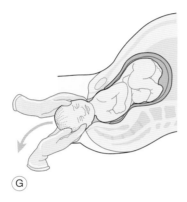

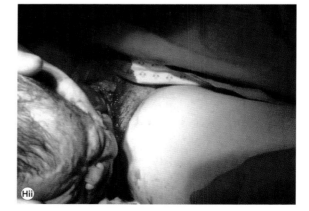

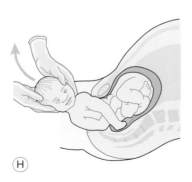

Fig. 38.5—cont'd

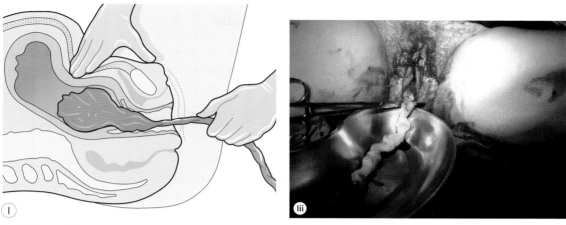

Fig. 38.5—cont'd

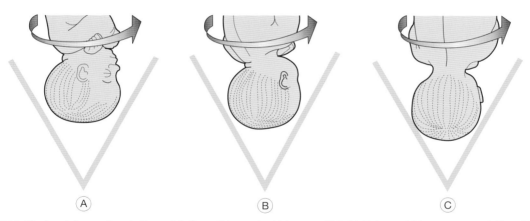

Fig. 38.6 The head descends onto the pelvic floor. This runs in a V shape, and it is this V shape which encourages rotation of the fetal head.

Clinical progress in labour

Labour is divided into three stages of unequal length **(Table 38.2)**. There is no 'normal' time for the length of labour. However, the mean length of established labour (i.e. from 4 cm dilated, with regular painful contractions), is 8 hours for primigravid women but can be up to 18 hours. The mean length for second and subsequent labours is 5.5 hours but can be up to 12 hours. Even after a labour of 40 hours the chance of a vaginal delivery is still around 50%. Fetal distress (hypoxia) is only partly related to the length of labour. The highest incidence of caesarean section for distress is in the first hour of labour, probably related to babies already compromised antenatally with some pre-existing problem. Even after 24 hours, however, the chance of fetal distress remains low. It is recognized that markedly prolonged labour is associated with subsequent maternal pelvic floor dysfunction and fistulae. There is therefore no 'optimal' length of labour and each mother should be assessed on an individual basis.

First stage

Progress in the first stage of labour is measured in terms of dilatation of the cervix and descent of the fetal head. Information about the labour is plotted on a partograph, which should be commenced when a woman is established in labour **(Fig. 38.8)**. It forms a graphic record of clinical findings and any relevant events. The purpose is to help early recognition of abnormal labour; to ensure appropriate transfer of care and aid continuity of care.

Vaginal examinations should be performed routinely every 4 hours depending on progress and, ideally, successive examinations should be carried out by the same person to minimize the subjective element in interpretation **(Table 38.3)**. The average rate of cervical dilatation

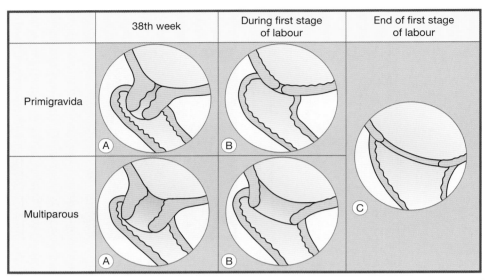

	38th week	During first stage of labour	End of first stage of labour
Primigravida	A	B	
Multiparous	A	B	C

Fig. 38.7 Cervical dilatation – primigravida versus multigravida. Note that in a multigravida, the cervix may dilate before efface-ment is complete.

Table 38.2

The three stages of labour

	Stage	Phases
First stage	From the onset of labour until the cervix is fully dilated, further subdivided into two phases:	(a) Latent – onset of contractions until the cervix is fully effaced (b) Active – cervical dilatation
Second stage	From full cervical dilatation until the head has delivered. It also has two phases:	(a) Propulsive – from full dilatation until head has descended onto the pelvic floor (b) Expulsive – from time the mother has an irresistible desire to bear down and push until the baby is delivered
Third stage	From delivery of the baby until expulsion of the placenta and membranes	

in primigravidae is around 1 cm per hour, although it is ac-cepted that ½ cm an hour can be normal for some women.

Descent of the fetal head is measured in labour by abdomi-nal examination, when the amount of the fetal head palpable above the pelvic brim (in fifths) is documented on the parto-graph. If only 2/5 or less of the fetal head is palpable abdomi-nally, then the head is determined to be 'engaged' **(Fig. 38.9)**.

On vaginal examination, the 'station' of the fetal head with respect to the ischial spines is recorded. Care should

be taken not to confuse increasing caput succedaneum (see below) with descent of the head itself. The ischial spines are designated station zero. When the head is above the spines, it is said to be at −1, −2, −3, or −4 cm. If the head is below the spines, the notation is +1, +2, +3, or +4 cm. If the head is at the level of the ischial spines, it must be engaged.

It is important to note that the 'position' of the head on vaginal examination is with reference to the occiput – for example, occipitoanterior (OA), right occipitotransverse (ROT) or left occipitoposterior (LOT).

'Caput' (succedaneum) is oedema of the scalp owing to pressure of the head against the rim of the cervix and is classified somewhat arbitrarily as '+', '++' or '+++'. 'Mould-ing' describes the change in head shape, which occurs during labour, made possible by movement of the individual scalp bones. It is arbitrarily termed '+' if the bones are op-posed, '++' if they overlap but can be reduced by digital pressure and '+++' if they overlap but cannot be reduced.

Second stage

This begins when the cervix is fully dilated. Progress is measured in terms of descent and rotation of the fetal head on vaginal examination. There are two distinct phases:

1. The propulsive/passive phase. This is from full dilata-tion until the head reaches the pelvic floor. During this time the head is relatively high in the pelvis, the position is typically occipitotransverse, the lower vagina is not stretched and the mother has no or little urge to push. In many respects it is a natural extension of the first stage of labour.
2. The expulsive/active phase. This begins when the fetal head reaches the pelvic floor and the mother usually has a strong involuntary desire to push.

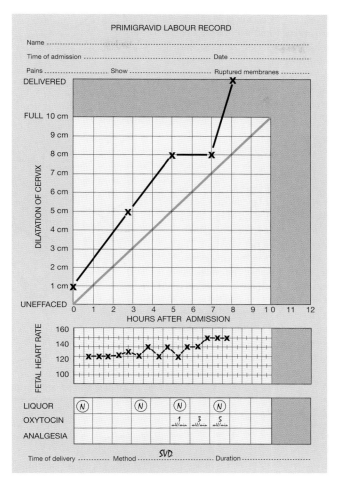

Fig. 38.8 **Partogram suitable for recording a primigravid labour.**

Table 38.3	
Vaginal examinations	
Findings on VE	**Details**
Presence or absence of meconium	Meconium staining might suggest fetal distress
Dilatation of the cervix	In centimetres from 0 to 10 cm
Station of the presenting part	In centimetres above or below the ischial spines
Position of the head	With reference to the occiput if cephalic, or sacrum if breech. A note should made of whether the head is flexed or deflexed
Presence of caput and/or moulding	If excessive, might suggest obstructed labour

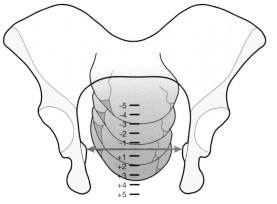

Fig. 38.9 **Descent of the head is described relative to the ischial spines.**

With pushing, the head usually delivers. Normally it does so in the occipitoanterior position. After delivery it restitutes, returning to an occipitolateral position by rotating with the shoulders as they descend into the pelvis. The birth attendant then applies lateral traction to the head, moving it in the direction of the mother's back to allow the birth of the anterior fetal shoulder (see above). At this point an oxytocic is injected intramuscularly into the mother's thigh to encourage a prolonged uterine contraction and minimize the chance of postpartum haemorrhage. The head is then lifted anteriorly to allow delivery of the posterior shoulder, after which the rest of the baby is delivered with lateral flexion of the fetal body. The umbilical cord is clamped and cut. If the baby does not require resuscitation, he or she may be placed on the mother's abdomen and skin-to-skin contact encouraged. If this is not the woman's preference, the baby should be wrapped in a warm towel and handed to the parents.

Third stage

The third stage of labour should be actively managed to minimize the risk of postpartum haemorrhage. This involves the use of an oxytocic (as above) and gentle controlled cord traction using the 'Brandt–Andrews' method **(Fig. 38.5l)**. Placental separation is recognized by apparent lengthening of the cord and a gush of dark blood per vaginam. The operator exerts traction on the cord while the other hand maintains pressure upwards on the fundus. The main risk of cord traction is uterine inversion and the fundus is continually 'guarded' to prevent this (see p. 371). Once the placenta passes the vulva it may be gently twisted to allow the membranes to peel off completely and the uterine fundus is rubbed up to ensure that the uterus is well contracted. The labia, vagina and perineum are inspected for tears and sutured if bleeding. Finally, the placenta is examined to ensure it is complete.

The normal blood loss at delivery is about 300 ml. The routine use of an oxytocic following delivery of the anterior shoulder reduces the risk of postpartum haemorrhage by about 60%.

Episiotomies and perineal tears

It was previously considered that the use of episiotomy reduced the incidence of anal sphincter tears. There is, however, little evidence to support this, and there is no evidence to support routine episiotomy in all deliveries as a preventive measure against third- or fourth-degree tears. Midline episiotomy in particular does not protect the perineum or sphincters during childbirth and may impair anal continence. If an episiotomy is to be performed, a right (or less commonly left) posterolateral episiotomy is preferred **(Fig. 38.10)**.

Restricting the use of episiotomy to specific fetal and maternal indications leads to lower rates of posterior perineal trauma, less need for suturing and fewer long-term complications. A spontaneous tear may be less painful than an episiotomy and may also heal better.

Possible indications for an episiotomy are as follows:

- a rigid perineum which is preventing delivery
- if it is judged that a large tear is imminent
- most instrumental deliveries (forceps or ventouse)
- shoulder dystocia (to permit access to the birth canal)
- vaginal breech delivery.

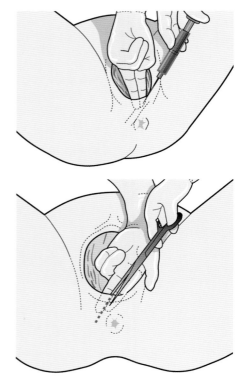

Fig. 38.10 If required, an episiotomy is usually carried out after infiltration of the perineum with local anaesthesia.

Table 38.4	
Classification of spontaneous perineal tears	
	Tear involves
First degree	Injury to the vaginal epithelium and vulval skin only
Second degree	Injury to the perineal muscles, but not the anal sphincter
Third degree	Injury to the perineum involving the anal sphincter complex
Fourth degree	Injury to the perineum involving the anal sphincter complex and anal/rectal mucosa

Prior to an episiotomy, local anaesthetic is injected into the subcutaneous tissues of the perineum and vagina (unless there is an effective regional block). A right mediolateral cut is made and pressure on the fetal head is maintained so that the delivery is slow and the head remains flexed, minimizing the possibility of the incision extending. Spontaneous tears are categorized into four degrees **(Table 38.4)**. An episiotomy is an iatrogenic second-degree tear. Anterior perineal trauma is classified as any injury to the labia, anterior vagina, urethra or clitoris and is described as such.

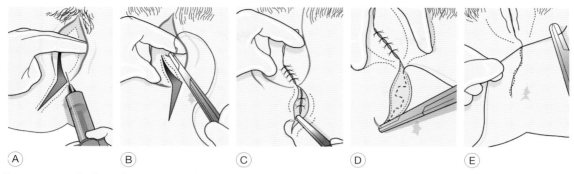

Fig. 38.11 Repair of a perineal tear or episiotomy (see text).

Repair of episiotomies and perineal tears

Repair should be with an absorbable synthetic material (Dexon or Vicryl), using a continuous subcuticular (possibly non-locking) technique to minimize short- and long-term problems **(Fig. 38.11)**. These newer materials result in less short-term pain and less analgesic requirements than do older materials such as catgut and non-absorbable sutures. Good perineal hygiene after delivery is likely to aid healing, and the use of ice packs and analgesia may be useful to alleviate discomfort.

Repair of episiotomy and first- or second-degree tears

The perineum is infiltrated with local anaesthetic **(Fig. 38.11A)** (unless an epidural is in place or there has been a pudendal block or perineal infiltration prior to delivery). The apex of the vaginal incision or tear is identified and the first suture placed just above this level **(Fig. 38.11B)** (care is needed because the rectum is just posterior to the vaginal wall).

A continuous locking suture is used to close the vaginal wall until the hymeneal edges are opposed. The suture can then be tied, or more simply locked, and the needle threaded between the opposed vaginal edges a few centimetres back, ready to close the perineal body **(Fig. 38.11C)**. The perineal body sutures should be interrupted. A continuous finer suture is then used for the skin **(Fig. 38.11D,E)**.

Repair of third- or fourth-degree tears

This should ideally be by an experienced clinician, in theatre, with good analgesia, good light, the appropriate instruments and an assistant. The anal mucosa (if involved) is repaired using interrupted dissolving sutures, with the knot of each suture placed in the anal canal. The internal sphincter is then identified and its ends approximated and sutured with a monofilament suture such as polydioxanone (PDS). Next, the ends of the external anal sphincter are identified and either approximated or overlapped, again with the monofilament suture. The rest is as described above for first- and second-degree tears. Antibiotics, laxatives and fibre are important to allow healing.

> **Key points**
>
> - The correct diagnosis of 'labour' is central to good management.
> - Labour is considered in three stages: the first from the onset of labour until the cervix is fully dilated, the second from then until delivery of the baby, and the third from that point until delivery of the placenta.
> - Compared to a multigravida, the labour of a primigravida is likely to be longer and more likely to result in both instrumental delivery and neonatal injury.

Monitoring of the fetus in labour

Introduction

The purpose of monitoring the fetus in labour is to try and identify those which might be at risk of hypoxic injury so that delivery can be expedited and potential problems prevented. This process of monitoring usually involves some form of fetal heart rate assessment either with intermittent auscultation or by continuous electronic measurement (cardiotocography; CTG) and analysis of the fetal ECG waveform. Intermittent auscultation of the fetal heart is appropriate for monitoring fetal condition in low-risk labour, with electronic fetal monitoring being used either in high-risk labour or if concern is raised by intermittent auscultation in low-risk patients. The CTG is good at identifying the normal healthy fetus but there is a high false positive rate and many fetuses labelled as 'distressed' are actually not hypoxic. As a consequence the rate of obstetric intervention may be increased in return for no neonatal benefit. Analysis of the ECG waveform in association with the CTG can improved its predictive ability for hypoxia.

Fetal physiology

Fetal oxygenation depends on a number of factors.

Maternal blood supply to the placenta

During a contraction, the intramural vessels supplying the placenta are constricted by the smooth muscle fibres of the uterus. Providing the contractions are not too long or too frequent, the placental blood supply has time to recover before the next contraction begins. In hyperstimulation, when the uterus is contracting too frequently, placental oxygenation may be impaired. In other circumstances there may be placental hypoperfusion, for example following the distal sympathetic blockade and associated hypotension which can occur with spinal or epidural anaesthesia.

Functional capacity of the placenta

A small, poorly formed placenta is less capable of adequate oxygen transfer than a larger placenta. In this condition, the fetus may already be growth restricted prior to the onset of labour and therefore more susceptible to a hypoxic stress. In abruptio placentae it is obvious that the resulting partial placental separation leaves a reduced surface area for vascular communication, and is therefore less efficient at oxygen exchange.

Fetal blood supply

This is dependent on adequate fetal cardiac output. The fetus responds to hypoxic stress with peripheral vasoconstriction and redistribution of the blood to the heart and the brain. Prolonged vasoconstriction may lead to damage in other organs, particularly the gastrointestinal tract (necrotizing enterocolitis), the lungs (respiratory distress) and kidneys (acute renal failure).

Hypoxia also leads to anaerobic metabolism and acidosis. Acidosis is therefore a reflection of the degree of oxygenation, and this forms the basis of intrapartum fetal blood sampling.

Risk assessment

Some form of monitoring is appropriate for all labours, but whether this should be continuous or intermittent is unclear. As noted above, the use of continuous electronic monitoring in 'low-risk' labours may increase the rate of

Babies at 'high risk' of distress in labour

Fetal factors

- Fetal growth restriction or any baby whose weight is estimated to be less that the 10th centile (see p. 283)

Placental factors

- Hypertension (see p. 291)
- Antepartum haemorrhage (see p. 277)

Obstetric factors

- Precipitate labour (see p. 349)
- Premature labour (see p. 299)
- Prolonged labour (see p. 349)
- Induced labours or those augmented with Syntocinon (see p. 354)
- Mothers with epidurals, a previous caesarean section or significant medical problems
- Those with meconium (fetal stool) stained liquor (see below)

intervention for no demonstrable neonatal benefit. It is therefore important to consider which babies are 'high risk' and which are 'low risk'. Some of these factors are outlined in **Box 39.1**. It is important to take these background factors into consideration before interpreting a heart rate problem.

Meconium staining of the liquor

Meconium (fetal stool) staining of the liquor is present in 15% of all deliveries at term and in about 40% at 42 weeks. The mechanism may be stimulation of the vagus (parasympathetic) nerves in utero causing the fetal gut to contract and the anal sphincter to relax. This often happens for no particular reason but it also may occur as a response to fetal hypoxia. While often not of clinical significance, the presence of meconium staining increases the likelihood that there is underlying fetal compromise. A normal cardiotocograph (CTG) provides reassurance, but an abnormal CTG becomes more significant in the presence of meconium and should lower the threshold for investigation or intervention.

As well as being a sign of fetal distress, meconium is found below the vocal cords postnatally in about one-third of cases in which it is present and may give rise to the meconium aspiration syndrome. This is a form of neonatal pneumonitis. Clinical features range from mild neonatal tachypnoea to severe respiratory compromise. The incidence is probably unrelated to fetal hypoxia (and indeed the majority of babies with meconium aspiration syndrome are not acidotic at delivery) but the syndrome is more likely to be severe if there is associated hypoxia/acidosis. It is also more severe when the meconium is thick. There is no evidence to support early delivery in the absence of fetal distress, as it is likely that the aspiration occurs in utero rather that at delivery itself.

Meconium can be graded as follows:

Grade 1: good volume of liquor stained lightly with meconium
Grade 2: reasonable volume of liquor with heavy suspension of meconium
Grade 3: thick undiluted meconium of 'pea-soup' consistency.

The higher the grade, the more likely it is to be associated with metabolic acidosis and the meconium aspiration syndrome. It is appropriate to consider continuous electronic fetal heart rate recording if meconium is found to be present.

Fetal heart rate recording

Intermittent monitoring

Assessment of the fetal heart rate can be used to provide some information about fetal well-being. In 'low-risk' labours, it is recommended to auscultate the fetal heart every 15 minutes before and after a contraction during the first stage of labour, and every 5 minutes between contractions in the second stage of labour. A baseline tachycardia or bradycardia, and the presence of decelerations are indications for further evaluation with continuous CTG monitoring. The heart can be auscultated using either a manual Pinard stethoscope or an electronic Doppler detector.

Continuous monitoring (cardiotocography)

A cardiotocograph (CTG) provides a continuous printed record of the fetal heart rate and uterine contractions. The contractions are registered by a pressure monitor supported on the mother's abdomen by an elastic belt, and the fetal heart rate is measured using either:

- an abdominal ultrasonic transmitter–receiver Doppler probe which detects fetal cardiac movements and hence the heart rate, or
- a clip, known as a fetal scalp electrode (FSE), which is attached to the baby's scalp and detects the R–R wave of the fetal ECG. It is usually used if the external abdominal monitoring is unsatisfactory.

The important features of a CTG are given in **Table 39.1**. Normally, the baseline fetal heart rate is between 110 and 150 beats per minute (bpm). This rate represents a balance between the sympathetic and parasympathetic systems. Sustained tachycardia is associated with prematurity, and the rate slows physiologically with advancing gestation. It may also be associated with fetal acidosis (probably as a response to increased sympathetic stimulation), maternal pyrexia, and the use of exogenous beta-sympathomimetics. Baseline bradycardia is associated with severe fetal

Table 39.1

Features of a cardiotocograph

Normal heart rate	110–150 bpm	Reassuring
Baseline variability	10–25 bpm	Reassuring
Accelerations		Reassuring
Decelerations	early (type 1)	These occur at the time of the contraction and are rarely of more than 40 bpm. They are probably related to parasympathetic stimulation associated with head compression, and are unlikely to be of clinical significance
	variable	These are variable in their timing in relation to the timing of the contraction. They are associated with cord compression and may indicate fetal hypoxia
	late (type 2)	These occur after the contraction, may be of low amplitude and are suggestive of fetal hypoxia

acidosis (e.g. abruption or uterine rupture) but is more commonly found with hypotension and maternal sedation. Congenital heart block is rare, but can occur especially in association with maternal systemic lupus erythematosus. Cardiac dysrhythmias are also rare but can cause extremes of heart rate, either fast or slow, with tachycardia usually being the more frequently encountered.

Baseline variability is the variation in the fetal heart rate from one beat to the next (the beat-to-beat variation) and is due to the balance between the parasympathetic and the sympathetic nervous systems. Since the nervous system of the baby develops as pregnancy advances, the beat-to-beat variability is reduced at earlier gestations. Baseline variability is described as normal, reduced or absent, and it gives a relatively good indication of well-being. The normal is 10–25 bpm. The commonest reason for loss of baseline variability is the 'sleep' or 'quiet' phase of the fetal behavioural cycle, which may last up to 40 minutes. Loss of variability is also associated with prematurity, acidosis and drugs (e.g. opiates or benzodiazepines). Fetal acidosis is much more likely if there is reduced variability in the presence of late decelerations.

Accelerations of the fetal heart rate with contractions are a sign of a healthy fetus but their absence in advanced labour is not unusual. Antenatally there should be at least two accelerations per 15 minutes, each with an amplitude greater than 15 bpm and lasting for at least 15 seconds.

Decelerations are of at least 15 bpm and last for more than 15 seconds. Early decelerations occur with contractions. If decelerations occur more than 15 seconds after the contraction they are termed 'late'. 'Variable' decelerations vary in both timing and shape.

- Early decelerations reflect increased vagal tone (intracranial pressure rises during a contraction) and are probably physiological.
- Variable decelerations may represent cord compression (particularly in oligohydramnios) or acidosis. A small acceleration at the beginning and end of a deceleration

(shouldering) suggests that the fetus is coping well with the stress of the intermittent compressions. Variable decelerations may resolve if the mother's position is changed.
- Late decelerations suggest acidosis. Shallow late decelerations may be particularly ominous.

A true sinusoidal trace is rare. This is a smooth undulating sine-wave-like baseline with no variability. It may represent fetal anaemia but can be a feature of fetal physiological behaviour. It should be considered to be serious until proven otherwise.

Fetal ECG

Analysis of the fetal ECG in labour can improve the specificity (i.e. reduce the number of false positives) of the CTG. A fetal scalp electrode (FSE) is required to obtain the ECG, the signal from which is a reflection of the electrical activity in the heart (the myocardium). The P wave corresponds to contraction of the atria, the QRS complex contraction of the ventricles and the T wave regeneration of myocardial membrane potentials prior to the next contraction.

Myocardial hypoxia leads to changes in the ECG waveform:

- An increased amplitude of the T wave. The ratio between the height of the T wave and the QRS amplitude (T/QRS ratio) gives an accurate measurement of changes in T wave height and its increase can be episodic (rises and returns within 10 minutes) or a rise in baseline (lasts for more than 10 minutes). The elevated T wave is the result of potassium release in association with the mobilization of stored glucose (glycogen).
- Changes in the shape of the ST segment, characteristically the appearance of a biphasic pattern thought to be the result of the depressant effect of hypoxia on myocardial function.

Used in conjunction with the CTG, fetal ECG analysis has been shown to result in fewer babies with severe metabolic acidosis at birth, fewer babies with neonatal encephalopathy, and fewer operative vaginal deliveries. The use of fetal ECG with CTG also reduces the need for fetal blood sampling (as described below).

Fetal blood sampling (FBS)

This is also known as fetal scalp sampling (FSS) and is a diagnostic test for fetal acidosis. As mentioned above, CTGs are used as a screening test to detect babies who may be developing 'distress' as measured by metabolic acidosis. CTGs are highly sensitive (good at detecting *true* positives) but very poorly specific (there are many *false* positives). In other words, when the CTG is normal the baby is very likely to be well, but the majority of abnormal CTGs occur in babies who are not distressed. CTGs used on their own lead to an approximately fourfold increase in caesarean section rates for presumed fetal distress, a figure much reduced if fetal blood sampling is used to identify a normal pH in the false positives.

Using an amnioscope, a tiny amount of blood is removed from the scalp (see below) and both pH and base excess are measured. Normal maternal pH is 7.38 but the normal range of fetal pH is broader, extending to as low as 7.20. In the presence of hypoxia the fetus compensates by anaerobic glycolysis. This leads to an accumulation of lactic acid and a fall in the pH. FBS carries a very small risk of fetal scalp haemorrhage and infection.

Indications for fetal blood sampling

1. Persistent late or variable decelerations on CTG
2. Persistent fetal tachycardia
3. Prolonged and persistent early decelerations
4. Significant meconium-stained liquor (Grade 2 or 3) along with any CTG abnormality
5. Prolonged loss of baseline variability.

FBS is contraindicated where there is a risk of infection transmitted from the mother (e.g. HIV, hepatitis B, herpes), a fetal bleeding diathesis (e.g. Von Willebrand's disease) and before 34' weeks gestation.

Method of fetal blood sampling

The mother is placed in the lithotomy position with 15° lateral tilt (or in the left lateral position if approaching full dilatation). An amnioscope appropriate for the dilatation is inserted and the scalp is dried with a sponge or swab on long sponge-holders. The scalp is then sprayed with ethyl chloride to induce hyperaemia and the area is covered with a thin layer of paraffin jelly (so that the blood will form a blob and not run). A blade is used to make a small nick in the scalp and the blob is touched with the capillary tube. Where possible, three samples are taken to ensure consistency of results.

Interpretation of results

The scalp blood pH reflects the state of the fetus only at the time of the sample, while the 'base excess' reflects a change over a longer period. The pH is plotted on a logarithmic scale, whereas base excess is on a linear scale, e.g. a fetus with a pH of 7.22 and a base excess of −12 mEq/l is more likely to be at risk than one with a similar pH and base excess of −6 mEq/l. The correlation between CTGs and scalp pH is not precise but as a general rule:

- If all four components of the CTG are normal, the risk of a pH <7.20 is ≈2%.
- With one or two components of the CTG abnormal, the risk of a pH <7.20 is ≈20%.
- With two to four components of the CTG abnormal, the risk of a pH <7.20 is ≈50%.

It is common practice to deliver the baby if the pH is <7.20, although it may be the rate of fall in pH rather than the absolute value which is relevant. See **Tables 39.2** and **39.3**.

Table 39.2		
pH results following fetal blood sampling		
pH		
>7.25	Normal	No action
7.20–7.25	Borderline	Repeat in 30–60 minutes if not delivered
<7.20	Abnormal	Deliver by forceps, ventouse or caesarean section as appropriate

Table 39.3	
Base excess results following fetal blood sampling	
Base excess	
< −6 mEq/l	Normal
−6.1 to −7.9 mEq/l	Borderline
≥ −8 mEq/l	Metabolic acidosis

Clinical examples of fetal monitoring scenarios with corresponding CTGs

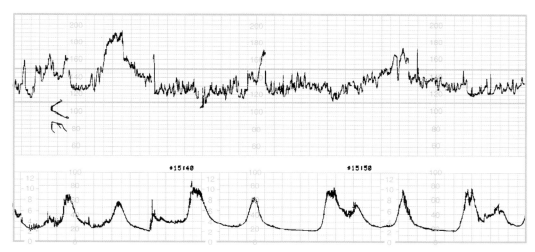

Fig. 39.1 A 29-year-old para 2, with a history of two previous normal deliveries, was admitted with apparently good contractions. The cervix was 3 cm dilated and fully effaced, but there was thick meconium staining. The CTG was reassuring, however, with a baseline of 130 bpm, good beat-to-beat variability and accelerations. She was given pethidine 100 mg for pain relief.

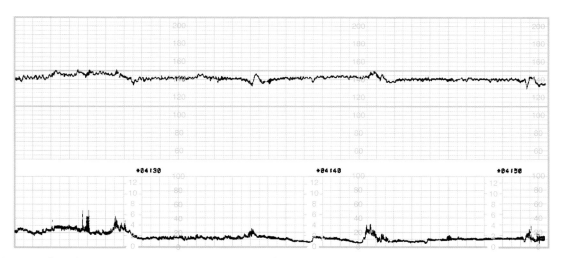

Fig. 39.2 After a further 2 hours, however, there was loss of baseline variability. Although there were no decelerations, it was recognized that meconium is a marker for fetal compromise and it was decided to perform fetal blood sampling. The pH was within the normal range at 7.31 and she went on to have a normal delivery 3 hours later.

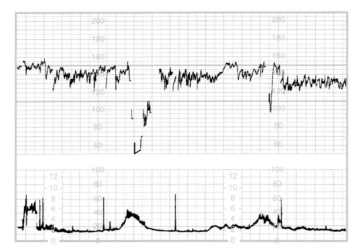

Fig. 39.3 A 40-year-old primigravida was admitted after spontaneous rupture of membranes. The liquor was clear and she was having mild contractions once every 8 minutes. The CTG baseline was 130–140 bpm with good reactivity but there were variable decelerations. These are not uncommon after membrane rupture as liquor cushions the baby and cord compression is less likely. Because the rest of the CTG was reassuring, she was allowed to establish in labour spontaneously. The decelerations resolved, but she required a caesarean section for failure to progress beyond 8 cm despite Syntocinon. The baby was in an occipitoposterior position.

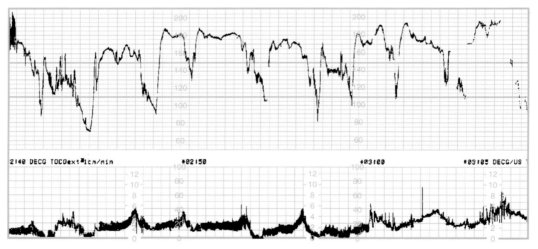

Fig. 39.4 This is the CTG of a 27-year-old primigravida who was induced at term +12 days as she was 'post-dates'. After prostaglandin gel was given vaginally, the cervix was suitable for membrane rupture and the induction was continued with Syntocinon. This trace is at 6 cm and it shows a baseline around 180 bpm with reduced variability and late decelerations. Fetal blood sampling showed a pH of 7.28, but on repetition 30 minutes later it was 7.19. By this stage the cervix was fully dilated and she had an uneventful ventouse delivery.

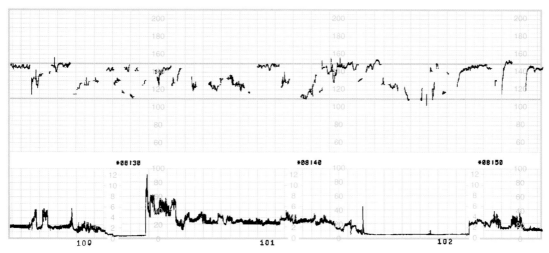

Fig. 39.5 This 19-year-old primigravida, who weighed 105 kg at booking, was admitted in early labour. The CTG shows poor pick-up from the abdominal Doppler probe and, after the membranes were ruptured, a scalp clip was applied. The subsequent traces were reassuring and she had a normal delivery.

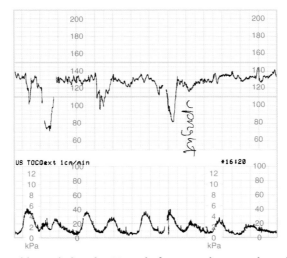

Fig. 39.6 A 26-year-old primigravida was induced at 33 weeks for worsening pre-eclampsia. The baby's estimated weight was on the 10th centile but liquor volume, biophysical profile and CTG were all normal. 8 hours after administration of the prostaglandin gel, with the cervix still closed, there were three unprovoked variable decelerations. While the relatively reassuring baseline variability might have warranted more conservative management in a normally grown term fetus, the underlying factors were felt sufficient to warrant caesarean section. The baby, weighing 1.6 kg, had Apgar scores of 9 and 10 at 1 and 5 minutes and made uneventful progress.

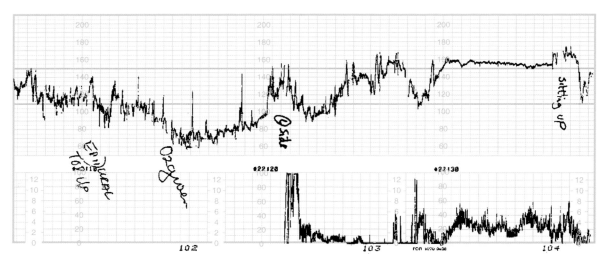

Fig. 39.7 This is the CTG of a 34-year-old primigravida at 4 cm who had just had an epidural sited. After epidural top-up there was a baseline bradycardia, which recovered to a tachycardia and settled again to normal. It is recognized that the peripheral hypotension associated with regional anaesthesia leads to placental hypoperfusion and fetal bradycardia. The bradycardia usually resolves spontaneously.

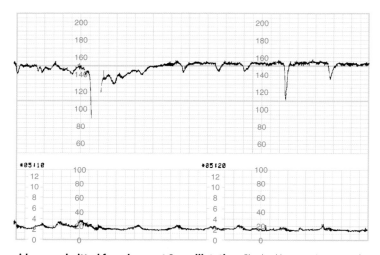

Fig. 39.8 This primigravida was admitted from home at 8 cm dilatation. She had been quite sore at home, but was not expecting to be at such an advanced stage of labour. The CTG had virtually no beat-to-beat variability and there were shallow late decelerations. A fetal blood sample showed a pH of 7.09 and a caesarean section was carried out. The baby had Apgar scores of 3 at 1 minute and 7 at 5 minutes, and weighed only 2.23 kg at 37 weeks' gestation. It made excellent progress.

Long-term prognosis following delivery

There are two key issues to be considered here:

- The first is whether a particular infant, born with apparent compromise, will later turn out to be neurologically normal, i.e. prospective prediction.
- The second is whether an infant, later discovered to be affected by cerebral abnormality, sustained its injury prior to the onset of labour or as the result of some intrapartum insult, i.e. retrospective evaluation.

Before considering these two overlapping issues, it should be noted that the term 'birth asphyxia' is best avoided as it is rarely possible to prove that 'asphyxia' occurred and even more difficult to time this to the birth.

Prospective prediction

The actual length of time and degree of hypoxia required to produce cerebral palsy in a previously healthy fetus are unknown but there are specific mechanisms which protect the fetus for considerably longer than an adult with similar blood gas concentrations. Nonetheless, hypoxia, whether of antenatal or intrapartum origin, can cause cerebral injury, and attempts have been made to correlate status at delivery with long-term neurological outcome. CTG abnormalities, Apgar scores, neonatal behaviour and neonatal brain imaging have all been evaluated.

CTGs and Apgar scores are of very limited value in assessing long-term prognosis. There is a high incidence of non-reassuring CTGs in what are later shown to be normal infants. The same is true for Apgar scores, which are intended as a guide to the need for resuscitation rather than a reflection of the degree of hypoxic injury. Low Apgar scores do not indicate the cause of the baby's poor condition, and are a reflection of its immediate status. Prolonged low values, however, are a more useful guide. Of those babies with an Apgar score <3 at 10 minutes, two-thirds usually die within 1 year, and of the survivors, 80% are normal.

Abnormal neonatal behaviour, referred to as 'neonatal encephalopathy', is considerably more useful. This is a clinically defined syndrome of disturbed neurological function occurring during the first week after birth characterized by difficulty with initiating and maintaining respiration, depression of tone and reflexes, altered level of consciousness, and seizures. There are three grades:

1. Hyper-alert and jittery with reduced tone and dilated pupils. This usually resolves within 24 hours without long-term sequelae.
2. Lethargic, with seizures and a weak suck. There is a 15–27% chance of severe sequelae.
3. Flaccid, no suck, no Moro reflex and prolonged seizures. The chance of severe sequelae is nearly 100%.

The prognosis is generally good if the baby does not develop Grade 3 neonatal encephalopathy, or if Grade 2 neonatal encephalopathy lasts less than 5 days.

Radiological assessment is also of value in assessing long-term neurological function. The prognosis is good if a CT or MRI scan appears normal but is less good if there is evidence of cerebral damage. This damage is most obvious in the periventricular area, an area particularly susceptible to insult, and appears radiologically as periventricular leucomalacia. Early cerebral oedema suggests a recent event, as oedema usually appears within 6–12 hours of an insult and clears by 4 days afterwards. Further clinical evaluation may be available from an electroencephalograph (EEG). The incidence of death or handicap is low if the EEG is normal. Often, however, despite these measures, the prognosis can not be defined with accuracy and only long-term follow-up will reveal the true clinical picture.

Retrospective evaluation

Cerebral palsy, which is characterized by non-progressive abnormal control of movement or posture, is usually not diagnosed until months or years after birth and it is often at this point that questions are asked about whether the cause lay in some difficulty with the delivery. In many instances it is impossible to say whether the cerebral insult was antenatal in origin or whether it truly occurred in labour, but this apparently academic point has two important implications. Firstly, if most cases of cerebral palsy are antenatal in origin, then no amount of intrapartum monitoring will affect the eventual outcome. Secondly, there may be major medicolegal ramifications. If a cerebral insult is found to have occurred as the result of negligence during labour, a potentially very large sum of money may need to be paid in compensation.

Epidemiological studies suggest that in about 90% of cases the cerebral injury is antenatal in origin, and that in the remaining 10% the problems may have been the result of either antenatal or intrapartum difficulties. In particular there is a strong association with prematurity, fetal growth restriction, intrauterine infection, fetal coagulation disorders, antepartum haemorrhage, and chromosomal or congenital anomalies. Many are idiopathic. Intrapartum complications appear to play only an infrequent role in the causation of cerebral palsy. Reduced CTG variability, meconium staining, low Apgar scores and neonatal encephalopathy may all reflect pre-existing cerebral injury from some earlier antenatal event.

There are many conflicting views about the criteria required to implicate intrapartum events as the cause of cerebral injury. One set of views is expressed in **Box 39.2**, but, while accepted by many, they are not the universal views of all clinicians.

In summary, therefore, research strongly suggests that the large majority of neurological pathologies causing cerebral palsy occur as a result of multifactorial and mostly unpreventable reasons during either fetal development or the neonatal period. This, however, should not be an excuse for careless intrapartum care and every effort should still be made to identify and act upon identifiable causes of potential cerebral injury.

Box 39.2

Criteria to define an acute intrapartum hypoxic event as the cause of later cerebral injury

- Evidence is required of a metabolic acidosis in an intrapartum fetal blood sample, umbilical arterial cord, or in very early neonatal blood. Metabolic acidaemia at birth is, however, comparatively common (2% of all births), and the vast majority of these infants do not develop cerebral palsy. An appropriate cut-off point that correlates with a risk of neurological deficit may be a pH of less than 7.00 and a base deficit of less than 16 mmol/l.
- There should be early onset of severe or moderate neonatal encephalopathy. It should be noted that over 75% of cases of neonatal encephalopathy have no other clinical signs of intrapartum hypoxia.
- Cerebral palsy should be of the spastic quadriplegic or dyskinetic type. Spastic quadriplegia and, less commonly, dyskinetic cerebral palsy are the only subtypes of cerebral palsy associated with acute hypoxic intrapartum events. Hemiplegic cerebral palsy, spastic diplegia, and ataxia do have this association.

Key points

- The purpose of monitoring the fetus is to try to identify those which might be of risk of hypoxic injury so that delivery can then be expedited and potential problems prevented. This process of monitoring usually involves some form of fetal heart rate assessment either with intermittent auscultation or by continuous electronic measurement (cardiotocography). Fetal blood sampling is also useful.
- Any interpretation of a CTG has to take account of the full clinical situation rather than the CTG in isolation.
- Meconium (fetal stool) staining of the liquor increases the chance that there is underlying fetal compromise. A normal CTG, however, is usually reassuring.
- The fetal ECG, when used in combination with the CTG, leads to fewer acidotic babies with fewer operative deliveries.
- Cerebral palsy is often the result of antenatal factors rather than intrapartum problems. This, however, should not be an excuse for careless intrapartum care and every effort should still be made to identify and act upon identifiable causes of potential cerebral injury.

40

Induction of labour

Introduction

Induction of labour is indicated when the risks of continuing the pregnancy are felt to be greater than the risks of ending the pregnancy. Induction is usually carried out in the interest of fetal well-being and less commonly for maternal reasons. The decision is often difficult, particularly at preterm gestations, and many factors, including the availability of neonatal facilities, need to be considered. Labour should not be induced until there has been a careful discussion with the mother about the pros and cons of the induction.

It should be noted that 'induction' is different from 'augmentation'. Induction refers to the process of starting labour and can only be applied to a mother who is not already in labour. Augmentation describes the process of accelerating labour after it has already started.

Fetal indications

- Post-dates – usually between 41 and 42 weeks' gestation (p. 243).
- Fetal growth restriction with risk of fetal compromise (based on estimated growth and fetal monitoring, see p. 286). There may be associated pre-eclampsia.
- Certain diabetic pregnancies (p. 254).
- Deteriorating haemolytic disease of the newborn (rare).

Maternal indications

- Pre-eclampsia. This is a condition in which both maternal and fetal interests are relevant. While it may, for example, be appropriate to induce for mild pre-eclampsia at term, the pre-eclampsia would need to be severe in a markedly preterm infant.
- Deteriorating medical conditions (cardiac or renal disease, severe systemic lupus erythematosus [SLE]).
- Antepartum haemorrhage.

The decision to induce labour depends on the balance between the risks of continuing fetal surveillance and the risks of induction and preterm delivery. Induction risks are largely related to the use of 'oxytocics', the preparations that are used to stimulate uterine activity. The side-effect of greatest concern is that of uterine hyperstimulation, which carries the risk of fetal compromise. The process of induction is also associated with increased obstetric intervention, particularly if carried out before 41+ weeks' gestation. Finally, induction may be unsuccessful and the obstetrician may feel compelled to undertake a caesarean section that would not otherwise have been necessary.

Before induction, the gestation should again be confirmed, the presentation checked and any contraindications (e.g. placenta praevia) excluded. It is important to note that real caution is required in those who have had a previous caesarean section or previous uterine surgery, as induction carries an increased risk of uterine scar rupture, and many clinicians would consider these as contraindications unless the cervix was very favourable. In addition, grand multiparity and a history of previous precipitate labour also carry increased risks of hyperstimulation.

The decision about which technique is the most appropriate depends on the cervix as assessed by the Bishop's scoring system **(Table 40.1)**, **(Box 40.1)**.

- If the score is ≤6, the cervix should be 'ripened' with prostaglandins (e.g. gel or pessary).
- If >6, either prostaglandins or artificial rupture of the membranes ± Syntocinon may be considered (there may be greater patient satisfaction with the former, but the latter may allow more control).

Unfavourable cervix

Prostaglandins

As discussed on page 320, prostaglandins promote cervical ripening and stimulate uterine contractility. They have been administered by the oral, parenteral and vaginal routes, as well as directly through the cervix and infused into the extra-amniotic space. The main side-effect is of

Table 40.1

Bishop's scoring system for cervical assessment

Score	0	1	2
Cervical dilatation (cm)	<1	1–2	3–4
Length of cervix (cm)	>2	1–2	<1
Station of presenting part (cm)	Spines –3	Spines –2	Spines –1
Consistency	Firm	Medium	Soft
Position	Posterior	Central	Anterior

Box 40.1

Overview of induction

- Confirm that the indications for induction are appropriate and that there are no contraindications
- Cervix unfavourable (Bishop's score ≤6) → 'ripen' with a vaginal prostaglandin preparation
- Cervix favourable (Bishop's score >6) → artificial rupture of the membranes ± Syntocinon

gastrointestinal upset with nausea, vomiting and diarrhoea, which may occur in up to 50% of instances depending on the route of administration. Vaginal preparations have fewer side-effects than do oral or parenteral preparations. Administration directly into the cervix has been associated with higher failure rates than have other routes.

Prostaglandin E_2 (PGE$_2$) is used in clinical practice. A gel or tablet is inserted into the posterior fornix and, if there is no uterine activity, the cervix is reassessed after 6 hours. If the Bishop's score is <7, further prostaglandin is given and the cervix reassessed again 6 hours later. Further doses may then be given or the patient left for 12–18 hours (e.g. overnight). If at any stage the Bishop's score is >6, an artificial rupture of the membranes may be performed, reassessment made in a further 2 hours and Syntocinon started if there is no further change. Prostaglandins should not be given if there is regular uterine activity. Misoprostol (a methyl ester of prostaglandin E$_1$) can also be used either orally or vaginally but carries a higher incidence of hyperstimulation than do preparations of PGE$_2$.

Sustained-release preparations are also available in the form of a polymer-based vaginal insert containing PGE$_2$, with retrieval thread. The preparation is placed in the posterior fornix for 12 hours, after which it is removed. This technique has the advantage that the insert can be removed if hyperstimulation develops, and trials indicate that it is as safe as other vaginal preparations. It has not, however, been shown to be superior to gel or tablets.

These preparations all cause uterine contractions and therefore have the potential to reduce uterine blood flow and compromise the fetus. Cardiotocography (CTG) monitoring is therefore indicated.

Favourable cervix

If the cervix is favourable, the choice is between:

- prostaglandins
- artificial rupture of the membranes
- artificial rupture of the membranes and Syntocinon.

It remains unclear which of these is the superior induction method, but there is some evidence that maternal satisfaction is greater with prostaglandins. The requirement for analgesia and the rates of postpartum haemorrhage may be lower in this group as well. On the other hand, almost 90% of women suitable for artificial rupture of membrane will enter labour spontaneously following the procedure.

Artificial rupture of the membranes (ARM)

Artificial rupture of the membranes (or 'amniotomy') may be used to induce labour in those with a sufficiently favourable cervix and is also used for augmentation of labour. It probably works by a combination of uterine decompression and local prostaglandin release. Another advantage is that it allows assessment of the colour of the liquor (see Meconium staining of the liquor, p. 332).

ARM has been advocated by some for all labours, spontaneous or induced. This is surrounded by a degree of controversy as it can be argued that there is less cushioning of the fetal head and therefore a greater incidence of fetal heart rate decelerations. Trials suggest that early artificial rupture of the membranes and Syntocinon probably do not confer benefit over conservative management in nulliparous women with mild delays in early spontaneous labour.

Before ARM, vaginal examination is performed. The fetal head should be well applied to the cervix to minimize the risk of cord prolapse. With asepsis, the tips of the index and middle fingers of one hand should be placed through the cervix onto the membranes **(Fig. 40.1)**. The amniotomy hook should be allowed to slide along the groove between these fingers (hook pointing towards the fingers) until the cervix is reached. The point is then turned upwards to break the membrane sac. Liquor is usually seen, but may be absent in oligohydramnios or with a well-engaged head. Cord prolapse should be excluded before removing the fingers and then the fetal heart should be rechecked. Absent liquor following artificial rupture of the membranes should be treated in the same way as meconium staining, with careful monitoring of the fetal condition.

Syntocinon

This may be used for induction after ARM with a favourable cervix, or for augmentation of a slow non-obstructed labour. It should only be started after membrane rupture, and continuous CTG monitoring is mandatory. The dose should be titrated against the contractions, aiming for not more than six to seven contractions every 15 minutes.

In induction, the use of Syntocinon immediately after ARM reduces the time to delivery, the rate of postpartum haemorrhage and the need for operative delivery. Nevertheless, without Syntocinon, labour will begin within 24 hours of ARM in nearly 90% of cases, so it is unclear whether these advantages outweigh the maternal inconvenience of an intravenous infusion, restricted mobility and continuous fetal monitoring. An individual approach is advised.

Other methods of induction

Membrane sweep

This involves performing a vaginal examination and inserting a finger through the internal cervical os to separate the membranes from the uterine wall, thus releasing endogenous prostaglandins **(Fig. 40.2)**. It is often uncomfortable for the mother. If a sweep is carried out once after 40 weeks' gestation, it doubles the incidence of spontaneous labour over controls, especially in those with a low Bishop's score. The risk of infection is considered to be minimal.

Anti-progesterones

Mifepristone, a progesterone antagonist, has been studied in early pregnancy and has been shown to increase uterine activity and lead to cervical softening. Research into its use as an induction agent later in pregnancy has shown promising results, but it is not yet in clinical use.

Extra-amniotic saline

This involves passing a Foley catheter through the cervix and infusing normal saline into the extra-amniotic space. The infusion volume should be limited to 1500 ml. Success at cervical ripening has been shown to be similar to that of PGE_2 but the process carries a small risk of introducing infection. It is a much cheaper technique than using PGE_2 and this, together with the fact that PGE_2 needs to be refrigerated, may make it a more suitable method for less affluent countries. It has not yet been compared in studies to misoprostol, a much cheaper prostaglandin preparation than PGE_2.

Failed induction

Despite the above techniques, induction of labour is sometimes unsuccessful. The plan then depends on the reason for the induction. If it was for some significant fetal or maternal indication, there is probably little choice but to consider caesarean section. If, on the other hand, the induction was for some less pressing reason (e.g. for post-dates), then it may be reasonable to consider a more conservative approach. This would depend on an informed discussion with the patient and her partner.

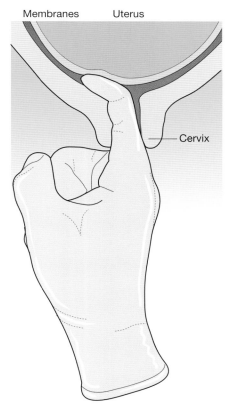

Fig. 40.2 A 'membrane sweep' may increase the incidence of spontaneous labour.

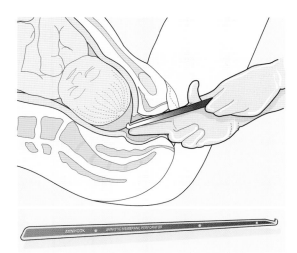

Fig. 40.1 Artificial rupture of the membranes can be used to induce or augment labour. (Redrawn after Greer IA, Cameron IT, Magowan BA et al. *Problem-Based Obstetrics and Gynaecology*. Churchill Livingstone, 2003.)

Key *points*

- The risks of induction need to be balanced against the risks of letting the pregnancy continue.
- The use of oxytocics and prostaglandins (especially misoprostol) carries the risk of uterine hyperstimulation. Close fetal monitoring is important.
- If the cervix is unfavourable, prostaglandins should be used for ripening. If favourable, artificial rupture of the membranes ± Syntocinon is favoured by most.

41
Pain relief in labour

Introduction

Although there is an acceptance, to a degree, that labour is a painful experience, we must guard against the inevitability that labour *should* be painful. Mothers may choose to suffer some pain, but the extent to which the mother should experience pain should ideally be agreed, mainly by the mother but in consultation with a midwife and/or obstetrician and/or anaesthetist.

The pain of labour can be severe. It is a complex mix of physiological, psychological and emotional factors and can be difficult to treat. Many different forms of analgesia have been suggested and each has varying efficacies, risk profiles and potential complications.

Pain is unpleasant for the mother, although there is often some amnesia, which can positively influence its perception in retrospect. It is also recognized that the childbirth experience is influenced by maternal expectations and preparation and by the severity of pain in labour. Influences of pain and pain relief, however, are not as powerful as the influence of the conduct of the caregiver.

Factors influencing pain

The severity of labour pain can vary depending on obstetric, psychological and emotional factors.

Pain scores have been shown to be higher in primigravid women than in multiparous women, especially if they have not had any antenatal preparation. Reports have also shown that primigravid women generally experience more sensory pain during early labour compared to multiparous women, who experience more intense pain much later in labour as a result of rapid descent of the fetus.

Long labours are perceived as being more painful. Labour is also reported to be more painful with fetal malposition, and, in particular, a woman whose baby is occipitoposterior may experience continuous backache.

Physiology of labour pain

There are two components to the pain of labour, visceral (relating to an organ, i.e. the uterus) and somatic (relating to other tissues).

Visceral labour pain occurs during the first stage of childbirth and is due to progressive mechanical dilatation of the cervix, distension of the lower uterine segment and contraction of the uterine muscles. Labour pain may also be as result of the myometrial and cervical ischaemia that occurs during contractions. Severity of this pain mirrors the duration and intensity of contractions. Visceral pain is transmitted by small unmyelinated 'C' fibres which travel with sympathetic fibres and pass through the uterine, cervical and hypogastric nerve plexuses into the main sympathetic chain. The pain fibres from the sympathetic chain then enter the white rami communicantes associated with the T10 to L1 spinal nerves and pass via their posterior nerve roots to synapse in the dorsal horn of the spinal cord. Chemical mediators involved in this pain transmission include bradykinin, leukotrienes, prostaglandins, serotonin, substance P and lactic acid. This pain is dull in character and is sensitive to opioid drugs.

Somatic labour pain occurs during the late first stage and the second stage of labour and is due to stretching and distension of the pelvic floor, perineum and vagina. It occurs as a result of descent of the fetus, and during this stage of labour, the uterus contracts more intensely in a rhythmic and regular manner. Somatic pain is transmitted by fine, myelinated, rapidly transmitting 'A delta' fibres. Transmission occurs via the pudendal nerves and perineal branches of the posterior cutaneous nerve of the thigh to S2 to S4 nerve roots. Somatic fibres from the cutaneous branches of the ilioinguinal and genitofemoral nerves also carry afferent fibres to L1 and, to some degree, L2.

All resulting nerve impulses (visceral and somatic) pass to dorsal horn cells and finally to the brain via the spinothalamic tract. Direct pressure of the fetus on the lumbosacral plexus also results in neuropathic pain during labour.

Psychology of labour pain

Maternal control makes labour a more positive experience. Attitudes to pain and pain relief in labour depend on personal aspirations, expectations, cultural factors, learned behaviours, peer group influences, desirability of the pregnancy, previous experiences of pain, pre-existing anxiety or depression, and preparation, education and communication.

Methods of pain relief

Non-pharmacological methods

Maternal support

Psychological support is extremely valuable and allows pharmacological intervention to be minimized. The continuous presence of a supportive companion, not necessarily a qualified practitioner, or the woman's partner is recommended. This is enhanced by a positive attitude from midwives or other professionals involved in the labour.

Environment

It is recommended that music of the mother's choice be played in labour, that light diet be offered and that the mother is encouraged to be mobile, to walk and to try to achieve comfortable positions; it is recognized that pain is increased by being flat on the back. Positions such as squatting, all fours, or a birthing chair may reduce the need for pharmacological pain relief.

Birthing pools (Fig. 41.1)

The use of warm baths and birthing pools has been shown to reduce pain and the need for regional analgesia. These should not be used within 2 hours of the administration of opioids or if the mother is drowsy.

Education

Maternal education has some effect in engendering calm and making expectations realistic; this thereby improves control, and reduces pain and distress in labour.

Breathing and relaxation techniques, massage, acupuncture, acupressure and hypnosis are used by many women, but have limited evidence to support their effectiveness. There is evidence that transcutaneous nerve stimulation (TENS) has no analgesic benefit, but its use is

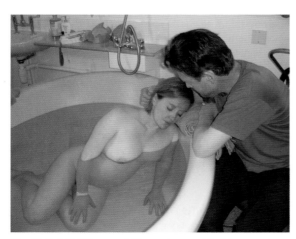

Fig. 41.1 A birthing pool. The environment for labour and delivery is important in reducing the need for pharmacological intervention. (With permission.)

not associated with harm. Injected water papules are not recommended.

Pharmacological methods

Inhaled analgesics

Entonox (a 50:50 mixture of oxygen and nitrous oxide) is commonly used by labouring mothers. Despite its widespread use, studies have shown that it is not a potent analgesic in labour; reassuringly, however, there is moderate evidence for its safety. Any pain relief it offers is limited, and it can lead to nausea, vomiting, drowsiness and light-headedness.

The anaesthetic gases isoflurane, desflurane and sevoflurane can be used safely at sub-anaesthetic concentrations with or without nitrous oxide to improve analgesic efficacy during labour. Although studies have shown that sevoflurane is superior to Entonox in providing pain relief, these gases are not widely available for use in the labour setting.

Systemic opioid analgesia

Systemic opioids have limited effect irrespective of the drug, the route or the method of administration. There is some limited evidence that intramuscular diamorphine gives more effective analgesia than other opioids, and it may have fewer side-effects. There is the potential for maternal nausea, vomiting and drowsiness, and short-term respiratory depression and drowsiness in the neonate. Antiemetics should be administered when parenteral opioids are used.

Pudendal analgesia

The pudendal nerve, derived from the second, third and fourth sacral nerve roots, supplies the vulva and perineum. It crosses the sacrospinous ligament behind the ischial spine along with the pudendal artery **(Fig. 41.2)**, and local infiltration at this point may provide useful perineal analgesia for a low-outlet forceps or ventouse delivery. A pudendal needle is inserted through the sacrospinous ligament and, after aspirating to ensure that the injection is not intravascular, a local anaesthetic is injected behind the ligament on that side. The injection is repeated on the other side and it is usual to infiltrate the perineum directly at the same time.

Regional analgesia

This refers to the delivery of analgesic drugs into the intrathecal (subarachnoid) space (cerebrospinal fluid) or into the epidural space **(Fig. 41.3)**. In obstetric anaesthesia, the introduction of drug to the intrathecal space tends to be known as 'a spinal' and the introduction of drug to the epidural space, as 'an epidural'.

In general, epidurals are used for analgesia in labour, and spinals as a form of anaesthesia for caesarean section and other operative procedures **(Table 41.1)**. The use of regional techniques for anaesthesia has resulted in a reduction in the use of general anaesthesia for caesarean section and other operative procedures. This in turn has

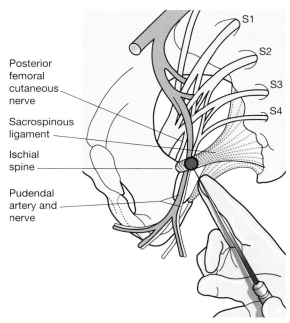

Fig. 41.2 The pudendal nerve runs behind the sacrospinous ligament.

Posterior femoral cutaneous nerve

Sacrospinous ligament

Ischial spine

Pudendal artery and nerve

S1
S2
S3
S4

Table 41.1	
Differences between epidural and spinal analgesia	
Epidural	**Spinal**
Extradural catheter placement	Subarachnoid injection
Cannula allows top-up for prolonged use	One-off injection lasting 2–4 hours
Analgesic effect may be patchy	Dense and relatively reliable anaesthetic blockade

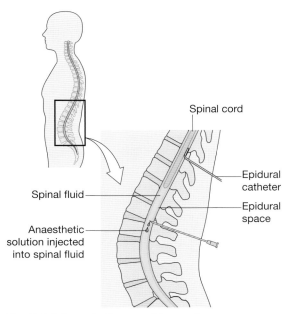

Fig. 41.3 Schematic diagram of the meninges.

Spinal cord

Spinal fluid

Anaesthetic solution injected into spinal fluid

Epidural catheter

Epidural space

be obstetric indications, e.g. in twin delivery to allow manipulation of the second twin if necessary. Epidurals do not cause a prolonged first stage, do not lead to an increased rate of caesarean section, and are not associated with long-term backache. They have, however, been associated with a prolonged second stage and a higher rate of instrumental delivery, but this may be less of an issue with some lower-dose regimens. The addition of opioid to the epidural solution allows less local anaesthetic use and therefore greater mobility. Continuous electronic fetal monitoring is recommended for at least 30 minutes after the initial epidural injection and after administration of each bolus thereafter. Epidural analgesia should be continued until after the third stage and for perineal repair if necessary.

Where labour proceeds to a trial of assisted delivery or caesarean section, or complications requiring operative intervention are encountered, the epidural can be topped up or a spinal can be used instead.

Side-effects of epidurals can arise from the mechanical nature of the technique, or from the drugs themselves. Neurological complications from mechanical insertion are rare, but inadvertent dural puncture may occur and ongoing CSF leakage following this can lead to a 'spinal headache'. This leakage can be sealed using a technique known as a 'blood patch'. Side-effects from the local anaesthetic and opioid are hypotension, urinary retention, pyrexia, pruritus, maternal respiratory depression and neonatal respiratory depression. The hypotension results from sympathetic blockade and peripheral vasodilation, and should be managed by lying the patient in the left lateral position, giving oxygen, and treating with either intravenous fluids or vasopressors.

Spinal anaesthesia

Spinals are rarely used primarily for analgesia, but are commonly used for anaesthesia before caesarean section, instrumental delivery, or the surgical management of postpartum complications such as a retained placenta or the repair of third- and fourth-degree tears **(Fig. 41.4)**. In obstetric anaesthesia, spinals are invariably carried out as a single shot which provides a dense block for 2–4 hours. As with epidurals, the addition of an opioid allows some sparing of the local anaesthetic volume (and therefore dose) which in turn allows some sparing of the side-effects of sympathetic block.

had an impact on maternal morbidity and mortality from anaesthetic causes.

Epidural analgesia for labour

There is good evidence that epidurals provide more effective pain relief than parenteral opioids. The main indication for epidural analgesia is maternal request, but there may

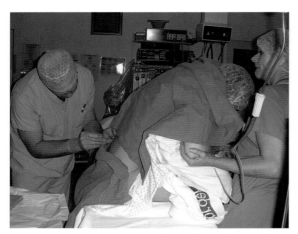

Fig. 41.4 Spinal anesthesia provides a dense block which is particularly useful for caesarean section and some instrumental deliveries.

Complications of spinal anaesthesia can again be considered as related to the procedure and related to the drugs. The mechanical complications are similar to those of the epidural. Hypotension also often occurs, and is managed as above. A high block (which blocks fibres above T4), however, can lead to bradycardia, which in turn compounds any hypotension. A total spinal is a rare complication in which local anaesthetic affects the brain directly and leads to unconsciousness.

Combined spinal–epidural (CSE) is a technique whereby the epidural space is accessed using an epidural needle and then a spinal needle is passed down the epidural needle and advanced to the intrathecal space. 'Spinal doses' of drugs are then given down the spinal needle and this needle is removed and an epidural catheter introduced down the epidural needle to the epidural space. The epidural catheter can then be 'topped up' as necessary. CSE is used when rapid-onset analgesia is needed but the procedure may be prolonged, such that epidural top-ups may be needed too, or when the patient's condition cannot risk the potential sympathetic block which might occur with a full spinal (cardiac disease) or a high motor block (respiratory disease); a smaller-dose spinal can then be used, with the facility to top this up epidurally.

General anaesthesia

General anaesthesia in pregnancy carries more risk than in the non-pregnant patient. As there is reduced gastro-oesophageal tone, increased intra-abdominal mass and reduced gastric emptying, regurgitation of gastric contents and aspiration of these to the lungs is more likely. In addition, as the gastric contents are more acidic in pregnancy, any aspiration is more likely to lead to pneumonitis. Difficult and failed intubation is more likely than in non-pregnant patients because of pregnancy-related obesity. Regional anaesthesia is therefore to be preferred if possible.

Key *points*

- Analgesia should be a balanced, well-informed decision dependent on what the mother wishes to endure and on the efficacy, risks and side-effects of the analgesic methods available.
- Non-pharmacological recommendations include psychological support from a birthing partner, a positive attitude from professionals, remaining mobile and finding comfortable positions, the use of warm baths and birthing pools, and other techniques of the mother's choice.
- Entonox is not a potent analgesic but there is moderate evidence for its efficacy. Systemic opioid analgesia also has limited effect.
- There is good evidence for the analgesic benefits of epidural analgesia compared to systemic opioids. A 'low-dose' local anaesthetic and opioid mixture may be optimal.

42

Precipitate labour and slow labour

Introduction

Abnormal uterine activity has no clear definition, partly because the range of normal uterine activity itself has no clear definition. It is tempting to refer to uterine 'overactivity' as that which results in labour progressing too quickly, and 'inadequate' uterine activity as that which is insufficient to provide adequate progress, but the rate of progress has no precise definition either. In practice, overactivity presents as rapid painful contractions often associated with fetal distress, and inadequate uterine activity as absent or slow cervical dilatation.

Precipitate labour results from uterine overactivity. Slow labour may result from inadequate uterine activity, cephalopelvic disproportion, or a combination of the two.

Cephalopelvic disproportion refers to how well the fetal head fits through the pelvis and may occur if the fetal head is too big or the pelvis too small. It is subdivided into 'true' cephalopelvic disproportion if the head is in the correct position and 'relative' cephalopelvic disproportion if the obstruction is caused by the head presenting in some less favourable position.

Precipitate labour

Spontaneous hypercontractility is rare, perhaps occurring in only 1:3000 pregnancies. The contractions may be excessively long or be excessively frequent and there is a risk of fetal hypoxia due to interference with the placental blood supply.

Uterine hyperstimulation occurs much more commonly, however, and by definition is caused by the use of oxytocics. Both Syntocinon (synthetic oxytocin that is administered by injection or infusion) and prostaglandins may be implicated. The choice of dosage regimens for each represents a compromise between efficacy and the risk of hyperstimulation. The appropriate dose of Syntocinon remains controversial, but there is good evidence for starting at a low dose, around 0.5–1 mU/min, and increasing over 4 or 5 hours to 12 mU/min. Whilst the licensed maximum dose is currently 20 mU/min, some clinicians support the use of regimens up to 40 mU/min.

With prostaglandins, hyperstimulation is also a significant risk but is less likely if their administration is intravaginal, rather than oral, intracervical or directly extra-amniotic.

Precipitate labour resulting from either spontaneous hypercontractility or uterine hyperstimulation may lead to fetal distress. Placental blood supply is via intramyometrial blood vessels which are constricted during the contraction, and excessively long or frequent contractions reduce the chance of recovery in the short times when blood flow is returned **(Fig. 42.1)**. Precipitate labour may also predispose to uterine rupture in parous women, particularly if there is a pre-existing caesarean section scar.

Management of precipitate labour is largely dependent on the fetal condition. If a Syntocinon infusion is running, it should be stopped and the mother given a tocolytic, e.g. a bolus of subcutaneous terbutaline or intravenous ritodrine. If severe fetal distress is apparent, it may be necessary to deliver the baby either instrumentally or by caesarean section, depending on the dilatation of the cervix. If a caesarean section is arranged, it is worth carrying out a vaginal examination prior to starting the operation, as the cervix may dilate rapidly during the time taken in the transfer to theatre, especially in a parous woman.

It is important to note that frequent uterine contractions are also a feature of placental abruption. Contractions with a frequency of more than one every 2 minutes are highly suggestive of this problem and these frequent contractions may increase the distress of a fetus already compromised by partial placental separation. The diagnosis of placental abruption is even more likely if there is associated lower abdominal pain, backache or vaginal bleeding. Tocolytics are contraindicated, as uterine relaxation may exacerbate the bleeding and precipitate further placental separation.

Slow labour

As discussed on page 327, it is important to monitor labour with a partogram in order to identify abnormalities in the progress of labour at the earliest stage. Early identification and correction of abnormal labour makes it more likely that the mother will achieve a vaginal delivery.

Slow labour is associated with:

- eventual fetal 'distress' and risk of fetal hypoxic injury
- an increased risk of intrauterine infection leading to fetal and maternal morbidity

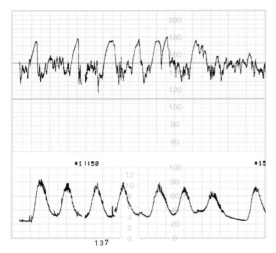

Fig. 42.1 Cardiotocograph trace in precipitate labour. There is hyperstimulation secondary to Syntocinon administration with five contractions occurring every 10 minutes. Despite this, there are reassuring fetal accelerations.

- maternal anxiety and longer-term 'psychological' scarring
- loss of confidence in those providing maternity care.

These in turn are associated with a greater chance of the mother being delivered by caesarean section or requiring an instrumental delivery. The causes of slow labour are summarized in **Table 42.1** and the outcome in **Table 42.2**.

Prolonged latent phase

Chapter 38 describes how the first stage of labour is divided into two parts, the latent phase (from the onset of contractions until the cervix is fully effaced) and the active phase (when the cervix begins to dilate). The latent phase is most likely to be prolonged in those whose cervix is unfavourable, and a prolonged latent phase is therefore much more common in primigravidae **(Fig. 42.2)**.

There is rarely any serious cause for a prolonged latent phase. Cephalopelvic disproportion usually presents at more advanced stages of cervical dilatation. Only very rarely are the symptoms mimicked by dehiscence of a previous caesarean section scar. With a prolonged latent phase, the mother often becomes weary and exhausted from what can sometimes be discomfort over a number of days. Within reason, it is important to resist the temptation to actively intervene by artificially rupturing the membranes or administering oxytocics, at least until the cervix is 2 or 3 cm dilated and fully effaced with a well-applied presenting part. These measures may actually increase the risk of further obstetric intervention in what might, with patience, have been an uneventful labour. Reassurance, encouragement and appropriate analgesia over this time are extremely important.

Prolonged active phase and secondary arrest

The active phase may be prolonged because of inadequate uterine activity or cephalopelvic disproportion **(Fig. 42.3)**.

Inadequate uterine activity

The uterus may be hypoactive or incoordinate. A hypoactive uterus is one with low resting tone and only weakly propagated contractions. There is often a longer interval

Table 42.1

Clinical classification of slow labour

Clinical features	Caused by
Prolonged latent phase	Idiopathic
Prolonged active phase and secondary arrest	Inadequate uterine activity: • Hypoactive • Incoordinate Obstruction (cephalopelvic disproportion): • True cephalopelvic disproportion (head too big or pelvis too small) • Relative cephalopelvic disproportion (malposition of the head increases the diameter of the presenting part)

Table 42.2

Outcome of delivery based on pattern of labour

	% of cases	Spontaneous vertex delivery %	Instrumental delivery %	Caesarean section %
Normal pattern	65–70	80	18	2
Prolonged latent phase	2–5	75	10	15
Prolonged active phase	20–30	55	30	15
Secondary arrest	5–10	40	35	25

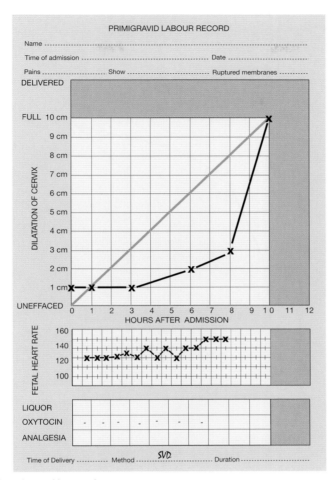

Fig. 42.2 Partogram with prolonged latent phase.

between contractions and the contractions are not particularly painful.

Incoordinate uterine activity may occur because of inadequate 'fundal dominance'. As noted on page 319, normal uterine contraction begins at a pacemaker point close to the junction of the uterus and the fallopian tube. It spreads from this point downwards, with its intensity maximal at the fundus (where the muscle is thickest), intermediate at the mid-zone and least at the lower segment. With incoordinate uterine activity, however, the intensity profile appears to be reversed, with the maximal intensity in the lower segment (where the muscle is thinnest) and weakest at the fundus. This is much less efficient. The resting tone is also found to be increased throughout and the threshold for pain is therefore reached earlier in the contraction.

Inadequate uterine activity has no specific cause, but is much commoner in primigravidae. It may simply be a developmental feature of the uterine muscle and there is evidence that many will resolve spontaneously given sufficient time. There is also some evidence that inadequate uterine activity is associated with cephalopelvic disproportion.

This is because cervical dilatation itself may improve uterine activity, but is less likely to occur if the presenting part is pressing less firmly on the cervix.

If progress is satisfactory, there is no need to consider treatment of inadequate uterine activity. Most will respond well to oxytocics, usually given by a stepwise i.v. Syntocinon infusion as described above. As labour is likely to be prolonged, care should be taken to make sure that the mother does not become dehydrated or ketotic, as this will further exacerbate the uterine problem.

Cephalopelvic disproportion (CPD)

This may occur because:

1. The baby's head is presenting in the optimal way but is too large relative to the pelvis ('true' cephalopelvic disproportion). It is diagnosed only if the head does not become engaged despite adequate uterine activity. It is not possible to predict CPD antenatally and even using the strictest antenatal criteria many of those considered to be at risk by clinical pelvic assessment will go on

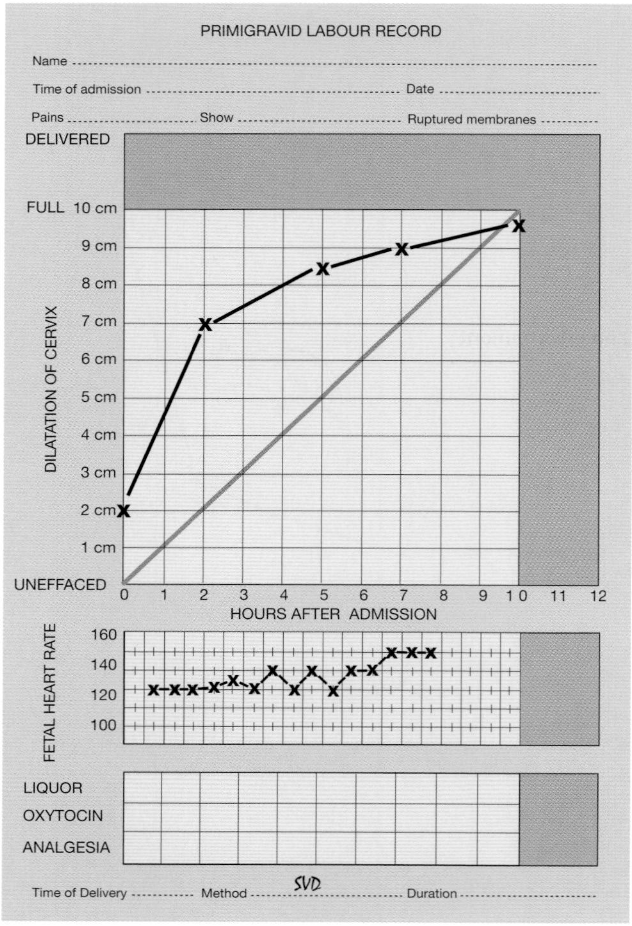

Fig. 42.3 Partogram with prolonged active phase.

to have a vaginal delivery. More complicated attempts to predict CPD using ultrasound measurements of the fetal head together with X-ray or CT pelvimetry measurements have also proved to be unreliable and only lead to unnecessary surgical intervention. Even short stature should not necessarily be regarded with suspicion, as these women are more likely to have smaller babies. The only true pelvimeter is labour.

2. There is a malpresentation or malposition of the baby's head so that a wider part of the head is being presented to the pelvis (p. 356). This is 'relative' cephalopelvic disproportion. It may occur with deflexed malpresentations (particularly of the brow and face, p. 357-8) but the most common cause of relative CPD occurs when the head rotates to the occipitoposterior (p. 359) rather than the occipitoanterior position. The first stage and second stage progress more slowly and, although spontaneous delivery is quite possible with the head coming out 'face to pubis', secondary arrest is not uncommon.

3. There is some form of pelvic abnormality. Major abnormalities are uncommon, particularly in affluent societies, and are usually associated with disease, injury or severe nutritional problems. The obstetric classification is based on the shape of the pelvic brim, as it is the pelvic inlet which seems to be the major determinant of successful delivery **(Fig. 42.4)**.

Pelves with normal shape and bone development

The round 'gynaecoid' pelvis is the commonest and, as would be teleologically predicted by the theory of natural selection; it is obstetrically ideal. The long oval 'anthropoid' pelvis is also relatively common but is associated with occipitoposterior presentation.

Pelves with abnormal shape and bone development

Defects of nutrition and environment

Minor The flat-brimmed 'platypelloid' pelvis and the triangular 'android' pelvis are considered to be minor variations associated with adverse nutrition in infancy and childhood. The flat-brimmed pelvis is found relatively more commonly in African women and the triangular pelvis in those from southern Europe.

Normal shape and bone development

Round gynecoid pelvis (A)

Long oval anthropoid pelvis (B)

Abnormal shape and bone development

Defects of nutrition and environment

Minor

Flat brimmed platypelloid pelvis (C)

Triangular android pelvis (D)

Major

Rickets (E)

Osteomalacia (F)

Disease or injury

Spinal - kyphosis or scoliosis (G)
Pelvic - tumours, fractures
Limbs - childhood polio or a congenitally
        dislocated hip

Congenital

Naegele's pelvis and (H)
Robert's pelvis

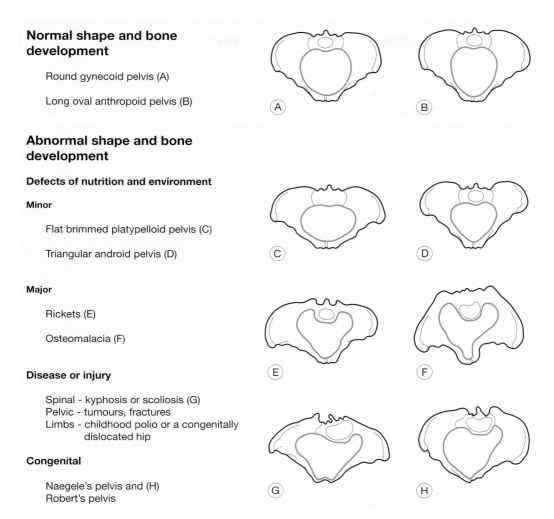

Fig. 42.4 Classification of pelvic shapes.

Major Rickets is caused by prolonged vitamin D deficiency in early life leading to poorly mineralized bones containing large areas of soft uncalcified osteoid. Weight bearing produces bony deformities by pushing the sacral promontory forward and pivoting the sacrum backwards. The result is a marked reduction in the anteroposterior measurement of the pelvic brim, with possible further mid-cavity narrowing in severe cases as the acetabula are also forced inwards. As the diet in many western countries contains adequate calcium and vitamin D, and many 'developing' countries have plenty of exposure to sunshine, rickets is uncommon. Osteomalacia – caused by adult calcium deficiency – is rare, except in certain parts of northern India and China.

Disease or injury

Abnormal pressure on the pelvis from kyphosis or scoliosis gradually moulds the pelvis into funnelled or asymmetric shapes. Asymmetrical weight bearing from polio or a congenitally dislocated hip may also mould the pelvis to

less favourable proportions. Pelvic fractures may leave the pelvis asymmetrical, and excessive bone formation at the fracture site may further narrow the passage.

Congenital malformations

Congenital absence of one or both sacral masses, (Naegele's pelvis and Robert's pelvis, respectively) results in direct fusion of the sacrum to the ilium and marked narrowing.

Management of slow labour

When progress is slow or when there is secondary arrest, it is important to distinguish whether the cause is inadequate uterine activity or cephalopelvic disproportion.

The strength of contractions is difficult to assess reliably. Direct intrauterine pressure monitoring is essentially only a research tool. Some idea of the strength can be gained through maternal observation and abdominal palpation. With an experienced observer, this can provide useful clinical information. In the presence of cephalopelvic disproportion there will be caput (a diffuse swelling of the scalp) and moulding (an alteration in the relation of the fetal cranial bones), and malposition or malpresentation may be identified by careful vaginal examination.

In practice, the clinical decision is whether or not to start a Syntocinon infusion. The main risks of starting Syntocinon are of:

- hyperstimulation of the uterus and subsequent fetal distress
- rupture of the uterus (this applies to multiparous mothers only and particularly to those with a previous caesarean section scar).

In primigravidae with slow progress or secondary arrest who do not have a prohibitive malpresentation (e.g. brow presentation) it is reasonable to start Syntocinon. This is not appropriate if there is suspected fetal distress and should only be after the membranes have been ruptured or have ruptured spontaneously. The aim is to titrate the infusion to the point where the contractions are coming at a frequency of three or four every 10 minutes. Vaginal examinations should be repeated every 2–3 hours after the infusion is started, to ensure adequate progress. If progress is still inadequate, then operative delivery will be required.

In parous women the decision is more difficult, mainly because of the risk of uterine rupture (p. 373). Rupture can occur suddenly and leads to expulsion of the fetus into the peritoneal cavity. Fetal death is common. If the mother has had a previous vaginal delivery, true cephalopelvic disproportion is extremely unlikely, but if the only previous delivery was an elective caesarean section (e.g. for breech presentation), there is no guide to the likelihood of true obstruction. Syntocinon should therefore be used only with caution and only in those women thought to have inadequate uterine activity with no evidence of obstruction. Vaginal examinations should again be repeated every 2–3 hours to ensure adequate progress, with a lower threshold for caesarean section in those thought to have some degree of cephalopelvic disproportion.

Key points

- Progress in labour requires adequate uterine activity and an appropriately proportioned fetal head compared to the size of the maternal pelvis.
- Precipitate labour is most commonly iatrogenic following oxytocic administration.
- Slow progress is often corrected with the use of Syntocinon, whether due to inadequate uterine activity or a small degree of cephalopelvic disproportion. Care must be taken to exclude a significant malpresentation before the infusion is started. Syntocinon carries a risk of uterine rupture in parous women only.

43

Malpresentations and malpositions

Introduction

In the third trimester of pregnancy, abdominal palpation should aim to define the lie, presentation, and position of the fetus, in that order. The *lie* refers to the long axis of the fetus in relation to the long axis of the uterus. Usually the fetus is longitudinal, but occasionally it may be transverse or oblique. The *presentation* is that part of the fetus which is at the pelvic brim, in other words the part of the fetus presenting to the pelvic inlet. Normal presentation is the vertex of the fetal head and the word 'malpresentation' describes any non-vertex presentation. This may be of the face, brow, breech, or some other part of the body if the lie is oblique or transverse.

The *position* of the fetus refers to the way in which the presenting part is positioned in relation to the maternal pelvis. Strictly speaking this refers to any presenting part, but here it will be considered in relation to those fetuses presenting head first (cephalic). As we have seen, the head is usually occipitotransverse at the pelvic brim and rotates to occipitoanterior at the pelvic floor. 'Malposition' is when the head, coming vertex first, does not rotate to occipitoanterior, presenting instead as persistent occipitotransverse or occipitoposterior.

Malpresentation

As described above, 'malpresentation' is a term used to describe any non-vertex presentation. Malpresentations include face presentation, brow presentation and breech presentation. When the fetus has a cephalic presentation, the presenting diameter is dependent on the degree of flexion or extension of the fetal head – deflexed and brow presentations offer a wide diameter to the pelvic inlet (**Table 43.1** and **Fig. 43.1**).

As the fetal neurocranium is made up of individual bony plates (the occipital, sphenoid, temporal and ethmoid bones) which are joined by cartilagenous sutures (the frontal, sagittal, lambdoid and coronal sutures), there is potential for the skull to be 'moulded' during labour. This allows the head to fit the birth canal more closely (**Fig. 43.2**). Moulding should be distinguished from caput, which refers to oedema of the presenting part of the scalp. Both moulding and caput can occur in any cephalic presentation, but are more likely to occur in malpresention.

Face presentation

This occurs in about 1:500 births (**Fig. 43.3A**). It is associated with anencephaly but this is a rare cause even in an unscreened population. Face presentation is usually only recognized after the onset of labour and, if the face is swollen (**Fig. 43.3B**), it is easy to confuse this presentation with that of a breech. The position of the face is described with reference to the chin, using the prefix 'mento-'.

The face usually enters the pelvis with the chin in the transverse position (mentotransverse) and 90% rotate to mentoanterior so that the head is born with flexion (**Fig. 43.3C**). If mentoposterior, the extending head presents an increasingly wider diameter to the pelvis, leading to worsening relative cephalopelvic disproportion and impacted obstruction (**Fig. 43.3D**). A caesarean section is usually required.

Brow presentation

This occurs in only approximately 1:1500 births and is the least favourable for delivery (**Fig. 43.4**). The supraorbital ridges and the bridge of the nose will be palpable on vaginal examination. The head may flex to become a vertex presentation or extend to a face presentation in early labour. If the brow presentation persists, a caesarean section will be required.

Breech presentation

Breech presentation describes a fetus presenting bottom-first. The incidence is around 40% at 20 weeks, 25% at 32 weeks, and only 3–4% at term. The chance of a breech presentation turning spontaneously after 38 weeks is less than 4%. Breech presentation is associated with multiple pregnancy, bicornuate uterus, fibroids, placenta praevia, polyhydramnios and oligohydramnios. It may also rarely be associated with fetal anomaly, particularly neural tube defects, neuromuscular disorders and autosomal trisomies. At term, 65% of breech presentations are frank (extended) with the remainder being flexed or footling (**Fig. 43.5**). Footling breech carries a 5–20% risk of cord prolapse (p. 368).

Table 43.1		
Presenting diameters of the fetal head		
	Presenting diameter	
Presentation		
Vertex	Suboccipito-bregmatic	9.5 cm
Deflexed OP	Occipito-frontal	11.5 cm
Brow	Mento-vertical	14 cm
Face	Submento-bregmatic	9.5 cm

Mode of delivery

There has been extensive debate about the safest route of delivery – whether it should be vaginal or by caesarean section. The risks of vaginal delivery are small, but include intracranial injury, widespread bruising, damage to internal organs, spinal cord transection, umbilical cord prolapse and hypoxia following obstruction of the after-coming head. The risks of caesarean section are largely maternal and related to surgical morbidity and mortality. There is now evidence that planned caesarean section is associated with less perinatal

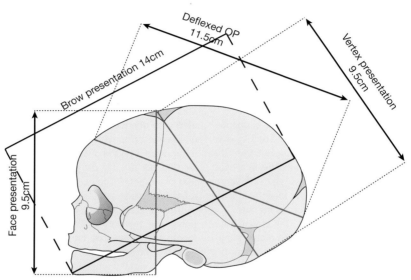

Fig. 43.1 The presenting diameter is dependent on the degree of flexion or extension of the fetal head.

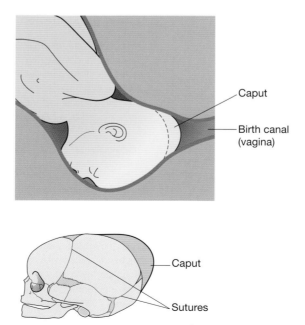

Fig 43.2 'Moulding' refers to the change in shape of the fetal skull during labour as it 'moulds' to the birth canal. Caput refers to oedema of the presenting part of the scalp.

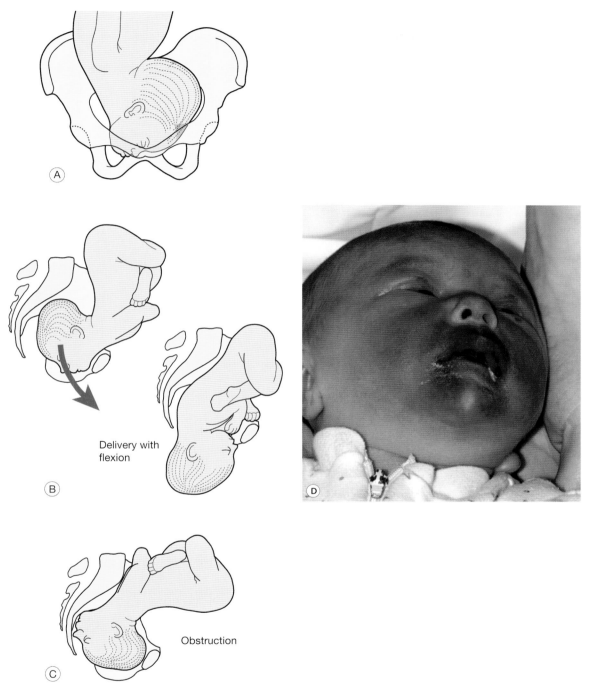

Fig. 43.3 Face presentation. (A) The head enters the pelvic brim in the transverse position. **(B)** Most rotate to the mentoanterior position and deliver without problems. **(C)** Those that rotate to mentoposterior will obstruct. **(D)** Face presentation is often associated with oedema and bruising. This baby recovered without problems.

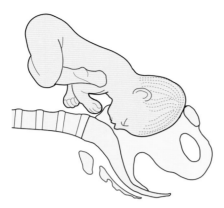

Fig 43.4 Brow presentation.

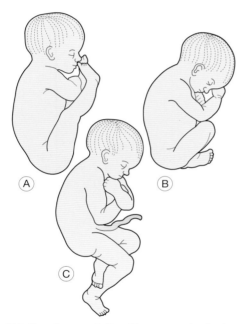

Fig. 43.5 Breech presentation. Those presenting by the breech may be **(A)** extended (or frank); **(B)** flexed; or **(C)** footling.

mortality and less serious neonatal morbidity than planned vaginal birth at term. The risks of serious maternal complications are much about the same, partly because planned vaginal delivery often ends with an intrapartum caesarean section and such caesarean sections carry greater risks than planned elective sections. The problem of delivery can be removed if it is possible to turn the baby prior to the onset of labour. This process is called external cephalic version.

External cephalic version (ECV)

All women with an uncomplicated breech pregnancy at term should be offered ECV. It is good practice to offer ECV from 36 weeks in nulliparous women and from 37 weeks in multiparous women. There is no point

in attempting ECV with a significant placenta praevia, as a caesarean section will still be required; other relative and absolute contraindications to ECV are outlined in **Box 43.1**.

Procedure

A cardiotocograph and ultrasound scan should be performed. Some obstetricians like the patient to be fasted and prepared for theatre, and although this is usually not necessary, it is reasonable to have access to theatre close at hand. ECV is most likely to be successful in parous women and when the presenting part is free, the liquor volume is normal, the head is easy to palpate and the uterus feels soft. A flexed breech is more likely to turn than an extended (frank) breech.

Ask the mother to lie flat with a 30° lateral tilt. The use of tocolysis to soften the uterus is associated with an increased success rate. Applying scanning gel to the abdomen allows easier manipulation and permits scanning during the procedure if required. Disengage the breech with the scan probe or hands, and then attempt to rotate in the direction in which the baby is facing (i.e. forward roll). Check the fetal heart every 2 minutes. If unsuccessful, a backward somersault can be tried. If the procedure is only partially successful (i.e. the fetus is converted to a transverse lie), return the fetus to breech rather than leave it transverse. Give anti-D 500 IU i.m. if rhesus negative. Perform a CTG after the procedure is completed. The success rate of version is ≈30% for primigravidae and ≈50% for parous women.

Caesarean section for breech presentation

The evidence quoted above considers term pregnancies only. It is probably also advisable to carry out a caesarean section in preterm deliveries, as there is the additional risk of the cervix closing around the neck after delivery of the breech. Whether caesarean section is also appropriate in extreme prematurity is more difficult to assess, as the delivery may still be traumatic for the baby. In this instance, the operation should be performed by an experienced obstetrician.

Vaginal delivery for breech presentation

This may occasionally be considered appropriate by some clinicians if the estimated fetal weight is <3.8 kg and there is no fetal compromise, pre-eclampsia or placenta praevia. Ideally the onset of labour should be spontaneous, the breech frank or flexed (but not footling) and the liquor volume normal. Those not assessed antenatally and presenting in advanced labour with an engaged breech usually deliver without adverse consequences.

The first stage is managed with caution. The role of epidural analgesia is particularly controversial – its use may facilitate manipulation of the fetus, but its presence may inhibit the desire to push, which is particularly important in breech delivery. Augmentation must only be used if disproportion has been excluded and even then with caution. There is no contraindication to a fetal 'scalp' electrode being applied to the breech, providing care is taken to avoid genital injury.

At full dilatation, the mother can be encouraged to push: the temptation to pull must be resisted. *Ideally, the baby should be left alone to delivery itself ('hands off'), taking care to ensure the back remains uppermost when advancing*. If there is undue delay, or there are concerns about fetal well-being (e.g. movements stopping, baby becoming floppy, no response to stimuli), assisted delivery can be used to encourage a more rapid delivery. The techniques of 'hands off' and 'assisted breech' are illustrated in **Figures 43.6 and 43.7**. Breech extraction may be considered when delivering the second twin (p. 311)

One of the key risks of breech delivery is that pulling may lead the head to extend and therefore become stuck at the pelvic brim. *The importance of maternal effort at this stage, rather than traction from below, cannot be overemphasized – it allows the head to flex and minimizes the risk of it becoming stuck at the pelvic brim*.

Should the head of a preterm breech become entrapped behind an incompletely dilated cervix, it should first be flexed as far as is possible to narrow the presenting diameter. Failing this, the options are then to incise the cervix at the 4 and 8 o'clock positions (risking massive, potentially fatal maternal haemorrhage) or to push the fetus back up and perform a caesarean section (very difficult). Because such interventions are very risky to the mother, it may be preferable to await spontaneous delivery.

All babies presenting by the breech should be examined for developmental dysplasia of the hip (p. 402) and Klumpke's paralysis (p. 403).

Transverse lie and oblique lie

These are uncommon, occurring in less than 1% of deliveries at term **(Fig. 43.8)**. Usually there is no specific cause, but abnormal lie is more common in multiparous women, multiple pregnancies, preterm labour and polyhydramnios. It may also be associated with placenta praevia, congenital abnormalities of the uterus, and lower uterine fibroids and other pelvic masses.

If transverse lie is identified antenatally, a scan should be undertaken to exclude placenta praevia, polyhydramnios, lower uterine fibroids and a pathologically enlarged fetal head. External cephalic version is usually possible (see above), and the mother should be reviewed a few days later to ensure that the lie is still cephalic. She should be advised to come to hospital if there is any suspicion of early labour, as it may still be possible to carry out an external cephalic version at that stage, providing the membranes are still intact. She should also particularly be advised to present if there is any suspicion of membrane rupture, as there is a risk of cord prolapse or prolapse of a limb **(Fig. 43.9A, B** and **c)**. In view of the small risk of cord prolapse, some clinicians advise that women with a transverse lie or unstable lie (see below) are admitted to hospital from 38 weeks' to await birth or until a longitudinal lie is maintained (Table 44.1).

If the lie is transverse in established labour, particularly after membrane rupture, a caesarean section will be required. These caesarean sections can be technically very difficult, and a vertical uterine incision may be necessary to allow adequate access for delivery.

Unstable lie

An unstable lie is one that varies from examination to examination. The options are:

- Manage conservatively, with repeated ECVs as required, and await the spontaneous onset of labour. Should the membranes rupture with the fetus in a non-cephalic presentation there may be a risk of cord prolapse, and, as described above, inpatient management is considered appropriate by some.
- Arrange to turn the baby to cephalic presentation and then induce labour. This is sometimes referred to as a 'stabilizing induction'. The disadvantage is that the induction itself is not without risks, and the lie may become unstable again even after the membranes have been ruptured.
- Carry out a caesarean section.

Malposition

Normally the head engages at the pelvic brim in the occipito transverse position, flexing as it descends into the pelvic cavity and rotating to occipitoanterior (OA) at the level of the ischial spines. The head then extends as it descends, distending the vulva until it is delivered. In about 10% of pregnancies, the fetal head enters the pelvis in a more occipitoposterior (OP) position than transverse or anterior, either by chance, or in association with an unfavourably shaped pelvis, particularly the long oval 'anthropoid' pelvis. The baby is then in a direct occipitoposterior position (DOP), or with the occiput to the right or left of the midline, referred to as right or left occipitoposterior (ROP or LOP).

As the breech descends with pushing, it rotates to the antero-posterior and advances over the perineum. It then rotates with the back uppermost. Any movement of the back posteriorly should be corrected.

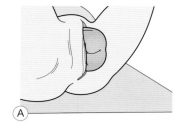

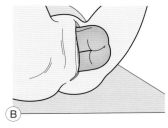

The legs will free themselves as the baby advances, and will hang down

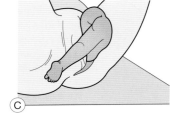

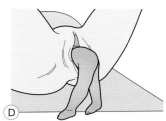

With pushing, the arms will deliver

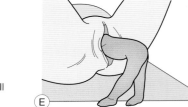

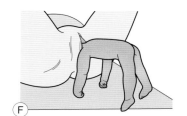

The breech should be allowed to hang in order for the head to flex, waiting for the nape of the neck to become visible

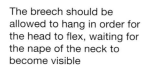

After delivery of the other arm, flexion of the baby's head is encouraged by placing the second and third fingers of the lower hand over the malar bones on the face, pulling them towards you....

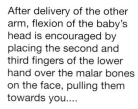

....while the second and third fingers of the other hand are used to push the occiput (back) of the head away from you. With maximum flexion, the head can then be delivered. An episotomy can be used if necessary

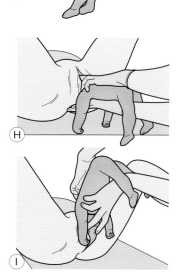

Fig. 43.6 'Hands off' vaginal breech delivery.

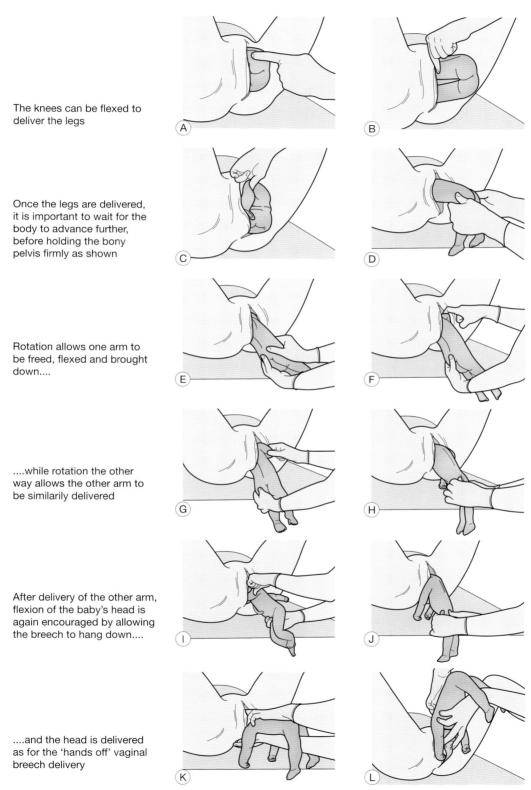

The knees can be flexed to deliver the legs

Once the legs are delivered, it is important to wait for the body to advance further, before holding the bony pelvis firmly as shown

Rotation allows one arm to be freed, flexed and brought down....

....while rotation the other way allows the other arm to be similarly delivered

After delivery of the other arm, flexion of the baby's head is again encouraged by allowing the breech to hang down....

....and the head is delivered as for the 'hands off' vaginal breech delivery

Fig. 43.7 Assisted vaginal breech delivery.

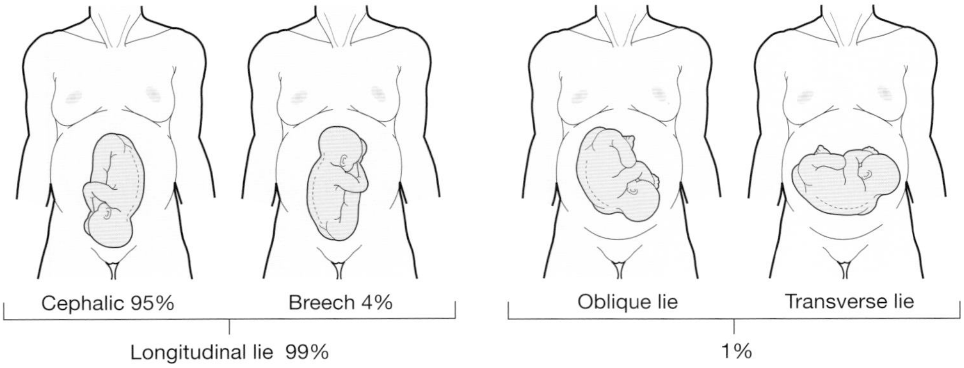

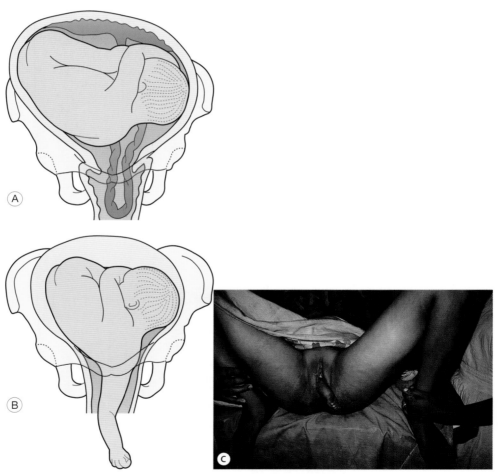

Fig. 43.8 Fetal lie at term.

Cephalic 95%   Breech 4%   Oblique lie   Transverse lie

Longitudinal lie 99%   1%

Fig. 43.9 Transverse lie is associated with (A) cord prolapse, (B) and (C) arm prolapse.

There are then three main possibilities **(Fig. 43.10C)**:

- the occiput will rotate anteriorly (through approximately 135°) to occipitoanterior, and then (usually) deliver normally (65%)

- it will partially rotate to occipitotransverse and not deliver (20%)
- it will rotate more posteriorly to occipitoposterior (15%).

Those that remain OP have greater difficulty negotiating the birth canal and are less likely to deliver spontaneously.

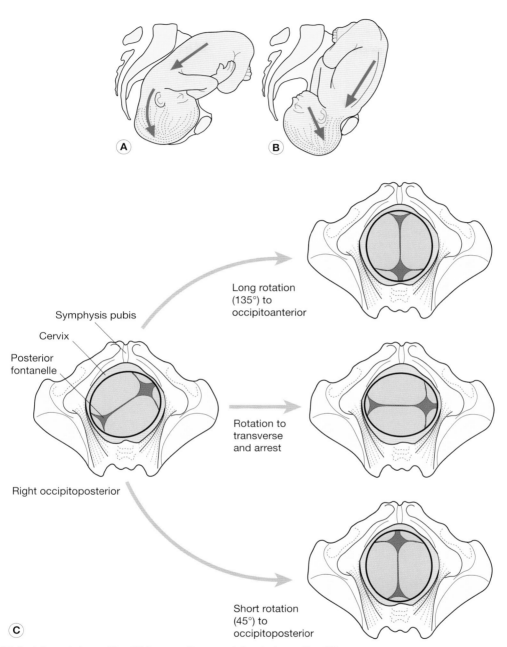

Long rotation
(135°) to
occipitoanterior

Symphysis pubis

Cervix

Posterior
fontanelle

Rotation to
transverse
and arrest

Right occipitoposterior

Short rotation
(45°) to
occipitoposterior

Fig. 43.10 Occipitoposterior position **(A)** Compared to an occipitoanterior position **(B).**

The normal mechanism of delivery involves extension of the head to OA, but extension is not possible in the OP position and a wider diameter is presented to the outlet **Table 43.1** and **Fig 43.10A** and **B**. With malposition, the first and second stages of labour are usually longer, partly because of the greater presenting diameter (relative cephalopelvic disproportion,) and partly because the head is less well applied to the cervix and therefore less able to encourage its dilatation. Back pain in labour appears to be more common with OP position. The mother is more likely to request an epidural, is more likely to experience secondary arrest due to relative cephalopelvic disproportion, and is more likely to require augmentation with Syntocinon.

If the cervix does not reach full dilatation despite Syntocinon, a caesarean section will be required. If full dilatation is reached, it is quite possible for a baby to deliver in the OP position (with the head coming out 'face to pubis'), but, not uncommonly, manual rotation, rotational ventouse, or Kielland's rotational forceps delivery will be required (p. 380).

Key *points*

- Normal presentation is with the vertex of the fetal head, and the word 'malpresentation' describes any non-vertex presentation. It may be of the face, brow, breech, or some other part of the body if the lie is oblique or transverse.
- Those who are presenting by the brow usually become obstructed, and those who are lying transversely always become obstructed.
- Babies presenting by the breech can often deliver vaginally, but there is a small risk of intrapartum injury.
- Babies with a face presentation usually deliver without significant problems.
- The term 'malposition' refers to the situation when the head, coming vertex first, does not rotate to occipitoanterior, and presents instead as persistent occipitotransverse or occipitoposterior. It is associated with prolonged labour and relative cephalopelvic disproportion.

44 Obstetric emergencies

Introduction

Worldwide, one woman dies every minute of every day from a complication of pregnancy. In developed countries, maternal death is uncommon, but evidence from the UK Confidential Enquiry into Maternal Deaths found substandard care in around two-thirds of cases. This is partly due to the fact that most obstetric emergencies are rare and often unfold with such rapidity that junior medical staff can find themselves facing potentially catastrophic conditions that they may never have seen before, let alone have managed.

This chapter will examine the obstetric emergencies listed below.

- unexpected collapse
- amniotic fluid embolism
- prolapsed umbilical cord
- retained placenta
- shoulder dystocia
- uterine inversion
- uterine rupture.

See also haemorrhage (p. 277), eclampsia (p. 296) and pulmonary embolism (p. 255):

Principles of management

Anticipation and preparation are essential – and they may lead to prevention. For example, if the mother has a history of postpartum haemorrhage, anticipation with i.v. access and blood sent for group and save in early labour may make an important difference to the outcome should the problem recur. If there are risk factors for shoulder dystocia, such as a presumed large fetus in a mother with diabetes and a long first stage of labour, it is important to ensure that an experienced midwife is allocated to care for her and that senior medical staff are present on the labour ward at the time of delivery.

In addition, as life-threatening emergencies are relatively rare, it is important that there should be regular 'fire drills' of obstetric emergencies to ensure that all staff are fully prepared, that equipment is fully functional and that supporting systems (portering, laboratory etc.) are prepared. It should also be remembered that emergencies can arise anywhere in the unit, not just in the labour ward.

The principles outlined in **Box 44.1** can be adapted for initial resuscitation in all obstetric emergencies which involve maternal compromise. Remember that there are often two lives at stake and in most emergencies minutes or even seconds count. Remember too, however, that panicking is never helpful. A good principle to remember is that the fetus rarely needs to be resuscitated directly – 'resuscitate the mother and you will resuscitate the fetus'. It should be noted that an obstetric emergency can cause profound lifelong psychological problems for both the mother and her partner. This can manifest itself as postnatal depression, post-traumatic stress syndrome and a real fear of becoming pregnant again. Counselling and debriefing after such experiences should be encouraged both whilst the woman is in hospital and some weeks later.

On identification of an emergency

1. Call for help. Emergency bleep the obstetrical emergency team. This should include a senior obstetrician and anaesthetist, the theatre team, a person skilled in neonatal resuscitation, the midwifery sister, a porter and the junior medical staff.
2. Ensure you have checked the environment is safe for you and apply ABC if appropriate:

   - Airway: Place patient head down, maintain airway patency, give O_2 (15 l/min) via facemask, attach pulse oximeter.
   - Breathing: Assess, monitor respiratory rate, ventilate if indicated.
   - Circulation: Insert two grey/brown i.v. cannulae, take full set of bloods (FBC, coagulation, crossmatch 6 units, urea and electrolytes, and liver function tests). In all cases of severe haemorrhage give 1 litre 0.9% saline or Hartman's solution stat.

3. Check maternal observations as appropriate, e.g. pulse, blood pressure, O_2 saturation monitoring, and bladder catheter for urinary output measurement.

At this point, see the appropriate management guidelines for the particular emergency (e.g. 4 Hs and 4 Ts, Box 44.2) as well as:

4. Considering an ECG, blood glucose measurements, central venous monitoring and an arterial line.
5. Using a compression cuff and warmer to give fluids if rapid administration is indicated.
6. Remembering to document fully in the notes all observations, procedures and actions with date, timings, a signature and a printed name.
7. Remembering the mother's partner. Although some partners might wish to wait outside, others may prefer to stay in the room.

Causes of collapse

4 Hs

- Hypoxia
- Hypovolaemia
- Hypo/hyperkalaemia
- Hypothermia

4 Ts

- Thromboembolism
- Toxic (including local anaesthesia)
- Tamponade
- Tension pneumothorax
  Also consider:
- Eclampsia (including magnesium toxicity)
- Amniotic fluid embolus

- Chemical pneumonitis is more likely than in the non-pregnant state, owing to the decreased pH of the stomach contents and the increased chance of inhaling the contents because of the changes outlined above.

It is therefore important, in the early stages of resuscitation, to:

- tilt the patient to the left by 15–30° (reduces aortocaval compression and increases potential cardiac output by 25%)
- apply cricoid pressure and intubate early, to avoid aspiration of gastric contents and to facilitate oxygenation
- involve a senior obstetrician and anaesthetist immediately or as early as possible (to facilitate intubation and early caesarean section where and when appropriate).

It is essential to perform a caesarean section early. The decision for peri-mortem caesarean section should be made by 4 minutes if there is no response to active resuscitation, and the delivery by 5 minutes (the '4-minute rule'). An anaesthetic is not required in order to proceed. This is primarily to save the life of the mother and forms part of the resuscitation technique. It makes CPR more efficient by:

- increasing venous return
- improving ease of ventilation
- allowing CPR to be carried out in the supine position
- reducing oxygen requirement after delivery.

Resuscitation

Resuscitation should have a strong focus on the ABC of Basic Life Support as noted in **Box 44.1**. The aim is to resuscitate the mother and then (and only then) to consider the welfare of the baby. Resuscitation in pregnancy has some differences from that in a non-pregnant person, as outlined below, but it is still essential to approach the problem by using ABC, and then consider possible causes. The four Hs and four Ts listed in **Box 44.2** are helpful.

The key resuscitation differences are that:

- The aorta and vena cava are compressed by the gravid uterus, impeding venous return and reducing cardiac output.
- There is an increased risk of aspiration of stomach contents due to relaxation of the oesophageal–gastric junction (progesterone effect) and the pressure of the uterus.
- Difficult intubation is more common in the pregnant than in the non-pregnant patient (1:300 vs 1:3000) – short neck and laryngeal oedema.

Amniotic fluid embolism

Epidemiology

This is one of the most catastrophic conditions that can occur in pregnancy. It is rare, with an incidence somewhere between 1:8000 and 1:30,000, and until recent years the mortality at 30 minutes was around 85%. Although improved ITU facilities and improved understanding of the condition have reduced this mortality, it still remains the third highest cause of maternal death within the UK.

Aetiology

The exact pathophysiology remains unclear. It was believed that some breakdown occurred in the physiological barrier separating the mother and fetus, allowing a bolus of amniotic fluid to enter the maternal circulation. This bolus moved to the pulmonary circulation and produced massive perfusion failure, bronchospasm and shock. More recently it has been suggested that the underlying mechanism may be an anaphylactoid reaction to fetal antigens entering the maternal circulation and individual variations in sensitivity to these antigens are reflected by the severity of the resulting clinical picture.

Risk factors

Amniotic fluid embolism can occur at any time in pregnancy but it most commonly occurs in labour (70%), after vaginal delivery (11%), and following caesarean section (19%). The following risk factors have been identified:

- multiparity
- placental abruption
- intrauterine death
- precipitate labour
- suction termination of pregnancy
- medical termination of pregnancy
- abdominal trauma
- external cephalic version
- amniocentesis.

Clinical features

The clinical picture usually develops almost instantaneously and the diagnosis must be considered in all collapsed obstetric patients. The mother may demonstrate some or all of the signs and symptoms listed in **Box 44.3** but classically a woman in late stages of labour or immediately postpartum starts to gasp for air, starts fitting and may have a cardiac arrest. There is often a profound disseminated intravascular coagulopathy (DIC) with massive haemorrhage, coma and death. There are inevitably signs of fetal compromise.

Diagnosis

The definitive diagnosis is usually at autopsy and is made by confirming the presence of fetal squames in the pulmonary vasculature. It is also possible to confirm the diagnosis in a surviving patient, again by finding fetal squames in washings from the bronchus or in a sample of blood from the right ventricle. In the acute situation, as there is no single clinical or laboratory finding which can diagnose or exclude amniotic fluid embolism, the diagnosis is made clinically by exclusion.

Management

This is primarily supportive and should be aggressive. There is, however, no evidence that any specific type of intervention significantly improves maternal prognosis. Initial therapy is aimed at supporting cardiac output and management of DIC. If the woman is undelivered, an immediate caesarean section may be appropriate, providing the mother can be stabilized.

A chest X-ray will often show pulmonary oedema, and an increase in right atrial and right ventricular size. The ECG demonstrates right ventricular strain and there is a metabolic acidosis (reduction of pO_2 and pCO_2).

In addition to the initial management of an obstetric emergency **(Box 44.1)**, therapy may include:

- aggressive fluid replacement
- maintenance of cardiac output with a dopamine infusion
- treatment of anaphylaxis with adrenaline (epinephrine), salbutamol, aminophylline and hydrocortisone
- treatment of DIC with fresh frozen plasma and cryoprecipitate
- treatment of haemorrhage after delivery with Syntocinon, ergometrine, carboprost (Haemabate) or misoprostol, and uterine massage (p. 280)
- early transfer to an ITU for central monitoring, respiratory support and other therapy as appropriate.

Prognosis

The outcome for the baby is very poor, with a perinatal mortality rate of approximately 60% and most survivors usually suffering neurological impairment. Maternal outcome in mothers who have suffered a cardiac arrest is complicated by the fact that many are left with serious neurological impairment.

Box 44.3

Symptoms and signs of amniotic fluid embolus

Symptoms

- Chills
- Shivering
- Sweating
- Anxiety
- Coughing

Signs

- Cyanosis
- Hypotension
- Bronchospasm
- Tachypnoea
- Tachycardia
- Arrhythmias
- Myocardial infarction
- Seizures
- Disseminated intravascular coagulopathy

Prolapsed umbilical cord (also p 359)

Definition

'Cord presentation' is defined as the presence of the cord between the presenting part and the membranes, prior to membrane rupture. 'Prolapsed umbilical cord' refers to the same situation after membrane rupture. The cord can remain in the vagina (occult prolapse) or can prolapse through the introitus with loops lying outside the vagina **(Figs 44.1 and 44.2)**. It is a true obstetric emergency requiring immediate action.

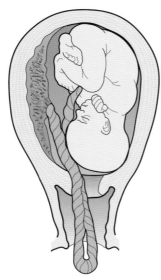

Fig. 44.1 Umbilical cord prolapsing through incompletely dilated cervix. This is due partially to a high presenting part.

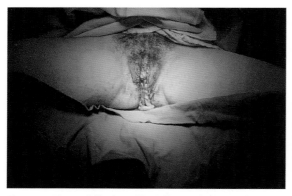

Fig. 44.2 The umbilical cord is visible at the introitus. This fetus requires immediate delivery. (Reprinted from *Picture Tests Obstetrics and Gynaecology*, Rymer J, Fig. 155, p. 78, 1995, by permission of the publisher Churchill Livingstone.)

Epidemiology

The incidence is related to presentation **(Table 44.1)**. Any obstetric condition that precludes a close fit between the fetus and the pelvic inlet makes a cord prolapse more likely, particularly breech presentation, malposition, preterm gestation, polyhydramnios, fetal growth restriction and placenta praevia. Other predisposing factors include a long umbilical cord, artificial rupture of the membranes, and being a second twin.

Clinical features/investigation

There are two main insults to the cord, both of which may lead to cessation of fetal blood flow and fetal death. Firstly there is direct compression by the fetal body against the maternal pelvis and secondly there is likely to be cord spasm from exposure to the cool external atmosphere or excessive handling of the cord.

Cardiotocography (CTG) usually indicates fetal compromise in the form of deep variable decelerations or a single prolonged deceleration **(Fig. 44.3)**.

In some instances the cord is clearly visible protruding through the vagina, but it may be found at a vaginal examination carried out in response to some CTG abnormality. It is important to routinely exclude cord prolapse following artificial rupture of the membranes or in the presence of variable decelerations of acute onset.

Management

It is important to act swiftly, providing the maternal condition is stable. If there is any possibility that a fetal heartbeat is still present, the baby should be delivered immediately. If the cervix is fully dilated, this should be by forceps or ventouse; if not, by immediate caesarean section. General anaesthesia is often required, but a spinal anaesthetic may be used by an experienced anaesthetist in some circumstances.

To protect the cord from occlusion during the transfer to theatre, the woman should be placed in the head-down position and a hand placed in the vagina to lift up the presenting part off the cord and prevent cord compression. An alternative is the knee–chest position **(Fig. 44.4)**. Another reasonable approach is to insert a Foley catheter and fill the maternal bladder with 500 ml fluid. The catheter can be spigotted and this will relieve the pressure on the cord. This

Table 44.1	
Incidence of cord prolapse in relation to presentation	
Presentation	**Incidence**
Vertex	0.4%
Frank breech	0.5%
Flexed breech	4–6%
Footling breech	15–18%

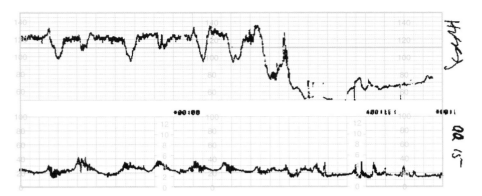

Fig. 44.3 In an occult umbilical cord prolapse the only indication may be CTG abnormalities which should mandate a vaginal examination.

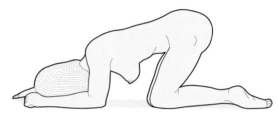

Fig. 44.4 The knee–chest position should be adopted on the way to theatre. Gravity ± an assistant's hand displace the presenting part away from the umbilical cord.

may be a useful approach when transporting the woman from a community setting. The bladder should be emptied before starting caesarean section. The cord should be kept within the vagina and handled as little as possible to avoid spasm. A tocolytic (e.g. terbutaline 0.25 mg s.c. or slow i.v.) should be given to minimize contractions.

If there is doubt as to fetal viability, for instance if the cord has prolapsed at home or silently on the antenatal ward, it is important to establish fetal viability before embarking on unnecessary surgical intervention. The absence of cord pulsation does not necessarily indicate fetal death, particularly if the prolapse is acute, and the fetal heart itself should be visualized directly by ultrasound. If fetal death has occurred, the mother should be allowed to labour and deliver spontaneously.

Prognosis

Fetal mortality has been reduced over the years with the increasing use of caesarean section and improvement in neonatal intensive care, but still remains around 10%.

Retained placenta (also p 280)

Definition

Retained placenta is defined as failure to deliver the placenta within 30 minutes of delivery of the fetus. A retained placenta increases the risk of postpartum haemorrhage by a factor of 10 owing to the inability of the uterus to contract down completely. This risk appears to be maximal at 40 minutes after delivery. Such haemorrhage can be severe and life-threatening, particularly if there has been a partial separation.

Epidemiology

Retained placenta occurs in 2–3% of all vaginal deliveries and is more likely with preterm gestations: if the baby is delivered before 37 weeks, the incidence increases by a factor of three, and if delivered at 26 weeks, the risk is increased by a factor of 20. It is also more common after a previous caesarean section, and rarely this can be associated with a morbidly adherent placenta.

Pathology

During normal childbirth, 90% of placentas are usually delivered within the first 15 minutes. Placental delivery is usually preceded by signs of placental separation, i.e. lengthening of the cord, a sudden small gush of dark blood and increased mobility of the uterus. Failure of the placenta to deliver may occur because of an unusually adherent unseparated placenta, or because the placenta has separated successfully but is retained within the uterus by a partially closed cervix. Failure of separation is much the more worrying of these two situations.

An adherent placenta is the result of abnormal placental implantation during the first trimester. Normally, the invading fetal trophoblast cells are arrested by the maternal decidual barrier, probably by the action of a specific form of leucocyte. If this maternal decidual layer is in some way ineffective, the trophoblast cells may invade further than usual and may extend through the myometrium or even as far as the outer serosal layer. The decidual barrier may be rendered ineffective by a number of factors, and is, for example, often thin and scarred following caesarean section. When over-invasion occurs, the placenta becomes abnormally adherent and is referred to as placenta accreta **(Box 44.4)**.

Table 44.2

Classification of abnormal placental attachment

Type	Incidence	Pathology
Placenta accreta	75–78%	Invades superficially into the myometrium
Placenta increta	17%	Invades deeply into the myometrium
Placenta percreta	5–7%	Invades through the myometrium and penetrates the outer serosal layer of the uterus. It may invade adjacent structures, including bladder and bowel

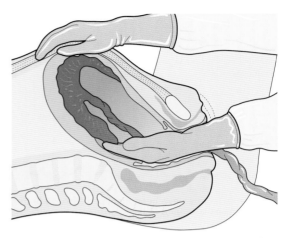

Fig. 44.5 Manual removal of the placenta. A cleavage plane is identified with the fingers, which then continue along the plane until the placenta is fully separated from the uterine wall.

Morbidly adherent placenta is subdivided into three subgroups: placenta accreta, placenta increta and placenta percreta, depending on the depth of invasion (see **Table 44.2**). There is loss of the physiological cleavage plane such that the placenta is unable to separate after delivery of the baby, and partial separation or iatrogenic effort at separation may lead to profound haemorrhage.

A particular problem is the increasing prevalence of mothers who have had previous caesarean sections. If there is a low anterior placenta in a subsequent pregnancy, there will be a significant risk of placenta accreta and subsequent haemorrhage.

Management

If the patient is bleeding heavily, a retained placenta is an obstetric emergency and treatment must be immediate. Aside from the initial resuscitation measures (above) the patient should be transferred to theatre for a manual removal of placenta.

If there is no bleeding, an initial conservative approach can be adopted. Intravenous access should be established and crossmatch arranged in case bleeding begins, and it is reasonable to wait an hour or so for spontaneous expulsion of the placenta to occur. In the interim the use of Syntocinon, the 'rubbing-up' of a contraction, or breastfeeding, with its resultant physiological release of oxytocin, may help to aid expulsion.

If the placenta is still retained after 1 hour, the mother should be transferred to theatre for regional or general anaesthesia. Then, under aseptic conditions, a hand is passed into the uterus through the cervix in order to identify the cleavage plane between the placenta and the uterine wall. During the procedure, the uterine fundus is supported through the abdominal wall using the opposite hand. The placenta can then be gently stripped off the uterine wall and delivered **(Fig. 44.5)**. Once it is out, a contraction should be 'rubbed-up' and a bolus of Syntocinon given i.v. to reduce the risk of postpartum haemorrhage due to an atonic uterus. The procedure must be covered with antibiotics as there is a significant association between manual removal of the placenta and postpartum endometritis.

If the cleavage plane cannot be found and the placenta is so firmly adherent to the uterine wall as to make removal impossible or dangerous (uterine rupture), the clinical diagnosis is 'placenta accreta'. Subsequent management then depends on the degree of haemorrhage. If there is persistent uncontrollable haemorrhage, a hysterectomy is often required. It may be possible to arrest the haemorrhage using tamponade techniques (using either a balloon or packing within the uterine cavity). If there is no active haemorrhage, suction curettage or conservative management are options. With conservative management, when the placenta is left in situ to be absorbed over time, there is a significant incidence of major complications from infection and bleeding.

Shoulder dystocia

Shoulder dystocia is one of the most frightening and threatening obstetric emergencies. There is a need to act quickly in order to prevent serious fetal morbidity and mortality.

Definition

The fetal anterior shoulder becomes impacted behind the symphysis pubis, preventing delivery. Clinically it is defined as difficulty delivering the shoulders requiring obstetric manoeuvres beyond episiotomy and moderate downward traction. Although the incidence overall is around 0.2%, it rises to 0.5% with a fetal weight of over 3.5 kg and 10% with a weight of over 4.5 kg. Shoulder dystocia accounts for 8% of all intrapartum fetal deaths.

Risk factors

Although risk factors have been identified **(Box 44.5)** they have only very limited predictive value. 50% of shoulder dystocia occurs in normal-sized fetuses and 98% of large fetuses do not have dystocia. It is estimated that 3695

Box 44.5

Risk factors for shoulder dystocia

Antepartum

- Macrosomia
- Past history of dystocia
- Diabetes
- Post-dates
- Obese mother
- High parity
- Male fetus

During first stage of labour

- Prolonged first stage
- Secondary arrest >8 cm
- Mid-cavity arrest

During second stage of labour

- Forceps/ventouse delivery
- Difficulty delivering chin

---

elective caesarean sections would have to be performed in non-diabetic mothers with babies estimated to weigh more than 4.5 kg in order to avoid one permanent brachial plexus injury.

Clinical features

The baby's head is often delivered as far as the chin and the fetal body is in the pelvis. The head often retracts tightly against the perineum and vulva – this is called the 'turtle sign' and should raise the possibility of an impending shoulder dystocia.

The umbilical cord is trapped and occluded between the fetal trunk and the maternal pelvis, leading to rapid fetal hypoxia and death. The pH drops by an estimated 0.04 per minute and it therefore takes around 7 minutes for the pH of a previously uncompromised fetus to fall below 7.00. It is estimated that 50% of deaths occur within 5 minutes.

Neonatal morbidity may result from brachial plexus damage due to excessive downward traction of the head during attempts at delivery. It is possible to damage nerve roots at the level of C5–T1, C5–6 (Erb's palsy, **Fig. 44.6**) or C7–T1 (Klumpke's palsy).

While the main concerns for shoulder dystocia relate to the fetus, there may also be maternal complications in the form of genital tract trauma and atonic postpartum haemorrhage. Uterine rupture is rare.

Management

This is an obstetric emergency where seconds count. The aim is to disimpact the anterior shoulder and allow the fetus to be delivered. The mnemonic 'HELPERR' is useful to help the clinician through a set of detailed manoeuvres in a calm logical way. Each manoeuvre is attempted for a maximum of 30 seconds before moving to the next **(Fig. 44.7)**.

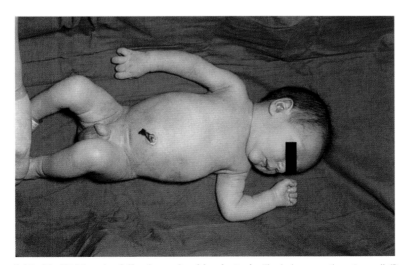

Fig. 44.6 There is a right-sided Erb's palsy following a shoulder dystocia. The baby was otherwise well. (Reprinted from *Picture Tests Obstetrics and Gynaecology*, Rymer J, Fig. 168, p. 85, 1995, by permission of the publisher Churchill Livingstone.)

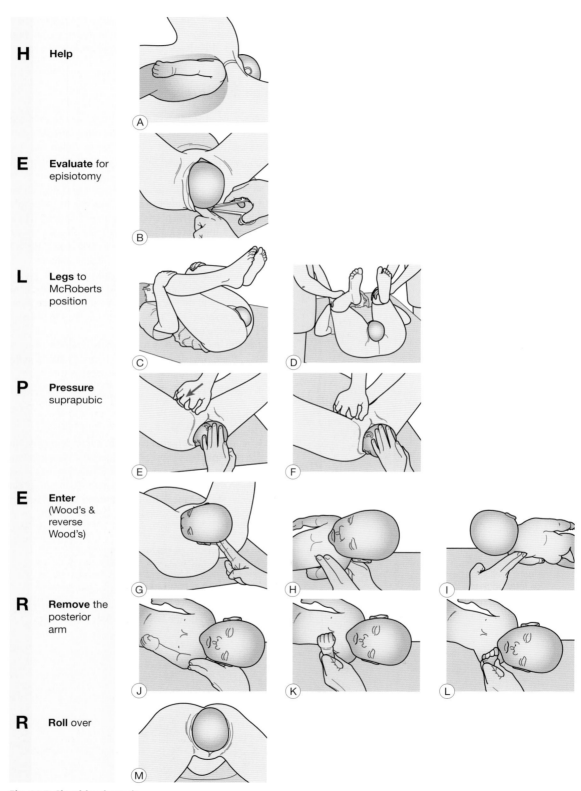

H   Help

E   **Evaluate** for episiotomy

L   **Legs** to McRoberts position

P   **Pressure** suprapubic

E   **Enter** (Wood's & reverse Wood's)

R   **Remove** the posterior arm

R   **Roll** over

Fig. 44.7 **Shoulder dystocia.**

H   As with all obstetrics emergencies the first response is to urgently bleep the emergency team. While waiting, use whatever help is available, including the birth partner.

E   This allows room for imminent internal manoeuvres and reduces the frequency of vaginal lacerations.

L   Known as McRoberts manoeuvre. With one midwife to each leg, the mother's legs are flexed hard against her abdomen and at the same slightly abducted outwards. This straightens the sacrum relative to the lumbar vertebrae and rotates the symphysis towards the maternal head, allowing the baby's shoulder to pass under by continuous traction on its head. This manoeuvre is successful in 40–60% of cases.

    Attempt delivery for 30 seconds before trying next manoeuvre (applies to each new manoeuvre below)

P   With the legs in the McRoberts position, suprapubic pressure is applied to posterior aspect of the anterior fetal shoulder at an angle of 45 degrees towards the fetal chest in an attempt to rotate the shoulder into the oblique and also to reduce the bisacromial diameter (Rubin I manoeuvre). This is used in conjunction with continuing head traction. If constant suprapubic pressure fails, the assistant can try a rocking movement.

E   There are three basic manoeuvres employed during attempts at internal rotation. The attendant's hand enters the vagina at the 5 and 7 o'clock position, depending where the fetal back is. The middle and index fingers are placed on the posterior aspect of the anterior shoulder and an attempt is made to rotate the shoulder forwards (Rubin II manoeuvre). If this fails, those fingers are kept static and the index and middle finger of the other hand are placed on to the anterior aspect of the posterior shoulder (Wood Screw manoeuvre). Both sets of fingers are again used to attempt rotation. If this fails the Reverse Wood Screw manoeuvre is attempted. The fingers on the posterior shoulder are withdrawn completely. The fingers on the anterior shoulder slide down the fetal back to lie against the posterior aspect of the posterior shoulder and rotation is attempted again.

R   The hand of the operator is passed into the hollow of the sacrum, fetal elbow identified, the forearm flexed and then delivered by sweeping it across the fetal chest and face. Fractures of the humerus are not uncommon with this manoeuvre.

R   It is possible to displace the anterior shoulder during the act of turning the mother over into the all fours position. If not, an attempt can be made to deliver the posterior shoulder first, i.e. the shoulder nearest the ceiling. It is possible to try all the above manoeuvres (except suprapubic pressure) again in this new position.

Fig. 44.7—cont'd

If all else fails, there are three 'last resort' measures. These are described in brief:

1. Symphysiotomy: the symphyseal joint is split with a scalpel, thereby increasing the pelvic diameters **(Fig. 44.8)**. Both legs must be supported during the process to prevent excessive abduction of the hips.
2. One or both clavicles of the fetus may be deliberately fractured to reduce the bisacromial distance.
3. The Zavanelli manoeuvre: this involves replacing the head with flexion and rotation, and then delivering by caesarean section. In the largest series to date, out of 59 such procedures 53 were successful. Generally, the fetal outcome is poor, often because this is a manoeuvre of last resort.

Shoulder dystocia remains an extremely serious, unpredictable and relatively rare event. Fetal survival and neurological normality are proportional to the speed of successful resolution.

Uterine inversion

Definition

Uterine inversion is rare, occurring in 1/2000–1/20,000 pregnancies, but as it may quickly lead to maternal death, it is an extremely significant third-stage complication. The uterus may undergo varying degrees of inversion and, in its extreme form, the fundus may pass through the cervix such that the whole uterus is turned completely inside out. As there is a rich vagal supply to the cervix, the inversion leads to profound vasovagal shock, and this may be exacerbated by massive postpartum haemorrhage secondary to uterine atony.

Pathology

Inversion occurs with active management of the third stage, that is to say it is usually iatrogenic, associated with cord traction before the uterus contracts **(Fig. 44.9)**. It is more likely with a fundal placenta and is found in association with the factors listed in **Box 44.6**.

Clinical presentation

With complete inversion, the uterus will appear as a bluish-grey mass protruding from the vagina, and in extreme cases there may also be vaginal eversion. The placenta remains attached in about 50% of cases. If the inversion is partial, the only obvious sign may be that of profound shock out of proportion to any blood loss. The diagnosis will require a vaginal examination although an abnormally shaped uterine fundus on abdominal palpation often suggests the diagnosis. Rarely, the presentation is sudden death following neurogenic shock **(Fig. 44.10)**.

Management

90% of patients will have immediate, potentially major life-threatening haemorrhage. In order to minimize vasovagal-induced shock and also haemorrhage, it is imperative to replace the uterus as quickly as is practicable. Immediate resuscitation is required **(Box 44.1)** and should involve all available obstetric and anaesthetic help. Simultaneous attempts should be made to replace the uterus either within the vagina or possibly back through the cervix if possible. No attempt should be made to separate the placenta, as this may exacerbate the haemorrhage.

One method of reduction is to grasp the uterine fundus with the fingers directed towards the posterior fornix and replace the uterus back into the vagina, pushing the fundus towards the umbilicus and allowing the uterine ligaments to pull the uterus back into position **(Fig. 44.11)**. Alternatively, the centre of the uterus may be indented with three or four fingers and only the centre of the fundus pushed up until it re-inverts. Once re-inversion has occurred, the hand inside the uterus should maintain pressure on the uterine fundus until oxytocics have been given in order to maintain a contracted uterine state and prevent recurrence.

Should these methods fail, O'Sullivan's hydrostatic technique should be employed. This involves passing 2 litres of warmed fluid into the vagina using either a ventouse cup or anaesthetic gas tubing. The resulting vaginal distension, especially at the vault, is extremely effective at allowing the uterus to return to the normal position. Up to 5 litres of fluid may be required to achieve uterine replacement. If successful, the fluid should be allowed to drain and oxytocics given as above.

Should all of these attempts fail, a laparotomy is required to aid re-inversion. An incision may be required at the rim of the inversion **(Fig. 44.12)**. Hysterectomy is an option.

Uterine rupture

Loss of the integrity of the wall of the uterus may occur either suddenly, or more gradually during the progress of labour. The uterine cavity may communicate directly with the peritoneal cavity (a complete uterine rupture; see **Fig. 27.5**) or be separated from the peritoneal cavity by the visceral peritoneum of the uterus (incomplete uterine rupture or uterine dehiscence).

A complete uterine rupture is a life-threatening emergency often resulting in fetal death, and may lead to maternal death from massive intra-abdominal haemorrhage. Early recourse to caesarean section in 'high-risk' parous labours with signs of obstruction is likely to reduce the incidence.

Epidemiology

This obstetric emergency is rare in multiparous women who have had previous vaginal deliveries and virtually unheard of in primigravidae. It does, however, complicate 0.6% of deliveries in those who have had a previous caesarean section, with the rupture occurring at the site of the caesarean section

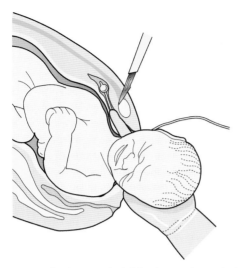

Fig. 44.8 Symphysiotomy. The left forefinger is shown displacing the urethra to the maternal left. A scalpel is positioned above the pubic symphysis and the joint divided anterior to posterior.

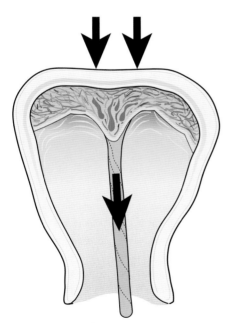

Fig. 44.9 Undue traction on a fundally sited placenta without guarding the uterus may result in uterine inversion.

Box 44.6

Factors associated with uterine inversion

- Previous history
- Fundal placental implantation
- Uterine atony
- Improper management of the third stage

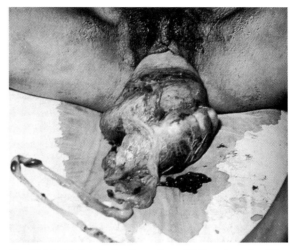

Fig. 44.10 A fatal uterine inversion with the placenta still attached. (Reprinted from *Williams Obstetrics*, Cunningham FG, Wenstrom KD, Gilstrap LC et al, Fig. 32-25, p. 768, 2001, with permission of The McGraw-Hill Companies.)

Pathology

With complete rupture, the fetus may be extruded into the abdominal cavity. As the rupture can extend laterally into the uterine arteries or broad ligament plexus of veins, there is often severe haemorrhage. Rarely, rupture may occur following direct abdominal trauma, for example a road traffic accident.

In caesarean section scar dehiscence, the fetal membranes remain intact. There is usually minimal bleeding and the rupture does not usually involve the entire scar length. Occasionally these are found incidentally at caesarean section carried out for other reasons.

Risk factors

There are many risk factors which increase the risk of uterine rupture **(Box 44.7)**, and most of the intrapartum causes are the consequence of increased force being applied to the uterine muscle.

Clinical features

The most common sign of uterine rupture is that of fetal compromise identified by acute onset of significant CTG changes. This occurs in 70%. Other features include

incision. This risk increases further when oxytocin is used injudiciously. Prostaglandin use is a particular risk and it is assumed that the consequent powerful contractions place a greater strain on the scar. The risk of rupture is increased yet again if the previous caesarean section was 'classical' rather than 'lower segment' (i.e. midline rather than low transverse uterine incision) and up to a third of pregnancies with classical incisions may be complicated by rupture even several weeks before term. Most obstetricians would offer those with a midline scar an early elective caesarean section.

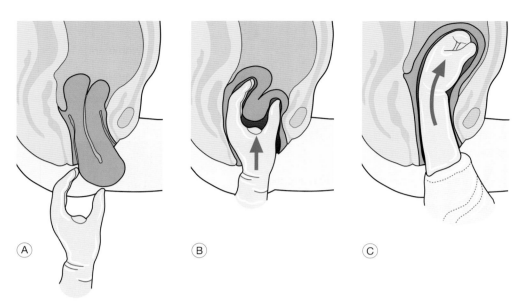

Fig. 44.11 Replacing an inverted uterus. (A) Recognition of uterine inversion. **(B)** Replacement of the uterus through the cervix. **(C)** Restitution of the uterus.

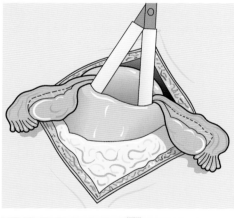

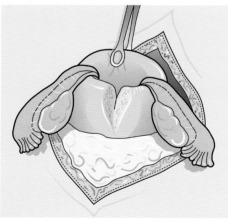

Fig. 44.12 It may be possible to reduce the inversion with division of the involuted rim at laparotomy.

Box 44.7

Risk factors associated with uterine rupture

Antepartum rupture (rare).

- Certain congenital malformations of uterus
- External trauma
- Classical caesarean section
- Previous uterine trauma/surgery
- External cephalic version

Intrapartum rupture

- Previous caesarean (esp. induction)
- Oxytocin in the multiparous mother
- Precipitate delivery
- Obstructed labour
- Operative vaginal delivery
- Shoulder dystocia
- Breech extraction
- Difficult manual removal of placenta (esp. accreta).

---

maternal tachycardia, vaginal bleeding (4%), abdominal pain (8%), and easily palpable fetal parts per abdomen. Occasionally, the fetal head is felt to have risen higher on vaginal examination. Dehiscence or rupture may occasionally be identified at a vaginal examination for postpartum haemorrhage. In severe instances there may be cardiovascular collapse.

Management

If uterine rupture is suspected, the initial drill of summoning immediate help and resuscitation is followed by an immediate emergency laparotomy to deliver the baby. At the time of laparotomy it may be possible to repair the defect, especially if this is simple dehiscence of a previous cae-sarean section scar. If there is massive haemorrhage (more likely if the rupture is complete), or if it does not involve a previous scar, or has led to extension of a scar, an emer-gency hysterectomy is likely to be required. Most cases of incomplete uterine rupture are not identified at the time of the acute rupture and only become apparent at caesarean section for fetal compromise.

Prognosis

With complete rupture and expulsion of the fetus into the abdominal cavity, the perinatal mortality rate approaches 75%. If untreated, most women would die from haemor-rhage and infection.

> **Key** *points*
>
> - Obstetric emergencies are rare and often unfold rap-idly. They are often very frightening for all concerned.
> - It is extremely important to be prepared to act promptly and to know exactly what to do and when to do it.
> - As these emergencies are rare, the labour ward team should participate in regular obstetrical emergency drills training.

Operative delivery

The phrase 'operative delivery' is used to describe both caesarean section and instrumental vaginal delivery. It may be indicated to expedite delivery in the presence of fetal distress, or for 'delay' or failed progress despite good contractions and maternal effort. The choice between caesarean and instrumental delivery depends partly on the stage of labour, with instrumental delivery possible only in the second stage; even then, specific criteria must be met. Caesarean section can be used in both the first and second stages of labour.

Instrumental vaginal delivery

The most common indications for instrumental delivery are presumed fetal distress and second-stage delay. The criteria in **Box 45.1** must be fulfilled before the procedure can be carried out.

Very careful assessment is required prior to instrumental delivery, beginning with abdominal palpation. There should be no head palpable above the symphysis although occasionally one-fifth is palpable in occipitoposterior positions. One of the most difficult parts of an instrumental delivery is being completely certain of the fetal position prior to applying the forceps or ventouse. If there is a suspicion from palpation of the sutures that the fetal head is occipitotransverse, it is often helpful to try to feel for an ear anteriorly under the symphysis pubis. Some obstetricians use transabdominal ultrasound to confirm the position of the fetal head.

Operative vaginal delivery requires a multidisciplinary approach to maximize the likelihood of success and minimize maternal and fetal trauma. In addition to the attending midwife, a practitioner experienced in neonatal resuscitation should be present and the anaesthetist is frequently involved in the provision of adequate analgesia. Umbilical artery and vein acid–base status should be routinely recorded immediately after delivery.

The choice is between forceps and the ventouse.

Forceps delivery

There are three main types of obstetric forceps **(Fig. 45.1)**:

- low-cavity outlet forceps (e.g. Wrigley's – history box), which are short and light, and are used when the head is on the perineum

History

Arthur Wrigley (1902–1983) was born in Lancashire and opposed the use of forceps when the fetal head was high. His own forceps, he said, were designed 'so that it is impossible to exert a tremendous pull'.

- mid-cavity forceps (e.g. Haig Ferguson, Neville–Barnes, Simpson's – history boxes) for use when the sagittal suture is in the anteroposterior plane (usually occipitoanterior)

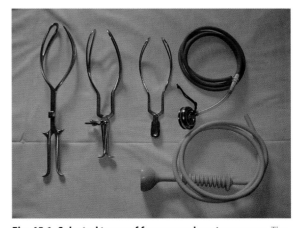

Fig. 45.1 Selected types of forceps and ventouse cups. The forceps, from left to right, are Kielland's, Haig Ferguson's and Wrigley's. The orange tubing is attached to an O'Neill occipitoanterior metal cup, and the blue ventouse is a 'Silc' cup.

Box 45.1

Criteria for instrumental vaginal delivery

- Consent from the mother obtained
- The cervix fully dilated with the membranes ruptured
- The head at spines or below, with no head palpable abdominally
- The position of the head known
- The bladder empty
- Analgesia satisfactory (perineal infiltration and pudendal blocks usually suffice for mid-cavity and ventouse deliveries but spinal or epidural analgesia is required for Kielland's rotational forceps)

History

James Haig Ferguson (1862–1934), from Edinburgh and related to Field Marshall Earl Haig, modified Simpson's forceps by shortening the handle and placing slots to allow the application of traction tapes; this increased fetal head flexion.

History

William Neville (d. 1904) and Robert Barnes (1817–1907), both from England, first displayed their forceps at the Obstetrical Society of London in 1867. The forceps were designed to grasp the moulded fetal head at or above the pelvic brim as an alternative to craniotomy or caesarean section.

History

James Young Simpson (1811–1870), from Edinburgh, had a huge impact on obstetric practice. In addition to his forceps, he introduced chloroform to obstetric anaesthesia (quoting Galen with 'pain is useless to the pained') and developed a forerunner to the ventouse.

■ Kielland's forceps (history box) for rotational delivery to an occipitoanterior or occipitoposterior position. The reduced pelvic curve allows rotation about the axis of the handle.

History

Christian Kielland (1871–1941) was born in Zululand and was of Norwegian descent. His design of straighter forceps permitted head rotation, and he set strict criteria for their use to ensure their safe use.

Low- or mid-cavity non-rotational forceps

The mother should be placed in the lithotomy position with her bottom just over the edge of the bed (the bottom half of the bed often lifts away). Using an aseptic technique, the perineum is cleaned and draped, the bladder emptied, and the vaginal examination findings rechecked. A pudendal block and perineal infiltration are inserted if required, and the forceps assembled discreetly in front of the perineum before application, care being taken to ensure that the pelvic curve will be sitting over the malar aspect of the baby's head, convex towards the baby's face. Traction is applied in conjunction with the uterine contractions and maternal effort, encouraged by the attending midwife. The rest of the technique is shown in **Figure 45.2**.

Rotational forceps

These forceps, known as Kielland's forceps **(Fig. 45.3)**, lack the pelvic curve of non-rotational forceps and can be applied directly to the baby's head, if occipitoposterior, to allow gentle rotation to occipitoanterior. After rotation, delivery is as for the mid-cavity forceps. If the baby's head is occipitotransverse, the blades may be applied directly or the anterior blade applied posteriorly before being 'wandered' past the baby's face to the anterior position **(Fig. 45.4)**. These forceps require considerable skill and may be associated with greater maternal injury than rotational ventouse. They should only be used by experienced obstetricians.

'Manual rotation' of the head is sometimes possible, and it is usual to use the right hand for left occipitotransverse (LOT) positions **(Fig. 45.5)** and the left hand for right occipitotransverse (ROT) positions. The head is grasped transversely and rotated with a pronation movement. Alternatively, it may be possible to achieve purchase on the head using the fingertips in the lambdoid sutures. Some operators prefer to rotate during a contraction to minimize the risk of pushing the head up out of the pelvis. If rotation is successful, it is almost always necessary to hold the new position with one hand while applying non-rotational forceps with the other to prevent the head rotating back again. Delivery with forceps is then completed in the usual way.

Ventouse

Whether to use ventouse or forceps remains an area for debate, but depends to a significant degree on operator experience and familiarity. Ventouse has the theoretical advantage that less pelvic space is required – with forceps the diameter of the presenting part includes both the fetal head and the width of the forceps, whereas with the ventouse it is only the diameter of the head which needs to be delivered.

The use of ventouse compared to forceps is associated with an increased risk of failure, less anaesthesia requirements, less maternal perineal or vaginal trauma, more cephalhaematomas, more retinal haemorrhages, and more low Apgar scores at 5 minutes. No differences between ventouse and forceps deliveries were found in the one study that followed-up mothers and children for 5 years. The use of a soft Silastic cup rather than a metal vacuum extractor cup is associated with more failures but fewer neonatal scalp injuries. Silastic cups are therefore often used for occipitoanterior deliveries and a metal occipitoposterior cup for transverse and posterior malpositions. Disposable cups are available; these produce a vacuum using a hand-powered pump. The same criteria for use apply to ventouse delivery as to forceps **(Box 45.1)**.

The cup should be placed in the midline overlying, or just anterior to, the posterior fontanelle in order to encourage flexion of the head. Failure to correctly position the cup is the commonest reason for ventouse failure. Suction is applied, care being taken to ensure that the vaginal skin is not included under the cup. Traction is also applied downwards as for forceps, but delivery is much more likely to be successful if traction is timed with contractions and maternal effort **(Fig. 45.6)**. The risk of significant fetal injury is increased with the duration of application (p. 403).

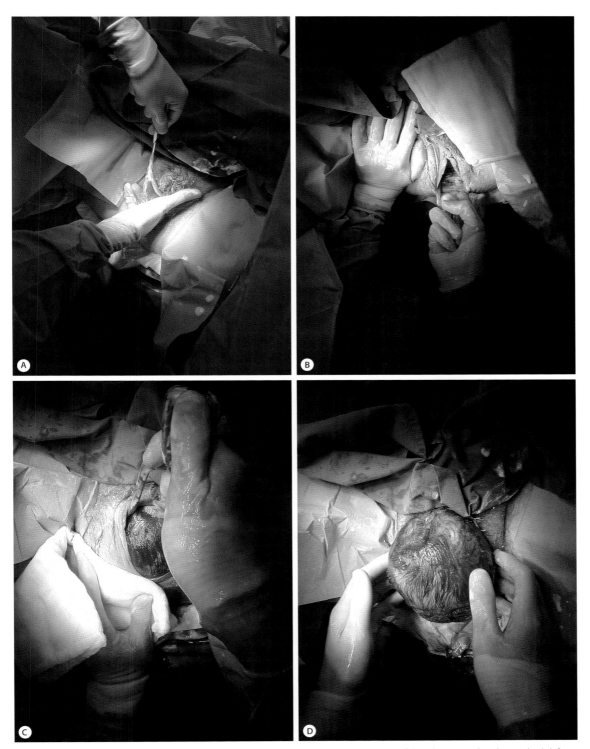

Fig. 45.2 Outlet forceps delivery with Wrigley's forceps. The handle in the operator's left hand is inserted to the mother's left side by placing the right hand into the vagina to prevent injury and slipping the blade between the hand and baby's head between contractions **(A).** Opposite hands are used to insert the right blade, and the blades are locked into position by lowering the handles and allowing articulation to occur gently. Traction is applied by pulling initially downwards at an angle of ≈60° (maternal pelvis to obstetrician's pelvis if the obstetrician is sitting **(B)**), with the direction of traction becoming horizontal and then upwards as the baby's head advances over the perineum **(C).** It is usual to perform an episiotomy as the vulva stretches, but occasionally, as here, this may not be necessary, especially in a parous woman. The forceps are removed after delivery of the baby's head and the remainder of the baby delivered as normal **(D).**

Although it has been suggested that ventouse should not be used at gestations of less than 36 weeks because of the risk of cephalhaematoma and intracranial haemorrhage, a case control study suggests that this restriction may be unnecessary. Nonetheless, caution is probably still required. There is minimal risk of fetal haemorrhage if the extractor is applied after fetal blood sampling or application of a spiral scalp electrode. No significant scalp bleeding was reported in two randomized trials comparing forceps and ventouse. The ventouse is contraindicated with a face presentation.

Forceps delivery before full dilatation of the cervix is contraindicated and ventouse delivery before full dilatation should only be considered in special circumstances and with a very experienced operator.

Caesarean section

Caesarean section (history box) may be:

1. pre-labour – this can be 'electively', for example with placenta praevia, severe fetal growth restriction, severe pre-eclampsia, transverse lie or breech presentations, or as an emergency, for example following a large abruption
2. in labour (i.e. 'emergency'), usually for the reasons listed under 'forceps', if the cervix is not fully dilated or the mother is unsuitable for vaginal delivery.

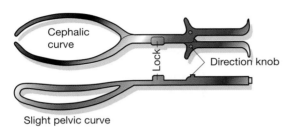

Fig. 45.3 Kielland's forceps for rotational delivery.

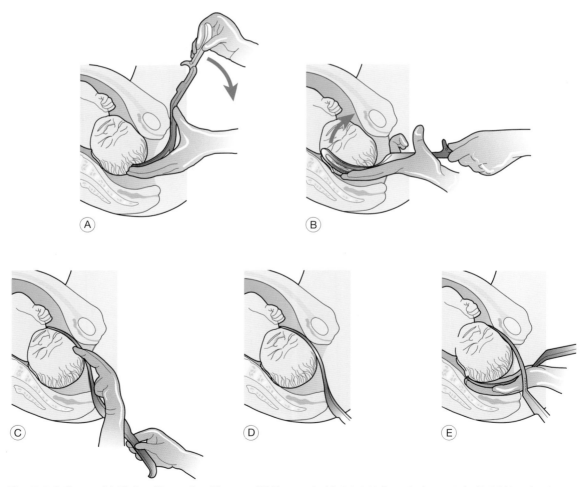

Fig. 45.4 Delivery with Kielland's rotational forceps. (A) The anterior blade is initially applied posteriorly. **(B,C,D)** It is then 'wandered' to the anterior position across the baby's face. **(E)** The posterior blade can then be applied and the baby's head rotated to the occipitoanterior position.

Maternal mortality is higher for emergency caesarean section than for elective. Overall there is also significant morbidity from thromboembolic disease, haemorrhage and infection. Deaths from thromboembolism have been dramatically reduced by the widespread use of appropriate thromboprophylaxis.

Lower uterine segment caesarean section is by far the most commonly used technique and has a lower rate of subsequent uterine rupture, together with better healing and fewer postoperative complications. A 'classical' caesarean section (vertical uterine incision) will provide better access for a transverse lie following ruptured membranes, or with very vascular anterior placenta praevias, very preterm fetuses (particularly after spontaneous rupture of the membranes [SRM]), or large lower-segment fibroids. The chance of scar rupture in subsequent pregnancies following a vertical uterine incision is, however, much greater than with the transverse incision.

Preparation includes obtaining maternal consent, intravenous access, group and save, sodium citrate ± ranitidine (to reduce the incidence of Mendelson's syndrome), appropriate thromboprophylaxis, antibiotic prophylaxis, anaesthesia (spinal, epidural or general), and bladder catheterization. The details of the operation are outlined in **Figure 45.7**.

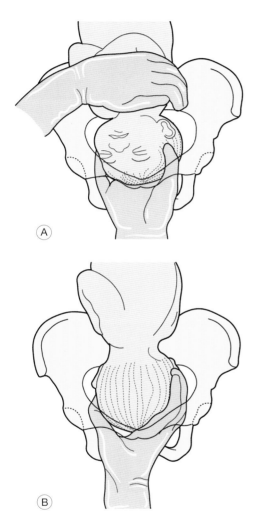

(A)

(B)

Fig. 45.5 Manual rotation from left occipitoposterior (LOP), as in A, to direct occipitoanterior (DOA) position, as in B, using the right hand.

> ### *h* *History*
>
> *Gaius Julius Caesar (100–44 BC). The name 'caesarean section' is probably derived from a Roman legal code called 'Lex Caesarea', which allegedly contained a law prescribing that the baby be cut out of its mother's womb in the case that she dies before giving birth. Caesar himself was not delivered this way.*

Caesarean section on maternal request

Women who have had a previous difficult delivery (e.g. instrumental delivery, shoulder dystocia, poor healing of episiotomy) may occasionally request an elective caesarean section. Although in many cases a more straightforward delivery may be anticipated next time around, careful consideration of the advantages and disadvantages of an elective delivery is required.

In general, women with a previous caesarean section for a non-recurrent indication, e.g. breech, fetal distress or relative cephalopelvic disproportion secondary to fetal malposition, should be offered a trial of labour, but repeat elective caesarean section may be considered.

Some women request an elective caesarean section for a first delivery where there is no obstetric or medical indication. Again, the advantages and disadvantages need careful consideration before an informed decision is reached.

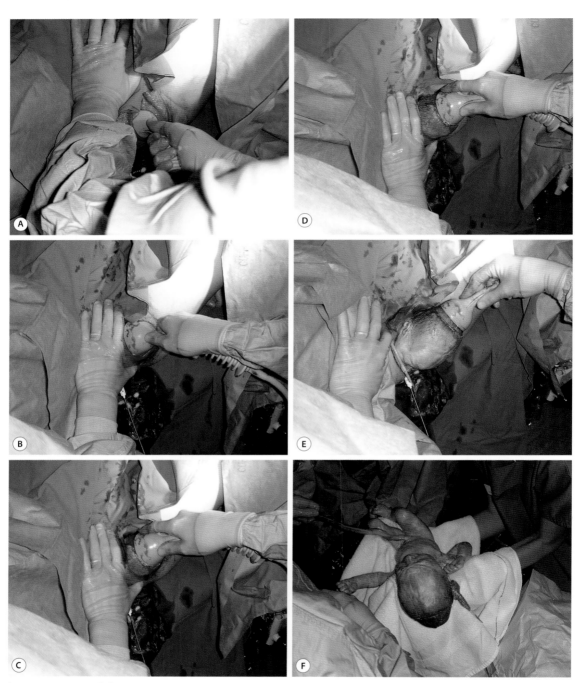

Fig. 45.6 Ventouse delivery. The ventouse cup is applied in the midline overlying, or just anterior to, the posterior fontanelle, care being taken to ensure that the vaginal skin is not included under the cup. Traction is then applied to coincide with maternal effort.

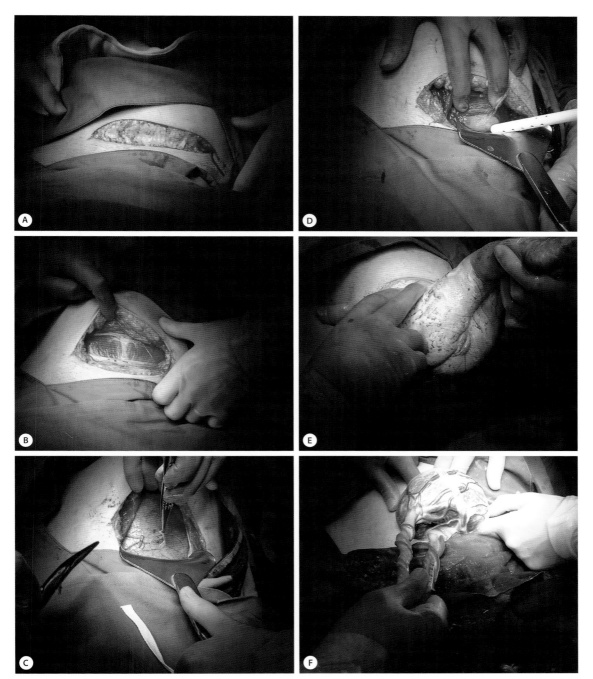

Fig. 45.7 Delivery by caesarean section. The table should be tilted 15° to the left side (to reduce aortocaval compression) and a lower abdominal transverse incision made, cutting through the fat **(A)** and the rectus sheath **(B)** to open the peritoneum. The bladder is freed **(C)** and pushed down, and a transverse lower segment incision is made in the uterus **(D).** If the presentation is cephalic, the head is then encouraged through the incision with firm fundal pressure from the assistant. Wrigley's forceps are occasionally required. If the baby is presenting by the breech, traction is applied to the baby's pelvis by placing a finger behind each flexed hip to deliver the bottom first **(E).** If transverse, a leg should be identified and pulled to deliver the baby (i.e. internal podalic version). After delivery Syntocinon is given intravenously and after uterine contraction the placenta is delivered **(F).**

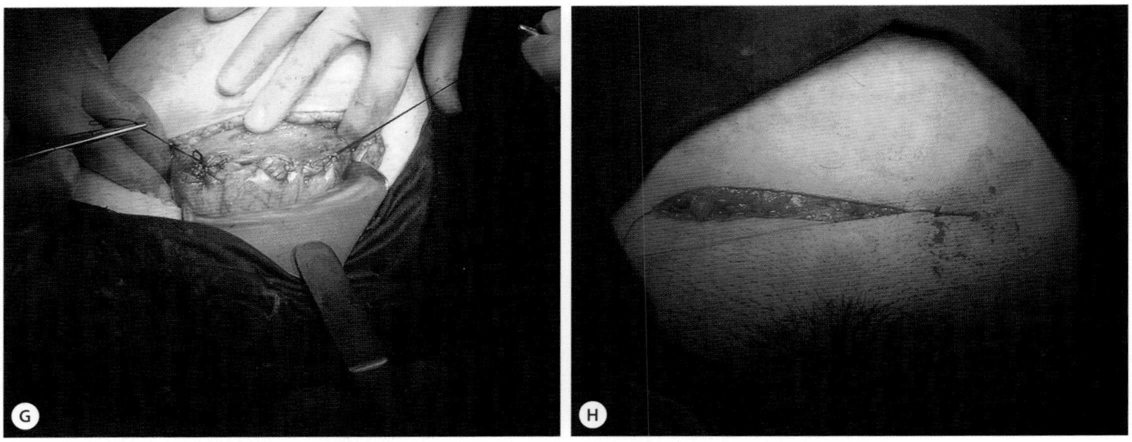

Fig. 45.7—cont'd Haemostasis is obtained with clamps and a check is made to ensure that the uterus is empty and that there are no ovarian cysts. The incision is closed with two layers of dissolving suture to the uterus, one layer to the rectus sheath **(G)** and one layer to the skin **(H).**

Key points

- Forceps may be low-cavity (outlet), mid-cavity or rotational (Kielland's).
- The use of ventouse compared to forceps is associated with less maternal perineal trauma, more cephalhaematomas and more retinal haemorrhages.
- Maternal morbidity is higher for emergency caesarean section than for elective.
- Evidence-based guidelines are available at www.rcog.org.uk and www.nice.org.

46 Stillbirth and neonatal death

Introduction

Loss of a baby at any stage of pregnancy is an extremely distressing event for parents. Among supporting staff, it may also engender feelings from profound sadness to a sense of personal failure. This sudden bereavement is a very challenging aspect of obstetric care through which to guide parents successfully, and this chapter will consider stillbirth and its immediate management.

Neonatal mortality, the loss of a live baby within the first 4 weeks of life, is also extremely tragic. This will also be considered in detail, focusing particularly on the differences between western care and care in less affluent countries.

The definitions of terms used in this chapter are in **Table 46.1**.

Stillbirth

Immediate management of in-utero fetal demise

In the absence of some obvious precipitating event, the diagnosis is often first suspected because of reduced fetal movements. Further suspicions are raised when the fetal heart is not heard with the Pinard stethoscope or Doppler probe, and the diagnosis of fetal death is usually confirmed by ultrasound scan. It is worth taking a short time to exclude any obvious fetal abnormality on the scan in case postmortem examination is declined, but, in reality, time is limited by the pressure to break the news. There is no easy way to do this, but it is essential to allow the parents to control the pace of subsequent events. The temptation to deliver a long speech on further management should be resisted until they are ready to begin asking the questions. The parents may need to be alone for a short time, and a room should be organized for them, ideally well away from the noise of a ward or clinic.

Labour will need to be induced. The technique is much the same as for any labour induction, although there is probably a useful role for 48 hours of pre-labour preparation with mifepristone. Some parents may not want this delay, while others may value a day or two at home before having to undergo such a physically and emotionally draining event.

All appropriate analgesia should be offered and experienced supportive midwifery care is vital. In general it is preferable to delay membrane rupture as long as reasonably possible, as the risk of chorioamnionitis is probably increased in comparison to live births. After delivery, the parents should be encouraged to see and hold their baby. This is a very impressionable time for the couple **(Box 46.1)**. Parents often find it useful to have photographs of the baby, as well as hand-prints, foot-prints and a lock of the baby's hair.

Some hospitals have a bereavement counsellor, whose role it is to explain the legal requirement of registration and discuss funeral arrangements, and some units are fortunate enough to have counsellors who will follow-up the parents at home. Most hospitals, however, do not. It is essential that the general practitioner and community midwife are informed before the woman is discharged from hospital. The couple should also be provided with a booklet containing information on, and contact numbers for, any local support groups, for example SANDS – the Stillbirth and Neonatal Death Society.

Investigation

All parents will ask the question 'why?' and most will want a full range of investigations to be carried out in order to establish both diagnosis and prognosis.

Maternal blood tests should be sent to look for:

■ Evidence of congenital infection with toxoplasmosis, rubella, cytomegalovirus or human parvovirus.
■ Lupus anticoagulant and antiphospholipid antibodies. These are associated with recurrent miscarriage, stillbirth, arterial and venous thrombosis, fetal growth restriction, pre-eclampsia and thrombocytopenia. There is now evidence that giving low-dose aspirin throughout pregnancy increases the incidence of live births.

Table 46.1

Definitions

Stillbirth	Any fetus born with no signs of life, after 24 weeks of gestation
Early neonatal death	Death in the first 6 days of life
Late neonatal death	Deaths from age 7 days to 27 completed days of life
Perinatal deaths	All stillbirths, plus deaths in the first week of life
Perinatal mortality rate (PNMR)	The number of perinatal deaths per thousand live and stillbirths
Post-neonatal death	Deaths at and beyond 28 days, but under 1 year
Infant death	Deaths at age under 1 year

- Diabetes, either with a random blood glucose or HbA_{1c}.
- Fetomaternal haemorrhage, with a Kleihauer test.
- Isoimmunization, either rhesus or non-rhesus.

A postmortem examination is extremely important. It is very rare for parents to regret this being carried out and it is not possible to have a useful postmortem at some later stage if the parents change their minds. The request must be handled as delicately as possible, and if the parents decline, it may be worth offering a more restricted postmortem, biopsies or radiological investigations.

The postmortem will include measurements of the baby's length and weight, and a detailed external inspection, particularly of the limbs and face. A systematic internal examination is then carried out to look for any malformations of the viscera, limbs or genitalia. Genetic advice may be sought and a karyotype is often checked using samples of skin or blood. Histology is usually carried out on significant organs, and X-rays taken if there is a suspicion of a skeletal dysplasia.

Placental examination, both macro- and microscopic, can provide useful information as to the cause of death. There may be a retroplacental clot indicating a placental abruption, or the aberrant vascular supply of vasa praevia. Atheromatous deposits throughout the placenta may be indicative of poor placentation and may explain fetal growth restriction or hypoxia as a cause of death.

Photographs are usually taken throughout as a record of any abnormality.

Causes of stillbirth

Rates in many western countries fell over the last half of the 20th century to a level around 6/1000 births, probably because of improved overall maternal health, better nutrition and wider education. An important, though probably lesser, contribution has been associated with improved obstetric care. Over the last decade, only minimal further progress

Box 46.1

A mother's story

When a child dies you can't, as with other deaths, adapt. You can't dismantle the connection you shared and eventually come to accept the world without them. For me, my child will always exist. Not because I dwell on his death, but because I was – I still am – his mother.

We already had one healthy son. When I found out I was pregnant for the second time, I was thrilled. I'd somehow imagined that I wouldn't have enough love for another child but it turns out that, where children are concerned, we do. On some deep level I trusted my body to bring this child into being – it was just a case of counting down the months. But then he ran into very serious problems. Sitting in the specialist's waiting room I looked at the walls covered with letters of thanks, photos of tiny babies that this man had saved. 'Maybe,' I thought, 'just maybe.'

'I'm sorry,' he said, 'I don't think he's going to make it.' A million moments pass us all the time – minutes of no import, filled with the ordinary everyday. And then one comes along and, on that pinprick of time, you trip and tumble. Then you fall and fall, because there is no floor. I know I wanted to give way, to allow the pain to become real. But I just froze. The baby was still in me, dying instead of growing. Things would have to happen – dreadful things – and I shut down. I lay for two days, waiting for him to die. Outside it was a blazing summer day, but we closed the curtains. On the Sunday morning I knew it was over. I didn't say at first, I needed time to absorb it. At lunchtime I told my husband 'I know he has died.'

The prospect of going through labour seemed macabre. Finally after 7 hours he arrived. How else can I describe it? He wasn't born, he was just there, silent and still, not breathing. I wanted to scream out 'Open your eyes!' But there was none of that and it just felt so wrong. His still-warm weight on me; knowing that those moments were all we had.

The despair that followed was deeper than I could ever have imagined. I came home without my baby, empty armed – and everything felt wrong. Upturned. When an adult dies there is a space in the house, but we hadn't even prepared the nursery. 'Keep talking,' we were advised, and we did. But what was there to talk about? Our son, after all, had no history; we'd made no memories with him. But we had had that love for him, the portion of love we'd set especially aside for our son. When I got pregnant again, the 9 months were nightmarish, charged with the fear that we'd lose this one too. When they handed him too me, he let out a cry and it was the most wonderful thing I have ever heard.

We're through it. It's not behind us, but it's with us. We have made it part of our lives, because he is part of our lives.

has been made, and the level now sits at 5.5/1000 births. More research is required to identify causes of stillbirth if we are to reduce this rate any further.

The obstetrical classification of stillbirths is summarized in **Table 46.2**. Congenital anomaly and the much larger 'unexplained' stillbirth categories are considered below. For antepartum haemorrhage, hypertension, medical disorders and isoimmunization, see relevant chapters.

Congenital abnormalities (see also p. 263)

These may or may not have been diagnosed antenatally **(Table 46.3)**. Despite antenatal screening for structural defects, many cardiovascular conditions remain unrecognized.

Table 46.2		
Obstetrical classification of stillbirth – Scottish figures 2006		
Classification	**Notes**	**Frequency**
Unexplained <2500 g	Often associated with prematurity	40%
Unexplained ≥2500 g		27%
Antepartum haemorrhage	Abruption and placenta praevia	11%
Congenital anomaly	Any structural, genetic or biochemical cause	11%
Hypertension of pregnancy		4%
Maternal disorder	e.g. maternal trauma, diabetes, surgery	4%
Trauma/ mechanical	e.g. uterine rupture, birth trauma, cord prolapse	3%
Miscellaneous		1%
Isoimmunization	Rhesus or non-rhesus	0%

Detailed ultrasound views of the heart can be difficult to assess with repeatable accuracy, and cardiac abnormalities make up the largest group of lethal congenital anomalies.

The incidence of neural tube defects (NTDs) among neonates seems to be falling. This can in part be explained by an increased number of earlier terminations following antenatal diagnosis with ultrasound, but there is probably a background reduction that is independent of this. As there is now good evidence that daily folic acid in the first weeks of pregnancy also reduces the incidence of NTDs, an argument can be put forward for routine supplementation of commonly eaten foodstuffs, for example bread or cereals.

Unexplained stillbirth

It is frustrating and disappointing that this group still accounts for so many stillbirths, and it remains difficult to know how to move forward in reducing the number. Whether a cause has been identified or not, all those who have lost a baby should be offered a follow-up appointment.

Follow-up and subsequent pregnancy

The appointment should be in a suitable clinic some 4–8 weeks after the delivery, depending on when any results are expected to be available. This enables the obstetrician to discuss all the factors involved, provide information on likely recurrence, and consider the appropriateness of any antenatal testing in a future pregnancy.

The consultation can be difficult, particularly in the 'unexplained' group. The chance of unexplained stillbirth in a subsequent pregnancy is low, probably less than 5%, and the couple should be reassured about this. In the absence of any identifiable cause, however, it is difficult to monitor

for problems. Screening for chromosomal abnormalities and carrying out an ultrasound scan for structural abnormality may provide reassurance, but it is likely that both of these would have been normal with the pregnancy that was lost. More frequent antenatal visits may also provide reassurance, particularly with growth scans every few weeks from 24 weeks onwards. It would also be relevant to check the liquor volume and umbilical artery Doppler flow as pregnancy advances.

Throughout, it is important to offer easy access to professional advice and support at times of anxiety, particularly if there are worries about fetal movements. There should be an easy point of contact at any time if problems do occur.

By 38–39 weeks, many couples will be extremely anxious, and are often keen to have labour induced. Induction carries the risks of fetal distress and hyperstimulation, and conservative management carries the risk, albeit small, of further in-utero demise. The pros and cons of these two should be discussed with the couple and an informed decision reached. Induction at this stage would not be an unreasonable course of action to minimize parental anxiety.

Neonatal mortality

Neonatal mortality is the loss of a live-born baby within the first 4 weeks of life. Perinatal mortality is the sum of stillbirths and early neonatal mortality (within the first 7 days from birth).

Western causes of neonatal mortality

These are outlined in **Figure 46.1**. Although only about 8% of babies are born prematurely, this group contains almost 80% of the perinatal deaths. The causes of death amongst this group are varied, but the majority are from:

- respiratory distress syndrome secondary to lung immaturity
- neonatal infection.

Advances in neonatal care have improved the survival of many premature infants, but particularly with the development of improved ventilation techniques and exogenous surfactant administration, it is now accepted practice to resuscitate babies at even earlier gestations than in the past. Survival below 24 weeks, however, is very rare **(Table 46.4)**.

Epidemiologists associate perinatal mortality with three factors: maternal age, parity and socioeconomic class. Although they are considered separately here, this is not so in practice. For example, higher parity is usually associated with increase in maternal age.

Maternal age

The safest time to have children has traditionally been between 25 and 29 years. The highest rates of neonatal mortality are in babies born to women under the age of 20

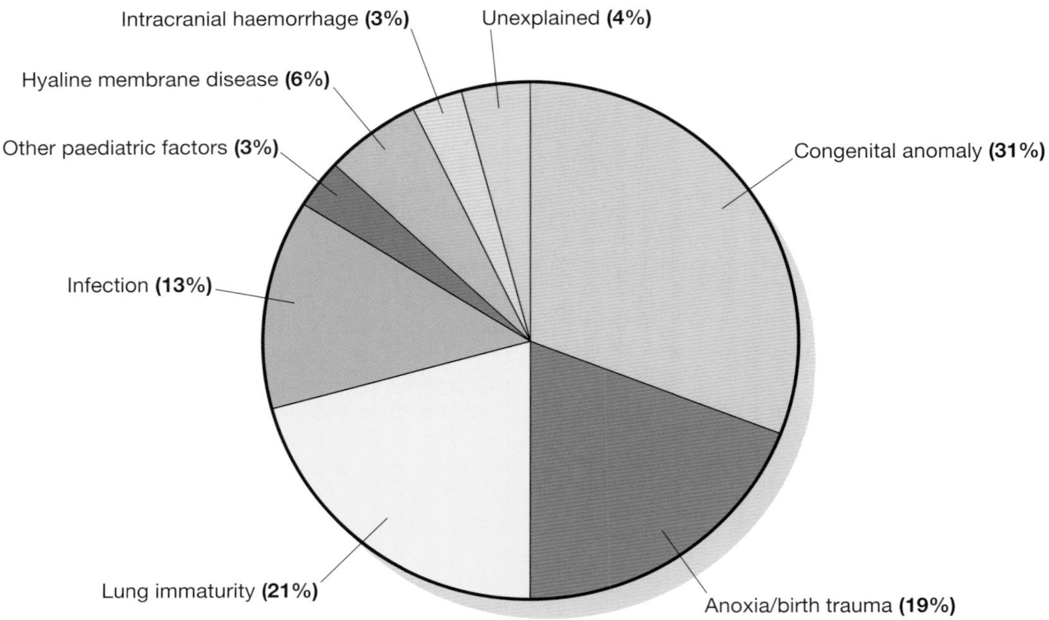

Fig. 46.1 Paediatric classification of neonatal deaths – Scottish figures 2006. The overall rate is 3.1/1000 live births.

Table 46.3		
Examples of potentially lethal congenital anomalies by system		
System	**Examples**	**Diagnosis**
CNS	Anencephaly	Ultrasound scan
Cardiovascular	Ventricular hypoplasia, valvular incompetence and arrhythmias	Ultrasound scan
Renal	Infantile polycystic kidney disease, posterior urethral valves, Potter syndrome	Ultrasound scan
Alimentary	Diaphragmatic hernia	Ultrasound scan
Chromosomal	Turner syndrome (45 XO), Down syndrome (47 +21), Edwards syndrome (47 +18) and Patau syndrome (47 +13)	While around two-thirds of fetuses with Down syndrome will look normal at 18 weeks, most of those with Edwards or Patau syndrome do show some abnormality, even though these are often not specific or diagnostic. An amniocentesis is therefore required to establish the diagnosis with certainty. (For screening, see p. 266)
Respiratory	Pulmonary hypoplasia (e.g. following very early preterm rupture of the membranes or Potter syndrome)	Ultrasound scan
Skeletal	Thanatophoric dysplasia, achondrogenesis, osteogenesis imperfecta type II	Ultrasound scan
Multiple abnormalities	• Cystic hygroma (particularly if associated with aneuploidy) • VATER association – this refers to a condition in which there are Vertebral, Anal, Tracheal, Esophageal and Renal lesions (Also extended to VACTERL by adding Cardiac and Limb abnormalities)	Ultrasound scan

Table 46.4	
Approximate neonatal mortality/1000 live births for western countries by gestation	
Gestation	**Neonatal mortality/1000 live births (approx.)**
24 weeks	420
28 weeks	80
32 weeks	20
36 weeks	3

Box 46.2
The 'two-thirds rule' of global infant mortality rates (this rule applies only to the world average)
■ More than seven million infants die each year between birth and 12 months
■ Almost two-thirds of infant deaths occur in the first month of life
■ Among those who die in the first month of life, about two-thirds die in the first week of life
■ Among those who die within the first week, two-thirds die in the first 24 hours of life

and over the age of 35. These increases at the extremes of reproductive life are due to:

■ the higher incidence of medical conditions and higher parity in women over 35
■ the lack of antenatal care and support that often occurs in women under the age of 20.

Parity

The safest pregnancies appear to be the second and third. First pregnancies are associated with a higher incidence of problems such as proteinuric hypertension and obstructed labour. As mentioned above, higher parity is often a reflection of increasing maternal age, and medical complications are more common.

Social class

There is a steady increase in neonatal mortality as social class falls.

Other factors

■ Reproductive history. The risk of a perinatal death is increased if the previous pregnancy ended in premature birth, miscarriage or perinatal death.
■ Ethnic factors are also important and are in themselves multifactorial. Some women from ethnic minorities may experience communication problems, may have had inadequate antenatal care, may be at increased risk because of consanguinity and are more likely to decline termination of a diagnosed lethal anomaly.

Perinatal mortality meetings

Most obstetric units hold regular perinatal mortality meetings. They are usually attended by all those involved in perinatal care and allow a multidisciplinary approach to the case review. In addition to striving for an accurate diagnosis, the meeting also addresses ways in which such a death may be prevented in the future. Providing this learning process is conducted in a non-judgemental atmosphere, it can be an extremely useful learning exercise for all concerned.

Comparison of perinatal mortality rates (PNMR) in different areas

International comparisons of PNMR can be misleading. For example:

■ Different countries have minor variations in the definition and therefore differences in inclusion criteria.
■ Countries such as Sweden have a more homogeneous population with an overall higher social class.
■ There may be different reproductive patterns – for example in China, where many couples have only one baby.
■ There may be differing rates of fetal abnormality, for example the UK has a high incidence of neural tube defects.
■ Differences can also be seen within a country. In the UK, again as an example, there is a tendency for the perinatal mortality rate to be lowest in the south-east and to increase towards the north-west. This trend runs in parallel with the proportion of lower social classes, which follows a similar distribution. In the lower social classes there is an increased incidence of low-birth-weight babies and congenital anomalies.

Worldwide perspective

Gathering information on perinatal morbidity and mortality in developing countries presents an exceptional challenge. The recording of statistics can be difficult due to geography, illiteracy, the high number of home births and because of the social acceptance of the death of a baby. As with maternal mortality, reduction in child mortality has been highlighted as one of the Millennium Development Goals (2000). This goal is aimed at all children under 5 years of age, of whom 10 million die each year. 8 million of these children die before their first birthday, so perinatal mortality figures and interventions to reduce perinatal mortality are attracting increasing attention.

The World Health Organization (WHO) estimates that 98% of perinatal deaths occur in under-resourced countries: every year, 3.3 million babies are stillborn, 3 million die in the first week of life and a further 1 million die before they are 4 weeks old **(Box 46.2)**. Of the stillborn babies, one third of deaths are probably due to intrapartum events and are potentially avoidable if prompt, good-quality obstetric care is available. It is a matter of concern that half of the world's women still give birth in their own home with no skilled birth attendant.

The highest rates of perinatal mortality are found in Africa, at 62 per 1000 total births, leading to nearly 2 million perinatal deaths a year. The worst affected parts of the continent are Middle and West Africa, where perinatal mortality rates in some countries are so high that over 1 in 10 babies are either stillborn or die within the first week of life **(Fig. 46.2)**.

Although the rate of perinatal mortality in Asia is lower, at 50/1000 total births, the higher population there means that its burden of perinatal deaths is far higher than that of Africa, with over 4 million deaths per year.

Interventions to reduce these numbers need not be complicated. Improved maternal nutrition, antenatal care and particularly availability of trained birth attendants can be of great benefit. Anecdotal evidence from WHO observers describes an incident in rural Sudan: a cyanotic, apnoeic newborn with a pulse was set aside to establish breathing on her own with no input from the birth attendants. The observers stepped in after 2 minutes, easily and successfully reviving the infant with stimulation and positive pressure ventilation. They were told that the baby would have been considered stillborn if she had died. In a rural part of India, where basic neonatal resuscitation techniques were taught to traditional birth attendants, the recorded stillbirth rate decreased from 18.6% to 9% over a 3-year period.

Global causes of neonatal deaths

Determining why newborns die in developing countries is difficult because most deaths occur at home, and families are often reluctant to seek outside help for a variety of sociocultural, logistical and economic reasons **(Fig. 46.3)**. The data, however, point to four main causes of neonatal death:

1. infection (tetanus, sepsis, pneumonia, diarrhoea)
2. complications during delivery (leading to birth asphyxia and birth injuries)
3. complications of prematurity
4. congenital anomalies.

Infections

Every year, an estimated 30 million newborns acquire a neonatal infection, and between one and two million of those infected die. The most common of these infections lead to neonatal tetanus, sepsis, pneumonia and diarrhoea, which together account for around 30% of neonatal deaths. Where hygiene is poor, newborns may become infected with bacteria leading to serious infections in the skin, umbilical cord, lungs, gastrointestinal tract, brain or blood.

Neonatal tetanus has been eliminated today in over 100 countries through immunizing mothers with tetanus toxoid, ensuring clean delivery practices, and maintaining clean care of the umbilical cord stump. Early and exclusive breastfeeding also contributes to reduced neonatal mortality from infections. Tetanus toxoid is one of the cheapest, safest, and most effective vaccines. It costs about US$1.20 – a sum that includes the purchase and delivery costs of three doses of vaccine. Three doses of tetanus toxoid ensure 10–15 years' protection for a woman and immunity for her newborns during the critical first 2 months of life. Five doses ensure a lifetime of protection for the mother, yet only around

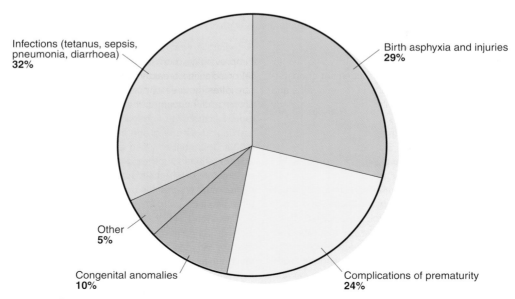

Infections (tetanus, sepsis, pneumonia, diarrhoea)
32%

Birth asphyxia and injuries
29%

Other
5%

Congenital anomalies
10%

Complications of prematurity
24%

Fig. 46.2 Neonatal mortality rate per 1000 live births in 2000.

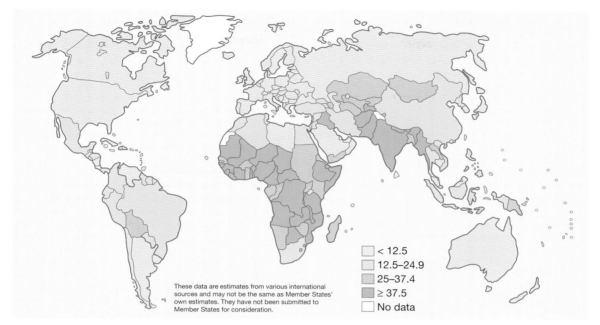

These data are estimates from various international sources and may not be the same as Member States' own estimates. They have not been submitted to Member States for consideration.

< 12.5
12.5–24.9
25–37.4
≥ 37.5
No data

Fig. 46.3 Global incidence of neonatal deaths (WHO) –1999. The overall rate is 31/1000 live births.

50% of pregnant women in developing countries are fully immunized.

Malaria is also associated with an increased risk of spontaneous miscarriage and stillbirths and is linked with maternal anaemia. These complications can be reduced by providing antimalarial treatment and iron supplements antenatally. Use of bed-nets impregnated with insecticide has also been proven to be effective in preventing malaria.

Complications during delivery

The WHO estimates that between four and nine million newborns suffer birth asphyxia each year. Of these, an estimated 1.2 million die and at least the same number develop severe consequences such as cerebral palsy and mental impairment. Prompt detection and management of obstetric complications could prevent many of these deaths and disabilities. Disabilities, in particular, can stretch already scarce resources for poor families.

Historically, skilled care at delivery has been associated with lower neonatal death rates. Skilled attendants at birth must be able to manage normal deliveries, and diagnose and manage, or refer, complicated cases. On average, around 60% of births occur in the home and only 50% of all births are attended by a health worker with appropriate skills. In other words, 53 million women each year give birth without the help of a trained professional. In some countries the incidence of skilled care at deliveries is much lower; 2% in Somalia, for example, and 9% in Nepal. Even in those cases where skilled healthcare is available, ongoing training and supervision of personnel and quality referral care for obstetric emergencies must be ensured.

Complications of prematurity

There is some evidence that the incidence of premature labour becomes less with improved maternal health.

Congenital anomalies

Congenital anomalies are the fourth most common cause of newborn deaths, a category that includes neural tube defects, cretinism, and congenital rubella syndrome. Cretinism can be avoided by providing mothers with adequate iodine, and congenital rubella syndrome can be prevented by immunizing mothers against rubella.

Cost-effective solutions

If improving newborn health were a matter of making medical or scientific breakthroughs, building expensive healthcare infrastructures, or purchasing expensive high-tech ventilators and incubators, then the reluctance to take up the cause of newborns might be more understandable. But it is not. Experience in developed nations has shown that neonatal and perinatal mortality rates fell most dramatically long before neonatal intensive care units came into existence, thanks to relatively simple, low-cost interventions such as better maternal and obstetric care, better routine newborn care, and the introduction of antibiotics **(Box 46.3)**.

Low-cost, proven interventions, such as the teaching of birth attendants in rural India described above, can be carried out entirely within the framework of existing maternal and child health programmes. Current reviews indicate that essential care during pregnancy, childbirth, and the newborn period costs an estimated US$3 a year per capita in low-income countries.

Box 46.3

Potential developments to improve perinatal care

Care during pregnancy

- Improve the nutrition of pregnant women
- Immunize against tetanus
- Screen and treat infections, especially syphilis and malaria
- Improve communication and counselling: birth preparedness, awareness of danger signs, and immediate and exclusive breastfeeding
- Monitor and treat pregnancy complications, such as anaemia, pre-eclampsia, and bleeding
- Promote voluntary counselling and testing for HIV
- Reduce the risk of mother-to-child transmission of HIV

Care at time of birth

- Ensure skilled care at delivery
- Provide for clean delivery: clean hands, clean delivery surface, clean cord cutting, tying and stump care, and clean clothes
- Keep the newborn warm: dry and wrap baby immediately, including head cover, or put skin-to-skin with mother and cover
- Initiate exclusive breastfeeding within the first hour
- Give prophylactic eye care, as appropriate

Key points

- The loss of a baby at any stage of pregnancy is an extremely distressing event for parents.
- A stillbirth may occur for a large number of reasons, including antepartum haemorrhage, congenital anomaly or hypertensive disorders of pregnancy. The majority, however, are unexplained.
- In western countries, the majority of neonatal deaths occur in association with prematurity. Worldwide, infection and birth injury are more common than the complications of preterm birth.

47

Neonatal resuscitation

Physiology

Clamping of the cord after delivery, leads to acute hypoxia. The latter is thought to be the major stimulant for a baby to start breathing. Physical stimuli such as cold air, rubbing, or physical discomfort may also provoke respiratory efforts. If the baby fails to start breathing, the baby's oxygen concentration falls further, the baby loses consciousness and enters 'primary apnoea'.

After 5–10 minutes of primary apnoea, spinal centres, which are normally suppressed by higher centres, begin to cause shuddering of the baby's body at a rate of approximately 12 per minute (agonal gasps). Once this gasping stops, the baby enters 'secondary' (or 'terminal') apnoea and without intervention the outcome is death.

The only way to tell whether a non-breathing newborn infant is in primary or secondary apnoea is by assessment of its response to resuscitation. If in primary apnoea, nearly all will start breathing within a few breaths; if secondary, the baby will usually gasp for some time before starting regular respiration. In reality, however, both are initially managed in the same way.

Practical aspects of neonatal resuscitation

Most babies born in primary apnoea will resuscitate themselves within 60–90 seconds given a clear airway. The basic approach to all resuscitation is therefore airway, breathing and circulation, but there are a number of additions which will be considered in more detail (Box 47.1).

Dry, wrap and keep the baby warm

Dry the baby immediately and then wrap in a warm dry towel. A naked, wet baby can still become hypothermic despite a warm room, especially if there is a draught. Cold babies have an increased oxygen consumption and are more likely to become hypoglycaemic and acidotic. They also have an increased mortality. If this is not addressed at the beginning of resuscitation, it is often forgotten. Most of the heat loss is by evaporation – hence the need to dry the baby and then to wrap the baby in a dry towel. Babies also have a large surface area-to-weight ratio: heat can be lost very quickly (Box 48.1).

Assessment

The Apgar score was proposed as a tool for evaluating a baby's condition at birth. Although the score, calculated at 1 and 5 minutes, may be of some use retrospectively, it is usually recorded subjectively (Table 47.1).

Acute assessment will categorize the baby into one of the three following colour groups:

- Pink, regular respirations, heart rate fast (>100 bpm). These are healthy babies and they should be kept warm and given to their mothers.
- Blue, irregular or inadequate respirations, heart rate slow (<100 bpm). If gentle stimulation does not induce effective breathing, the airway should be opened. If the baby responds, no further resuscitation is needed. If not, progress to lung inflation.
- Blue or white, apnoeic, heart rate slow (<60 bpm). Whether an apnoeic baby is in primary or secondary apnoea, the initial management is the same:

Open the airway, and look to see whether the chest is rising or falling. A reassessment of any heart rate response then directs further resuscitation. Reassess heart rate and respiration at regular intervals throughout, e.g. every 30 seconds. Depending upon the assessment, resuscitation follows: airway, breathing and circulation, with the use of drugs in a few severe cases.

Airway

Position the baby with the head in the neutral position (i.e. the face is parallel to the ceiling). Overextension may collapse the newborn baby's pharyngeal airway just as will flexion (Fig. 47.1).

A folded towel placed under the neck and shoulders may help to maintain the airway in a neutral position and a jaw thrust may be needed to bring the tongue forward and open the airway, especially if the baby is floppy. Suction of the airways with a soft catheter should only be carried out under direct vision of the cords.

Meconium-stained liquor in various guises is relatively common. Fortunately, though, meconium aspiration is a rare event and often occurs in utero before delivery. If the baby is vigorous, no specific action (other than drying and wrapping the baby) is needed. If the baby is not vigorous, inspect the oropharynx with a laryngoscope and aspirate any particulate meconium seen using a soft catheter.

Box 47.1

Neonatal resuscitation

- Get help
- Start the clock
- Dry, wrap and keep the baby warm
- Assess colour, tone, respirations and heart rate
- Commence resuscitation:
  - Airway
  - Breathing (lung inflation and ventilation)
  - Circulation
  - Drugs

History

Virginia Apgar (1909–1974), from New York City, was an anaesthetist who devised this system of early neonatal evaluation.

Table 47.1

The Apgar scoring system

Feature	Score		
	0	1	2
Colour	White	Blue	Pink
Tone	None	Poor	Good
Heart rate	<60 bpm	60-100 bpm	>100 bpm
Respiration	None	Gasping	Vigorous
Response to simulation	None	Minimal	Vigorous

If the baby is not breathing and you have the skill, intubate the baby with an endotracheal tube (ideally with a meconium aspirator attached) and use this to suck out the trachea. If you are unable to intubate, call for assistance from someone who has the skill. While waiting for them to arrive, suck out the oropharynx with a wide-bore suction catheter, as above, and then provide intermittent positive pressure ventilation.

Breathing

The first five breaths should be inflation breaths. These should be 2- to 3-second sustained breaths using a continuous gas supply, a pressure-limiting device, and a mask. If no such system is available, a 500 ml self-inflating bag and a blow-off valve set at 30–40 cm H_2O pressure can be used. Use a transparent, soft, reformable mask big enough to cover the nose and mouth of the baby **(Fig. 47.2)**. The use of oxygen probably carries no benefit over air in term babies.

The chest may not move during the first one to three breaths as fluid is displaced. Once the chest is inflated, reassess the heart rate. Assess air entry by chest movement, not by auscultation. In fluid-filled lungs, breath sounds may be heard without lung inflation. If the heart rate responds, it is safe to assume that the chest has been inflated successfully.

A Guedel airway may be used to help maintain the airway **(Fig. 47.3)**. It should be inserted under direct vision with a laryngoscope as shown. The correct size of airway should reach from the middle of the chin to the angle of the jaw. The correct way to support the mask is also illustrated. Once the chest is inflated, ventilation is continued at a rate of 30–40 ventilations per minute. Continue to reassess that the airway is clear and that the chest is inflating.

Circulation

If the heart rate remains slow (less than 60 bpm) once the lungs are inflated, cardiac compressions must be started. The most efficient way of doing this in the neonate is to encircle the chest with both hands, so that the fingers lie behind the baby and the thumbs are apposed on the sternum just below the inter-nipple line **(Fig. 47.4)**. Compress the chest briskly to one-third of its diameter. Current advice is to perform three compressions for each inflation of the chest.

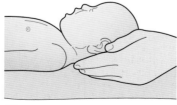
(A)   Too flexed

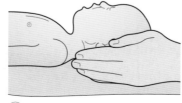
(B)   Neutral (correct position)

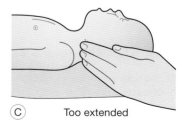
(C)   Too extended

Fig. 47.1 Head position.

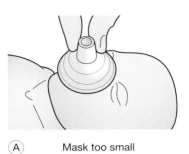 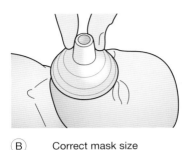 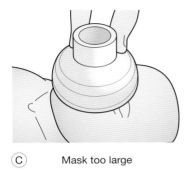

| (A) Mask too small | (B) Correct mask size | (C) Mask too large |

Fig. 47.2 Mask positioning.

The purpose of cardiac compression is to move a small amount of oxygenated blood or drugs to the coronary arteries in order to initiate cardiac recovery. There is therefore no point in cardiac compression before the lungs have been inflated. Similarly, compressions are ineffective unless interposed breaths are of good quality and inflate the chest. The emphasis must be upon good-quality breaths followed by effective compressions. Once the heart rate is above 60 bpm and rising, cardiac compression can be discontinued.

Drugs

If, after adequate lung inflation and cardiac compression, the heart rate has not responded, drug therapy should be considered. The most common reason for failure of the heart rate to respond, however, is failure to achieve lung inflation. Airway and breathing must be reassessed as adequate before proceeding to drug therapy. Venous access will be required via an umbilical venous line, as drugs should be given centrally.

- Adrenaline (epinephrine) can be given in the presence of profound unresponsive bradycardia or circulatory standstill.
- A bolus of dextrose can be used if there is hypoglycaemia.
- Very occasionally, hypovolaemia may be present because of known or suspected blood loss (antepartum haemorrhage, placenta or vasa praevia, unclamped cord) or be secondary to loss of vascular tone following asphyxia. Volume expansion with normal saline may be appropriate. If blood loss is acute and severe, non-crossmatched O-negative blood should be given immediately. Most newborn or neonatal resuscitations do not require fluid unless there has been known blood loss or septicaemic shock.
- Occasionally, a baby who has been effectively resuscitated and is pink, with a heart rate over 100 bpm, may not breathe because of the effects of maternal opiates. If respiratory depressant effects are suspected, the baby should be given naloxone intramuscularly. The effect will only last a few minutes and naloxone should not be considered a drug of resuscitation.

Response to resuscitation

Often, the first indication of success will be an increase in heart rate. Recovery of respiratory drive may be delayed. Babies in terminal apnoea will tend to gasp first as they recover, before starting normal respirations. Those who were in primary apnoea are likely to start with irregular but more normal breaths, which may commence at any stage of resuscitation.

Tracheal intubation

Most babies can be adequately resuscitated using a mask, and research suggests that if this is applied correctly, only 1 in 500 babies actually need to be intubated. However, endotracheal intubation remains the gold standard in airway management. It is especially useful in prolonged resuscitations, preterm babies and cases of meconium aspiration. It should be considered if mask ventilation has failed, although the most common reason for failure with mask inflation is poor positioning of the head with consequent failure to open the airway.

Preterm babies

The more preterm a baby is, the less likely it is to establish adequate respirations. Preterm babies (esp. less than 32 weeks) are also likely to be deficient in surfactant. The effort required to breathe is greater and yet the muscles are less developed. One must anticipate that babies born before 32 weeks may need help to establish prompt aeration and ventilation.

Preterm babies are more likely to become cold (higher surface area:mass ratio) and more likely to be hypoglycaemic (fewer glycogen stores). The temperature of very preterm babies can be maintained if they are immediately placed in a plastic bag (without drying) under a radiant heater on the Resuscitaire, leaving the face exposed and covering the head with a hat.

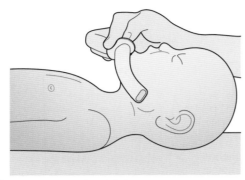

(A) Correct size of Guedel airway

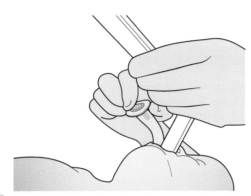

(B) Insertion with a laryngoscope

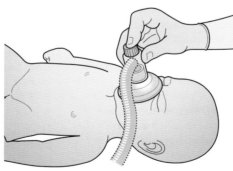

(C) Keeping a seal with the mask

Fig. 47.3 Maintaining the airway.

Action in the event of poor initial response to resuscitation after five inflation breaths

Consider the following:

- Is the baby in the neutral position?
- Is there a good seal on the mask?
- Do you need jaw thrust?

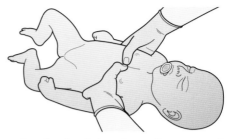

Fig. 47.4 Two-hand technique for cardiac compressions.

- Check for airway obstruction.
- Consider Guedel airway.
- Is mask ventilation effective? Observe the chest wall movement and consider endotracheal intubation.
- Is the endotracheal tube in the trachea or right main bronchus? Auscultate both axillae and observe movement.
- Does the baby have a pneumothorax? This occurs spontaneously in up to 1% of newborns but those requiring action in the delivery unit are exceptionally rare. Auscultate the chest for asymmetry of breath sounds. If a tension pneumothorax is thought to be present clinically, a 21-gauge butterfly needle should be inserted through the second intercostal space in the mid-clavicular line. Remember that you may well cause a pneumothorax during this procedure.
- Does the baby remain cyanosed despite breathing with a good heart rate? There may be a congenital heart malformation, which may be duct dependent, or there may be persistent pulmonary hypertension of the newborn.

Discontinuation of resuscitation

The outcome for a baby with no cardiac output after 15 minutes of effective full resuscitation is likely to be very poor. The decision to discontinue resuscitation should be taken by a senior member of the team, ideally a consultant. This means that help must have been called.

Key *points*

- Dry the baby and keep it warm.
- Good airway management and good ventilation are the mainstays of successful resuscitation.

48

Neonatal care

Introduction

Good-quality neonatal care is extremely important, and may have key implications for the rest of a baby's life. Those born prematurely need skilled intensive support, and those born with presumed hypoxia need appropriate resuscitation. The early neonatal period is often the time when congenital abnormalities become apparent and precise diagnosis and management can make a difference to the quality of life, or even influence whether the baby will live or die. The aim of this chapter is not to provide a comprehensive guide to neonatal care, but rather to highlight some of the more common neonatal problems which can occur.

It is essential that the obstetrician, midwife, paediatrician, neonatologist and neonatal nurse collaborate closely as a team. High-quality communication is essential if decision-making is to be optimized.

The transition at birth

The apparent ease with which most babies make the transition from fetal to neonatal life conceals a host of complex physiological changes in virtually every system. Several relatively common neonatal disorders are related to difficulties with this transition.

Respiratory system

The fetal lung at term contains about 100 ml of liquid. This equals the functional residual capacity and in a sense the fetal lung can be said to form around a liquid cast of the future air spaces. Lung fluid is formed by alveolar cells, and fluid is essential for normal lung growth and development.

The fluid must be cleared at birth to make way for air, and failure to do so leads to breathlessness. This is known as transient tachypnoea of the newborn (TTN). It may last for a day or two, and is commoner after elective caesarean section.

Respiratory distress syndrome (RDS) is caused by a deficiency of surfactant and is commoner in preterm infants (0.1% at term vs 30% at 28 weeks). Surfactant, a complex lipoprotein consisting largely of phosphatidyl choline, is synthesized by type II pneumocytes within the alveoli and is important in allowing the alveolus to expand. Hypoxia, acidosis and hypothermia reduce surfactant production; antenatal steroids increase production and thereby reduce the incidence of RDS. Clinically there is tachypnoea, grunting and intercostal recession commencing within the first 4 hours of life, and the chest X-ray demonstrates a generalized reticulogranular appearance referred to as like 'ground glass' **(Fig. 48.1)**. Treatment is with oxygen ± supportive ventilation and often includes giving artificial surfactant through an endotracheal tube.

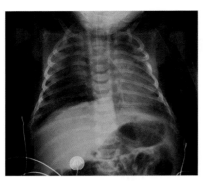

Fig. 48.1 Respiratory distress syndrome following emergency caesarean section. The mother had diabetes, which predisposes to respiratory distress syndrome. Note the ground-glass appearance of the lungs.

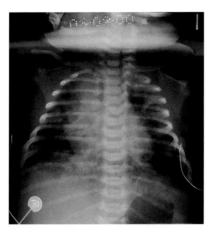

Fig. 48.2 Meconium aspiration syndrome. Note the widespread patchy shadowing in both lungs.

Meconium aspiration syndrome is also a potentially serious respiratory complication. In utero, meconium is usually retained within the colon. Although it may be passed through the sphincter under physiological conditions, particularly after 40 weeks, it also has an association with fetal hypoxic stress. Meconium is irritative to the neonatal lungs and may lead to a pneumonitis, the meconium aspiration syndrome **(Fig. 48.2)**. Clinical features range from mild neonatal tachypnoea to severe respiratory compromise. The incidence is probably unrelated to fetal pH (and indeed the majority of babies with meconium aspiration syndrome are not acidotic at delivery) but the syndrome is more likely to be severe if there is associated acidosis. It is also more severe when the meconium is thick. Treatment is with oxygen, mechanical ventilation and, if very severe, extracorporeal membrane oxygenation.

Cardiovascular system

The switch from fetal to neonatal circulation is normally made rapidly after birth. The key event is relaxation of the smooth muscle in the pulmonary blood vessels, which is triggered by the entry of oxygen into the lung with the first breath (note this paradoxical response to oxygen, which is the opposite to that of all other blood vessels).

In some babies, especially when there has been prolonged fetal hypoxia, this circulatory switch does not occur and may itself lead to further hypoxia. This condition is known as persistent fetal circulation and is difficult to distinguish clinically from congenital cyanotic heart disease.

Genitourinary system

Although the fetal kidney is important in maintaining the amniotic fluid volume, it has a negligible role in the excretion of waste products. After birth, the kidney must excrete all the body's waste as well as conserve fluid. In a baby born at term, the kidney is just able to manage this role although there is always an initial rise in the blood urea and creatinine concentrations. The maximum urine osmolality which the newborn can attain is about 600 mOsm/kg (compared with 1800 mOsm/kg in the adult) and it is therefore not surprising that dehydration and electrolyte disturbances are common complications of neonatal illness.

Gastrointestinal system

The fetus swallows amniotic fluid at about the same rate as it is produced, and deficiencies in fetal swallowing result in polyhydramnios. If there has been polyhydramnios, the baby should be examined for swallowing problems and should have an orogastric tube passed in order to exclude complete oesophageal atresia.

Haematological system

The term fetus has a high haemoglobin concentration, at around 18 g/dl. This is a response to the low arterial oxygen tension (3–4 kPa) which characterizes the latter part of intrauterine life. Once the oxygen tension rises after birth, this high haemoglobin is no longer needed, and falls to around 10 g/dl by about 8 weeks of age.

The white cell count at birth is high (12–20 ×10^9/l) and polymorphs predominate. By 4 days of age, it is usually in the range 7–12 ×10^9/l and is mainly lymphocytic.

Routine care at birth

There are several routine observations and procedures to perform on the newborn shortly after birth, but, providing the baby does not need to be resuscitate, none of them should be allowed to prevent the mother from seeing and holding her baby as soon as possible.

Assessment

The baby's condition at 1 and 5 minutes of age is assessed by means of the Apgar score (**Table 47.1**). The purpose of this is to have a reasonably objective record of how

Heat balance at birth

Mechanisms of heat loss (in priority order)

- Evaporation of water from wet skin
- Convective loss due to air currents
- Radiation to cold surfaces
- Conductive loss to cold mattress

Mechanisms of heat gain

- Oxidation of brown fat (plentiful in newborn)
- Muscular activity
- Radiant heater over cot or Resuscitaire
- Warm mattress

Table 48.1

Some dimensions of an average male* infant at 40 weeks

Weight	3500 g
Length	50 cm
Head circumference	35 cm
Brain weight	400 g (12% of body weight)
Blood volume	280 ml (80 ml/kg)

*Females are about 10% smaller.

the baby initially responded to the challenge of extrauterine life. It serves as a guide to the need for resuscitation, but, unless the score fails to improve with resuscitation, it has very little predictive value for later disability (p. 402). A low Apgar score is not synonymous with birth asphyxia. It could, for example, be a reflection of a pre-existing fetal problem or of sedation caused by the maternal drug administration.

Preventing hypothermia

Newborn babies can lose heat faster than they can generate it **(Box 48.1)**. Hypothermia is dangerous and must be prevented. The delivery room must be warm and draughts kept to a minimum. The baby should be dried at once – especially the top of the head, from which most heat is lost – and wrapped in dry towels or blankets. If resuscitation is required, it should be performed under a radiant heater. Increasingly, neonatologists are putting babies into polythene bags even prior to intubation, to minimize evaporative losses and improve temperature control.

Examination

Providing all appears well, all that is needed in the labour ward is a brief examination for any obvious external abnormalities. A full routine examination should be deferred until later.

Weighing and measuring

Weight, length, and head circumference measurements provide an assessment of how well the baby has grown in utero and are a baseline against which to judge subsequent growth. **Table 48.1** gives some normative term data and such data are also available for neonates born at earlier gestations.

The umbilical cord

The cord should be checked to see whether it contains the usual two arteries and one vein. A single artery has a 20% association with congenital abnormalities, mainly of the genitourinary system. A plastic cord clamp should be fixed so as to leave about 2 cm of cord proximally. Subsequent care of the cord is controversial. Some authorities advocate no specific measures, whereas most like to apply an antiseptic agent, such as chlorhexidine powder. If the baby is likely to need intensive care, the cord should be left longer, to allow arterial and venous cannulation.

Preventing haemorrhagic disease of the newborn

Vitamin K does not cross the placenta well and newborn babies have low serum concentrations and poor stores. They do not have gut bacteria to synthesize it for them, and human milk is a relatively poor source of the vitamin. Lack of vitamin K leads to shortage of clotting factors II, VII, IX and X, and about 1 in 1000 breast-fed babies will experience serious bleeding, a condition known as haemorrhagic disease of the newborn. The classical form occurs between days 1–7, although an early form occurs in infants born to mothers taking anticonvulsants and a late (and sometimes more serious form) may also occur, even up to 12 weeks after delivery. Bottle-fed babies are at less risk because formulae are supplemented with vitamins.

Almost complete protection is provided by the administration of vitamin K 1 mg i.m. at the time of birth, and possibly less-complete protection is provided by giving vitamin K 2 mg orally twice in the first week (with a further oral dose at 1 month). Some epidemiological studies have found an association between i.m. vitamin K (as opposed to oral vitamin K) and childhood leukaemias, resulting in a swing away from treatment. Many large subsequent studies have failed to prove the connection.

Perinatal asphyxia

Evolution has equipped the fetus with a remarkable ability to tolerate asphyxia without adverse consequences, to the extent that sometimes 10 or 15 minutes of absolute anoxia can be compatible with normal survival. In practice, absolute anoxia only occurs with rare events such as massive placental abruption or cord prolapse. Asphyxia may lead to cerebral palsy, essentially a motor disorder affecting posture and movement which is variably accompanied by mental impairment, epilepsy or sensory defects. Despite popular belief, it is likely that less than 10% of cerebral palsy is caused primarily by perinatal asphyxia.

Neonatologists are wary of making a diagnosis of perinatal asphyxia unless there is a good antenatal history (e.g. abruption) together with neonatal 'depression' (e.g. poor Apgar scores) and evidence of subsequent multiorgan failure. Such multiorgan failure may present with seizures, cerebral oedema, oliguria, haematuria, coagulopathy, jaundice or occasionally pulmonary haemorrhage. The question of predicting the likelihood of neurological injury following a specific birth and the question of whether a subsequent developmental abnormality was caused by a specific intrapartum insult is seldom straight forward.

Neonatal examination

Sometime during the first day or two of life all newborn babies should be carefully and systematically examined, for the reasons outlined in **Box 48.2**. The technique for this examination must be learned, as must the range of normal findings. It is probably better to follow an anatomical progression from head to toe **(Table 48.2)** rather than to adopt a system-orientated approach.

Developmental dysplasia of the hip

Developmental dysplasia of the hip (previously referred to as 'congenital dislocation of the hip') has an overall incidence of approximately 1%, but is commoner in breech presentation, oligohydramnios, firstborn females and those with a family history. Early neonatal diagnosis carries an excellent prognosis as most respond to several months in a versatile harness (the Pavlik harness – pronounced 'Pau-lick'). Those in whom the diagnosis is delayed rarely attain normal hip development. Clinical screening with Ortolani's test (history box) may miss a significant proportion of cases. Ultrasound is likely to detect

a greater proportion and, although commonly used only in higher-risk neonates, it may become part of the routine screening process.

History

Marino Ortolani (1904–1983) was professor and chief of paediatrics in Ferrara, Italy, whose clinic became an international centre for the detection, treatment and prophylaxis of congenital luxations of the hip.

Biochemical screening

As well as screening by physical examination, babies in the UK are screened biochemically for a number of different disorders by performing a heel-prick blood sample on about the 7th day of life. The disorders assessed vary in different regions, but may include phenylketonuria, congenital hypothyroidism and cystic fibrosis.

Physical birth injury

Serious physical injury to the baby during birth is rare in western practice. Injuries are most likely to occur when there is absolute or relative disproportion between the size of the baby and the maternal pelvis, or following malpresentation or instrumental delivery. Preterm babies are more easily damaged than those at term.

Box 48.2

Reasons for performing the routine newborn examination

- To detect abnormalities for which early diagnosis and treatment offer an improved prognosis, e.g. congenital hip dysplasia
- To detect abnormalities early in order to plan therapy, follow-up or genetic counselling, e.g. cardiac abnormalities, Down syndrome
- To reassure parents that their baby appears to have no serious problem
- It is an opportunity to provide health education

Table 48.2

Key abnormalities in routine newborn examination

Head	Abnormal size or shape
	Raised anterior fontanelle tension
Face	Dysmorphic features, facial nerve palsy
Eyes	Asymmetry, lens opacities
Mouth	Cleft-palate, thrush
Jaw	Micrognathia
Neck	Goitre, sternomastoid nodules
Chest	Breathlessness
Heart	Murmurs or signs of overactivity
Abdomen	Enlarged kidneys or other masses
Umbilicus	Signs of sepsis
Groins	Herniae
Genitalia	Ambiguity of sex. Undescended testes or urethral abnormalities in the male, bulging of the hymen or bleeding in the female
Anus	Imperforate
Spine	Abnormal curvature or any surface lesion
Hips	Signs of dysplasia
Feet	Talipes (twisting of feet and ankles)
CNS	Abnormal tone, lack of movement or reduced responsiveness

Nerve palsies

These are due either to overstretching of the nerve or to direct external pressure on the nerve. In more than 85% of instances, the nerve fibres remain intact and full recovery occurs. Nerve disruption may result in permanent disability.

Brachial plexus

Erb's palsy is caused by injury to roots C5 and C6 and produces a limp arm, held alongside the body with the forearm pronated – 'waiter's tip' posture. Klumpke's palsy is rarer, involves C8 and T1, and mainly affects the wrist extensors and the small hand muscles. Injury to the phrenic nerve is rare. It is associated with brachial plexus injury and can cause marked respiratory difficulty (Fig 44.6).

Facial nerve

This is a lower motor neuron lesion due to compression of the facial nerve by maternal pelvic bones or forceps. Minor, transient cases are quite common, but permanent weakness is seen in only about 5% of instances.

Skeletal injury

Although the skull often undergoes marked distortion during delivery, fractures are very uncommon and usually cause little trouble. Fractures of the clavicle are not infrequently seen even after normal delivery and usually heal very well, although sometimes with massive callus formation. Fractures of other bones are rare and suggest significant trauma at delivery.

Soft tissue injury

This is rarely of any serious consequence but may be distressing for parents as well as for whoever conducted the birth.

Caput succedaneum

Essentially oedema of the 'presenting' scalp, this disappears rapidly after birth and requires no treatment.

Chignon

This is the name given to the swelling produced by a ventouse vacuum extractor. There are usually no complications, but infection and necrosis of the skin can occur.

Cephalhaematoma

Bleeding between a skull bone and its overlying periosteum occurs in about 1% of babies. The lesion is confined to the margins of the bone by attachment of the periosteum, which prevents the amount of blood loss from becoming significant **(Fig. 48.3)**. It is almost always parietal, but can occasionally be occipital. Palpation around the edge of the lesion often gives the impression of an associated depressed fracture, but this is an illusion. In 5% of cases there is an inconsequential linear fracture of the underlying bone. Spontaneous regression occurs and no treatment is required.

Subaponeurotic haemorrhage

This is much rarer than cephalhaematoma, but may lead to serious blood loss and can be fatal. There is bleeding into the potentially very large space between the skull and the overlying occipitofrontalis aponeurosis **(Fig. 48.3)**.

Sternomastoid tumour

This is a fibrous lump in the sternomastoid muscle, probably secondary to compression of the muscle leading to ischaemia. It settles spontaneously but can cause torticollis.

Congenital abnormalities

Approximately 2% of newborn babies have a serious abnormality detectable at, or soon after, birth. Some of the more serious abnormalities may have been identified antenatally following appropriate screening, particularly neural tube defects, renal agenesis, diaphragmatic hernias and some cardiac problems. In addition to these major abnormalities, 2–3% more babies may have some minor abnormality.

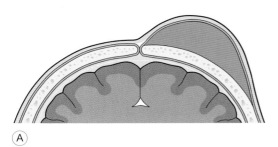
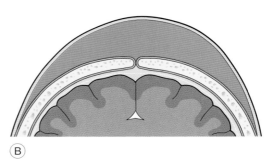

(A) (B)

Fig. 48.3 Comparison of cephalhaematoma and subaponeurotic haemorrhage. (A) The space under a cephalhaematoma is relatively small and major blood loss is unlikely. **(B)** There is a much larger potential space under the aponeurosis, and there may be serious blood loss.

Advantages of human milk

- It contains IgA, lactoferrin and other proteins which protect against infection
- It is not allergenic
- It is easily digested and meets the nutritional needs of the newborn
- It is normally uncontaminated by pathogens
- It partially protects against necrotizing enterocolitis

Table 48.3

Recommended feed volumes for term newborn infants	
Day 1	60 ml/kg
Day 2	75 ml/kg
Day 3	90 ml/kg
Day 4	120 ml/kg
Day 5	150 ml/kg

Congenital abnormalities are discussed in more detail in Chapter 31.

Feeding

At term, human milk has considerable advantages over a cow's milk-based formula (see **Box 48.3**). In addition, breastfeeding is psychologically advantageous to both mother and baby, and also confers physiological and disease-prevention benefits on the mother. Mothers should be encouraged to put the baby to the breast soon after birth, and thereafter the baby should be fed on demand. In many high-income countries, the prevalence of breastfeeding remains low, and marketing from artificial-feed companies is intense.

Correct reconstitution of powdered milk formulae is essential for safe artificial feeding, as babies do not tolerate excessive osmolar loads (see **Table 48.3**). Whichever way the baby is fed, a close watch must be kept on the adequacy of weight gain. Between 170 g and 200 g per week is appropriate for a term neonate during the first few weeks of life.

Special formulae are available for preterm babies, and have higher levels of protein, sodium, calcium and phosphate. Preterm babies should gain weight at about 12 g/kg/day. 'Special' milks, such as those based on soya, should only be used when there are clear medical indications.

Signs of illness

Newborn babies have a very limited number of ways to show that they are ill **(Box 48.4)**. These signs may be subtle

Box 48.4

Signs of illness in the newborn

- Excessive sleepiness and lack of interest in feeding
- Slow feeding
- Diminished or, occasionally, excessive crying
- Poor muscle tone, with limbs held extended rather than flexed
- Skin pallor or slaty-grey coloration with mottling
- Temperature instability
- Vomiting and abdominal distension
- Episodes of apnoea
- Tachypnoea and tachycardia
- Grunting respirations

and most often are first noticed by the mother or the nursing staff. The signs may occasionally be non-specific, so that a baby with an infection may initially be clinically indistinguishable from one with a metabolic disorder or even cardiac disease. This, coupled with the speed with which newborn babies deteriorate during serious illness, means that a very high index of suspicion and a low threshold for investigation are appropriate.

When a baby shows some of the features listed in **Box 48.4**, infection is by far the likeliest cause and the following approach should be pursued:

- Take a history, considering particularly:
  - maternal health during pregnancy
  - risk factors for infection, such as prolonged rupture of the membranes, maternal illness, or nursery contact with sick babies
  - family history of neonatal illness or neonatal death.
- Examine the baby. As well as assessing the severity of illness, the examination should seek signs of superficial infection, which might have led to septicaemia, and signs of organ dysfunction.
- Investigate as follows:
  - blood culture
  - full blood count and film
  - blood glucose
  - arterial blood gas, if the baby is breathless or seriously ill
  - C-reactive protein
  - urine culture
  - swabs, from any inflamed lesions
  - chest X-ray
  - stool culture, if stools abnormal
  - lumbar puncture, if sepsis is suspected and the source is unclear.
- Treat. If infection seems a possibility, broad-spectrum antibiotic therapy should be started, for example a combination of ampicillin and gentamicin or a third-generation cephalosporin. The results of investigations will allow the rationalization of treatment.

Jaundice

Clinically apparent jaundice (serum bilirubin greater than about 75 mmol/l) affects more than half of all newborns during the first week of life.

Physiological jaundice

Almost all jaundiced babies will have a harmless physiological jaundice which is part of the normal transition from fetal to postnatal life. The fetal liver does not handle unconjugated bilirubin but rather leaves it to cross the placenta to be conjugated and excreted by the mother. Following birth, the neonatal liver must handle all of the unconjugated bilirubin produced but cannot do so immediately. During the first few days of life, liver function improves rapidly, but, while this is happening, the serum unconjugated bilirubin invariably rises.

Unconjugated bilirubin can cross the blood–brain barrier and is toxic to the central nervous system, especially the basal ganglia and the auditory pathways. Bilirubin encephalopathy, or kernicterus, may lead to an athetoid cerebral palsy, deafness, and may even be lethal. The unconjugated serum bilirubin concentration probably needs to exceed 500 mmol/l in order to injure the brain of a healthy term infant and this never occurs with physiological jaundice.

Pathological jaundice

The main problem with physiological jaundice is that it makes it difficult to spot the very few infants with pathological jaundice due to the causes in **Box 48.5**. Some of these conditions are important in their own right, while others pose a risk of kernicterus. Jaundice which fulfils any of the criteria listed in **Box 48.6** should be regarded as potentially pathological.

Most of the pathological causes of jaundice are easy to understand and it is relatively easy to reach a diagnosis if a systematic approach is adopted. **Box 48.7** lists the main tests to be performed.

Breast milk jaundice

Breast milk jaundice is still not completely understood but it is thought that compounds in the milk of some women interfere with conjugation of bilirubin in the baby's liver. It is a harmless condition but problematic because there is no specific test for it. It presents as persistent jaundice which is mainly unconjugated in nature. Other more serious causes of persistent jaundice, such as hypothyroidism or hepatitis, must be excluded before the diagnosis of breast milk jaundice can be safely accepted.

Obstructive jaundice

The diagnosis must be considered in any baby who is still jaundiced at 2 weeks of age and is an important diagnosis to make. The history of pale stools and dark urine should

---

Box 48.5

Major pathological causes of neonatal jaundice

1. Excessive production of bilirubin:
   a. Intravascular haemolysis due to rhesus or ABO incompatibility or inherited red cell defects
   b. Bruising
   c. Polycythaemia
2. Diminished conjugation:
   a. Breast milk jaundice
   b. Hypothyroidism
   c. Hepatic enzyme deficiencies
   d. Inborn errors of metabolism
   e. Hepatitis from various causes
3. Obstruction:
   a. Atresia of intra- or extrahepatic bile ducts
   b. Congenital bile duct cyst

Box 48.6

Indicators that jaundice may be pathological

- Becomes apparent during the first day of life
- Rises faster than 75 mmol/l/day
- Exceeds 250 mmol/l
- Persists beyond 10 days of age
- Is associated with pale stools, dark urine or bilirubinuria

---

Box 48.7

Investigation of suspected pathological jaundice

1. Mother's blood group, baby's blood group and Coombs' test – to look for rhesus or ABO incompatibility
2. Haemoglobin and blood film – to look for anaemia and signs of haemolysis
3. Unconjugated and conjugated serum bilirubin concentrations – to estimate the risk of encephalopathy and to look for signs of obstruction
4. Liver function tests – for evidence of liver disease
5. Test urine for reducing substances (? galactosaemia)
6. Check thyroid screening result and repeat if indicated

---

be sought and the urine tested for bilirubin. If obstructive jaundice is suspected, the biliary tree should be investigated using ultrasound, radioisotope scans and possibly liver biopsy. Most cases of biliary atresia can be treated, at least partially, by surgical anastomosis of the liver to the small bowel. Long term, liver transplantation will be required by many survivors of neonatal surgery.

Jaundice due to haemolysis

Some of the pathological causes of neonatal jaundice can raise the serum concentration of unconjugated bilirubin to levels at which encephalopathy might occur. This is most likely with rhesus disease but occasionally happens with ABO incompatibility or other haemolytic disorders. The use of anti-D immunoglobulin to treat rhesus-negative women after childbirth or obstetric procedures has made rhesus disease quite rare. ABO incompatibility usually exists when a group O mother has a group B or A baby (see Ch. 37).

Treatment of pathological jaundice

Above an age-specific bilirubin threshold, phototherapy is indicated. This involves the use of high-intensity light in the 450 nm wavelength to convert stable lipid-soluble unconjugated bilirubin into unstable water-soluble isomers which can be excreted in the bile without the need for conjugation. It takes about 12–24 hours to have an effect on the rate of rise of the bilirubin. If the bilirubin rises above a further threshold despite phototherapy, an exchange transfusion is required.

Low-birth-weight infants

Although low-birth-weight (LBW) babies account for only 10% of all births in the UK, they account for around 70% of the perinatal mortality. Approximately two-thirds of LBW babies are preterm **(Fig. 48.4)** and the rest are term but small-for-gestational age (SGA).

Prematurity-related problems

Survival increases from approximately 5% at 23 weeks' gestation to 95% at 31 weeks. About 25% of these survivors have some disability – including cerebral palsy, short stature, respiratory difficulties, visual impairment and poor school performance. It is now well established that corticosteroids given to mothers who subsequently deliver preterm are effective in reducing the incidence of respiratory distress syndrome by around 50% as well as the risk of periventricular haemorrhage. Whether or not to start resuscitation with an extremely premature infant (less than 24 weeks) can sometimes be a difficult question and, ideally, discussions with the prospective parents should have taken place beforehand in order to gauge their wishes.

The problems of prematurity are outlined in **Table 48.4**.

Problems with being small for gestational age

By definition, 10% of babies are small for dates, the majority for no pathological reason. Around a third, however, have fetal growth restriction as defined as 'a baby which has failed to reach its genetic growth potential', and are more at risk of peripartum hypoxia and neonatal hypoglycaemia. The implications of fetal growth restriction are discussed further on page 287.

Infection

Although the fetus is generally isolated from the external bacteriological environment, some pathogens are occasionally able to cross the placenta and infect the baby. This may sometimes lead to permanent damage, and the details of some of these conditions are discussed on page 273.

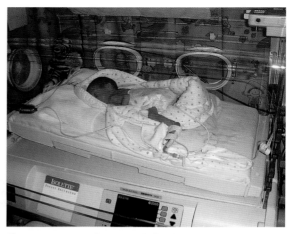

Fig. 48.4 A 26-week preterm infant has immature lungs, skin, central nervous system, gastrointestinal system and genitourinary system, and is also more prone to infection.

Newborn babies are immunocompromised relative to older children for the reasons shown in **Box 48.8** and are therefore at increased risk of infection. Neonatal infections may be with organisms from the birth canal, such as group B β-haemolytic streptococci, or from the neonatal environment, for example *Escherichia coli*, *Proteus* species, *Staphylococcus aureus* and *S. epidermidis*. The risks are of pneumonia, meningitis, pyelonephritis and osteomyelitis, and a low index of suspicion is important for these conditions.

Some common minor infections are considered below.

Conjunctivitis

'Sticky eyes' are common and most cases respond rapidly to topical antibacterial treatment. Infection with gonorrhoea and chlamydia, however, may be more serious.

- Gonococcal ophthalmia usually presents as a fulminant, unilateral or bilateral, purulent infection during the first few days of life. The maternal history may give a clue. Prompt diagnosis and treatment with systemic and local penicillin is needed to prevent corneal damage and permanent visual impairment.
- Chlamydial eye infections usually present as sticky eyes which do not settle with conventional antibacterial agents. The diagnosis is best made from corneal brushings but can be made from an ordinary eye swab if the laboratory is asked to look specifically for the organism. Treatment is with tetracycline eye drops and systemic erythromycin to clear the organisms from the upper respiratory tract, from where they may go on to cause pneumonia. Systemic tetracycline is never given to babies or young children because it stains dental enamel and interferes with its development.

Table 48.4

The problems of prematurity

Skin	Extremely preterm infants have a very high surface area to mass ratio and thin skin, and are extremely liable to hypothermia. This means that it is vitally important to deliver in a warm room with heated towels for drying and some method to keep the baby warm during resuscitation, e.g. an overhead heater. Survival is directly related to the temperature of the infant on admission to the neonatal intensive care unit
Lung	At 23–24 weeks the respiratory epithelial cells start to differentiate into type I (gas exchange) and type II (surfactant production) pneumocytes. Surfactant levels at this gestation are therefore very low but can be increased by antenatal glucocorticoids (see RDS, p. 399). Respiratory support is often by mechanical ventilation, either 'conventional' or with 'high-frequency oscillation', and exogenous prophylactic surfactant administration. A large proportion of extremely preterm infants develop chronic lung disease of prematurity (bronchopulmonary dysplasia), with continuing requirements for respiratory support
Central nervous system	The subependymal germinal matrix lies close to the ventricular space and contains the developing brain cells of the premature infant. Bleeding from this very vascular area may occur with preterm birth, giving rise to periventricular haemorrhage. A major intraventricular haemorrhage may lead to hydrocephalus and cortical damage. The extremely preterm infant is also prone to ischaemic brain injury from low arterial oxygen tension, hypotension, or reduced cerebral blood flow. Subsequent periventricular cysts (periventricular leucomalacia) may form and, if this happens, long-term neurological sequelae are likely The location of brain injury in the white matter adjacent to the lateral ventricles means that the subsequent disability is mainly motor and often affects the lower limbs. This presents as a spastic diplegia with relative sparing of the intellect and affects about 10% of babies with birth weights below 1500 g
GI system	Structurally the bowel is well developed by the end of the second trimester but there is functional immaturity. Motility and food absorption are both reduced and early enteral feeding may not be tolerated. Parenteral nutrition may be needed during the early days and weeks, but this may lead to numerous problems, both from the need to maintain adequate venous access and the tolerability of the amino acid and lipid solutions Necrotizing enterocolitis (NEC) is not uncommon in premature infants, and is characterized by ischaemic bowel necrosis. Although the aetiology is unclear, it typically presents after the introduction of enteral feeds and is postulated to be an abnormal reaction to bowel colonization
Liver	There may be jaundice, poor clotting, poor glucose control and a limited ability to excrete waste products
Blood	There is reduced immunoglobulin and white cell function, so the risk of sepsis is increased. Furthermore, frequent use of multiple, broad-spectrum antibiotics renders the tiny baby more prone to infection with sub-pathogenic bacteria such as *Staphylococcus epidermidis*, and fungi, especially *Candida albicans*
Eye	Early vasoconstriction damage to the retina occurs as a result of high oxygen pressure and other factors. The incidence of this is reduced by using ventilation at lower P_{O_2} levels. Secondary proliferation of weaker, potentially haemorrhagic, vessels occurs, a condition referred to as retinopathy of prematurity. Regular ophthalmological review is vital as early laser or cryotherapy treatment of these new vessels can preserve vision

Box 48.8

Immunological deficiencies among normal infants

1. Complete lack of IgM and IgA – only humoral activity is IgG from mother
2. Low numbers of neutrophils with poor chemotactic and killing powers
3. Poor local inflammatory response allows spread of organisms to circulation

Candida

'Thrush' infections are common either in the mouth or in the nappy area and are caused by a yeast, *Candida albicans*. In the mouth, the appearance is of adherent white patches of exudate. In the nappy area, inflammation may be confused with other causes of nappy rash, although satellite lesions around the main area of erythema are suggestive of candida. Treatment is with topical nystatin or one of the more modern antifungal agents, such as miconazole.

Skin sepsis

Skin sepsis is relatively common and is usually due to staphylococci, although streptococci and other organisms may be involved. Paronychia, pustules and periumbilical infection are the most likely manifestations. Blistering and desquamation are seen with some strains of staphylococci. All suspected staphylococcal or streptococcal infections should be taken very seriously and a low threshold for systemic treatment is appropriate.

Urinary tract infection

Urinary tract infection in babies is more common in boys than in girls and is usually caused by *E. coli* and other Gram-negative organisms. Screening can be performed using bag specimens but diagnosis is best confirmed by suprapubic aspiration. Because of the association with congenital abnormalities of the urinary tract, an ultrasound scan or other imaging techniques should be considered.

Meningitis

Neonatal meningitis is most commonly caused by group B β-haemolytic streptococci or *E. coli* and has a high morbidity and mortality. A very low threshold for investigation and treatment is appropriate.

Key *points*

- Good-quality neonatal care is extremely important, and may have key implications for the rest of a baby's life.
- Those born prematurely need skilled intensive support, and those born with presumed hypoxia need appropriate resuscitation.
- The early neonatal period is often the time when congenital abnormalities become apparent, and precise diagnosis and management can make a difference to the quality of life, or even influence whether the baby will live or die.

Index

Page numbers in **bold** refer to figures, tables or boxes.